Handbook of
Child Abuse Research and Treatment

Issues in Clinical Child Psychology

Series Editors: **Michael C. Roberts,** *University of Kansas–Lawrence, Kansas*
Lizette Peterson, *University of Missouri–Columbia, Missouri*

BEHAVIORAL ASPECTS OF PEDIATRIC BURNS
Edited by Kenneth J. Tarnowski

CHILDREN AND DISASTERS
Edited by Conway F. Saylor

CONSULTING WITH PEDIATRICIANS: Psychological Perspectives
Dennis Drotar

HANDBOOK OF ADOLESCENT HEALTH RISK BEHAVIOR
Edited by Ralph J. DiClemente, William B. Hansen, and Lynn E. Ponton

HANDBOOK OF CHILD ABUSE RESEARCH AND TREATMENT
Edited by John R. Lutzker

HANDBOOK OF CHILD BEHAVIOR THERAPY
Edited by T. Steuart Watson and Frank M. Gresham

HANDBOOK OF CHILDREN'S COPING:
Linking Theory and Intervention
Edited by Sharlene A. Wolchik and Irwin N. Sandler

HANDBOOK OF DEPRESSION IN CHILDREN AND ADOLESCENTS
Edited by William M. Reynolds and Hugh F. Johnston

INTERNATIONAL HANDBOOK OF PHOBIC AND ANXIETY
DISORDERS IN CHILDREN AND ADOLESCENTS
Edited by Thomas H. Ollendick, Neville J. King, and William Yule

MENTAL HEALTH INTERVENTIONS WITH PRESCHOOL CHILDREN
Robert D. Lyman and Toni L. Hembree-Kigin

SCHOOL CONSULTATION: Conceptual and Empirical Bases of Practice
William P. Erchul and Brian K. Martens

SUCCESSFUL PREVENTION PROGRAMS FOR CHILDREN
AND ADOLESCENTS
Joseph A. Durlak

A Continuation Order Plan is available for this series. A continuation order will bring delivery of each new volume immediately upon publication. Volumes are billed only upon actual shipment. For further information please contact the publisher.

Handbook of
Child Abuse Research
and Treatment

Edited by

John R. Lutzker

University of Judaism
Los Angeles, California

Plenum Press • New York and London

Library of Congress Cataloging-in-Publication Data

Handbook of child abuse research and treatment / edited by John R.
Lutzker.
        p.   cm. -- (Issues in clinical child psychology)
     Includes bibliographical references and index.
     ISBN 0-306-45659-1
     1. Child abuse--Psychological aspects. 2. Child abuse-
-Prevention. 3. Abusive parents--Behavior modification. 4. Abused
children--Rehabilitation.   I. Lutzker, John R., 1947-
II. Series.
     HV6626.5.H36   1997
     362.76'7--dc21   97-39967
                                                                CIP

ISBN 0-306-45659-1

© 1998 Plenum Press, New York
A Division of Plenum Publishing Corporation
233 Spring Street, New York, N.Y. 10013

http://www.plenum.com

10 9 8 7 6 5 4 3 2 1

Printed in the United States of America

In memory of Abe and Anne Lutzker,
who knew only nurturing.

Contributors

Robert T. Ammerman, MCP ♦ Hahnemann School of Medicine, Allegheny University of the Health Sciences, Pittsburgh, Pennsylvania 15212

Sandra T. Azar, Frances L. Hiatt School of Psychology, Clark University, Worcester, Massachusetts 01610

Kathryn M. Bigelow, University of Kansas, Lawrence, Kansas 66045

Karen S. Budd, Department of Psychology, DePaul University, Chicago, Illinois 60614

Kathleen Coyle Coolahan, University of Pennsylvania, Philadelphia, Pennsylvania 19104

Ronald M. Doctor, California State University, Northridge, California 91330

John Fantuzzo, University of Pennsylvania, Philadelphia, Pennsylvania 19104

Maurice A. Feldman, Department of Psychology, Queen's University and Ongwanada Centre, Kingston, Ontario, Canada K7L 3N6

Sara Gable, Human Development and Family Studies Extension, University of Missouri at Columbia, Columbia, Missouri 65211

Ronit M. Gershater, University of Kansas, Lawrence, Kansas 66045

Brandon F. Greene, Behavior Analysis and Therapy Program, Southern Illinois University, Carbondale, Illinois 62901

W. Rodney Hammond, National Center for Injury Prevention and Control, Centers for Disease Control, Atlanta, Georgia 30341-3724

David J. Hansen, Department of Psychology, University of Nebraska, Lincoln, Nebraska 68588

Rochelle F. Hanson, Center for Sexual Assault/Abuse Recovery and Education, University of Florida, Gainesville, Florida 32607

Debra B. Hecht, Department of Psychology, University of Nebraska, Lincoln, Nebraska 68588

Stella Kilili, Behavior Analysis and Therapy Program, Southern Illinois University, Carbondale, Illinois 62901

David Kolko, University of Pittsburgh Medical Center, Western Psychiatric Institute and Clinic, Pittsburgh, Pennsylvania 15213

Allison F. Lauretti, Frances L. Hiatt School of Psychology, Clark University, Worcester, Massachusetts 01610

Lori M. Lundquist, Department of Psychology, University of Nebraska, Lincoln, Nebraska 68588

John R. Lutzker, Department of Psychology, University of Judaism, Los Angeles, California 90077-1599

Elizabeth N. Miller, Graduate School of Applied and Preventive Psychology, Rutgers University, Piscataway, New Jersey 08855

Joel S. Milner, Department of Psychology, Northern Illinois University, DeKalb, Illinois 60115

Margaret S. Mitchell, College of Charleston, Charleston, South Carolina 29401

William D. Murphy, Department of Psychiatry, University of Tennessee, Memphis, Tennessee 38105

Lizette Peterson, Department of Psychology, University of Missouri at Columbia, Columbia, Missouri 65211

Elsie M. Pinkston, School of Social Service Administration, University of Chicago, Chicago, Illinois 60637

Anna-Lee Pittman, Department of Psychology, University of Western Ontario, London, Ontario, Canada N6A 5C2

Sharon G. Portwood, University of Missouri–Kansas City, Kansas City, Missouri 64110

Christina L. Pouquette, Frances L. Hiatt School of Psychology, Clark University, Worcester, Massachusetts 01610

Tania Y. Povilaitis, Frances L. Hiatt School of Psychology, Clark University, Worcester, Massachusetts 01610

N. Dickon Reppucci, University of Virginia, Charlottesville, Virginia 22903

Michaelle Ann Robinson, Center for Persons with Disabilities, Utah State University, Logan, Utah 84322-6800

Malcolm D. Smith, School of Social Service Administration, University of Chicago, Chicago, Illinois 60637

Kristin D. Stockman, Department of Psychology, DePaul University, Chicago, Illinois 60614

Sebastian Striefel, Center for Persons with Disabilities and Psychology Department, Utah State University, Logan, Utah 84322-6800

Cynthia Cupit Swenson, Department of Psychiatry and Behavioral Sciences, Family Services Research Center, Medical University of South Carolina, Charleston, South Carolina 29425

Randi M. Tolliver, Department of Psychology, Northern Illinois University, DeKalb, Illinois 60115

Pat Truhn, Center for Persons with Disabilities, Utah State University, Logan, Utah 84322-6800

Alexander J. Tymchuk, Department of Psychiatry, School of Medicine, University of California, Los Angeles, California 90024-1759

Linda A. Valle, Department of Psychology, Northern Illinois University, DeKalb, Illinois 60115

Jody E. Warner-Rogers, MRC Child Psychiatry Unit, London SE5 8AF, England

Barbara Hanna Wasik, School of Education, University of North Carolina, Chapel Hill, North Carolina 27599

Carolyn Webster-Stratton, Parenting Clinic, Family & Child Nursing, University of Washington, Seattle, Washington 98105-4631

Andrea DelGaudio Weiss, University of Pennsylvania, Philadelphia, Pennsylvania 19104

Christine Wekerle, Department of Psychology, York University, North York, Ontario, Canada M3J 1P3

David A. Wolfe, Department of Psychology, University of Western Ontario, London, Ontario, Canada N6A 5C2

Sandy K. Wurtele, Psychology Department, University of Colorado, Colorado Springs, Colorado 80933-7150

Betty R. Yung, School of Professional Psychology, Wright State University, Dayton, Ohio 45407

Preface

Child abuse and neglect (CAN) came to the forefront in the 1960s. At first, theories were spun, usually dealing with the intrapsychic reasons why a parent might engage in such terrible behavior. The 1970s brought theory that tended to deal increasingly with sociocultural and ecological explanations for CAN. It was not until the 1980s and 1990s, however, that treatment strategies, research, and legal issues emerged.

This book represents a state-of-the-art compilation from the leading figures of today's work in theory, research, and treatment. In addition, this volume presents treatises on cultural issues in CAN, youth violence, sexual abuse, and child developmental factors in CAN.

The topics covered in this book are based upon empirical research. Although CAN has been professionally discussed since the 1960s, empirically based work in the field has been somewhat scarce. Thus, this volume fills a void.

It is hoped that this book can be used as a text and reference source for many disciplines. It should be useful in psychology, psychiatry, social work, public health, pediatrics, child development and early childhood education, and law.

My own work in CAN began in 1979. Since then, I have been involved in two large-scale research and service projects aimed at the treatment and prevention of CAN. I have found that the problem appears treatable and preventable if the appropriate resources are available, if the services and research are properly evaluated, and if staff are trained to measurable performance criteria. Again, this empirical bias can be seen throughout the volume.

Countless individuals always need to be acknowledged in writing or editing a book. First, I would like to thank the staffs of Project 12-Ways and Project Safe-Care. They have taught me so much over the years and have been creative and flexible in exploring and providing our ecobehavioral model. My doctoral student working on Project SafeCare, Ronit Gershater, has been very helpful, as has my colleague, Ron Doctor. Of particular note, the work and help of my doctoral student and Program Manager of Project SafeCare, Kathryn M. Bigelow, has been invaluable, as has the assistance of Randi Sherman. Joshua D. Wilner was most helpful with the indices.

My initial plans for an edited book on child abuse and neglect were modest. I am fortunate that Lizette Peterson and Michael Roberts, two cherished colleagues and editors of this series for Plenum, took me aside at a conference and convinced me that a handbook would make more of an impact.

The editing of this book and the chapters I have contributed were supported, in part, by a grant from the California Wellness Foundation. That grant, for Project SafeCare, enabled us to systematically replicate our ecobehavioral model for CAN.

In other books I have written, I have acknowledged my family. They, of course, provide support, but they are colleagues as well. My wife, Sandra, is a sounding board for my professional dilemmas; my son Dov has provided legal insights, and my son Tov provides immeasurable computer assistance. And I love them!

—J.R.L.

Contents

Part III. Treatment

Part VI. Conclusion

Part I

Theory, Law, and Standards

After the initial exposure of child abuse and neglect (CAN) to the public and to professionals in the 1960s, theories of how such a phenomenon could occur began to be spun. As will be seen in Chapter 1, by Azar, Povilaitis, Lauretti, and Pouquette, none were completely adequate and some were far from adequate. Azar and associates examine the etiological models of CAN, provide a historical overview, and attempt to integrate current theories into a meta model of CAN.

Legal issues must be considered in any examination of CAN. Portwood, Reppucci, and Mitchell, in Chapter 2, note that civil and criminal penalties can apply to adults involved in CAN. They discuss the relatively limited powers of the state in changing family structure and modifying family behavior and provide an important review of standards of parenting and of the definition of minimally adequate parenting. Portwood and colleagues remind us of the need for better training of professionals in reporting and assessing CAN. Finally, these authors review the role of the child as a witness.

In Chapter 3 Greene and Kilili stress the need for developing observable, reliable, and valid measures of parenting adequacy. As an example, they describe the validation of a measure of home cleanliness, an issue often important in the determination of neglect.

Thus, Part One covers theory, law, and standards, issues that are inherent in work described in the subsequent sections of this book.

1

The Current Status of Etiological Theories in Intrafamilial Child Maltreatment

SANDRA T. AZAR, TANIA Y. POVILAITIS, ALLISON F. LAURETTI, and CHRISTINA L. POUQUETTE

Child maltreatment is a major social problem affecting over a million children and their families each year (National Center on Child Abuse and Neglect, 1992). Effective treatment development for both perpetrators and victims of this problem rests on the availability of well-articulated and validated theories of etiology. Such theories allow for empirical documentation of causal factors and ultimately, more precisely targeted interventions. The goal of this chapter is to assess progress in the development of etiological models of intrafamilial child maltreatment. The chapter begins with a historical overview of the forces that operated to slow theory building in early phases of this field and ones that are now more fostering of theory development. We then examine the foundations of current theories about each form of child maltreatment, highlighting the definitions and assumptions that models have adopted and the basic dimensions on which they differ. The chapter ends with a preliminary attempt to integrate current theorizing into a meta-model that would be useful in treatment development.

SANDRA T. AZAR, TANIA Y. POVILAITIS, ALLISON F. LAURETTI, and CHRISTINA L. POUQUETTE • Frances L. Hiatt School of Psychology, Clark University, Worcester, Massachusetts 01610.

Handbook of Child Abuse Research and Treatment, edited by Lutzker. Plenum Press, New York, 1998.

FORCES INFLUENCING MODEL DEVELOPMENT

Society's initial outrage at the identification of child abuse as a social problem impelled it to take legal actions to protect children, but this emotional atmosphere did not encourage careful scientific inquiry into the etiology of the problem (Azar, Fantuzzo, & Twentyman, 1984; Gelles, 1983). Treatment took precedence over defining the disorder and searching for causes, limiting the knowledge base from which model building could take place. The epistemologies and emphases of the disciplines that dominated the field early in its history (law, medicine, and psychodynamic psychiatry) also slowed the development of an empirical knowledge base upon which to build theory.

In the late 1970s, such professionals as social learning theorists, sociologists, and developmental psychologists began to enter the field, bringing strong empirical traditions and rich theoretical backgrounds to bear on the problem. Unfortunately, a lack of research funding hampered their efforts. In addition, many methodological issues from earlier decades remained unresolved (e.g., the lack of operational definitions; Azar, 1988; Plotkin, Azar, Twentyman, & Perri, 1981). Consequently, growth in the field's knowledge base was slow.

Recently, however, the picture has begun to change. The number of maltreated children has startled society, and preliminary solutions have proven to be ineffective (e.g., foster care, legal sanctions). Federal task forces have called for more careful theory-guided research (National Research Council, 1993; The U.S.

Definitions
Assumptions
    —Defect
    —Deficit
    —Disruption
    —Mismatch between typical modes of responding and that which is more appropriate or effective
      in a given situation
Levels of analysis
    —Biological
    —Personality–emotional
    —Experiential–learning
    —Societal–cultural
Complexity
    —Single factor models
    —Lists of factors
    —Integrated models
Model form (modified version of Handlon, 1960; Wiener & Cromer, 1967)
    —Model 1: Abuse is a class with a single member, this member having a single cause.
    —Model 2: Abuse is a class with a single member, having multiple factors constituting the
      radical cause.
    —Model 3: Abuse is a class with several members, all members having the same single cause.
    —Model 4: Abuse is a class with several members, each having a single or multiple causes that
      are not necessarily unique to that member.
    —Model 5: Abuse is a class with several members, each member having a single unique cause.
    —Model 6: Conditional statements in ordered series predicting points in the development of
      disorder.

Figure 1. Dimensions on which models differ.

Advisory Board on Child Abuse and Neglect; 1993). Although growth has been slow, enough data have accumulated in at least two of the areas (physical and sexual abuse) to contribute to more sophisticated model development.

Over time, theories of maltreatment have shifted from single cause models (e.g., stress) to more recent integrated perspectives (e.g., cognitive–behavioral perspectives, social–ecological frameworks). These newer approaches hold the most promise for intervention development. Data in the areas of neglect and emotional maltreatment, however, have continued to lag behind. Our discussion of theory in these two forms of maltreatment will, therefore, be more limited.

DIMENSIONS ON WHICH MODELS VARY

Models of intrafamilial child maltreatment vary on a number of dimensions, including definition of the behavior in question, assumptions regarding its origins, level of identification of its determinants (e.g., intra-individual, social group, culture), complexity (single cause versus multiple causes), and form of antecedent–consequence relationships (Azar, 1991; Figure 1). When developing frameworks, theorists implicitly or explicitly make decisions on all five dimensions. In this section, each form of maltreatment will be considered separately, examining these dimensions and assessing progress.

PHYSICAL CHILD ABUSE[1]

Definitions

Perhaps the most important factor in determining a model's direction is how it defines the phenomenon in question. For example, some models begin with the premise that physical child abuse is an aggressive act and, thus, can be explained by existing models of aggression (e.g., mediational models, Bandura, 1983; frustration–aggression models, Miller, 1941). Others see the context in which it occurs, the family, as having special meaning and, therefore, invoke processes in social groups and families (e.g. general social systems theory, Straus, 1973). Such conceptualizations have resulted in explanatory models that often combine all forms of family violence.

Some models have moved away from aggression as an organizing construct and classified physical abuse within broader categories (e.g., conflict strategies, use of power). For example, resource theory (Goode, 1971) sees violence as a resource for obtaining dominance, a resource that is used only when others are lacking.

Moving even further from a narrow focus on aggression are theories that view physical abuse as one of many possible interpersonal behaviors, some of which facilitate transactions (e.g., produce good child outcome) and others of which do not. Such models attempt to delineate why one behavior is chosen over another (e.g., differential modeling experiences, attributional biases). For instance, in some recent models, abuse is at one end of a continuum of normal parenting with the other

[1] This section relies heavily upon Azar (1991).

end being optimal parenting (Azar, 1986, 1989; Wolfe, 1987). Here, abuse is viewed as part of a constellation of parental behaviors that negatively affect child outcome. Developmentally based, these models are intrinsically models of parenting adequacy. This view will form the core of the meta-model that will be outlined later in this chapter.

Other theorists, while conceiving of physical abuse as part of a constellation of aberrant parenting behavior, see it as discontinuous with "normal" parenting. Physical punishment is not viewed as on the same continuum with abuse, and the processes leading to abuse are seen as more trauma-based than those posited in the continuum view (e.g., disturbed attachment; Carlson, Cicchetti, Barnett, & Braunwald, 1989).

The definition of physical child abuse sets the stage for the other aspects of a model. Because definitions of all forms of maltreatment have not been given much attention, research has focused on narrowly defined cases (i.e., identified families), limiting the nature of the models produced.

Assumptions

Along with classifying physical child abuse, theories make assumptions about its origins that further determine theory development (Wiener & Cromer, 1967). First, there can be an assumption of *defect* (i.e., some malfunction such that the individual [parent, child or both] cannot benefit from his or her experiences). Impairment is thought to be permanent or of such a deeply based nature that it would be highly resistant to treatment (e.g., neurological defects, Elliot, 1988; arousal problems, Vasta, 1982; mental retardation, Schilling, Schinke, Blythe, & Barth, 1982). Typically, defect models do not provide avenues for treatment development and have not had much empirical support. Consequently, such models have not held much appeal for professionals, except perhaps in some legal contexts (e.g., termination of parental rights). They do have popular appeal in that society may prefer to distance itself from all maltreating parents by seeing them as defective.

The second assumption possible is that physical abuse is linked to some *deficiency*—the absence of some function—that is amenable to change. Models of this sort became prevalent when social learning theorists entered the field. Such a perspective is implicit in education-based social work responses to abuse and in recent behavioral interventions aimed at skill deficits.

The third possible assumption is that abuse involves a *disruption*. That is, some external factor interferes with appropriate parental functioning. Such views arrived with the movement of social psychologists and sociologists into the field. In models with this assumption, individual or culture-based stressors are posited as causal (Garbarino, 1976). Interventions are then aimed at reducing such stress (e.g., day care, economic subsidies).

The last possible assumption attributes disorder to differences or *mismatches between typical modes of responding and that which is more appropriate or effective in a given situation* (e.g., an overreliance on coercive transactions to elicit child compliance, Wolfe, 1987). The emphasis is on transactional problems (response–environment fit). This assumption places the problem in a transaction, not an individual. Models emphasizing societal validation of violence as a response to conflict or those positing a mismatch between the needs of families and societal/culture based supports would fit here (e.g., Levinson, 1988; Steinmetz & Straus, 1974). Interventions would require broad social changes that may pose a threat to strongly held social values.

Recently, models of physical child abuse have begun to combine assumptions (Cicchetti & Rizley, 1981; Wolfe, 1987). It is not clear whether this approach will be useful.

Levels of Analysis

Models differ as to where they direct the search for causal mechanisms—in biological, personality–emotional, experiential–learning, and societal–cultural levels of analysis. Early theories focused on variables within the individual. More recent transactional views have attempted to integrate multiple levels of analysis. For example, Belsky's model (1980) suggests causes in multiple ecological systems: what parents bring to parenthood (e.g., preparation), factors in the family's immediate context (e.g., child care needs), factors in larger social settings (e.g., work), and culture based values/beliefs. Variables within each system interact with variables in other systems to produce specific family transactions. The model does not, however, specify whether disturbances in only one system or in more than one are required for abuse to occur; this lowers its usefulness for treatment development.

Complexity

Over time in all fields, the complexity of models evolves. As noted earlier, integration has begun to occur in theories of physical abuse. These efforts, however, are in their earliest stages and typically are merely lists of the components of single-factor theories with little attempt to specify contingent relationships among factors or prioritize their contribution to etiology. In some cases, too many components are posited to result in testable models (Gelles & Straus, 1979). Some theorists have argued that integration may not be possible and others have suggested that mid-level theories, moderate in complexity, may have the greatest ultimate utility (Gelles, 1983).

Model Form

The final dimension on which models differ is in their structure (i.e., the form of antecedent–consequence relationship posited). Using a formal analysis framework delineated by Handlon (1960), progress and conceptual problems hindering model development can be seen. In applying this framework, more basic problems quickly become apparent (Figure 1). First, elaborate theories are still rare, and thus, what we call theories and how we group them may be open to question. Indeed, many would not meet strict criteria for being deemed theories (e.g., operational definitions of components, testable hypotheses). Second, because all forms of maltreatment involve transactions rather than one individual's behavior, simple linear relationships might not be the most appropriate explanatory format. Wiener and Cromer's (1967) addition of type 6 models to Handlon's framework may ultimately prove to be more appropriate. Here, abuse would be seen as the end point of a transactional process (see Wolfe, 1987 for an example). Third, most models of physical child abuse view it as a class with a single member or combine it with other forms of family violence, limiting attempts at models 3 to 5.

Until the last decade or so, it was type 1 models that dominated the field ("If A, then X"). Here, each case of physical child abuse is seen as equivalent to every other case and having its origin in a single factor, something about the perpetrator, the victim, or the context in which they interact. Early type 1 models were typically "borrowed" from other areas (e.g., behavioral models of family [Patterson & Reid, 1967]). With more data, models specific to physical child abuse have emerged.

Perpetrator models are the most common type 1 model. In the extreme, these models posited that child maltreaters were psychotic or suffered from personality disorders, with factors in the perpetrator's early history being crucial (e.g., a lack of empathic caregiving; Steele, 1980). Their underlying constructs (e.g., disrupted identification processes), however, have not been amenable to empirical validation, and specific diagnoses have not differentiated maltreaters. The idea of negative early parental role models, however, has been retained in more recent frameworks.

Until recently, among the least adequately developed of the perpetrator theories have been biological approaches. These efforts have included early attempts at ethological models (e.g., "critical period" attachment views, Klaus & Kennell, 1976) and recent explanations of physical abuse involving nonspecific neurological problems (Elliot, 1988) and physiological reactivity (Frodi & Lamb, 1980). Although the biological bases of these disturbances have not been documented, these ideas have been retained in more behavioral form in recent frameworks (e.g., "conditioned arousal," behavioral system views of attachment). Sociobiological concepts, such as inclusive fitness, have also been invoked, although they do better at explaining abuse where a stepparent is involved (Burgess & Draper, 1989; Daly & Wilson, 1981).

In the last few years, perpetrator theories have become more sophisticated. For example, Azar (1986, 1989) has suggested parental social–cognitive disturbances (e.g., disturbed schema involving children, problem-solving deficits) are present in perpetrators that result in negative interpretations of child behavior. These, ultimately, lead to abusive transactions and to an environment that does not support children's overall development. Along the same lines, Newberger and Cook (1983) have explained abuse using a developmental model of "parental awareness," where less sophisticated levels of perspective-taking ability and conceptions of children are conducive to maladaptive parenting. Research focusing on parent and child disturbances in emotion recognition and expression (Camras, et al., 1990) is also promising and may, ultimately, result in fine-tuned emotion-based theory. Perpetrator theories that are well specified and validated may prove very useful for treatment development.

In addition to a focus on perpetrators, studies have attempted to identify characteristics of abused children that either produce abuse directly or hasten an abusive cycle in a "vulnerable" parent. For example, such children may begin life with characteristics which make them seem more aversive (e.g., handicaps, difficult temperament; Belsky, 1980; Parke & Collmer, 1975), or through modeling or reinforcement processes, "difficult" child behavior may occur, maintaining an abusive pattern (Azar, 1989; Wolfe, 1987). No single child factor, however, distinguishes physically abused children, and prospective work suggests that any differences observed are more likely to have resulted from the abuse itself than to be causal (Pianta, Egeland, & Erickson, 1989). Overall, child-based theories have met with great resistance. They are seen as "blaming the victim." However, transactional views of children's development (where both participants play a part in outcomes) are dominant in developmental literature. Thus, a model without a child component may be less useful, although such elements might be relegated to a lower priority than parental or contextual ones.

In the final kind of type 1 model, environmental factors are seen as impinging on families' general ability to function, or to function in certain ways. In the extreme, such models would argue that any parent, given the right circumstances, could be physically abusive. For example, associations have been found between abuse and both stress (Egeland Breitenbucher, & Rosenberg, 1980) and lack of social support (Salzinger, Kaplan, & Artemyeff, 1983), although it is not clear why only *some* parents experiencing these conditions become aggressive. Other models view as causal society's validation of the use of violence (Gelles 1983; Gelles & Straus, 1979). Again, most parents do not engage in physical child abuse; therefore, societal values alone cannot account for abuse.

In summary, no single factor appears to account for significant amounts of physical abuse. These early views, however, stimulated research and many of their components have been incorporated in more recent type 2 models, which posit multiple routes to the development of physically abusive behavior. At first, these newer models were merely lists of the single factors posited in the early theories, without providing any organizing links between them. More recent attempts have provided global organizing frameworks or have even posited staged processes. An example is Belsky's (1980) ecological framework described earlier. Another is that of Azar and Twentyman (1986), who outlined five areas of parental skill deficit that increase abuse risk: parenting skills (e.g., too narrow a repertoire), cognitive dysfunctions (e.g., unrealistic expectations regarding children), and impulse control, stress management, and social skills problems. Over time, these deficits result in a four-stage sequence of responses leading to an abusive incident (Figure 2; Azar, 1989).

Other type 2 models provide global contingent factors (i.e., "if high levels of A and low levels of B, then X"). For example, Cicchetti and Rizley's (1981) transactional model posits that risk involves both transient and enduring factors that may be potentiating (increase risk) or compensatory (buffering or protective in nature). When potentiating factors are more frequent than buffering ones, abuse is likely.

Stage 1: The parent holds unrealistic standards regarding what are appropriate behaviors in children.
Stage 2: They encounter a child behavior that fails to meet their standards.
Stage 3: The parent misattribtues negative intent to the behavior and does not question her interpretations or blames herself when her interventions do not change the child's response.
Stage 4: The parent overreacts perhaps after making some poorly skilled effort to change the child's behavior, and punishes the child excessively.

Figure 2. Physical abuse: A four-stage process.

This model nicely emphasizes risk over time and links potential causal elements to child outcome. Unfortunately, it does not prioritize the factors it specifies.

Wolfe's (1987) transitional model also explicitly includes time. Initially, this model described an escalation theory, whereby the abusive parent over-relies on coercion to elicit child compliance (Wolfe, Kaufman, Aragona, & Sandler, 1981). Although such strategies are effective at first, children eventually habituate to them and increasingly higher levels of coercion are required to produce an impact, culminating in physical abuse. In a recent reformulation, Wolfe (1987) provides three stages in the development of these abusive patterns and the destabilizing and compensatory factors that might facilitate or inhibit movement through them. (This reformulation in some ways foreshadows a type 6 model.) Although similar to Cicchetti and Rizley's (1981) model, this one is more firmly based in social learning theory and, therefore, a deficiency assumption is made throughout.

As noted earlier, the development of models beyond type 2 is more limited. Most require differentiated views of physical child abuse. While there were some early efforts in this direction (e.g., Merrill, 1962), the typologies produced were not empirically validated. A more recent attempt at classifying physical child abuse is that of Gelles and Straus (1979) who posit two defining dimensions: expressive/instrumental and legitimacy/illegitimacy. *Expressive violence* is physical abuse that serves to reduce perpetrators' tension level, whereas *instrumental violence* involves violent acts intended to produce a response in others (e.g., discipline that becomes excessive). *Legitimacy* involves a continuum in the use of physical force in situations where it is approved or required by society. The resulting four-cell taxonomy may ultimately prove useful to developing models that differentiate between types of physical abuse.

Based on actual observations of abusive parent–child interaction patterns, Oldershaw, Walters, and Hall (1989) posited a typology with three subgroups: Hostile, Emotionally Distant, and Intrusive. This empirically defined typology could serve as a foundation for more complex theories.

A third alternative has been suggested by Azar and Siegel (1990). They argue that abuse that emerges in different developmental periods (e.g., in infancy versus adolescence, or across more than one period) may have different antecedents and, thus, may require different models. Using tasks required of parents in each period of childhood, they outlined potential causal factors that either cut across developmental phases or vary with children's needs. For example, they posit unrealistic expectations regarding children's behavior that may play a causal role across development, and behavioral skills that may be important in one phase, but not in others (e.g., verbal negotiation skills with teens). This framework will form the core for the meta-model that will be described later.

INTRAFAMILIAL SEXUAL ABUSE

Although sexual contact between children and adult family members has always been a taboo in most cultures, the study of the causes of sexual abuse is a much younger field than that of physical abuse. At the same time, perhaps because of this taboo and a bias toward seeing the victims of this form of abuse as more psychologically damaged (Vitulano, Lewis, Doran, Nordhaus, & Adnopoz,

1986), research in this area has progressed more rapidly. Current frameworks for understanding etiology, however, are still somewhat simplistic. These frameworks are usually lists of single factors that differentiate perpetrators of incest. The narrowness of the samples studied (e.g., fathers/stepfathers, incarcerated perpetrators) may also limit the generalization of the models produced (Williams & Finkelhor, 1990).

Definitions

A common definition of sexual abuse has been sexual exploitation involving physical contact between a child and another person (Cohen & Mannarino, 1993). Exploitation implies an inequality of power between the child and the abuser on the basis of age, physical size, and/or the nature of the emotional relationship. Physical contact includes anal, genital, oral, or breast contact. As with physical abuse, models of incest either have separated it from other forms of child abuse and other sexual offenses (e.g., rape) or, at the other extreme, have combined it with these other disturbances. Attempts have also been made to explain parent (stepparent) incest separately from sexual offenses within the family carried out by other family members (e.g., siblings). Finally, including exploitation as a defining quality has also directed some theorizing to the realm of power and its misuse both within and outside the family and directed it away from the sexual nature of the act.

Assumptions

In examining the four types of assumptions inherent in models of incest, patterns similar to the early stages of model development in physical abuse can be detected. The major portion of work to date has emphasized defects or deficits within the perpetrator. One defect-based model describes deviant sexual arousal and interests gained through conditioning and social learning (Laws & Marshall, 1990). Neuropsychological correlates of violence and aggression, in general, and of sex offending, in particular, have also been found. The biological bases for such models are supported primarily by inappropriate sexual behavior shown in individuals suffering from central nervous system degeneration, as in Alzheimer's disease or brain injuries (Golden, Jackson, Peterson-Rohne, & Gontkovsky, 1996). However, psychopathology models, another form of defect models, have not been supported; the majority of incestuous fathers do not manifest severe psychiatric problems (Williams & Finkelhor, 1990). Despite limited evidence, defect models remain popular because society would prefer to see perpetrators as untreatable and have them locked away as criminals.

Deficiency models have also been postulated. For example, perpetrators have been described as having empathy deficits and problems in emotional recognition skills, freeing them to engage in behavior harmful to children (Marshall, Hudson, Jones, & Fernandez, 1995; Monto, Zgourides, Wilson, & Harris, 1994). Cognitive disturbances regarding the meaning of their behavior have also been identified in offenders, which may also free them to act. For example, child molesters perceive more benefits to children from sexual contact, greater complicity on the child's part, and less responsibility on the adult's part, all of which may play a facilitating role in child molesting (Abel & Rouleau, 1995; Stermac & Segal, 1989). Deficits in social skills (Stermac Segal, & Gillis, 1990) and in establishing intimacy in adult relationships have also been found; these may lead to high levels of emotional loneliness (Marshall, 1989; Seidman, Marshall, Hudson, & Robertson, 1994). Although each of these individual factors has some validity standing alone, some combination may provide a more comprehensive picture of the origins of sexual abuse.

Disruption models of sexual abuse have been less prevalent. Unlike physical abuse, sexual abuse occurs across all social classes, suggesting that environmental stress does not play as strong a role as it may in neglect or emotional abuse. Haugaard (1988), however, refers to a chaos explanation where risk for sexual abuse may occur when there is a lack of external regulation in a community, such as in postwar disorganization. Generally, the sociopolitical atmosphere surrounding sexual abuse (the need to see perpetrators as disturbed) may prevent implicating external factors. One exception is exploring the effects of alcohol consumption, which may be viewed as more within perpetrators' control (Koss & Gaines, 1993).

Models that focus on missocialization processes may be examples of "mismatch" models in this area. Finkelhor (1984) suggests that abuse should be described as a problem within masculine socialization, with men learning to focus on sex as part of their gender identities and to see younger and smaller persons as their appropriate sexual partners. In addition, he notes that our culture teaches us that children and females are less powerful and the risk of sexual abuse may increase if this view is internalized too strongly. Thus, in the extreme, what society may teach some men is a "mismatch" with what would be more appropriate—the avoidance of using children for sexual gratification. Supporting such views is interesting social psychological research indicating that males have a greater tendency than females to interpret friendliness on the part of members of the opposite sex as indicative of sexual attraction (Abbey, 1982, 1987). In addition to missocialization, alcohol consumption may increase disinhibition and misattributions in individuals prone to sexual aggression (Crowe & George, 1989). Such findings provide the beginnings for more integrative theories using multiple assumptions.

Levels of Analysis

Biological (e.g., neuropsychological problems), personality–emotional (e.g., lack of empathy), experiential–learning (e.g., transmission of sex offending in boys through modeling), and societal–cultural factors (e.g., societal values) have all been given attention in theories in this area and have been examined at each level of analysis: intra-individual, social group, and cultural group. For example, when misuse of power is considered the defining element of sexual abuse, models have focused on power relationships either within the family, between genders, or within the larger society (Finkelhor, 1981; Solomon, 1992).

Complexity

As with physical abuse, sexual abuse models have evolved to embody a range of complexity. Early on, descriptive models identifying single factors that differentiated sexual abusers from nonabusers were common. When a variety of factors were identified (i.e., social isolation, lack of empathy, history of abuse), models combining these factors began to appear. Although these continue to dominate the field, few attempts to integrate them have been made. Examples of each will be provided below.

Model Form

Almost all models of etiology for this form of maltreatment are type 1 frameworks. Sexual abuse is seen as having its origin in a single factor, typically within perpetrators. In his review, Haugaard (1988) groups models into four general categories: individual deviance explanations (defect-deficiency models), chaotic explanations (i.e., models citing a lack of external regulation, a disruption view), feminist perspectives (focusing on inequality of the sexes), and the functional explanation, where incest serves a purpose within the context in which it occurs (e.g., acting as a compensatory factor if a couple is having marital problems).

Intergenerational transmission has also been posited. It seems that prior abuse or mistreatment may place a victim at greater risk for perpetrating sexual offenses (Renshaw, 1994). Ryan (1989) suggests past victims may offend to gain some sense of personal control lost as a result of their own abuse. Insecure attachment has also been posited as the mechanism whereby the experience of abuse translates into perpetration (Alexander, 1992), and may be a precursor of intimacy deficits noted by Marshall (1989). Such deficits in turn may lead to aggression and a tendency to pursue sexual contacts to find intimacy, even with inappropriate partners.

Sociobiological perspectives have also been posited. Higher rates of incest have been found for nonbiological fathers and for biological fathers who did not participate in crucial early socialization and nurturing activities, such as diapering and feeding (Daly & Wilson, 1985; Parker & Parker, 1986).

Single-factor models focusing on children have not developed in this area. In the past, psychoanalytic perspectives hinted that victims may contribute to their abuse by being seductive (Diamond, 1989). Few researchers today focus on the personality characteristics of victims, although behavioral characteristics of victims may place them at risk. For example, exploration of factors that make a child vulnerable, more accessible, and less able to prevent abuse or to report it (e.g., handicapped children) has continued.

Overall, no single factor seems acceptable as an explanation for the etiology of sexual abuse. Consequently, listlike frameworks (type 2 models) have appeared. Finkelhor's (1984) sociological model describes four preconditions essential to the occurrence of sexual abuse (although they may not play a causal role): (1) motivation to sexually abuse a child (e.g., emotional needs, sexual arousal by children); (2) weakened internal inhibitions that would normally prevent such abuse; (3) few external barriers to abuse (i.e., easy assessibility to locations where the offense could occur); and (4) the perpetrator's ability to overcome the resistance of the child. While each may contribute to abuse, this framework does not prioritize them.

A few early attempts to define types of incest perpetrators were made. For example, Rist (1979) identified three types of incestuous fathers: the socially isolated man who is highly dependent on his family for interpersonal relationships, the father who has a psychopathic personality and is indiscriminate in choosing sexual partners, and the father who has pedophilic tendencies and is sexually involved with several children, including his daughter. This emphasis on patterns of offending has formed the basis for later empirically based higher-level models.

Hall and Hirschmann (1991, 1992), for example, have attempted to integrate factors found in the literature into a model of all forms of sexual aggression against both adults and children. Their quadripartite model emphasizes the presence of deviant patterns of sexual arousal, a level of cognitive distortion great enough to counteract environmentally based information, deviant appraisal patterns, and loss of affective control, all of which combine to increase risk for sexual aggression. When the affect is depression, the target of the sexual aggression is likely to be a child, whereas when it is anger, it is more often an adult. Personality factors are seen as further mediating risk.

Marshall and Barbaree (1990) have also made an attempt to integrate empirical findings. Their model posits biological, early experiential (e.g., poor attachment), sociocultural, and transitory situational factors that combine to explain cases where both sexual abuse and aggression occur.

Recent theorizing has emphasized a person-by-environment transactional model. Holman and Stokols (1994) cite the role of sociocultural and physical environmental factors in moderating the occurrence and long-term consequences of sexual abuse. Although they are similar to Marshall and Barbaree in their articulation of important factors, they organize these factors within phases: pre-abuse, abuse, and post-abuse. Thus, their framework has relevance both to the occurrence of abuse and to potential outcomes in the child. The framework also adds greater emphasis to physical and macrolevel factors (e.g., the residential environment of the child, neighborhood, and community).

As can be seen in our discussion, the field is beginning to move away from single-factor frameworks to more unified versions. This movement has been facilitated by a stronger empirical data base where single factors are validated and combined to produce more complex models for testing. This kind of progress has yet to occur in development of theories of neglect and emotional abuse.

NEGLECT

The diversity of behaviors that are labeled neglectful has made model building particularly difficult (Figure 3; Zuravin, 1991). Neglect has received less research attention than the other forms of maltreatment discussed thus far. Unlike children suffering from physical and sexual abuse, neglected children are often seen by the nursing and social work professions, both of which have only recently developed research traditions. In addition, in many cases, neglect is linked to poverty; this fact adds a sociopolitical element that may be less palatable to a scientific community that attempts to be apolitical. Neglect may also be thought of as the least "compelling" type of child maltreatment and may not arouse as high a level of societal outrage as do other forms (e.g., sexual abuse). In addition, it involves behaviors that tend to be viewed as chronic, with perpetrators viewed as more dispositionally disturbed. Intervention may, therefore, be viewed as more futile than with other types of child maltreatment and, thus, model building may be seen as less important. Complicating theory development

Refusal to provide physical health care
Delay in providing physical health care
Refusal to provide mental health care
Delay in providing mental health care
Supervisory neglect
Custody refusal
Custody-related neglect
Abandonment/desertion
Failure to provide a permanent home
Personal hygiene neglect
Housing hazards
Housing sanitation
Nutritional neglect
Educational neglect

Figure 3. Subtypes of neglect (Zuravin, 1991).

further is the difficulty posed by measuring acts of omission (e.g., failing to provide medical care), which is more difficult than assessing observable and quantifiable acts of commission.

In devising perpetrator models, the question of who is labeled the neglector is open to debate. Mothers are typically the ones so labeled, even if a father or another caretaker is present.

The nature of neglect also depends on the child's developmental level. Behaviors that might be neglectful of an infant may not be neglectful of an adolescent. The issue of how chronically the parental omission needs to occur before it is considered neglectful has also not been adequately addressed. The etiology of chronic neglect may be quite different from neglect that occurs in response to a parental stress (e.g., in response to a recent job loss). Finally, the relevance of intent in defining neglect, and how this might be determined has not received much attention. Wolock and Horowitz (1977) in their definition of housing sanitation problems (e.g., spoiled food, dirty dishes), for instance, require that they be parent induced in order to be considered neglect.

The lack of theory in this area is striking, given that neglected children typically outnumber those who have encountered the other forms of maltreatment. Incidence rates in one study (Sedlak, 1990) were 14.6 per 1,000 children compared to 4.9 per 1,000 for physical abuse and 2.1 per 1,000 for sexual abuse. There are no estimated rates for emotional maltreatment of children, although if substantiated cases are examined, it accounts for only 6% or less of cases compared to 45% for neglect (National Center on Child Abuse and Neglect, 1992). Furthermore, in the long run, neglect may have the most far-reaching implications for children's social, emotional, and physical outcomes.

Definitions

As noted above, models may vary with the subtype of neglect being addressed. Neglect of health care and hygiene may result from basic knowledge deficits in parents (e.g., how to take a child's temperature), whereas abandonment could originate in a myriad of other factors besides lack of knowledge (e.g., substance abuse, severe psychopathology). Types of neglect that have been addressed include failure to provide medical care, supervision, nutrition, personal hygiene, emotional nurturing, education, and safe housing (Gaudin, 1993).

The definitions of neglect have focused on the types of outcomes seen. For example, neglect is often considered one cause of failure to thrive and has been cited in the category of feeding problems in some discussions. Failure to attend to medical needs has been considered in the larger category of treatment noncompliance. The former classification might lead to models regarding parent–infant transactional problems, whereas the latter might focus models on understanding motivational deficits.

Assumptions

Because mothers are identified as perpetrators, models have focused especially on characterological or personal deficits of neglectful women. For example, they have been described as having severe defects in ego and general personality development (e.g., immaturity, narcissism, Cantwell, 1980; Meier, 1964; Young, 1964). As with physical and sexual abuse, more fundamental defects have also been posited (e.g., psychoses and mental retardation). More recently, however, factors more amenable to change have been emphasized, including lack of knowledge about children's development, poor parental judgment, and motivational problems (Cantwell, 1980; Polansky, Chalmers, Buttenwieser, & Williams, 1981).

In an elaborate personality-based explanation, Galdston (1968) argued for what might be conceived of as a relational disturbance underlying neglect. He suggested that neglect results from a failure to perceive the child as one's own, such that mothers cannot accommodate the child in any way. Such a parent is seen as self-centered. Other potential mechanisms have been suggested that may account for this perceptual problem (e.g., attachment disturbances, Crittenden, 1993; information processing problems, Azar, Robinson, Hekimian, & Twentyman, 1984).

Contextual factors have also been highlighted as causal elements. Some of these factors are low family income and educational level (Garbarino, 1991; Polansky et al., 1981; Polansky, Gaudin, Ammons, & David, 1985), lack of social support, and high life stress (Gaudin et al., 1993). The direction of causality is, however, open to question. Although it has been found that lack of resources (e.g. food stamps, housing, employment, available day care; Pelton, 1994) can affect parental functioning, it is possible that neglectful mothers are less able to balance the resources they do have. For example, it has been found that neglectful parents tend to belong to significantly fewer formal organizations than nonneglectful parents (Young, 1964) but it is not known whether this external factor causes inappropriate parental functioning or whether both poor parenting and lack of such contacts are related to some other third element (e.g., poor social skills).

Although there do not appear to be formal models emphasizing mismatches between typical modes of responding and that which is more appropriate or effective in a given situation, it appears that our culture, with its emphasis on obtaining material goods (e.g., owning your own home, TV, expensive cars), could contribute to the neglect of children, as many parents emphasize these material factors over the kind of self-sacrificing often required to raise children. Economic conditions may also create a situation wherein neglect may be unavoidable (e.g., parents who are unable to afford child care being forced to leave children home alone while at work). Promoting some forms of neglect may also be a recent increased emphasis in our culture on children doing for themselves without the assistance of parents, often placing greater demands upon young children. This belief may be particularly appealing in families where both parents work and where there are single parents who are highly stressed. It also may be possible that neglectful parents internalized from their own childhoods a maladaptive schema or working model of relationships, where children are seen as existing to meet adult needs.

Belsky's (1980) integrative framework mentioned earlier in describing physical abuse is one of the few that considers neglect to be multidetermined, including child, parent, family, community, and societal factors. For example, neglectful parents may enter parenthood with a template that children are to meet parent needs, and may also have a predisposition toward depression, limiting their level of initiation with their children and others. As contextual stress increases and familial supports decrease or are taxed, neglect may occur.

Levels of Analysis

As with the other types of maltreatment, causes for neglect have been suggested at all levels of analysis. These include biological (e.g., mental retardation), personality–emotional (e.g., ego deficiency), experiential (e.g., attachment during the first year of life), and sociocultural (e.g., poverty, social isolation). Early research focused on variables within the individual; the second wave has focused more strongly on sociocultural forces (e.g., poverty). Only recently there is beginning to be an emphasis on the interaction of factors at more than one level of analysis.

Complexity

Models of neglect often have not been separated from those of physical abuse, and they have traveled the same path of model development. Unfortunately, although more complex models of parental aggression have begun to emerge, similar complexity has been lacking for neglect. Presently, frameworks have progressed only to lists that describe single factors distinguishing chronically neglectful mothers, and this may not be applicable in less chronic situations or with fathers. A sampling of such frameworks is provided in the next section.

Model Form

Structurally, almost all models of neglect are either type 1 frameworks (i.e., "If A, then X") or weak type 2 models (i.e., "If A or B, then X"). Polansky, (Polansky et al., 1981), one of the few theorists in this area, adopted a personality theory perspective, arguing for enduring character disorders as causes of neglect. His view is similar to that of theorists who tried to explain child maltreatment more generally (Galdston, 1968). Polansky saw the majority of neglectful mothers' behavior as resulting from their own early histories of inadequate parental care. Based on two extensive studies, he developed a list of types of women who are likely to neglect their children: the impulse ridden, individuals with mental retardation, women in reactive depression, those with a borderline personality disorder or even a psychosis (which he saw as rare), and the apathetic-futile type. The most pervasive of perpetrators was the last type, who appears passive, withdrawn, and lacking in expression and whom he considered the most chronically immature. This is a type

2 model, in that any one of these character problems might result in neglect. Evidence that such disturbances alone would lead to neglect is limited, however.

In a more complex model, Crittenden's (1993) information-processing perspective focuses on four stages of responses required for successfully meeting children's needs where failures may result in neglect. These stages are (1) perception of essential aspects of children's states, (2) accurate interpretation of the meaning of these perceptions, (3) selection of adaptive responses, and (4) responding in ways that meet children's needs. The neglect observed may have different qualities (e.g., severity) depending upon which and how many of these stages are failed. Underlying these problems in information processing are four factors: excluding the perception of child cues to avoid rejection (defensive exclusion), faulty attributions leading to role reversal, a limited repertoire of childrearing responses, and a chaotic living environment produced by the parent where children's needs are ignored or go unnoticed. All of these factors are described as having their roots in poor early parental attachment relationships (an experiential assumption where the parent failed to have their own needs met in childhood). Azar (1986, 1989) posited a similar model to describe maltreating parenting more generally, including neglect, but used a social cognitive perspective. She argued for a set of cognitive distortions underlying social information-processing difficulties in childrearing situations that interact with contextual stress and behavioral skills deficits to result in abuse or neglect. This model and its recent elaboration (Azar & Siegel, 1990) will be discussed in detail later in this chapter.

Gaudin (Gaudin, Polansky, Kilpatrick, & Shilton, 1993) takes a different perspective, placing more emphasis on environmental factors. His starting point is the strong relationship between child neglect and poverty. In designing his research, he attempts to distinguish between poor neglectful and nonneglectful parents. He argues that it is the interaction of poverty with intense perceptions of social isolation that produces neglect. These last two models represent more transactional views.

Garbarino (1977) has also argued for an exclusively environmental explanation for child maltreatment (both physical abuse and neglect). He postulates three environmental conditions as crucial to maltreatment: (1) a cultural context that condones violence in general, (2) families who experience stress in their life circumstances combined with social isolation, and (3) consensual values concerning family autonomy and parental ownership of children. This model differs from the others because all three conditions are needed for abuse-neglect to occur.

Subcultural explanations for neglect have not received much attention. It can easily be seen, however, that differences in values between cultures may result in practices that might be labeled neglectful (e.g., the importance of school attendance, views on how independent children should be). Mismatches between practices that are acceptable in one culture and not in another may explain some neglectful situations. For example, a mother interviewed by the first author in an urban high-rise apartment was charged with neglect for letting her young children wander outside the building alone. She explained that in her home culture, adults see it as their responsibility to monitor unattended children and she expected others would watch her children.

As data have accumulated regarding the pervasive impact of neglect, more attention has begun to focus on model building in this area. Soon, more complexity may emerge here, as well as for emotional maltreatment, discussed next.

EMOTIONAL MALTREATMENT

Of the four types of child maltreatment discussed in this chapter, emotional abuse has received the least attention. This is surprising, as some theorists believe it is at the core of other forms of maltreatment (Hart, Germain, & Brassard, 1987). The paucity of research in this area may be due to the greater ease with which more readily identifiable forms of abuse can be studied (Egeland & Erickson, 1987) and lack of consensus on both conceptual and operational definitions (McGee & Wolfe, 1991). As a result, our discussion of this area is speculative.

Definitions

The main definitional dilemmas involve a delineation of behaviors that form the basis of emotional maltreatment, and the question as to whether it is a separate entity or in fact core to the other forms of maltreatment, or both. Hart and associates (1987) offer one of the most inclusive conceptual definitions of emotional maltreatment. They posit that it consists of acts of omission or commission deemed to be psychologically damaging to children, including those acts which pose a threat, either immediately or ultimately, to children's behavioral, cognitive, affective, or physical functioning. Thus, all forms of maltreatment would be considered emotional maltreatment. Other writers, in discussing definitional issues, argue that such inclusive conceptual definitions are problematic due to redundancy. McGee and Wolfe (1991) posit that psychological maltreatment consists of any communication pattern between adult and child that has the *potential* to undermine the child's social, emotional, cognitive, or social–cognitive development. They argue for including only those forms of nonphysical acts or omission which might cause nonphysical damage to children.

Following from conceptual problems, operational definitions have also been difficult. McGee and Wolfe (1991), for example, provide a substantial list of behaviors: rejecting, degrading, terrorizing, isolating, missocializing, exploiting, and denying emotional responsiveness. The consequences of having such a wide range of definitions has been discussed by Garbarino and Vondra (1987), who argue that narrow definitions capture only the most severe forms of emotional maltreatment, whereas more broad ones are likely to characterize all parents at one time or another. In contrast, Egeland and Erickson (1987) argue that caregivers who are psychologically unavailable provide the most damaging form of maltreatment, but this would be overlooked by narrow definitions. Underlying this discussion is a debate as to whether maltreaters are on the same continuum with other parents. We will return to this issue as we consider an overarching model of maltreatment.

Assumptions

Defect models have not developed in this area as they have been in other areas, although when emotional maltreatment is viewed as core to the other forms of maltreatment, the same models might be discussed here. Deeply rooted impairments, such as neurological disturbances, that may influence parents' emotional regulation and their perception of affect in others, have not yet been posited, although they may be viable explanations for the failures in caregiving observed.

Early theorizing in this area discussed parental psychiatric disturbances (e.g., depression, personality disorders, or alcoholism). In her review of studies of emotional neglect, Shakel (1987) describes studies in which parents were viewed as recreating patterns of emotional neglect and stimulus deprivation that they experienced as children. They let their own needs take precedence, fail to achieve a feeling of competence as parents, and are unable to provide adult role models for their children. Shakel, however, points out that these responses may result from parental stress or their social situation and, thus, emotional abuse may be explained just as easily by external factors.

Deficiencies in the behavioral or cognitive area may also explain emotional maltreatment (Azar, 1989). For example, psychologically maltreating parents may not have the ability to interact with their children in a normal and supportive manner as a result of poor modeling experiences with their own parents. Similarly, it may be assumed that such parents may not have the problem-solving skills necessary to correct their children's misbehavior in any manner other than a verbally abusive one. That is, they have more restricted repertoires, dominated by verbally coercive approaches. Finally, a cognitive perspective might focus on the self-efficacy of such parents. For example, these parents may perceive parenting failures more negatively and as personal failures. Bugenthal and Shennum (1984) have focused on perceptions of control in parents at risk for maladaptive parenting responses; they argue that such parents perceive their children as having more control than they do. Emotional maltreatment may, therefore, be an attempt to rectify a perceived power differential. Depression may also be present in such parents, leading to misperceptions that children are negatively evaluating them. Indeed, there are some data that maltreating parents see their children as intentionally acting to annoy them (Azar, 1989). If additional perspective-taking deficits are present, then these parents would not be able to accurately appraise the impact of their words.

Contextual factors may also influence the occurrence of emotional maltreatment. For example, in divorcing families, single-parent families, and other highly stressed families, parental functioning has been found to be negatively affected (Belsky & Vondra, 1989) and in the extreme, emotional unavailability and higher levels of verbally abusive behavior may result.

Levels of Analysis

Little research exists on emotional maltreatment and, therefore, there are limitations in the approaches people have taken to positing etiological factors. Sociobiologists have explored animal models of caregiver rejection of offspring. For example, rhesus monkeys deprived early in development of contact with maternal caretakers and contact with peers show higher levels of inadequate caretaking behaviors (Suomi, 1978). Lack of exposure to specific types of caregiving behavior during critical periods of childhood have been implicated (e.g., nursing and ventral contact). How deprivation of these experiences translates into inadequate caregiving with their own offspring and whether the mechanisms are biological is not clear as yet. A list of potential biological mechanisms might be generated (e.g., emotional regulation difficulties, neurological difficulties influencing responsivity, hormonal changes).

Theories of etiology involving the personality and emotional characteristics of the psychologically maltreating parent are the most common. The best known of these is in the work of Egeland and Erickson (1987), who described what they called the "psychologically unavailable" mother (similar to Polansky's apathetic-futile neglectful mother category), whose children show the worst outcomes. These women were withdrawn, displayed flat affect, and appeared depressed compared to control mothers and mothers who engaged in other forms of abuse. They also identified a group of mothers who engaged in constant harassment and degradation of their children. Core to these responses are parental emotional states (Pianta, Egeland, & Erickson, 1989). Similarly, Belsky and Vondra (1989) suggest that parenting behaviors (including psychologically abusive ones) may be influenced by characteristics of the individual. It is posited that the origins of such responses are within the parent's early developmental history and may affect parenting behaviors directly and indirectly by influencing the broader context in which the parent–child relationship exists, such as marital relations and social networks. Indeed, Lesnik-Oberstein, Koers, and Cohen (1995) found that psychologically abusive mothers had negative childhood upbringings and recalled less caring mothers and overcontrolling fathers. They also reported having partner relationships that were less affectionate and more verbally and physically aggressive. It appears that the high levels of subjective distress that result are described as spilling over into parenting in the form of hostile feelings.

Complexity and Form

As can be seen by the limited discussion above, theories of emotional maltreatment are limited. Most are merely extensions of theories designed to explain physical child abuse (indeed there is often an overlap between the two). For example, Lesnik-Oberstein, Koers, and Cohen (1995) posit that factors at many systemic levels (individual, family, community, subcultural) contribute to the occurrence of psychological maltreatment. They suggest that three main factors—parental hostility, parental inhibition of overt aggression, and focusing of parental aggression on children—are each the outcome of a network of other subfactors. For example, low parental inhibition of overt aggression is the outcome of six elements: preconventional cognitive developmental level of moral reasoning, low cultural inhibition of overt aggression, lack of insight into their own past abuse, alcohol or drug abuse, absence of a supportive partner or social network, and low level of empathy. The type of child abuse (physical versus emotional) that occurs depends upon the ratio of parental hostility to parental inhibition of aggression. They suggest that low coping skills, a negative developmental history, and a high level of stress lead to a high level of parental hostility, which predisposes the parent to psychological abuse.

Egeland and Erickson (1987), mentioned earlier, posit that the responses of psychologically unavailable mothers come from a combination of a mother's own unmet emotional needs and low levels of social support. In more recent work, Pianta, Egeland, and Erickson (1989) suggest that these psychological characteristics of maltreating parents are more central to the cause of all forms of maltreatment than are all other external factors.

Integrated models have also been posited (e.g., ones that parallel Belsky's (1980) ecological framework or developmental ones that link children's developmental stage [Erikson's (1950) stages]) to vulnerabilities of children in the parenting they receive [Hart, Germain, & Brassard, 1987]. Although these preliminary attempts to posit such models seem viable, they may be premature, given the very limited data base available. Less complex models of emotional maltreatment that are empirically validated may make more sense at this point in development of the field. The findings from these simple attempts ultimately would be integrated into more complex frameworks.

Conclusions

In the material presented here, one can see the beginnings of more complex views of etiology (model types 3 to 6) that will, one hopes, stimulate new research. With validation of these new perspectives should come more fine-tuned treatment efforts and better control of this social problem. Given the overlap between forms of maltreatment and the similarity of many of the factors that appear to be associated with each, it might be useful for the field to attempt to integrate models across forms. We make a preliminary attempt to do this in the last section by integrating three different frameworks to explain child maltreatment. These frameworks include the specification of cognitive–behavioral skills problems that are linked to multiple forms of maltreatment, factors that would lead to failures in meeting the developmental requirements of children, and systemic factors that would act as setting events for maltreatment to occur.

AN INTEGRATED META-MODEL OF CHILD MALTREATMENT

In positing a meta-model of child maltreatment, a number of basic criteria might be considered. As noted earlier, one of the major goals of theory is to inform treatment development. Thus, a meta-theory should posit factors that are amenable to change or that are of such a nature that intervention can allow for some "prosthetic" strategies (i.e., defects that families could work around). An argument has also been made that theories of etiology in child maltreatment need to be linked to factors that relate to child outcome (Azar, 1989, 1991). It is the negative impact of parental behavior on children's outcomes that is of most concern to mental health professionals. Finally, although theories that see abusive and neglectful parents as distinct from other parents make sense in environments where categorical classification is crucial (e.g., determining fit versus unfit parents in termination of parental rights hearings in the legal system), treatment does not typically involve families where such sharp distinctions are required. Thus, a meta-model might best begin with a continuum view. Such a model would consequently be a model of parenting competence and thus, would approach the issue of maltreatment from a broader perspective than that undertaken to date.

Based on these criteria, a number of factors emerged from our review across the forms of maltreatment that would be the most fruitful for inclusion in a meta-model of child maltreatment and that would lead most directly into intervention development. These include parent-based cognitive disturbances and behavioral skill deficits and disrupting socioenvironmental conditions. In positing a model, these must be considered in the context of children's needs at various stages of development and the tasks that all parents face at each of these stages (adult development). When children's needs are violated to such an extent that poor outcome is likely, parenting incompetence might legitimately be viewed as of concern to society and targeted for intervention, whether or not it meets legal criteria for maltreatment. Inherent in this perspective is a continuum view of parenting, with factors that lead to a continuum of risk.

Five general domains of parental disturbance might be posited: (1) cognitive disturbances, (2) parenting skill problems, (3) impulse control problems, (4) stress management problems, and (5) social skill problems (Azar & Twentyman, 1986). In turn, these may be seen as also playing a role in systemic difficulties that foster further child risk. For example, poor parental social skills would lead to fewer friends, perceptions of low intimacy, poor marital relationships, higher levels of distress, poorer life adjustment, higher levels of negative arousal, and a lower mood state, all of which have been identified as descriptive of maltreaters across types. The disturbances outlined may have their origins in the parents' own childhood experiences, mainly through the modeling provided by their adult role models, but may also evolve under situational strain (e.g., mood disturbances, marital violence).

Children, for their part, at various points in their development demand the successful completion of specific parental tasks. Both parents (and children) also need specific types of systemic supports in order for their skills to be refined and to be carried out without obstacles. For example, the parent of an infant must have a high tolerance for infant crying and the parent of a newly mobile toddler needs to have the capacity to monitor safety issues in the home. The ability to marshal a cadre of friends and/or relatives supports both of these capacities. Social support helps with child care, providing additional assistance when the infant is inconsolable, or when the toddler is in need of monitoring while the parent is engaged in other tasks (e.g., cooking dinner). The level and type of ftustration tolerance and monitoring skills needed for infants and toddlers, however, is different from that required for teenagers. At this later point in development, good communication skills and accurate understanding of adolescents' need for autonomy are required to provide an optimal environment for development. However, the *quality* of verbal communication skills (e.g., modeling of negotiation skills) required with teenagers may be crucial, whereas, with an infant, the *amount* of communication (e.g., level of verbal stimulation) may be more important. All of the above tasks may be more difficult to carry out effectively if the parent is under extreme environmental stress. For example, if poverty is an issue, the parent may have a more difficult time reducing environmental risks (e.g., with a toddler, preventing lead paint poisoning because of limits on housing quality available, or, with a teenager, gang membership), such that even higher levels of monitoring skills are likely to be less effective. Thus, under some environmental contingencies, parental skill levels must be of an even higher quality than is typical in more benign contexts, what Cauce (1995) has called "precision parenting in an unforgiving environment." We also know that cognitive processing narrows under stress and this would mean the presence of the cognitive disturbances posited would be even more detrimental to functioning.

Azar and Siegel (1990) posit a framework for child abuse and neglect that argues for a set of unique tasks that parents must accomplish at each level of a child's development, as well as ones that cut across development. They also outlined period-specific child-based and contextual obstacles to accomplishing these tasks successfully and the interactional and child outcomes to be expected when they fail. A preliminary list of types of skills problems that might emerge and the child outcomes seen has been compiled (Azar, Miller, & Breton, in press). Much as Crittenden (1993) has argued for neglect, the foundational disturbance in this approach is an information-processing one. Difficulties at this fundamental level would short-circuit all subsequent responses that parents would make. That is, if one misperceives child or situational cues in childrearing, then the responses that follow would by definition be maladaptive or dissynchronous with children's needs. Effective parents are seen as approaching interactions with their children with developmentally sensitive schemata (expectations) (Azar, 1986, 1989). That is, such parents have accurate perceptions of their children's capabilities, as well as what their own role should be in moving them forward developmentally (Miller, 1988). Indeed, such accurate perceptions have been associated with optimal parenting and child outcome and inaccurate perceptions have been linked to maltreatment (Abel & Rouleau, 1995; Azar, Robinson, Hekimian, & Twentyman, 1984; Azar & Rohrbeck 1986). Parents with inaccurate perceptions come to hold children more responsible for their mishaps, aversive behavior, and the parent's own loss of control. In addition, inherent in their schemata regarding parent–child relationships is an expectation that children will provide parents with comfort and care rather than the other way around. In the extreme, the expectancies may be so distorted that the parent may expect sexual gratification from the child.

Along with accurate standards, effective parents also have an adequate-enough repertoire of childrearing strategies and problem-solving skills to allow them to adapt their responses appropriately to any given situation and to the skill level of their children. For example, the effective parent recognizes that explanations may be very effective with an adolescent or school-aged child, but will be less appropriate as the sole strategy with a toddler. Likewise, strategies that are effective when the child is in good health may fail when the child is tired or ill. Unlike effective parents, maltreating ones have been seen as possessing a narrow repertoire of childrearing skills (mostly negative strategies), as well as poor problem-solving ability (Azar, Robinson, Hekimian, & Twentyman, 1984; Hanson, Pallotta, Tishelman, Conaway, & MacMillan, 1989). Consequently, they are more likely to fail at crucial tasks required of parents; this leads to increased frustration levels, lowered beliefs in self efficacy, and perhaps, a perception that the child has more power than they do (Bugenthal & Shennum, 1984). Effective parents also have a positive bias in their interpretations of events involving their children that, together with their developmentally sensitive schemata and parenting skills, allows them to maintain a relatively positive affective state and to make adaptive and positive responses, even when aversive child behaviors are involved. For example, when such parents find that their 3-year-old has spilled milk, they will draw on their understanding that 3-year-olds have trouble holding onto objects (i.e., a schemata regarding the motor skills of 3-year-olds) and will make attributions to developmental factors (e.g., "She's only 3.") or external factors outside both their own and their children's control, thus reducing stress and frustration. Their script regarding parenting is one in which parents are to be patient in such situations and, at the same time, they are forgiving of themselves when they experience frustration. Abusive parents have a negative bias and will often attribute their children's mishaps to spitefulness or their own inadequacy to get their children to "mind" them (Larrance & Twentyman, 1983). Such attributions by abusive parents further contribute to their becoming overly frustrated and feeling ineffective in encounters with their children. Thus, appropriate schemata, adaptive attributions, and a wide repertoire of childrearing strategies and problem-solving skills combine to produce a situation in which parents are attuned to the developmental needs of their children, can discriminate situations where intervention is required and where it is not, and are capable of meeting parenting tasks more calmly, flexibly, and successfully. Lack of complexity and precision in cognitive processing may contribute to parental maltreating behavior, dissatisfaction in their roles as parents, inept parenting more generally, and poor child outcomes.

Because contextual stress may interfere further with cognitive processing, a positive affective state, and parents' capacity to respond optimally, parents who are effective also have skills that help them to handle stress well when it does occur, to develop buffers for themselves against its negative consequences, and when possible, to anticipate and prevent stressors from occurring in the first place. For example, parents with optimal skills may anticipate an impending financial strain and adjust their budget accordingly, or when faced with a marital breakup, have adequate social skills and friends to provide support and to help them with parenting (e.g., alternative child care). Such support networks have the added positive effect of providing information to fine-tune parental schemata and introduce new behavioral strategies through the feedback and role modeling they provide. Unlike effective parents, maltreating parents are more impulsive in their responses (Rohrbeck & Twentyman, 1986), and this impulsivity, together with poor problem-solving capacities and poor social skills, results in their experiencing many life stressors and having fewer social supports to help them (Salzinger, Kaplan & Artemyeff, 1983). Contextual stress and a small social support network surrounding the family also provides the child with less opportunity to have alternative models and situations crucial to further development.

Thus, overall, this model provides explanations for both parental maladaptive behaviors and poor outcomes in children. As stated, this model provides explanations for three of the forms of child maltreatment (physical abuse, neglect, and emotional abuse), and for many factors associated with sexually abusive behavior as well (e.g., offender cognitive distortions, social skill deficits, and impulse control problems). Although other models have posited such a developmental perspective, arguing for debilitating and compensatory factors in families at risk for abuse and/or factors at multiple levels of analysis, this social cognitive model prioritizes the area most in need of intervention and thus allows for a more targeted intervention strategy. Its continuum perspective allows for the development of prevention efforts as well.

FUTURE DIRECTIONS

Progress has begun to be made in the development of more complex models of child maltreatment. Ultimately, well-validated models for specific types of maltreatment or for maltreatment more globally would enhance both intervention and prevention efforts, which until recently have had a "shot-gun" quality. More directive and empirically based interventions (e.g., behavioral and cognitive behavior approaches have shown the best outcomes.

ACKNOWLEDGEMENT
The writing of this chapter was supported by a NIMH FIRST Grant Award (NIMH grant #MH46940) to the first author.

REFERENCES

Abbey, A. (1982). Sex differences in attributions for friendly behavior: Do males misperceive females' friendliness? *Journal of Personality and Social Psychology, 42*(5), 830–838.

Abbey, A. (1987). Misperceptions of friendly behavior as sexual interest: A survey of naturally occurring incidents. *Psychology of Women Quarterly, 11*, 173–194.

Abel, G. G., & Rouleau, J. L. (1995). Sexual abuses. *Psychiatric Clinics of North America, 18*(1), 139–153.

Alexander, P. C. (1992). Application of attachment theory to the study of sexual abuse. *Journal of Consulting and Clinical Psychology, 60*(2), 185–195.

Azar, S. T. (1986). A framework for understanding child maltreatment: An integration of cognitive behavioral and developmental perspectives. *Canadian Journal of Behavioral Science, 18*, 340–355.

Azar, S. T. (1988). Methodological considerations in treatment outcome research in child maltreatment. In G. T. Hotaling, D. Finkelhor, J. T. Kirkpatrick, & M. A. Straus (Eds.), *Coping with family violence* (pp. 288–299). Newbury Park, CA: Sage.

Azar, S. T. (1989). Training parents of abused children. In C. E. Schaefer & J. M. Briesmeister (Eds.), *Handbook of parent training* (pp. 414–441). New York: Wiley.

Azar, S. T. (1991). Models of child abuse: A metatheoretical analysis. *Criminal Justice and Behavior, 18*, 30–46.

Azar, S. T., Fantuzzo, J. W., & Twentyman, C. T. (1984). An applied behavioral approach to child maltreatment: Back to basics. *Advances in Behavior Research and Therapy, 6*, 3–11.

Azar, S. T., Miller, L. P., & Breton, S. (in press). Cognitive behavioral group work and physical child abuse. In K. C. Stoiber & T. Kratochwill (Eds.), *Group intervention in the school and the community.* New York: Allyn & Bacon.

Azar, S. T., Robinson, D. R., Hekimian, E., & Twentyman, C. T. (1984). Unrealistic expectations and problem solving ability in maltreating and comparison mothers. *Journal of Consulting and Clinical Psychology, 52*, 687–691.

Azar, S. T., & Rohrbeck, C. A. (1986). Child abuse and unrealistic expectations: Further validation of the Parent Opinion Questionnaire. *Journal of Consulting and Clinical Psychology, 54*, 867–868.

Azar, S. T., & Siegel, B. (1990). Behavioral treatment of child abuse: A developmental perspective. *Behavior Modification, 14*, 279–300.

Azar, S. T., & Twentyman, C. T. (1986). Cognitive behavioral perspectives on the assessment and treatment of child abuse. In P. C. Kendall (Ed.), *Advances in cognitive behavioral research and therapy* (Vol. 5, pp. 237–267). New York: Academic Press.

Bandura, A. (1983). Psychological mechanisms of aggression. In R. G. Green & E. J. Donnerstein (Eds.), *Aggression: Theoretical and empirical review* (pp. 1–40). New York: Academic Press.

Belsky, J. (1980). Child maltreatment: An ecological integration. *American Psychologist, 35*, 320–335.

Belsky, J., & Vondra, J. (1989). Lessons from child abuse: The determinants of parenting. In D. Cicchetti & V. Carlson (Eds.), *Child maltreatment* (pp. 153–202). New York: Cambridge University Press.

Bugenthal, D. B., & Shennum, W. A. (1984). "Difficult" children as elicitors and targets of adult communication patterns: An attributional-transactional analysis. *Monographs of the Society of Research in Child Development, 49* (Serial No. 205,1).

Burgess, R. L., & Draper, P. (1989). The explanation of family violence: The role of biological, behavioral, and cultural selection. In L. Ohlin & M. Tonry (Eds.), *Family violence* (pp. 59–116). Chicago: University of Chicago Press.

Camras, L., Ribordy, S., Hill, J., Martino, S., Sachs, V., Spacarelli, S., & Stefani, R. (1990). Maternal facial behavior and the recognition and production of emotional expression by maltreated and nonmaltreated children. *Developmental Psychology, 26,* 304–312.

Cantwell, H. B. (1980). Child neglect. In C. H. Kempe & R. E. Helfer (Eds.), *The battered child* (pp. 183–197). Chicago: University of Chicago Press.

Carlson, V., Cicchetti, D. Barnett, R., & Braunwald, K. G. (1989). Finding order in disorganization. In D. Cicchetti & V. Carlson (Eds.) *Child maltreatment* (pp. 494–528). New York: Cambridge University Press.

Cauce, A. M. (1995, June). *Slouching toward cultural competency in research.* Presented at the Family Process Institute, Ogunquit, ME.

Cicchetti, D., & Rizley, R. (1981). Developmental perspectives on the etiology, intergenerational transmission, and sequelae of child maltreatment. *New Directions for Child Development, 11,* 31–56.

Cohen, J. A., & Mannarino, A. P. (1993). A treatment model for sexually abuse preschoolers. *Journal of Interpersonal Violence, 3,* 115–131.

Crittenden, P. M. (1993). An information processing perspective on the behavior of neglectful parents. *Criminal Justice and Behavior, 20,* 27–48.

Crowe, L. C., & George, W. H. (1989). Alcohol and human sexuality: Review and integration. *Psychological Bulletin, 105*(3), 374–386.

Daly, M., & Wilson, M. J. (1981). Child maltreatment from a sociobiological perspective. *New Directions for Child Development, 11,* 93–112.

Daly, M., & Wilson, M. (1985). Child abuse and other risks of not living with both parents. *Ethology and Sociobioloay 6,* 197–210.

Diamond, D. (1989). Father–daughter incest: Unconscious fantasy and social fact. *Psychoanalytic Psychology 6,* 421–37.

Egeland, B., Breitenbucher, M., & Rosenberg, D. (1980). Prospective study of the significance of life stress in the etiology of child abuse. *Journal of Consulting and Clinical Psychology 48,* 194–205.

Egeland, B., & Erickson, M. F. (1987). Psychologically unavailable caregiving. In M. Brassard, R. Germain, & S. Hart (Eds.), *Psychological maltreatment of children and youth* (pp. 110–120). New York: Pergamon.

Elliot, F. A. (1988). Neurological factors. In V. B. VanHasselt, R. L. Morrison, A. S. Bellack, & M. Hersen (Eds.), *Handbook of family violence* (pp. 359–382). New York: Plenum Press.

Erikson, E. H. (1950). *Childhood and society.* New York: Norton.

Finkelhor, D. (July 1981). *Common features of family abuse.* Paper presented at the Research Conference on Family Violence, Durham, NH.

Finkelhor, D. (1984). *Child sexual abuse.* New York: Free Press.

Frodi, A. M., & Lamb, M. (1980). Child abuser's responses to infant smiles and cries. *Child Development, 51,* 238–241.

Galdston, R. (1968). Dysfunctions of parenting: The battered child, the neglected child, the exploited child. In J. G. Howells (Ed.), *Modern perspectives of international child psychiatry* (pp. 571–588). Edinburgh: Oliver & Boyd.

Garbarino, J. (1976). A preliminary study of some ecological correlates of child abuse: The impact of socioeconomic stress on mothers. *Child Development, 47,* 178–185.

Garbarino, J. (1977). The human ecology of child maltreatment: A conceptual model for research. *Journal of Marriage and Family, 39,* 721–735.

Garbarino, J. (1991). Not all bad developmental outcomes are the result of child abuse. *Development and Psychopathology, 3,* 45–50.

Garbarino, J., & Vondra, J. (1987). Psychological maltreatment: Issues and perspectives. In M. Brassard R. Germain, & S. Hart (Eds.), *Psychological maltreatment of children and youth* (pp. 25–44). New York: Pergamon.

Gaudin, J. M. (1993). Effective intervention with neglectful families. *Criminal Justice and Behavior, 20,* 66–89.

Gaudin, J. M., Polansky, N. A., Kilpatrick, A. C., & Shilton, P. (1993). Loneliness, depression, stress and social supports in neglectful families. *American Journal of Orthopsychiatry, 63,* 597–605.

Gelles, R. J. (1983). An exchange social control theory. In D. Finkelhohr, R. J. Gelles, G. T. Hotaling, & M. A. Straus (Eds.) *The dark side of families* (pp. 151–165). Beverly Hills, CA: Sage.

Gelles, R. J., & Straus, M. A. (1979). Determinants of violence in the family: Toward a theoretical integration. In W. R. Burr, R. Hill, F. I. Nye, & I. L. Reiss (Eds.), *Contemporary theories about the family* (pp. 549–581). New York: Free Press.

Golden, C. J., Jackson, M. L., Peterson-Rohne, A., & Gontkovsky S. T. (1996). Neuropsychological correlates of violence and aggression: A review of the clinical literature. *Aggression and Violent Behavior, 1,* 3–25.

Goode, W. J. (1971). Force and violence in the family. *Journal of Marriage and the Family, 33,* 624–636.

Hall, G. C. N., & Hirschman, R. (1991). Toward a theory of sexual aggression: A quadripartite model. *Journal of Consulting and Clinical Psychology, 59*(5), 662–669.

Hall, G. C. N., & Hirschman, R. (1992). Sexual aggression against children: A conceptual perspective of etiology. *Criminal Justice and Behavior, 19*(1), 8–23.

Handlon, J. (1960). A metatheoretical view of assumptions regarding the etiology of schizophrenia. *Archives of General Psychiatry, 3,* 43–60.

Hansen, D. J., Pallotta, G. M., Tishelman, A. C., Conaway, L. P., & MacMillan, J. M. (1989). Parental problem-solving skills and child behavior problems: A comparison of physically abusive, neglectful, clinic, and community families. *Journal of Family Violence, 4,* 353–368.

Hart, S. N., Germain, R. B., & Brassard, M. R. (1987). The challenge: To better understand and combat psychological maltreatment of children and youth. In M. Brassard, R. Germain, & S. Hart (Eds.), *Psychological maltreatment of children and youth* (pp. 3–24). New York: Pergamon.

Haugaard, J. J. (1988). The use of theories about the etiology of incest as guidelines for legal and therapeutic interventions. *Behavioral Sciences and the Law, 6*(2), 221–238.

Holman, E. A., & Stokols, D. (1994). The environmental psychology of child sexual abuse. *Journal of Environmental Psychology, 14,* 237–252.

Klaus, M. H., & Kennell, J. H. (1976). *Maternal–infant bonding.* St. Louis, MO: Mosby.

Koss, M. P., & Gaines, J. A. (1993). The prediction of sexual aggression by alcohol use, athletic participation and fraternity affiliation. *Journal of Interpersonal Violence, 8,* 94–108.

Larrance, D. T., & Twentyman C. T. (1983). Maternal attributions in child abuse. *Journal of Abnormal Psychology, 92,* 449–457.

Laws, D. R., & Marshall, W. L. (1990). A conditioning theory of the etiology and maintenance of deviant sexual preferences and behavior. In W. L. Marshall, D. R. Laws, and H. E. Barbaree (Eds.), *Handbook of sexual assault* (pp. 209–229). New York: Plenum Press.

Lesnik-Oberstein, M., Koers, A. J., & Cohen, L. (1995). Parental hostility in psychologically abusive mothers: A test of the three-factor theory. *Child Abuse & Neglect, 19,* 33–49.

Levinson, D. (1988). Family violence in cross cultural perspective. In V. B. VanHasselt, R. L. Morrison, A. S. Bellak, & M. Hersen (Eds.), *Handbook of family violence* (pp. 435–455). New York: Plenum Press.

Marshall, W. L. (1989). Intimacy, loneliness, and sexual offenders. *Behavior Research and Therapy, 27*(5), 491–503.

Marshall, W. L., & Barbaree, H. E. (1990). An integrated theory of the etiology of sexual offending. In W. L. Marshall, D. R. Laws, & H. E. Barbaree (Eds.), *Handbook of sexual assault* (pp. 257–275). New York: Plenum Press.

Marshall, W. L., Hudson, S. M., Jones, R., & Fernandez, Y. M. (1995). Empathy in sex offenders. *Clinical Psychology Review, 15*(2), 99–113.

McGee R. A., & Wolfe, D. A. (1991). Psychological maltreatment: Toward an operational definition. *Development and Psychopathology, 3,* 3–18.

Meier, E. G. (1964). Child neglect. In N. E. Cohen (Ed.), *Social work and social problems.* New York: National Association of Social Workers.

Merrill, E. J. (1962). Physical abuse of children: An agency study. In V. DeFrancis (Ed.), *Protecting the Battered Child* (pp. 17–28). Denver, CO: American Humane Association.

Miller, N. E. (1941). The frustration-aggression hypothesis. *Psychological Review, 48,* 337–342.

Miller, S. (1988). Parents' beliefs about children's cognitive development. *Child Development, 59,* 259–285.

Monto, M., Zgourides, G., Wilson, J., & Harris, R. (1994). Empathy and adolescent male sex-offenders. *Perceptual and Motor Skills, 79*(3), 1598.

National Center on Child Abuse and Neglect. (1992, April). *National child abuse and neglect data system: Working paper 1, 1990 summary data component* DHHS Publication No. (ACF) 92-30361. Washington, DC: U.S. Government Printing Office.

National Research Council (1993). *Understanding child abuse and neglect.* Washington, DC: National Academy Press.

Newberger, C. M., & Cook, S. J. (1983). Parental awareness and child abuse and neglect: A cognitive developmental analysis of urban and rural samples. *American Journal of Orthopsychiatry, 53,* 512–524.

Oldershaw, L., Walters, G. C., & Hall, D. K. (1989). A behavioral approach to the classification of different types of abusive mothers. *Merrill-Palmer Quarterly, 35,* 255–279.

Park, R. D., & Collmer, C. W. (1975). Child abuse: An interdisciplinary analysis. In E. M. Hetherington (Ed.), *Review of child development research* (Vol. 5, pp. 509–590). Chicago: University of Chicago Press.

Parker, H., & Parker, S. (1986). Father–daughter sexual abuse: An emerging perspective. *American Journal of Orthopsychiatry, 56,* 531–549.

Patterson, G. R., & Reid, J. (1967). Reciprocity and coercion: Two facets of social systems. In C. Nueringer & J. Michael (Eds.), *Behavior modification in clinical psychology* (pp. 133–177). New York: Appleton-Century-Croft.

Pelton L. (1994). The role of material factors in child abuse and neglect. In G. B. Melton & F. D. Barry (Eds.), *Protecting children from abuse and neglect* (pp. 131–181). New York: Guilford Press.

Pianta, R., Egeland, B. & Erickson, M. F. (1989). The antecedents of maltreatment: Results of the mother–child interaction research project. In D. Cicchetti & V. Carlson (Eds.), *Child maltreatment* (pp. 203–253). New York: Cambridge University Press.

Plotkin R. C., Azar, S. T., Twentyman, C. T., & Perri, M. G. (1981). A critical evaluation of the research methodology employed in the investigation of causative factors of child abuse and neglect. *International Journal of Child Abuse and Neglect, 1,* 449–455.

Polansky, N. A.; Chalmers, M. A., Buttenwieser, E., & Williams, D. P. (1981). *Damaged parents: An anatomy of child neglect.* Chicago: University of Chicago Press.

Polansky, N. A., Gaudin, J. M., Ammons, P. W., & David, K. B. (1985). The psychological ecology of the neglectful mother. *Child Abuse & Neglect, 9,* 265–275.

Renshaw, K. L. (1994). Child molesters: Do those molested as children report larger numbers of victims than those who deny childhood sexual abuse? *Journal of Addictions and Offender Counseling, 15*(1), 24–32.

Rist, K. (1979). Incest: Theoretical and clinical views. *American Journal of Orthopsychiatry, 49*(4), 680–691.

Rohrbeck, C. A., & Twentyman, C. T. (1986). A multimodal assessment of impulsiveness in abusing, neglectful, and nonmaltreating mothers and their preschool children. *Journal of Consulting and Clinical Psychology, 54,* 231–236.

Ryan, G. (1989). Victim to victimizer: Rethinking victim treatment. *Journal of Interpersonal Violence, 4*(3), 325–341.

Salzinger, S., Kaplan, S., & Artemyeff, C. (1983). Mother's personal social networks and child maltreatment. *Journal of Abnormal Psychology, 92,* 68–72.

Schilling, R. F., Schinke, S. P,. Blythe B., & Barth, R. P. (1982). Child maltreatment and mentally retarded parents. *Mental Retardation, 20,* 201–209.

Sedlak, A. J. (1990). *Technical amendment to the study findings: National incidence and prevalence of child abuse and neglect, 1988.* Rockville, MD: Westat.

Seidman, B. T., Marshall, W. L., Hudson, S. M., & Robertson, P. J. (1994). An examination of intimacy and loneliness in sex offenders. *Journal of Interpersonal Violence, 9*(4), 518–534.

Shakel, J. A. (1987). Emotional neglect and stimulus deprivation. In M. Brassard, R. Germain, & S. Hart (Eds.), *Psychological maltreatment of children and youth* (pp. 100–109). New York: Pergamon.

Solomon, J. C. (1992). Child sexual abuse by family members: A radical feminist perspective. *Sex Roles, 27*(9–10), 473–485.

Steele, B. F. (1980). Psychodynamic factors in child abuse. In R. E. Helfer & C. H. Kempe (Eds.), *The battered child* (pp. 86–103). Chicago: University of Chicago Press.

Steinmetz, S. K., & Straus, M. A. (1974). *Violence in the family.* New York: Harper.

Straus, M. A. (1973). A general systems theory approach to a theory of violence between family members. *Social Science Information, 12,* 105–125.

Stermac L. E., & Segal, Z. V. (1989). Adult sexual contact with children: An examination of cognitive factors. *Behavior Therapy, 20*, 573–584.

Stermac, L. E., Segal, Z. V., & Gillis, R. (1990). Social and cultural factors in sexual assault. In W. L. Marshall, D. R. Laws, & H. E. Barbaree (Eds.), *Handbook of sexual assault* (pp. 143–159). New York: Plenum Press.

Suomi, S. J. (1978). Maternal behavior by socially incompetent monkeys: Neglect and abuse of offspring. *Journal of Pediatric Psychology, 3*, 28–34.

The U. S. Advisory Board on Child Abuse and Neglect (1993). *The continuing child protection emergency: A challenge to the nation.* Washington, DC: Administration for Children, Youth, and Families, U.S. DHHS.

Vasta R. (1982). Physical child abuse: A dual-component analysis. *Developmental Review, 2*, 125–149.

Vitulano, L. A., Lewis, M., Doran, L. D., Nordhaus, B., & Adnopoz, J. (1986). Treatment recommendation, implementation, and follow-up in child abuse. *American Journal of Orthopsychiatry, 56*, 478–480.

Wiener, M., & Cromer, W. (1967). Reading and reading difficulty: A conceptual analysis. *Harvard Educational Review, 37*, 620–643.

Williams, L. M., & Finkelhor, D. (1990). The characteristics of incestuous fathers: A review of recent studies. In W. L. Marshall, D. R. Laws, & H. E. Barbaree (Eds.), *Handbook of sexual assault* (pp. 231–255). New York: Plenum Press.

Wolfe, D. A. (1987). *Child abuse: Implications for child development and psychopathology.* Newbury Park, CA: Sage.

Wolfe, D. A., Kaufman, D., Aragona, J., & Sandler, J. (1981). *The child management program for abusive parents.* Winter Park, CO: Anna.

Wolock, I., & Horowitz, B. (1977). *Factors relating to levels of child care among families receiving public assistance in New Jersey. Final report to the National Center on Child Abuse and Neglect DHEW Grant 90-C-418).* Washington, DC: National Clearinghouse on Child Abuse and Neglect Information.

Young, L. (1964). *Wednesday's children.* New York: McGraw Hill.

Zuravin S. J. (1991). Research definitions of child physical abuse and neglect: Current problems. In R. H. Starr & D. A. Wolfe (Eds.), *The effects of child abuse and neglect* (pp. 100–128). New York: Guilford Press.

2

Balancing Rights and Responsibilities
Legal Perspectives on Child Maltreatment

SHARON G. PORTWOOD, N. DICKON REPPUCCI, and MARGARET S. MITCHELL

The topic of child abuse and neglect has reached such a prominent place in the American consciousness that few are unaware of the potential dangers that children face at the hands of adults, including teachers, child care personnel, strangers, community leaders, and, all too often, members of a child's own family. Indeed, one need only tune in to network television on any night to encounter at least one more story involving the victimization of a child. Although the laws of all 50 states now provide for both criminal and civil prosecution of child abuse and neglect (Bulkley, Feller, Stern, & Roe, 1996), there remains a great deal of misunderstanding and often a lack of knowledge regarding legal responses to cases in which a child is alleged to have been abused or neglected. Cases such as the infamous 1984 McMartin Preschool trial, which extended over five years and resulted in the defendants' acquittal on all charges, render suspect the degree to which not only the general public, but also those professionals regularly involved in the resolution of these cases (particularly mental health professionals) understand the relevant legal context. The purpose of this chapter is not only to illuminate those rules and guidelines that dictate the parameters of legal responses to allegations of child maltreatment, but also to provide insight into many of the controversies that arise when a case of maltreatment is submitted to legal authorities. Following an overview of the legal principles that guide the courts in resolving controversies involving children, current procedures and relevant research relating to each stage of the legal process, from identification of potential cases of child maltreatment to potential outcomes, both inside

---

SHARON G. PORTWOOD • University of Missouri–Kansas City, Kansas City, Missouri 64110. N. DICKON REPPUCCI • University of Virginia, Charlottesville, Virginia 22903.   MARGARET S. MITCHELL • College of Charleston, Charleston, South Carolina 29401.

Handbook of Child Abuse Research and Treatment, edited by Lutzker. Plenum Press, New York, 1998.

and outside the courtroom, will be addressed. Throughout this discussion, issues related to the rights of both children and defendants will be highlighted.

As noted, child maltreatment cases may arise under criminal laws subjecting an offender to criminal penalties, as well as under civil laws which may entitle a party successful in prosecuting such an action to monetary damages. In addition, allegations of child abuse or neglect may arise in divorce and child custody cases. Regardless of the nature of the claim, the courts attempt to balance the potentially competing rights of the child and the parents, as well as the interests of the State, which, under the *parens patriae* doctrine, is empowered to protect children. In cases of child abuse and neglect, this traditional triangular framework may be expanded to add the rights of the defendant, who may or may not already be represented as the child's parent. As noted by many commentators (e.g., Mnookin, 1979; Reppucci, Weithorn, Mulvey, & Monahan, 1984), this delicate balancing test creates the potential for various unsatisfactory outcomes which, in many cases, require that the interests of at least one entity—child, family (defendant), or State—yield to the rights of another. Historically, the rights of the child have been subordinated to the paternalistic and protectivist roles of parent and State, as well as to the legal rights of alleged offenders who are not related to the child.

Despite the fact that by 1967, all states had enacted child protection laws (Starr, 1988), early Supreme Court decisions that continue as the foundation for current court doctrine (e.g., *Meyer v. Nebraska*, 1923; *Pierce v. Society of Sisters*, 1925; *Prince v. Massachusetts*, 1944) emphasize the right of family autonomy, that is, the right of parents to raise their children as they see fit. The right of the State to intervene in the family, and thus violate family autonomy, derives from its police power, through which it is empowered to act to promote the public welfare, and from the concept of *parens patriae*, which is the limited power of the State "to protect or promote the welfare of certain individuals, including children, who lack the capacity to act in their own best interest" (Rosenberg & Hunt, 1984). The exercise of the *parens patriae* power is limited by three principles: (1) *parens patriae* is founded on the presumption that children do not possess the mental competence and maturity of adults; (2) before intervening in the family, the State must establish that a child's parents or guardians are incapable of or unwilling to care for the child; and (3) the State's power should be exercised solely to promote the best interest of the child (Mnookin, 1978). Thus, while attempting to afford due consideration to the "interests" of the child, the State nonetheless defers to the "rights" of the parents. While at least some courts have recognized that a child's rights may outweigh those of his or her parents in cases of suspected abuse, the Supreme Court has declined to impose an affirmative duty on the State to protect children from their parents (*DeShaney v. Winnebago County Department of Social Services*, 1989). In *DeShaney*, the Court instead noted that the individual states could, if they desired, place responsibility for such a failure to act on the State and its officials by enacting appropriate provisions in their tort laws.

The fundamental and often overriding right of parents to raise their children free of State interference is based on the premise that the private, autonomous family is the institution best suited to care for children (Reppucci & Crosby, 1993). This premise arises from two further presumptions: (1) parents will act in their child's best interests, and (2) parents have the maturity, experience, and judgment that a child lacks (Reppucci & Crosby, 1993). The clear violation of this first presumption in those cases in which a parent is shown to have abused his or her child is what serves as a justification for legal intervention (Haugaard & Reppucci, 1988). Despite the current state of the law, which continues to defer to the rights of the parents, an advocacy movement fueled largely by mental health professionals has begun to challenge the power of parents and the State over the lives of children—especially adolescents (Scott, Reppucci, & Woolard, 1995). In response to this movement, many commentators (e.g., Barnett, Manly, & Cicchetti, 1993; Goldstein, Freud, & Solnit, 1973; Nelson, 1984) have observed an overall trend toward a prevailing belief that the rights and protection of children supersede the right of family privacy in situations in which children are at risk of mental or physical injury.

Wadlington, Whitebread, and Davis (1983) identify three possible meanings of the term "children's rights": (1) "the extension of broad freedom of personal action and decision-making to children," (2) the "increased protections from governmental intrusion in matters of parental (and thus family) decision-making for children," and, (3) the pronouncement of "statements of fundamental principles to be used judicially as guidelines for interpreting or applying various laws or procedures" (p. 47). The first of these again recognizes that the rights of parents and children are not necessarily synonymous. As stated, the general deference that courts have extended to families in matters involving their children is based, in part, on the presumption that this is the best way to ensure that the best interests of the child are served. Indeed, this "best interests" standard has been the driving force behind legal responses to cases of alleged abuse or neglect. Unfortunately, this standard is a very subjective one: the best interest of the child "is not demonstrable by scientific proof, but is instead fundamentally a matter of values" (Mnookin, 1978, pp. 163–164). We simply do not have the ability to predict accurately in every case what alternative is best for the specific child (Reppucci & Crosby, 1993). Accordingly, our legal system continues to struggle to protect children from maltreatment within the confines of traditional legal doctrines and with the assistance of relatively little solid, empirical evidence on relevant topics.

ISSUES OF DEFINITION AND IDENTIFICATION

Overview

At present, four categories of child maltreatment are generally recognized: physical abuse, sexual abuse, psychological abuse (or emotional maltreatment), and neglect. Popular definitions of these concepts, and child maltreatment as a whole, have been based on various factors: the form, intensity, and frequency of the act; the physical or psychological consequences to the victim; the intent of the perpetrator; mitigating situational influences; and, community standards (Emery, 1989). Legal definitions of child abuse and neglect are typically delineated in criminal offense and child protection statutes and/or juvenile or family court jurisdiction acts. However, more important than any variation in the source of these definitions are the variations in the definitions themselves; the language used differs widely between states (Bulkley, 1985). While some commentators (e.g., Bulkley, 1985) have noted a trend toward providing more specific definitions of prohibited acts, others (e.g., Burns & Lake, 1983; Kim, 1986) have not been so optimistic. After surveying North

American legislation, Burns and Lake (1983) found that few jurisdictions set forth precise definitions of forms of child maltreatment, instead concluding that most definitions are covered in "common-sense evidentiary expressions which legislators feel that no reasonable person could misinterpret" (p. 45). Likewise, Atteberry-Bennet (1987) noted that although legislative definitions are frequently designed to reflect the spirit of public and professional opinions, they typically require a significant degree of interpretation. Illustrative of the terms most often left to interpretation are "emotional abuse," "mental injury," or impairment of "emotional health," which few states even attempt to define (Melton & Davidson, 1987). Those states that do provide statutory or regulatory definitions of psychologically abusive behaviors include some of the following terms: "rejection, intimidation, or humiliation of the child; chaotic, bizarre, hostile, or violent acts producing fear or guilt on the part of the child; lack of nurturance, intimacy, affection, and acceptance; damage to the child's intellectual or psychological capacity or functioning and impairment of the child's ability to function within a normal range of performance and behavior" (Melton & Davidson, 1987, p. 173). Unfortunately for those who seek to apply these definitions, these terms themselves are subject to multiple interpretations.

One common theme found in statutory definitions of child maltreatment is that of harm or threatened harm by acts or omissions (Kim, 1986; Roscoe, 1990). For abuse, the critical factor appears to be a nonaccidental injury, while neglect encompasses harm to a child's health or welfare due to negligent treatment through omission of health and welfare responsibilities (Roscoe, 1990). Despite the emphasis the law places on whether the perpetrator intends to harm the child, research examining the attitudes of legal professionals, mental health professionals, medical professionals, educators, and laypersons indicates that there is little consensus either between or within these groups as to the weight that should be afforded the intent factor in determining whether a particular act constitutes maltreatment (Portwood, 1996). Moreover, all groups rated this factor as substantially less important to such a determination than are actual physical or psychological harm to the child, possible physical or psychological harm to the child, whether the act is sexual in nature, the seriousness of the act, and the frequency of the act, even though none of these factors receives precedence over intent in the written law (Portwood, 1996).

Other criteria, beyond intent, upon which legal definitions usually depend are the ages of the child and the perpetrator and the type of act involved (Haugaard & Reppucci, 1988). Typical of state legal definitions are the relevant provisions of the State Code of Virginia, which define an "abused or neglect child" as any child:

1. Whose parents or other person responsible for his care creates or inflicts, threatens to create or inflict, or allows to be created or inflicted upon such child a physical or mental injury by other than accidental means, or creates a substantial risk of death, disfigurement or impairment of bodily or mental functions;
2. Whose parents or other person responsible for his care neglects or refuses to provide care necessary for his health; . . .
3. Whose parents or other person responsible for his care abandons such child;
4. Whose parents or other person responsible for his care commits or allows to be committed any sexual act upon a child in violation of the law; or

5. Who is without parental care or guardianship, caused by the unreasonable absence or the mental or physical incapacity of the child's parent, guardian, legal custodian or other person standing in loco parentis. (*Va. Code* §§ 16.1-228, 63.1-248.2).

Despite the fact that legal definitions of child maltreatment are often criticized as too broad, there is some indication that people involved in the area of child protection favor such expanded definitions, which necessarily include a variety of acts (Cohen & Sussman, 1975). However, others (e.g., Giovannoni, 1991) have commented that what those within the legal system desire is not so much a definition as a standard for ascertaining when a child has been abused.

Both empirical studies and commentaries (e.g., Barnett et al., 1993; Nagi, 1977) indicate that there is a great deal of dissatisfaction among professionals in the child protection field regarding imprecise definitions of maltreatment. In fact, one consequence of the ambiguity arising from current legal definitions is a divergence of views among various professionals coming into contact with abused children. These differences are clear within, as well as between, professional groups and the general public. However, recent research indicates that there is a growing consensus among professionals as to the factors that are important in making a determination of maltreatment, as well as whether particular acts should be deemed abusive (Portwood, 1996). Portwood (1996) found that, consistent with previous findings (e.g., Giavannoni & Becerra, 1979), lay persons view acts as more abusive than do professionals, with the exception of teaching professionals. However, even this gap appears to be closing, with a potentially dangerous trend emerging toward identifying any act involving a child as abusive (Portwood, 1996).

Obstacles to Developing Clear Legal Guidelines

Although the need for a clear, objective legal definition of maltreatment is great, problems of subjectivity will no doubt continue to plague both courts and legislatures as a result of a number of as yet unresolved problems. At the most fundamental level, maltreatment is generally viewed as harmful or improper behavior (Haugaard, 1991). Clearly, deeming an act to be either "harmful" or "improper" involves value judgments. In addition, if "harm" is to be used as the standard, characteristics of the individual child (e.g., temperament, developmental level, resiliency) immediately take on a prominent role, making it difficult to formulate general criteria by which all children can be assessed. Although some acts are easily perceived as harmful when directed at very young children (e.g., not preparing regular meals), these same acts may not present any danger to older children; the opposite is also true (e.g., bathing, sleeping in the same bed). Such developmental considerations have been shown to influence some professionals' definitions (Baily & Baily, 1986). Moreover, a conceptualization of maltreatment based on harm to the child means judging the effects of particular acts on a particular child; this task is made even more difficult by the fact that effects may not become apparent for many years (Haugaard & Reppucci, 1988).

Focusing on the "impropriety" of behavior necessarily invokes some societal standard. Those attempting to formulate an objective definition of child maltreatment cannot ignore the broader cultural context in which that behavior occurs;

nonetheless, the influence of culture and the role it plays in individuals' assessments of whether an act is abusive has often been overlooked. Both within and between cultural groups, important differences exist in patterns of childrearing, the extent to which childhood is viewed as a developmental stage deserving of special consideration, the conditions deemed necessary for proper development, and the "rights" afforded to children (Eisenberg, 1981). Instead of a universal standard for either optimal child care or for child maltreatment, there is great cross-cultural variability in beliefs and behaviors regarding childrearing (Korbin, 1977, 1991). There are also problems presented by great variations in socioeconomic status within our society. There is a general consensus that under current definitional standards, socioeconomic factors have resulted in African-American children's being overrepresented as victims of abuse, whereas white children have been underrepresented (Garbarino & Ebata, 1983; Wilson & Saft, 1993). Spearly and Lauderdale (1983) obtained results which support the notion that nonwhite abusive families, particularly African-Americans, have been overrepresented because of a higher incidence of poverty and a greater prevalence of fatherless homes and working mothers. Particularly in the arena of neglect, low socioeconomic status may result in circumstances which, when not viewed in their appropriate context, suggest a failure to provide on the part of a child's parent or caretaker (e.g., worn clothing, unbalanced meals).

Given the many factors that contribute to value judgments of parental behavior, serious questions arise as to the acceptance of community standards as an appropriate means of defining child abuse. In applying such a standard, the critical question is "Which community will provide those standards?" or, given that current laws are seen as reflecting community standards, "Which community *is* providing those standards?"

INITIAL RESPONSES TO CASES OF SUSPECTED MALTREATMENT

Reporting Suspected Cases of Maltreatment

Since 1974, legislation in all 50 states has mandated reporting of suspected cases of child abuse and neglect (Kean & Dukes, 1991). These statutes detail who must (or may) report suspected incidents of child maltreatment, what must be reported, whether certain information qualifies as a privileged communication, sanctions for failure to report, and reporting procedures (Aber & Reppucci, 1992). The primary purpose of these mandatory reporting laws is to ensure that children are as safe and well cared for as possible, as well as to promote children's basic rights to food, clothing, shelter, and education (Brooks, Perry, Starr, & Teply, 1994). Among those professionals who are required by all states to report child maltreatment are physicians, nurses, emergency room personnel, coroners, medical examiners, dentists, mental health professionals, social workers, day care personnel, and law enforcement officers (Abrahams, Casey, & Daro, 1992; Brooks et al., 1994; Bulkley et al., 1996). Some states go so far as to require *any* person who suspects child maltreatment to report to a designated authority those facts known to her or him (Bulkley et al., 1996). Further, legislation may subject to civil and/or criminal liability a mandated reporter who knowingly fails to report a suspected case of abuse or neglect; such liability may also arise as the result of a negligent failure to report (Bulkley et al., 1996).

Despite these broad mandates, many commentators (e.g., Finkelhor, 1993; Haugaard & Reppucci, 1988) believe that overall reporting rates are low. Perhaps because of the reluctance of those professionals in a unique position to identify child maltreatment to report suspected cases, most reports come from private citizens (Barnett et al., 1993; Knudsen, 1988). Accordingly, it is nonprofessionals who are most often identifying, and thus defining, those acts that constitute child maltreatment. Delays in reporting, refusals to report, and/or decisions not to report perhaps indicate an ambiguity in the definitions of abuse held by both professionals and members of the general public. Surveys have, in fact, shown that physicians, who are often specifically targeted by mandatory reporting requirements due to the fact that they are frequently the first people outside the family to observe serious cases of child maltreatment, are much more willing to diagnose than to report child maltreatment (Kim, 1986). Teachers, too, tend to hold two definitions of abuse: a multidimensional theoretical concept that is actually broader than legal definitions and a much more narrow concept of "punishable" or "reportable" abuse (Pelcovitz, 1980; Tite, 1993). A reluctance to report may also be attributable to concerns about the well-being not only of the child but also of the other individuals involved (Zellman, 1992). Clearly, the interests of a number of people are at stake whenever an individual evaluates whether to report his or her suspicions of maltreatment. In addition to the welfare of the child, the impact of such a report on the child's family, on the perpetrator of the alleged abuse, and on the reporter may all factor into the ultimate decision (Brooks et al., 1994).

Some (e.g., Abrahams et al., 1992; Wurtele & Schmitt, 1992) have suggested, based on findings that mandated reporters have incorrect suppositions about their responsibilities in relation to reporting, that there may be an overall lack of knowledge about reporting laws and the behavioral process that accompanies them. Many people are aware that legal consequences attach to a failure to report; in fact, affected professionals may be more aware of the negative consequences of reporting than of the professional interests served by legislation on reporting (Brooks et al., 1994; Pollak & Levy, 1989). There is a common misperception that in order to report, an indiviudal must have solid evidence of dubious treatment. To the contrary, the decision to report is only the initial step in addressing a case of child abuse and neglect and the substantiation of suspicions is not within the duties of mandated reporters; reporters are required only to have a reasonable suggestion of maltreatment (Wurtele & Schmitt, 1992).

A survey of day-care employees provided further evidence of widespread misconceptions regarding reporting requirements (Wurtele & Schmitt, 1992). Although the majority of participants were aware of the reporting mandates, many falsely believed all citizens to be mandated reporters. As the researchers noted, such a misconception could discourage the accurate production of reports because of an inference that others will fulfill reporting obligations, in an alternative application of Latane and Darley's (1968) theory of diffusion of responsibility.

Many considerations, including perceived socioeconomic status of the family and age, gender, and race of the child, parent, and reporter, may factor into the decision of whether to report a suspected case of child maltreatment (Warner & Hansen, 1994). A number of studies indicate that reporting decisions may vary according to the type of maltreatment that is believed to exist in the particular situation. Saulsbury and Campbell (1985) observed that of three general categories of maltreatment—physical abuse, sexual abuse, and neglect—sexual abuse was most likely to be reported by physicians, whereas cases of neglect were the least likely to be reported. In a survey of physicians, psychologists, psychiatrists, social service personnel, and child care employees, Zellman (1992) found that sexual abuse was not only more likely to be reported, but was also believed to be more serious than both physical abuse and neglect. It was this perceived seriousness of the act, along with comprehension of reporting laws, that most affected actual reporting behavior. In contrast with the findings of Zellman (1992) and Saulsbury and Campbell (1985), Winefield and Bradley (1992) found reports of physical abuse to be the most prevalent, followed by allegations of sexual abuse, neglect, and emotional abuse.

Pollak and Levy (1989) hypothesized that issues of countertransference underlie decisions not to report and may contribute to a lack of appropriate reporting among those professionals subject to mandates. Pollak and Levy defined countertransference as conscious and unconscious emotional components which are the result of past personal experiences and that affect attitudes toward those individuals who will be affected by a report (e.g., the child, family, suspected perpetrator). Countertransference is said to occur when such emotions are manifested as deviations from what would be viewed as standard reporting behavior; for example, fear, guilt, sympathy, and anger may arise from a professional's expectations. Potential support for this hypothesis is found in a survey of school districts in 29 counties across the United States, in which teachers admitted to having reservations about reporting based on perceived legal consequences of producing an unsubstantiated report, possible disruption of the relationship between teachers and children or parents, and parents' refuting reports (Abrahams et al., 1992).

As a whole, the research related to mandated reporting shows a need for training of affected professionals on the specifics of reporting requirements and appropriate evaluation criteria. One might argue, however, that the effectiveness of any training efforts would be severely hampered by the lack of clear guidelines in exisiting reporting laws. Nonetheless, training could have a positive impact on general reporting behaviors and thus promote the best interests of children by ensuring not only that reports are made in appropriate situations, but that they are made in a manner that ensures they will be addressed in an efficient manner. For example, teachers and child care employees report a tendency to make reports to school personnel rather than child protection authorities (Abrahams et al., 1992), which practice may impede further investigation and intervention by creating an additional opportunity for "case-screening" by other mandated reporters.

A final and largely unexplored topic related to reporting is the extent to which children report or even possess the skills necessary to report their own abuse. An obvious but often overlooked fact is that children must themselves identify an act as abusive before reporting it to an adult. Reppucci and Haugaard (1989) have noted this dilemma in the context of programs aimed at training children to repel or report sexual abuse. Such programs assume, without empirical support, that a child possesses the ability first to recognize that he or she is in an abusive situation, then to believe that he or she can and should take some sort of action, and finally to implement specific self-protective skills. In fact, the limited research in this area suggests that few young children are capable of either defining maltreatment or identifying an act as abusive (Miller-Perrin & Wurtele, 1989).

Emergency Placement Determinations

Once an allegation of child maltreatment is made, state legislation typically provides that under certain circumstances abused or neglected children may be taken into custody immediately (Portwood & Reppucci, 1994). Despite the courts' continued policy of nonintervention in deference to the right of family autonomy, at least one appellate court has held that the parental liberty interest in keeping the family unit intact is not a clearly established right when there is a reasonable suspicion that a parent may be abusing a child (*Myers v. Morris,* 1987). The guiding principle in such emergency placement is that the option selected should constitute the least drastic alternative and that every effort should be made to prevent removal and to support continued placement in the home.

Decisions to Prosecute Suspected Cases of Maltreatment

After a report of suspected child maltreatment is lodged, social service and/or child protective agencies typically handle the determination of whether that report can be substantiated; only if a case is deemed "valid" by these agencies may it proceed to a court of law (Cross, DeVos, & Whitcomb, 1994; Winefield & Bradley, 1992). According to the 1988 National Incidence Survey, the substantiation rate for reported cases of child maltreatment in the United States in that year was 53% (cited in Winefield & Bradley, 1992). Critics of the method by which this rate was calculated urge that a more representative rate is in the range of 40 to 42% (Besharov, 1993). Regardless of this discrepancy, it appears that substantiation rates have increased since the establishment of reporting mandates (Tjaden & Thoennes, 1992). Some aspects of cases that relate to their likelihood of substantiation include the age of the victim, with age correlating positively with corroboration of the report; whether the victim had been the subject of previous reports; occupational status of the alleged offender; severity of the alleged maltreatment; and the professional identity of the individual or individuals initiating the report (Winefield & Bradley, 1992). Interestingly, there is some empirical evidence that policy considerations, as well as legal factors (e.g., the amount of evidence required), play a role in rates of substantiation (Flango, 1991).

While substantiation is typically a predicate to legal prosecution, substantiation by no means ensures that prosecution will follow. According to Tjaden and Thoennes's 1992 report of findings by the National Center on Child Abuse and Neglect, fewer than half of those cases that are confirmed result in criminal prosecution. While this figure might suggest that a majority of offenders are not being confronted by the courts, the reality is that alternative or mandatory treatment is often substituted for criminal penalties such as probation or incarceration (Fridell, 1991; Tjaden & Thoennes, 1992). Typical of such alternative programs is the Sacramento County Child Sexual Abuse Treatment Program which is made available to perpetrators of child maltreatment who admit responsibility for their abusive or neglectful actions provided the offender is a member of the victim's family, has no documented history of criminal or violent behavior, and is deemed emotionally and mentally stable enough to participate successfully (Fridell, 1991).

COURTROOM PROCEEDINGS

Because acts viewed as more severe will necessarily be deemed to justify more intrusive forms of intervention, serious cases of abuse—at least those in which sufficient evidence is available—will be directed to the court system. Although most cases of suspected abuse or neglect are resolved without court intervention (Miller, Shireman, Burke, & Brown, 1982), 15% to 20% of child protection cases prompt action by the courts (Rosenberg & Hunt, 1984). Given that the number of reports of suspected child maltreatment in the United States had risen to 2.7 million by 1991 (National Center for Child Abuse and Neglect, 1993), the number of formal court cases of abuse and neglect are clearly in the hundreds of thousands. Once legal proceedings are instituted, two critical concerns arise regarding the child's role in the courtroom: (1) Is the child capable of serving as a witness? and (2) Will testifying result in trauma to the child? These concerns have spawned many recent reforms in courtroom procedures in an effort to protect children and improve the reliability of their testimony. We now examine those issues that arise when a child is called upon to testify in legal proceedings and the steps undertaken by courts to facilitate such testimony.

Children as Witnesses

At the outset, it is important to note that many children who do not serve as witnesses at trial are nonetheless primary sources of information against an accused. In fact, children are questioned an average of 11 times prior to testifying in court (Ceci & Bruck, 1993a). Accordingly, general issues regarding children's ability to provide accurate reports of incidents of maltreatment are relevant not only to an ultimate determination of guilt or innocence in the courtroom, but at each stage of the proceedings, beginning with the investigation and all-important determination of whether there is sufficient evidence to justify criminal prosecution.

At each of these stages, there are many concerns regarding the child's role as a witness, particularly when the child is of preschool age. These concerns relate not only to the effect of testifying on the child, but also to the merit to be afforded the child's testimony. Primary among these concerns is the fear that the child is not reporting what he or she remembers, but what he or she has been told or otherwise led to believe by an adult. For example, there is a general fear that misleading questioning by investigators leads to false allegations and improper convictions (Goodman & Clarke-Stewart, 1991). Others contend that parents could prompt their children to give false accounts which the child might eventually come to believe, as, for example, in a hotly contested child custody case (Haugaard, 1993; Haugaard & Reppucci, 1992; Yuille, Hunter, Joffe, & Zaparniuk, 1993). Whether the empirical evidence supports such claims has been the subject of much debate.

Although there is some contradictory evidence (Luus & Wells, 1992), surveys of the general public have suggested that adults are skeptical of children's capacities as witnesses (Perry & Wrightsman, 1991; Leippe & Romanczyk, 1987). Ross, Dunning, Toglia, and Ceci (1989) found that adults believe that compared to adult witnesses, children are less likely to be accurate and more likely to be open to suggestion. Jury simulation studies also indicate that child witnesses are deemed less credible than their adult counterparts (Goodman, Golding, & Haith, 1984; Goodman, Golding, Helegson, Haith, & Michelli, 1987). Judges, psychologists, police officers, and attorneys have all expressed concerns regarding the accuracy of children's testimony (Goodman & Reed, 1986).

Despite the apparent consensus that child witnesses are inferior to their adult counterparts, ineffective prosecution of child abuse cases has generated several changes in the legal system. Foremost among these is the shift in legal presumptions away from viewing children as incompetent to instead deeming children competent to serve as witnesses, with the question of credibility going to the jury (Perry & Wrightsman, 1991). Under Rule 601 of the Federal Rules of Evidence, children are presumed competent; thus, as with adult witnesses, the jury is to consider the abilities of the particular child in determining his or her credibility. Even where competence is not presumed, the majority of states allow a child to testify provided his or her competence is demonstrated to the court (Whitcomb, 1992). Other standards, beyond age, generally applied in competency determinations include an understanding and appreciation of the oath to tell the truth, sufficient mental capacity to recall an event independently, and the ability to articulate such recollections and answer questions concerning the event (Bulkley, 1988; Weithorn, 1984).

Once the question of competence has been resolved, either by proof or by presumption, the child is treated as is any adult witness in that the sole issue for determination is whether his or her testimony is credible. The judge or the jury may choose to accept or reject the child's testimony, in whole or in part, based on its assessment of whether the child is telling the truth. Typically, this determination has two components: (1) the question of memory and the extent to which children can accurately recall legally relevant information; and (2) the question of suggestibility, that is, whether the child is telling the truth or simply reciting what he or she has been coached into reporting, and possibly even accepting as true.

Children's Memory

Based on the empirical research, there is an apparent consensus that memory skills improve with age (Cohen & Harnick, 1980; Kail, 1989; Schneider & Pressley, 1989). Much of the early research into the accuracy of children's recollections was limited by its focus on school-aged children (Ceci & Bruck, 1993b), more recent investigations have included those children who are most likely to serve as witnesses in abuse proceedings—preschoolers. In a 1993 analysis, Gray found that children below age 8 were involved in 45% of sexual abuse cases; 19% of these witnesses were age 5 or below. Current research indicates that there are situations in which the recall of even preschoolers is accurate. For example, preschoolers exhibit clear recall for action-related events (Davies, Tarrant, & Flin, 1989); for events in which the child is a participant (Rudy & Goodman, 1991); when recognition, rather than free recall, is used as a standard (Ceci, Ross, & Toglia, 1987; Cole & Loftus, 1987); and when specific questions are asked and the task does not emphasize verbal skills (Marin, Holmes, Guth, & Kovac, 1979; Nurcombe, 1986). These findings further suggest that children's errors in reporting are more often acts of omission rather than commission; in other words, although children may recall less than adults, what they do recall may be quite accurate (Goodman & Helegson,

1985). As many commentators (e.g., Marin et al., 1979) have noted, the primary problem may be not young children's ability to remember, but their ability to report their recollections in an accurate and meaningful way.

Perhaps the major obstacle to applying most of the existing research to assessments of child witness competence is the fact that most studies have examined children's short-term recall of objects rather than actions and of peripheral rather than central events (Ceci & Bruck, 1993b). Clearly, the results of such studies do not automatically generalize to cases of alleged maltreatment, in which children are likely to have longer exposure to the information to be recalled and to be direct participants in, rather than bystanders to, the event of interest (Ornstein, Larus, & Clubb, 1991; Goodman & Reed, 1986). Some initial attempts at examining children's mnemonic accuracy in more legally relevant contexts have shown promising results. For example, Ornstein, Gordon, and Larus (1992) examined 3- and 6-year-olds' memory for a visit to their pediatrician for a physical examination. During an immediate memory test, both age groups remembered most features of the examination, even though the older group performed somewhat better. Although the mnemonic performance of 3-year-olds decreased at one- and three-week intervals, the performance of the 6-year-olds remained constant. Both groups also gave accurate responses to misleading questions; however, 3-year-olds again performed less well. In examining children's recall of inoculation and venipuncture procedures, Goodman, Aman, and Hirshman (1987) found that 5- and 6-year-olds answered questions more accurately than 3- and 4-year-olds; however, neither group exhibited any apparent decrease in general recall at delays of up to 9 days. In the study perhaps most closely approximating the characteristics of an abuse incident, Saywitz, Goodman, Nicholas, and Moan (1989) compared recollections of groups of 5- and 7-year-old girls, half of whom had a scoliosis exam and half of whom had a genital exam. Between one and four weeks following their exam, participants were asked suggestive and nonsuggestive questions that were both abuse- and nonabuse-related. Although older children's responses to suggestive nonabuse questions and nonsuggestive abuse questions were more accurate than those of the younger group, there were essentially no differences in the accuracy of the two age groups on suggestive abuse questions.

In summary, it is important to note that although children do exhibit some problems with memory, these same problems are also exhibited by adults to some degree (Goodman & Helegson, 1985). Nonetheless, the general skepticism regarding children's capacities, along with the increasing frequency with which children are being called upon to testify, demands much more work regarding the accuracy of their testimony.

Children's Suggestibility

Underlying the general skepticism surrounding children's testimony is not only a concern that children are less capable of remembering legally relevant information, but also a fear that they are more suggestible and easily misled than adults. To date, the research regarding children's suggestibility has been contradictory. Although some researchers (e.g., Berliner, 1985; Goodman, Rudy, Bottoms, & Aman, 1990) have characterized children as resistant to suggestion, unlikely to lie, and reliable as witnesses in regard to acts perpetrated on their own bodies, others (e.g., Gardner, 1989; Underwager & Wakefield, 1989) describe children as having difficulty distinguishing fantasy from reality, being easily influenced by authority figures, and, thus, being unreliable as witnesses in legal proceedings. It has been suggested that this controversy may be attributable to inconsistencies in the interpretation of data rather than in the data itself, as studies on both sides of the debate are plagued by methodological problems such as relatively small sample sizes, confounds (e.g., linguistic complexity of questions), and the artificiality of study conditions (Ceci, 1991; Ceci & Bruck, 1993b).

In an especially clever study designed to explore children's suggestibility in a context that could give rise to an allegation of sexual abuse, Rudy and Goodman (1991) left pairs of children, ages 4 and 7, in a trailer with a strange adult. One child was selected at random to play a game with the adult that involved being dressed in a clown costume, lifted, and photographed, while the other child observed. Approximately 10 days later, participants were interviewed about the event using suggestive and nonsuggestive questions about the adult's actions. Misleading information that could lead to an allegation of abuse was incorporated into questions (e.g., "He took your clothes off, didn't he?"; "He kissed you, didn't he?"). From a finding that younger and older children had similar high rates of accuracy on misleading questions suggestive of abuse, Rudy and Goodman (1991) concluded that children are less susceptible to suggestion regarding a personally experienced event and highly resistant to suggestions indicating abuse.

After reviewing the suggestibility literature, Ceci and Bruck (1993b) concluded that there do appear to be significant age differences in suggestibility; preschool-age children are disproportionately more suggestible than either school-aged children or adults. From a series of four studies designed to assess preschoolers' susceptibility to misleading postevent suggestions and to determine whether some of the variables that have been identified as susceptibility to suggestion also account for preschoolers' vulnerability to misinformation, Ceci, Ross, and Toglia (1987) concluded that young children's memory is comparable to that of adults when there is no biasing. However, preschoolers' memories are more susceptible to misleading postevent information than are the memories of older children, even after other sources of variance are considered. Some of this susceptibility may be explained by young children's tendency to conform to the wishes of an adult.

Along with cognitive factors, such as mnemonic accuracy, social and motivational factors appear to play an important role in determining the extent of a child's suggestibility. Of particular concern in legal contexts is the fact that when asked the same question more than once, children often change their response, presumably because they interpret the repetition of the question as their inability to give an acceptable response initially (Moston, 1987; Poole & White, 1991). This tendency may have particularly serious repercussions for the child involved in a case of alleged maltreatment because, again, he or she will typically be interviewed many times, often by several adults, during the course of an investigation (Ceci & Bruck, 1993a).

Much more research is needed to delineate the extent to which children's suggestibility represents their response to adult interviewers, given initial evidence that supports the notion that children are susceptible to misinformation presented by an adult. For example, young children view adults as credible and competent sources of information, placing much more faith in statements made by adults than in those made by peers (Ackerman, 1983). Not only do young children perceive adults as cooperative conversational partners who will attempt to communicate with the child to the best of their ability, but children in turn attempt to be cooperative in their interactions with adults, often supplying a questioner with the type of information the child thinks is being requested (Ervin-Tripp, 1978; Read & Cherry, 1978) or trying to please the adult interviewer.

When questioned by adults, children may also attempt to make their answers consistent with what they see as the intent of the questioner rather than consistent with the child's actual knowledge (Ceci & Bruck, 1993b). For example, a majority of children ages 5 and 7 attempted to answer even nonsensical questions (e.g., "Is milk bigger than water?") when they were posed by adults (Hughes & Grieve, 1980). In courtroom settings, attorneys may ask equally confusing questions, injecting age-inappropriate vocabulary, complex syntax (e.g., pronouns with unclear referents), and general ambiguity into their examination (Walker, 1993), thus eliciting suboptimal testimony from the child witness. Attorneys may also confuse young witnesses through the use of leading questions, that is, those requiring only a "yes" or "no" answer ("He took your clothes off, didn't he?"). Findings by Portwood and Reppucci (1996) indicate that there may be an important distinction between children's susceptibility to direct suggestions and their susceptibility to indirect suggestions; thus, the need to question children in a manner that minimizes the potential for an adult to influence the child's response, even unintentionally, may be even more crucial than many commentators (e.g., Doris, 1991; Goodman & Bottoms, 1993; Perry & Wrightsman, 1991) have emphasized. Equally important to continuing efforts to delineate the determinants of children's suggestibility is the role that research can play in developing and improving procedures for obtaining accurate testimony from children.

Summary

Courts would no doubt welcome conclusive research regarding the capacities of child witnesses and methods of assessing the capacities of a specific child in particular. However, many obstacles, including the difficulty in testing children under conditions that simulate the trauma of abuse,make it virtually impossible to develop a study that can resolve the global question of whether preschoolers are suggestible. Although a growing consensus of findings indicates that young children are likely to resist misinformation about an event involving their own bodies (a finding which, if accepted by a court, would satisfy the "preponderance of the evidence" standard applied in civil suits), the fact that even a small percentage of children incorporate such misinformation into their reports defeats any attempt to establish criminal liability "beyond a reasonable doubt."

Courtroom Reforms

Several procedural reforms have been instituted at least partly because of the increase in the number of children testifying in a legal arena. Some researchers have suggested that the stress of testifying in a courtroom may equal the trauma of the abuse itself (Crosby & Reppucci, 1993), sparking numerous attempts to protect children involved in litigation. As has been emphasized, any legal resolution of alleged maltreatment entails an attempt to balance the rights of the child or children against the rights of the accused. At first blush, it might appear that the rights of an accused must necessarily bend to concerns for the child. The need for continued attention to defendants' rights becomes especially salient, however, in cases of alleged sexual abuse, given the devastating effects that such allegations have on the defendant, even when he or she is later adjudicated innocent (Davis & Reppucci, 1992). The principle of defendants' rights is based on the Sixth Amendment of the U.S. Constitution, which provides that citizens subject to prosecution in criminal courts retain the right to a public trial and the right to confront and challenge the accusations of the witnesses against them. To date, the majority of courtroom reforms have focused on limiting face-to-face contact between the defendant and the child. However, the courts must balance the need to protect child witnesses against the defendant's constitutional right to confront the witnesses against him or her. The Supreme Court, as well as the lower courts, has recognized three purposes behind this constitutional right: (1) to bind witnesses to testimony under oath, (2) to afford the defendant an opportunity to cross-examine, and (3) to allow the judge and/or jury to observe the witness's demeanor (Portwood & Reppucci, 1994). If the defendant is to be denied this right to confront his or her accuser, certain standards enumerated by the Supreme Court in *Ohio v. Roberts* (1980) must be met. In *Roberts,* the Court held that hearsay statements do not violate the right to confrontation provided the witness is "unavailable" (either actually, that is, deceased or beyond the court's subpoena power, or figuratively, that is, incompetent to testify) and the statement possesses a sufficient guarantee of trustworthiness. With these guidelines in mind, many states have adopted the use of two-way closed circuit television or videotaped statements in lieu of live child testimony and/or admission of certain (out-of-court) hearsay statements (Crosby & Reppucci, 1993).

Alternatives to "Live" Testimony

In *Coy v. Iowa* (1989), the Supreme Court first considered the constitutionality of procedures designed to protect alleged victims of child abuse by limiting face-to-face confrontation with the defendant. Although the Court rejected the Iowa statute, which provided that the witness would be separated from the defendant by a screen, on the ground that there was no showing that these particular witnesses required special protection, subsequent cases have supported courtroom reforms. In *Maryland v. Craig* (1990), the Court sanctioned the use of testimony by an alleged victim via one-way closed-circuit television, citing the *amicus curiae* brief filed by the American Psychological Association and the research referenced in it to support the majority's finding that the State does have a compelling interest in protecting child witnesses from physical and psychological harm. The Court held that the interest of alleged child abuse victims may outweigh the defendant's Sixth Amendment rights provided there is a "specific finding of necessity." While these cases suggest that the Court is amenable to the use of certain procedural safeguards when child victims are required to testify, their holdings may be limited to cases of *sexual* abuse.

Although numerous criticisms have been levied at the use of videotaped testimony, "[t]he major threat of videotaping is that in states that do not require the

defendant's presence during the child's testimony, the jury may draw inappropriate inferences about the defendant's guilt, because of the harm that it appears the
court is suggesting will be caused by the child's seeing the defendant" (Haugaard
& Reppucci, 1988, p. 363). Clearly, this same threat is posed where the court or leg-
islature has taken other steps to shield a child witness from a defendant. Perhaps
in deference to this criticism, videotaped testimony appears to be used relatively
infrequently in those states where it is authorized (Whitcomb, 1985).

Hearsay Exceptions

Under general evidentiary rules, hearsay testimony (i.e., matters that the witness did not experience firsthand but rather were told to him or her by another
[such as the testimony of an adult as to the content of a child's statements regarding an abuse incident]) may be admitted if the child is found "unavailable" and
the testimony has some indicia of reliability (Federal Rule of Evidence 803). When
a child does not testify at trial, his or her hearsay statements automatically violate
the Sixth Amendment rights afforded criminal defendants *unless* the statements
meet the criteria for an established exception to the hearsay rule, such as a statement made for the purpose of medical diagnosis or treatment (Federal Rule of Evidence 803(4)). However, a growing number of states have expanded the scope of
such exceptions by way of special hearsay statutes applicable to child maltreatment cases (Bulkley et al., 1996; Haugaard & Reppucci, 1988). Among the factors
to be considered in determining whether there is sufficient indicia of the reliability of the statement to justify its admission into evidence are the general character
of the child, whether he or she has a motive to lie, the spontaneity of the statement, the timing of the statement, the person(s) to whom the statement was made,
and the number of individuals who heard the statement (Bulkley et al., 1996). Although such hearsay testimony can be severely damaging to a defendant, his or
her situation is not substantially improved when the child is allowed to testify in
person (Patterson, 1992).

POTENTIAL LEGAL OUTCOMES

As noted, child abuse and neglect cases can be instituted in either or both
criminal and civil courts of law. The major distinction between these two systems
is the burden of proof or standard against which the evidence will be weighed by
the judge or jury. In criminal courts, the State must establish guilt "beyond a reasonable doubt," whereas in civil courts, a complaining party need only prove his
or her case by a "preponderence" or greater weight of the evidence. The fact that
child custody disputes arise in civil court, in which the reduced standard is applied, exposes an alleged perpetrator to a greater risk of an adverse finding and
perhaps less attention to his or her individual rights because here, the "best interests of the child" are paramount (Patterson, 1992). The potential outcomes of criminal and civil proceedings also differ substantially. A guilty verdict in criminal
court may result in a fine and/or imprisonment. A verdict against a civil defendant
typically results in an award of damages or, in a custody dispute in family court,
the loss of custody, visitation privileges, or even parental rights.

When the court determines that a parent or guardian has abused or neglected a child, several alternative placements may be considered. For example, the court may allow the child to remain with the parents subject to certain conditions, or may transfer legal custody to the grandparents, other relatives, a child welfare agency, or public or private social services. Transfer of custody to a public service agency typically results in the child's being placed in temporary or permanent foster care. In the most extreme cases, the court may pursue termination of parental rights.

Termination of Parental Rights

Although the Supreme Court has recognized a fundamental right of parenthood, the Court has also recognized that parental rights are not absolute (*Prince v. Massachusetts,* 1944). In extreme cases in which parental rights conflict with the best interests of the child, parental rights may be terminated. In termination cases, despite the circumstances or the consequences to the parents, who may themselves be victims of circumstances beyond their control, the best interests of the child are paramount. However, because parental rights are fundamental, they cannot be terminated absent a showing of a compelling state interest. Courts will apply a strict scrutiny test to any termination standard, requiring that any infringement on the right of family autonomy serve an important state interest. In addition, clear and convincing evidence is required for a termination of parental rights.

One of the primary bases for seeking a termination of parental rights is to emancipate the child for legal adoption (Portwood & Reppucci, 1994). In essence, violation of the biological family is simply a means of placing the child in an intact family. Because adoption is controlled by the laws of the various states, a full discussion of the procedures and guidelines is beyond the scope of this chapter. However, it should be noted that although a court may serve as an overseer in adoption proceedings, primary determinations of parental fitness have been left largely to social service agencies.

CONCLUSIONS

The courts, as well as all of those who comprise the legal system, face many challenges when presented with cases involving child abuse and neglect. These individuals must first ascertain whether an act or omission should be characterized as abuse or neglect such that intervention, and the violation of family autonomy which it entails, is merited. When a case is referred to legal authorities, these authorities continue to give great consideration to the rights of the parents, attempting to keep the family intact. Although recent cases have held that when there is a threat of danger to the child, his or her rights may supersede the parents' right to privacy, the courts have remained hesitant to place the rights of children before those of parents or other adults accused of abuse or neglect. Moreover, the typically extended period of time between the initiation of a report of suspected abuse until final resolution of the case—in one system an average of five years (Poitrast, 1992)—threatens to keep both children, families, and/or defendants in a state of limbo, in which the interests of none are served.

Overall, actions by the courts in the past decade are suggestive of a move toward increasing consideration of children's rights Nonetheless, there is little, if any, indication that the Supreme Court is willing to abandon more traditional views that defer to the rights of parents and afford them great autonomy in all matters concerning their children. Although the legal system continues in its commitment to serving the best interests of children, the lack of scientific knowledge regarding how best to serve or even identify these interests severely hampers any ability to protect children from future harm. Arguably, a child's best interests are not susceptible to scientific proof, as they are a matter of values rather than empirical fact (Mnookin, 1978). However, to the extent that the laws that affect children are based on erroneous assumptions, researchers can assist in exposing errors and formulating more appropriate policies and procedures to address cases of child maltreatment (Melton, 1987; Woolard, Reppucci, & Redding, 1996).

REFERENCES

Aber, M., & Reppucci, N. D. (1992). Child abuse prevention and the legal system. In D. Willis, E. W. Holden, & M. Rosenberg (Eds.), *Prevention of child maltreatment: Developmental and ecological perspectives* (pp. 249–266). New York: Wiley.

Abrahams, N., Casey, K., & Daro, D. (1992). Teachers' knowledge, attitudes, and beliefs about child abuse and its prevention. *Child Abuse & Neglect, 16*, 229–238.

Ackerman, B. (1983). Speaker bias in children's evaluation of the external consistency of statements. *Journal of Experimental Child Psychology, 35*, 111–127.

Atteberry-Bennett, J. (1987). *Child sexual abuse: Definitions and interventions of parents and professionals.* Unpublished doctoral dissertation, University of Virginia, Charlottesville.

Baily, T. F., & Baily, W. H. (1986). *Operational definitions of child emotional maltreatment: Final report.* National Center on Child Abuse and Neglect (DHHS 90-CA-0956). Washington, DC: U.S. Government Printing Office.

Barnett, D., Manly, J. T., & Cicchetti, D. (1993). Defining child maltreatment: The interface between policy and research. In D. Cicchetti & S. L. Toth (Eds.), *Child abuse, child development, and social policy* (pp. 7–73). Norwood, NJ: Ablex.

Berliner, L. (1985). The child and the criminal justice system. In A. W. Burgess (Ed.), *Rape and sexual assault* (pp. 199–208). NY: Garland.

Besharov, D. J. (1993). Overreporting and underreporting are twin problems. In R. J. Gelles & D. R. Loseke (Eds.), *Current controversies on family violence* (pp. 257–272). Newbury Park, CA: Sage.

Brooks, C. M., Perry, N. W., Starr, S. D., & Teply, L. L. (1994). Child abuse and neglect reporting laws: Understanding interests, understanding policy. *Behavioral Sciences and the Law, 12*, 49–64.

Bulkley, J. (1985). Analysis of civil child protection statutes dealing with sexual abuse. In J. Bulkley (Ed.), *Child sexual abuse and the law* (5th ed.). Washington, DC: American Bar Association.

Bulkley, J. (Ed.). (1988). *Child sexual abuse and the law.* Washington, DC: American Bar Association.

Bulkley, J. A., Feller, J. N., Stern, P., & Roe, R. (1996). Child abuse and neglect laws and legal proceedings. In J. Briere, L. Berliner, J. A. Bulkley, C. Jenny, C., & T. Reid, *The APSAC handbook on child maltreatment* (pp. 271–296). Thousand Oaks, CA: Sage.

Burns, G. E., & Lake, D. E. (1983). A sociological perspective on implementing child abuse legislation in education. *Interchange, 14*(2), 33–49.

Ceci, S. J. (1991). Some overarching issues in the children's suggestibility debate. In J. Doris (Ed.), *The suggestibility of children's recollections* (pp. 1–9). Washington, DC: American Psychiatric Association.

Ceci, S. J., & Bruck, M. (1993a). Child witnesses: Translating research into policy. *Social Policy Report, 8*(3). Society for Research in Child Development.

Ceci, S. J., & Bruck, M. (1993b). The suggestibility of the child witness: A historical review and synthesis. *Psychological Bulletin, 113*, 403–404.

Ceci, S. J., Ross, D. F., & Toglia, M. P. (1987). Suggestibility of children's memory: Psycholegal implications. *Journal of Experimental Psycholgy, 116*, 38–49.

Cohen, R. L., & Harnick, M. A. (1980). The susceptibility of child witnesses to suggestion: An empirical study. *Law and Human Behavior, 4,* 201–210.

Cohen, S., & Sussman, A. (1975). *Reporting child abuse and neglect: Guidelines for legislation.* Cambridge: Ballinger.

Cole, C. B., & Loftus, E. F. (1987). The memory of children. In S. J. Ceci, M. Toglia, & D. Ross, (Eds.), *Children's eyewitness memory* (pp. 178–208). New York: Springer-Verlag.

Coy v. Iowa, 108 S.Ct. 2798 (1989).

Crosby, C. A., & Reppucci, N. D. (1993). The legal system and adolescents. In P. Tolan & B. Cohler (Eds.), *Handbook of clinical research and practice with adolescents* (pp. 281–384). New York: Wiley.

Cross, T. P., DeVos, E., & Whitcomb, D. (1994). Prosecution of child sexual abuse: Which cases are accepted? *Child Abuse & Neglect, 18,* 663–677.

Davies, G. M., Tarrant, A., & Flin, R. (1989). Close encounters of a witness kind: Children's memory for a simulated health inspection. *British Journal of Psychology, 80,* 415–429.

Davis, S., & Reppucci, N. D. (March, 1992). *Accusations of child sexual abuse: A study of process and consequences.* Paper presented at the Biennial Meeting of the American Psychology/Law Society, San Diego, CA.

DeShaney v. Winnebago County Department of Social Services, 489 U.S. 189 (1989).

Doris, J. (Ed.). (1991). *The suggestibility of children's recollections.* Washington, DC: American Psychological Association.

Eisenberg, L. (1981). Cross-cultural and historical perspectives on child abuse and neglect. *Child Abuse & Neglect, 5,* 299–308.

Emery, R. E. (1989). Family violence. *American Psychologist, 44,* 321–328.

Ervin-Tripp, S. (1978). "Wait for me, Roller Skate!" In S. Ervin-Tripp & C. Mitchell-Kernan (Eds.), *Child discourse* (pp. 165–188). New York: Academic Press.

Finkelhor, D. (1993). The main problem is still underreporting, not overreporting. In R. J. Gelles & D. R. Loseke (Eds.), *Current controversies on family violence* (pp. 273–287). Newbury Park, CA: Sage.

Flango, V. E. (1991). Can central registries improve substantiation rates in child abuse and neglect cases? *Child Abuse & Neglect, 15,* 403–413.

Fridell, L. A. (1991). Intrafamilial child sexual abuse treatment: Prosecution following expulsion. *Child Abuse & Neglect, 15,* 587–592.

Garbarino, J., & Ebata, A. (1983). The significance of ethnic and cultural differences. *Journal of Marriage and the Family, 45,* 773–783.

Gardner, R. (1989). *Sex abuse hysteria: Salem witch trials revisited.* Longwood, NJ: Creative Therapeutics Press.

Giovannoni, J. (1991). Social policy considerations in defining psychological maltreatment. *Development and Psychopathology, 3,* 51–59.

Giovannoni, J. M., & Becerra, R. M. (1979). *Defining child abuse.* New York: Free Press.

Goldstein, J., Freud, A., & Solnit, A. (1973). *Beyond the best interest of the child.* New York: Free Press.

Goodman, G. S., Aman, C., & Hirshman, J. (1987). Child sexual and physical abuse: Children's testimory. In S. J. Ceci, M. P. Toglia, and D. F. Ross (Eds.), *Children's eyewitness memory.* New York: Springer-Verlag.

Goodman, G. S., & Bottoms, B. L. (Eds.) (1993). *Child victims, child witnesses: Understanding and improving testimony.* New York: Guilford.

Goodman, G., & Clarke-Stewart, A. (1991). Suggestibility in children's testimony: Implications for sexual abuse investigations. In J. Doris (Ed.), *The suggestibility of children's recollections* (pp. 92–117). Washington, DC: American Psychological Association.

Goodman, G. S., Golding, J. M., & Haith, M. M. (1984). Jurors' reactions to child witnesses. *Journal of Social Issues, 40,* 139–156.

Goodman, G. S., Golding, J. M., Helegson, V. S., Haith, M., & Michelli, J. (1987). When a child takes the stand: Jurors' perceptions of children's eyewitness testimony. *Law and Human Behavior, 11,* 27–40.

Goodman, G. S., & Helegson, V. S. (1985). Child sexual assault: Children's memory and the law. *University of Miami Law Review, 40,* 181–208.

Goodman, G., & Reed, R. (1986). Age differences in eyewitness testimony. *Law & Human Behavior, 10,* 317–332.

Goodman, G. S., Rudy, L., Bottoms, B., & Aman, C. (1990). Children's concerns and memory: Issues of ecological validity in the study of children's eyewitness testimony. In R. Fivush & J. Hudson (Eds.), *Knowing and remembering in young children* (pp. 249–284). New York: Cambridge University Press.

Gray, E. (1993). *Unequal justice: The prosecution of child sexual abuse.* New York: Macmillan.

Haugaard, J. J. (1991). Defining psychological maltreatment: A prelude to research or an outcome of research? *Development and Psychopathology, 3,* 71–77.

Haugaard, J. J. (1993). Young children's classification of the corroboration of a false statement as the truth or a lie. *Law and Human Behavior, 17,* 645–659.

Haugaard, J. J., & Reppucci, N. D. (1988). *The sexual abuse of children.* San Francisco: Jossey-Bass.

Haugaard, J., & Reppucci, N. D. (1992). Children and the truth. In S. Ceci, M. DeSimone, & M. E. Putrick (Eds.), *Cognitive and social factors in early deception* (pp.29–46). New York: Erlbaum.

Hughes, M., & Grieve, R. (1980). On asking children bizarre questions. *First language, 1,* 149–160.

Kail, R.V. (1989). *The development of memory in children* (2nd ed.). New York: Freeman.

Kean, R. B., & Dukes, R. L. (1991). Effects of witness characteristics on the perception and reportage of child abuse. *Child Abuse & Neglect, 15,* 423–435.

Kim, D. S. (1986). How physicians respond to child maltreatment cases. *Health and Social Work, 11,* 95–106.

Knudsen, D. D. (1988). *Child Protective Services: Discretion, decisions, dilemmas.* Springfield, IL: Thomas.

Korbin, J. (1977). Anthropological contributions to the study of child abuse. *Child Abuse & Neglect, 1,* 7–24.

Korbin, J. E. (1991). Cross-cultural perspectives and research directions for the 21st century. *Child Abuse & Neglect, 15*(Suppl. 1), 67–77.

Latane, B., & Darley, J. M. (1968). Group inhibition of bystander intervention in emergencies. *Journal of Personality and Social Psychology, 10,* 215–221.

Leippe, M. R., & Romanczyk, A. (1987). Children on the witness stand: A communication/persuasion analysis of jurors' reactions to child witnesses. In S. J. Ceci, M. P. Toglia, & D. F. Ross (Eds.), *Children's eyewitness memory* (pp. 155–177). New York: Springer-Verlag.

Luus, C. A., & Wells, G. L. (1992). The perceived credibility of child eyewitnesses. In H. Dent & R. Flin (Eds.), *Children as witnesses* (pp. 73–92). West Sussex, England: Wiley.

Marin, B. V., Holmes, D. L., Guth, M., & Kovac, P. (1979). The potential of children as eyewitnesses: A comparison of children and adults on eyewitness tasks. *Law and Human Behavior, 3,* 295–305.

Maryland v. Craig, 497 U.S. 836 (1990).

Melton, G. (1987). *Reforming the law: Impact of child development research.* New York: Guilford Press.

Melton, G. B., & Davidson, H. A. (1987). Child protection and society: When should the state intervene? *American Psychologist, 42,* 172–175.

Meyer v. Nebraska, 262 U.S. 390 (1923).

Miller, B., Shireman, J., Burke, P., & Brown, H. F. (1982). System responses to initial reports of child abuse and neglect cases. *Journal of Social Service Research, 5,* 95–111.

Miller-Perrin, C. L., & Wurtele, S. K. (1989). Children's conceptions of personal body safety: A comparison across ages. *Journal of Clinical Child Psychology, 18,* 25–35.

Mnookin, R. (1978). Children's rights: Beyond kiddie libbers and child savers. *Journal of Clinical Child Psychiatry, 7,* 163–167.

Mnookin, R. H. (1979). *Child, family and state: Problems and materials on children and the law.* Boston: Little, Brown.

Moston, S. (1987). The suggestibility of children in interview studies. *First Lanuage, 7,* 67–78.

Myers v. Morris, 810 F.2d 1437 (8th Cir. 1987), *cert. denied,* 108 S.Ct. 97, 484 U.S. 828, 98 L.Ed.2d 58.

Nagi, S. Z. (1977). *Child maltreatment in the United States.* New York: Columbia University Press.

National Center for Child Abuse and Neglect. (1993). National Child Abuse and Neglect Data System, 1991; Summary data component.

Nelson, B. (1984). *Making an issue of child abuse: Political agenda setting for social problems.* Chicago: University of Chicago Press.

Nurcombe, B. (1986). The child as witness: Competency and credibility. *Journal of American Academy of Child Psychiatry, 25,* 473–480.

Ohio v. Roberts, 448 U.S. 56 (1980).

Ornstein, P. A., Gordon, B. N., & Larus, D. M. (1992). Children's memory for a personally experienced event: Implications for testimony. *Applied Cognitive Psychology, 6,* 49–60.

Omstein, P. A., Larus, D. M., & Clubb, P. A. (1991). Understanding children's testimony: Implications of research on the development of memory. *Annals of Child Development, 8,* 145–176.

Patterson, D. H. (1992). The other victim: The falsely accused parent in a sexual abuse custody case. *Journal of Family Law, 30,* 919–941.

Pelcovitz, D. A. (1980). *Child abuse as viewed by suburban elementary school teachers.* Saratoga, CA: Century Twenty-One.

Perry, N. W., & Wrightsman, L. S. (1991). *The child witness: Legal issues and dilemmas.* Newbury Park, CA: Sage.

Pierce v. Society of Sisters, 268 U.S. 510 (1925).

Poitrast, F. G. (1992). Protecting seriously mistreated children: Time delays in a court sample. *Child Abuse & Neglect, 16,* 465–474.

Pollak, J., & Levy, S. (1989). Countertransference and failure to report child abuse and neglect. *Child Abuse & Neglect, 13,* 515–522.

Poole, D. A., & White, L. T. (1991). Effects of question repetition on the eyewitness testimony of children and adults. *Developmental Psychology, 27,* 975–986.

Portwood, S. G. (1996). *Child maltreatment: Coming to terms with issues of definition.* Unpublished doctoral dissertation, University of Virginia, Charlottesville.

Portwood, S. G., & Reppucci, N. D. (1994). Intervention vs. interference: The role of the courts in child placement. In J. Blacher (Ed.), *When there's no place like home.* Baltimore: Paul H. Brookes.

Portwood, S. G., & Reppucci, N. D. (1996). Adults' impact on the suggestibility of preschoolers' recollections. *Journal of Applied Developmental Psychology, 17,* 175–198.

Prince v. Massachusetts, 321 U.S. 158 (1944).

Read, B., & Cherry, L. (1978). Preschool children's productions of directive forms. *Discourse Processes 1,* 233–245.

Reppucci, N. D., & Crosby, C. A. (1993). Law, psychology and children: Overarching issues. *Law and Human Behavior, 17,* 1–10.

Reppucci, N. D., & Haugaard, J. J. (1989). Prevention of child sexual abuse: Myth or reality? *American Psychologist, 44,* 1266–1275.

Reppucci, N. D., Weithorn, L. A., Mulvey, E. P., & Monahan, J. (Eds.). (1984). *Children, mental health, and the law.* Beverly Hills, CA: Sage.

Roscoe, B. (1990). Defining child maltreatment: Ratings of parental behaviors. *Adolescence, 99,* 517.

Rosenberg, M. S., & Hunt, R. D. (1984). Child maltreatment: Legal and mental health issues. In N. D. Reppucci, L. A. Weithorn, E. P. Mulvey, & J. Monahan (Eds.), *Children, mental health, and the law* (pp. 79–101). Beverly Hills, CA: Sage.

Ross, D. F., Dunning, D., Toglia, M. P., & Ceci, S. J. (1989). Age stereotypes, communication modality, and mock jurors' perceptions of the child witness. In S. J. Ceci, D. F. Ross, & M. P. Toglia (Eds.), *Perspectives on children's testimony* (pp. 37–56). New York: Springer-Verlag.

Rudy, L., & Goodman, G. S. (1991). Effects of participation on children's reports: Implications for children's testimony. *Developmental Psychology, 27,* 527–538.

Saulsbury, F., & Campbell, R. (1985). Evaluation of child abuse reporting by physicians. *American Journal of Diseases of Children, 139,* 393–395.

Saywitz, K., Goodman, G, Nicholas, G., & Moan, S. (1989). Children's memory for a genital exam: Implications for child sexual abuse. Symposium presented at the biennial meeting of the Society for Research in Child Development, Kansas City, MO.

Schneider, W., & Pressley, M. (1989). *Memory development between 2 and 20.* New York: Springer-Verlag.

Scott, E. S., & Reppucci, N. D., & Woolard, J. L. (1995). Evaluating adolescent decision-making in legal contexts. *Law and Human Behavior, 19,* 219–242.

Spearly, J. L., & Lauderdale, M. (1983). Community characteristics and ethnicity in the prediction of child maltreatment rates. *Child Abuse & Neglect, 7,* 91–105.

Starr, R. H. (1988). Physical abuse of children. In V. B. Van Hasselt, R. L. Morrison, A. S. Bellack, & M. Hersen (Eds.), *Handbook of family violence* (pp. 119–148). New York: Plenum Press.

Tite, R. (1993). How teachers define and respond to child abuse: The distinction between theoretical and reportable cases. *Child Abuse & Neglect, 17,* 591–603.

Tjaden, P. G., & Thoennes, N. (1992). Predictors of legal intervention in child maltreatment cases. *Child Abuse & Neglect, 16,* 807–821.

Underwager, R., & Wakefield, H. (1989). *The real world of child interrogations.* Springfield, IL: C. C. Thomas.

Va. Code §16.1-228 (West, 1995 Supplement), and *Va. Code* §63.1-248.2 (West, 1995 Supplement).

Wadlington, W., Whitebread, C. H., & Davis, S. M. (1983). *Children in the legal system: Cases and materials.* Mineola, NY: Foundation Press.

Walker, A. G. (1993). Questioning young children in court. *Law and Human Behavior, 17,* 59–81.

Wamer, J. E., & Hansen, D. J. (1994). The identification and reporting of physical abuse by physicians: A review and implications for research. *Child Abuse & Neglect, 18,* 11–25.

Weithorn, L. A. (1984). Children's capacities in legal contexts. In N. D. Reppucci, L. A. Weithorn, E. P. Mulvey, & J. Monahan (Eds.), *Children, mental health, and the law* (pp. 25–55). Beverly Hills, CA: Sage.

Whitcomb, D. (1985). Prosecution of child sexual abuse: Innovations in practice. In *Research in brief.* Washington, DC: National Institute of Justice.

Whitcomb, D. (1992). Legal reforms on behalf of child witnesses: Recent developments in the American courts. In H. Dent & R. Flin (Eds.), *Children as witnesses* (pp. 156–165).

Wilson, M. N., & Saft, E. W. (1993). Child maltreatment in the African-American community. In D. Cicchetti & V. Toth (Eds.), *Child abuse, child development, and social policy* (pp. 249–300). NY: Ablex.

Winefield, H. R., & Bradley, P. W. (1992). Substantiation of reported child abuse or neglect: Predictors and implications. *Child Abuse & Neglect, 16,* 661–671.

Woolard, J. L., Reppucci, N. D., & Redding, R. (1996). Theoretical and methodological issues in studying children's capacities in legal contexts. *Law and Human Behavior, 20,* 219–228.

Wurtele, S. K., & Schmitt, A. (1992). Child care workers' knowledge about reporting suspected child sexual abuse. *Child Abuse & Neglect, 16,* 385–390.

Yuille, J. C., Hunter, R., Joffe, R., & Zaparinuk, J. (1993). Interviewing children in sexual abuse cases. In G. S. Goodman & B. L. Bottoms (Eds.), *Child victims, child witnesses: Understanding and improving testimony* (pp. 95–115). New York: Guilford Press.

Zellman, G. L. (1992). The impact of case characteristics on child abuse reporting decisions. *Child Abuse & Neglect, 16,* 57–74.

3

How Good Does a Parent Have to Be?

Issues and Examples Associated with Empirical Assessments of Parenting Adequacy in Cases of Child Abuse and Neglect

BRANDON F. GREENE and STELLA KILILI

INTRODUCTION

This chapter is concerned with assessment in cases of child abuse and neglect. The topic is almost as old as the problem of child maltreatment itself. Indeed, assessment strategies, in one form or another, have been the basis for estimating the incidence and prevalence of child maltreatment, testing hypotheses about the psychological nature of perpetrators and victims, creating models that describe potential causes of child maltreatment, and for deriving strategies to prevent it. In short, assessment of child maltreatment actually encompasses a broad spectrum of well-established strategies and practices, each uniquely responsive to particular questions about the problem.

However, as will be discussed in subsequent sections, most assessment strategies neither effectively probe some of the most fundamental concerns nor inform some of the most critical decisions that arise in individual cases of child abuse and neglect. That is, whenever a case of child abuse or neglect is alleged, professionals in the child welfare system will be concerned with (1) whether the allegation is justified, (2) whether it is necessary to take the child into protective custody, (3) if, when, where, and under what conditions parents will be allowed to visit children whom the state places in foster care, (4) whether the family is making incremental

BRANDON F. GREENE and STELLA KILILI • Behavior Analysis and Therapy Program, Southern Illinois University, Carbondale, Illinois 62901.

Handbook of Child Abuse Research and Treatment, edited by Lutzker. Plenum Press, New York, 1998.

progress in correcting the circumstances that required state intervention, and (5) whether progress is ultimately sufficient to enable the family to remain intact.

At the core of many of these concerns is the question of whether parenting is adequate. That is not a question that typically can be raised and answered only once in the course of serving a case. That is, parenting skills are amenable to change. Therefore, when serving a family with a history of child maltreatment, professionals must repeatedly question and probe the adequacy of parenting, quickly recognize when small changes occur, and reinforce change that is adaptive.

Why are current assessment practices generally unresponsive to the ongoing question about the adequacy of parenting? To understand their limitations, it is first necessary to understand what competent (or at least adequate) parenting is.

WHAT IS COMPETENT PARENTING?

Most of us probably think of competent parents as adults who are highly responsive to children, who actively seek numerous opportunities within and outside of the home for children to fulfill their potential, who provide safe but reasonable limits, and who maintain their allegiance even when children transgress social norms. The reality, of course, is that parenting can be much less than this before its adequacy is ever questioned by the child welfare system. That is, in actual cases involving child maltreatment, the touchstone for parental fitness or competence is not an exemplary standard; rather, it is a standard of *minimal adequacy*. This practice stems from the culture's long-standing misgivings with state intervention in matters of individual and family autonomy, and respect for the importance of maintaining the relationship between parents and children whenever possible (Goldstein, Freud, & Solnit, 1973; Mnookin, 1985).

For example, the child welfare system in Illinois outlines what it regards as "minimum parenting standards" (Illinois Department of Children and Family Services, 1985). The enumeration of these standards (see Table 1) serves to establish the broad terms of an implied contract between family and state whereby the state agrees to (1) respect the autonomy of the family if the standards are not violated, and (2) limit the areas and extent to which improvements in parenting may be required before state intervention ceases and/or custody of the children is restored. Thus, they are intended to focus the caseworker's attention on the essentials of parenting and to avoid demands for changes which may be arbitrary, that divert limited resources, and that ultimately compromise an appropriate resolution to the case (Stein, Gambrill, & Wiltse, 1978).

However, the general descriptions and examples of parenting in Table 1 are standards only in the broadest sense of the word. That is, they have no operational definitions, no quantitative criteria, litmus test, or established assessment strategies to determine whether parenting meets, approximates, or exceeds the minimum in any particular case. Of course, it is not reasonable to expect that a particular assessment or battery of assessments will render a precise formula that distinguishes adequate from inadequate parenting. Furthermore, ultimate judgments about the adequacy of parenting are, appropriately, social judgments often made in a court of law. Nevertheless, reliable assessments should directly inform such judgments and closely guide the recurring clinical questions about whether

Table 1. IDCFS Minimum Parenting Standards

I. Income and money management standards
  A. Income: The family has income sufficient to meet the family's basic needs for food, shelter, clothing, education, and health care.
    Indicator areas
    1. Employability of parents
    2. Employment history
    3. Income earned from employment
    4. Income (cash) from other sources (e.g., public benefits)
    5. In-kind value of rent subsidies, food stamps, etc.
    6. Parental ability to access community resources to secure or supplement income as required
  B. Money management: The parent demonstrates money management skills necessary to meet the needs of the children.
    Indicator areas
    1. Budgeting skills
    2. Shopping skills
    3. Menu planning skills
    4. Expenditure history (what is spent for what)
    5. Nonessential expenditures (alcohol, drugs, tobacco)
    6. Banking skills
    7. Knowledge of free/low cost community resources for securing food, clothing, health care, etc.
II. Physical care standards
  A. Food: The parents obtain and provide the quantity and quality of food necessary to assure the adequate health and development of individual family members.
    Indicator areas
    1. Presence of sufficient quantities of nutritional food (age-appropriate to the child)
    2. Number of meals prepared each day
    3. Nutritional balance of daily/weekly menu
    4. Shopping patterns (frequency)
    5. Meal preparation skills
    6. Cooking equipment present/usable
    7. Food storage hygiene
    8. Kitchen/cooking area hygiene
  B. Shelter: The parents provide a structurally safe and protective living residence.
    Indicator areas
    1. Electrical safety (outlets, wiring, etc.)
    2. Properly operating, safe heating source
    3. Roof, walls, doors, and windows are in adequate repair and exterior doors and windows can be locked
    4. Operating plumbing, water, and toilet facilities (or access to such in a safe external source)
    5. Adequate sanitary conditions
    6. Adequate furniture and room space (particularly bedding and sleeping arrangements)
    7. Garbage disposal methods
    8. "Child safe" storage of medicines, cleaning supplies, etc.
  C. Clothing: Parents provide and maintain clothing which is of sufficient quantity and quality
    Indicator areas
    1. Presence and utilization of clothing (particularly seasonally appropriate clothing such as boots, gloves, jackets, and coats)
    2. State of repair of clothing
    3. Cleanliness of clothing (e.g., laundering patterns)
    4. Shopping/access skills for obtaining clothing
  D. Personal hygiene: The parents assure the personal hygiene of children
    Indicator areas
    1. Bathing/washing frequency (age appropriate)
    2. Dental care patterns

(continued)

Table 1. (*Continued*)

3. Hair care patterns (washing/brushing)
4. Presence and utilization of personal hygiene supplies (e.g., soap, shampoo, combs/brushes, towels, washcloths, deodorant, baby supplies, etc.)

  E. Medical care: The parents provide necessary medical care to children
    Indicator areas
    1. Examination frequency
    2. Immunizations
    3. Presence and utilization of home health care supplies (e.g., bandages, antiseptics, etc.)
    4. Regular appointments, treatment if needed due to special health issues
    5. Parental knowledge/competence (re: medical needs of children)
    6. Access skills for obtaining emergency medical care

III. Affection standards
  A. Spouse-to-spouse: The parents demonstrate or model positive affection in their relationship
    Indicator areas
    1. Method/frequency/duration of positive physical interaction
    2. Method/frequency/duration of positive verbal expressions of affection
    3. Method/frequency/duration of negative physical conduct
    4. Method/frequency/duration of verbally negative conduct

  B. Parent-to-child: The parents demonstrate positive affection toward the child
    Indicator areas
    1. Method/frequency/duration of positive physical interaction
    2. Method/frequency/duration of positive verbal expressions of affection
    3. Method/frequency/duration of negative physical conduct
    4. Method/frequency/duration of verbally negative conduct

  C. Sibling-to-sibling: The interaction between siblings demonstrates positive, age-appropriate affection
    Indicator areas
    1. Method/frequency/duration of positive physical interaction
    2. Method/frequency/duration of positive verbal expressions of affection
    3. Method/frequency/duration of negative physical conduct
    4. Method/frequency/duration of verbally negative conduct

  D. Other adult-to-child: Interaction between non-parental adults and the child(ren) demonstrates positive age-appropriate affection
    Indicator areas
    1. Method/frequency/duration of positive physical interaction
    2. Method/frequency/duration of positive verbal expressions of affection
    3. Method/frequency/duration of negative physical conduct
    4. Method/frequency/duration of verbally negative conduct

IV. Educational standards
  A. Social education: The parent demonstrates the ability to educate the child in social interaction skills
    Indicator areas (age-appropriate)
    1. Health care and hygiene skills
    2. Clothing procurement and care skills
    3. Personal interaction and problem-solving skills
    4. Nutrition/eating skills
    5. Transportation skills
    6. Child care skills
    7. Safety/security skills

  B. Academic education: The parent demonstrates an ability to foster the child's achievement of age-appropriate academic skills
    Indicator areas (age-appropriate)
    1. Preschool, day-care participation
    2. Reading/writing/math skills
    3. School enrollment
    4. Homework patterns and parent interaction

Table 1. (*Continued*)

___

    5. Presence of educational toys
    6. Parental visits/communication with school personnel
    7. School attendance patterns
    8. Special diagnostic testing, if needed
V. Guidance standards
  A. The parent demonstrates positive methods of providing age-appropriate guidance to the child
    Indicator areas
    1. Frequency/methods for providing advice/feedback to the child
    2. Level of understanding regarding child development process, issues, and limitations
    3. Patterns/sources/methods of providing supervision for the child
    4. Methods/patterns/sources of discipline
    5. The ability to access community resources to secure professional guidance counseling as required

___

Source: Child Welfare Services Practice Handbook, Illinois Department of Children and Family Services, 1985.

parenting improves as a function of services. Unfortunately, current assessment practices do neither.

Although current assessments have utility and validity for certain purposes, they are not responsive to questions of parenting adequacy. Accordingly, in the sections that follow, some of the major practices in the assessment of child maltreatment are considered for their usefulness in informing judgments about the adequacy of parenting. The discussion is not intended to be exhaustive of the pertinent literature. Rather, it is intended only to review the primary functions and characteristics of various assessment practices and to discuss why these do not suffice to inform judgments of parenting adequacy.

WHAT ARE THE LIMITATIONS TO CURRENT ASSESSMENT STRATEGIES AND PRACTICES?

Assessment of Incidence and Prevalence

Epidemiological estimates of the incidence and prevalence of child abuse and neglect describe how pervasive the problem is. Of course, such assessment information was never intended to bear on questions of parenting competence in particular cases. For example, knowing that child abuse and neglect is estimated to affect 2.7 million children nationally (National Center for Child Abuse and Neglect, 1992) is not especially pertinent to decisions about parenting competence in a particular case. However, an analysis of these estimates by types of child maltreatment provides an indication of the areas of parenting where the demand for individual assessments may be great. For example, neglect accounts for the largest proportion, or approximately half, of child maltreatment (National Center for Child Abuse and Neglect, 1992).

Such national statistics are consistent with reports in Illinois of 75,534 families involving 136,255 children (Illinois Department of Children and Family Services, 1994). Approximately 35% of these reports of abuse and neglect were substantiated and, as depicted in Figure 1, neglect, particularly environmental neglect, accounted for the largest proportion of reported cases.

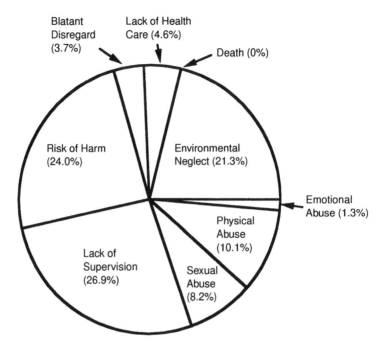

Figure 1. Types of child abuse and neglect reported in fiscal year 1994 in the State of Illinois. (*Source*: Child Abuse and Neglect Statistics, Annual Report, Fiscal Year 1994, Illinois Department of Children and Family Services.)

Psychological Assessments

One of the most extensive areas of research in child abuse and neglect has involved the psychological assessment of perpetrators. That was inevitable after Kempe and associates (Kempe, Silverman, Steele, Droegemueller, & Silver, 1962) defined the "battered child syndrome" not only in terms of the trauma experienced by the child, but with reference to presumed defects in the character of the abuser. Thus ensued decades of search and research for every conceivable malady, affliction, or perturbation that might distinguish the psychological profile of abusers. The search has been less than fruitful. At best, the evidence for a set of distinctive psychological characteristics among abusers is equivocal (National Research Council, 1993).

Nevertheless, it continues to be common practice for child welfare specialists and courts to seek the testimony of "experts" who base their opinions of parenting adequacy on psychological testing. The practice may have its roots in the mystique and presumed relevance of psychological opinion, the dubious assumption that psychological assessment results are predictive of minimally adequate parenting, or the absence of any better alternative. In any case, the practice may become more widely challenged as more direct measures of parenting competence are developed and as evidence mounts that psychological conditions or diagnoses (e.g., mental retardation) do not necessarily preclude such competence (cf. Greene, Norman, Searle, Daniels, & Lubeck, 1995).

Assessment of Correlates and Contributing Conditions

An extensive body of assessment information bears on the relationship between child abuse and conditions such as socioeconomic status, unemployment, substance abuse, social isolation, and various sources of family stress (National Research Council, 1993). Such findings may certainly inform public policy, but their relevance to an assessment of whether parenting is adequate in individual cases is remote. That is, there are many adults who provide adequate parenting despite being unemployed, uneducated, poor, and socially isolated. Some may even abuse substances. Therefore, although these conditions may be markers of difficulties in parenting among the general population, their presence in a particular case is not necessarily an indication of a failure or inability to meet minimum parenting standards.

Behavioral Assessment

The hallmark of a behavioral approach to assessment is its emphasis on reliable and direct observation of precisely defined behaviors. It would seem that such an approach would be ideally suited to the task of operationally defining and quantifying the minimum parenting standards outlined in Table 1. Indeed, an extensive literature exists involving the behavioral assessment of parent and child relations. The enduring work of Patterson (1982), Wahler (1969), and their colleagues is particularly notable. However, the assessment targets in this and related research were not explicitly selected or intended to reflect minimally adequate parenting, per se. Rather, such assessments typically have targeted certain classes of parental behavior involved in managing difficult or oppositional children (e.g., providing differential reinforcement, administering timeout). Thus, it remains an untested possibility that an assessment of these or related classes of behavior may be informative to a judgment of whether parenting is minimally adequate.

Summary

The concept of minimum parenting standards will probably always elude explicit definition and quantification. What constitutes minimally adequate parenting is ultimately a social judgment subject to varied interpretations over time and with the particular circumstances of individual cases. However, although an assessment should explicitly inform this judgment, familiar assessment practices either cannot be or have not been adapted to this purpose.

Nevertheless, the concept of minimally adequate parenting implies that (1) there may be dimensions of parenting or child care which are essential, (2) proficiency in parenting falls along a continuum of each dimension, and (3) parenting adequacy begins to be questionable at some points or within some range of that continuum.

Some dimensions of parenting may be more amenable to quantification than others. For example, it may be technically easier to quantify the adequacy of physical care, such as the sufficiency of nutritious food, than the adequacy of affection or emotional support that parents offer to children. Nevertheless, in principle, each dimension of parenting could be operationalized and quantified along a continuum.

Points, or at least a range of points, may be indicative of problems in parenting. The sections that follow describe a case example and an experiment that illustrate two different strategies for quantifying the continuum of parenting adequacy in two areas identified in Illinois' minimum parenting standards.

QUANTIFYING THE CONTINUUM OF COMPETENT PARENTING ON THE BASIS OF ESTABLISHED STANDARDS: THE EXAMPLE OF NUTRITIOUS MEALS

Greene et al. (1995) reported an experimental case study of a developmentally disabled mother (IQ = 71) and her son who had been repeatedly hospitalized for failure to thrive. There is evidence that such parents are at particular risk for losing custody of their children, in part because of cultural biases regarding their parenting ability (Taylor, Norman, Murphy, Jellinek, Quinn, Poitrast, & Goshko, 1991).

The child was ultimately placed in foster care and the child welfare agency contracted for services with Project 12-Ways. Project 12-Ways operates under the auspices of the Behavior Analysis and Therapy Program at Southern Illinois University and provides in-home parent training and other services to families with a history of child abuse and neglect (Lutzker, 1984).

Over a period of two years, the parent was instructed in a broad range of child care skills (Greene et al., 1995). Of particular interest here is the assessment conducted to determine the adequacy of the food that the parent provided.

Assessment and training initially emphasized bottle feeding and related aspects of care. However, as the child developed and began to consume regular food, it was necessary to assess the quality of his diet. The framework for doing so was the recommended daily allowance (RDA) for the four major food groups (dairy, vegetable, meat, and bread).

Specifically, during his period in foster care, the child visited the parent at her home. The parent prepared meals while Project 12-Ways staff and the parent herself recorded the quantity of servings of each food group. That quantity was later analyzed in relation to the RDA for the food group. Thus, on any given day the child might receive the exact RDA (a proportion equal to 1), or a quantity less than or in excess of the RDA (i.e., a proportion less than or greater than 1, respectively). Figure 2 is a graphic depiction of the proportion of the RDA in each food group that the child received during a sample of meals from baseline, training, and follow-up phases.

The details of each phase are not important for this discussion (cf. Greene et al., 1995). However, it is evident that there are periods when the serving was noticeably less than or exceeded the RDA.

There are several key points to discuss. First, we are not suggesting that any variance from the RDA constitutes child maltreatment. Presumably, although continuous and marked variances could be cause for concern, there is no simple algorithm that can be applied to the data which renders a judgment about the adequacy either of the child's diet specifically or of this area of parenting in general. We are suggesting, however, that the data depicted in Figure 2 are relevant and vital to an informed judgment which experts and others in the child welfare system may be asked to make in cases such as this where the child's nutrition has been seriously deficient.

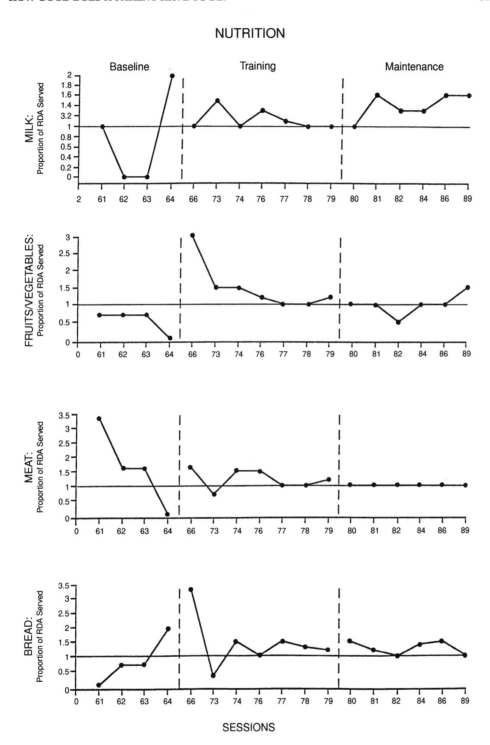

Figure 2. The proportion of the recommended daily allowance (RDA) for each food group that the mother served the child during meals she prepared for him. The solid horizontal lines indicate the RDA for each food group.

Second, we have found that continuous, systematic assessment of any dimension of parenting is essential to an informed judgment. In this case, for example, there were professionals from many agencies who were periodically present in the home with the mother and child. There was a tendency among some to form pervasive opinions about the quality of parenting based on brief, episodic observations. Thus, if on any particular day or meal the child's diet was noticeably unbalanced, there was a tendency among professionals to make sweeping conclusions about the overall adequacy of nutrition that the parent provided. A series of continuous and quantified observations of the sort depicted in Figure 2 provides a more appropriate basis for forming opinions.

Third, the data in Figure 2 reflect only one dimension of the adequacy of nutrition. The figure reflects only what the parent served, not what the child consumed or whether that nourishment was sufficient to promote adequate growth. (In the actual study [Greene et al., 1995], however, the child's height and weight were also examined over an extended period. By the end of service his growth met the norms for his age.)

Fourth, when an assessment suggests that the quality of any aspect of parenting appears to be deficient, we prefer to correct the problem whenever possible, not to indict the parent. That is, in general, the proper use of the data is to develop and evaluate services that can improve the quality of parenting, not to provide sophisticated evidence of its inadequacy. Should reasonable efforts fail to improve parenting, however, we recognize that the data may inform other courses of action.

This case illustrates the possibility of assessing the adequacy of some aspects of parenting on the basis of established or recognized standards (e.g., the RDA). Of course, not all aspects of parenting will be amenable to such an assessment where no comparable standard exists. In these cases, however, it may be possible to establish an appropriate and reasonable standard. That is, perhaps assessments can be developed to quantify some aspects of parenting outlined in Table 1, to establish norms for each assessment on the basis of the general population or particular groups within the general population, and to use those norms to establish a continuum along which the adequacy of parenting can be identified in particular cases. The experiment described in the subsequent sections is illustrative.

QUANTIFYING THE CONTINUUM OF COMPETENT PARENTING ON THE BASIS OF NORMATIVE DATA: THE EXAMPLE OF HOME CLEANLINESS

The impetus for this study was our concern in Project 12-Ways with the problem of child neglect. Both abuse and neglect are harmful to children, but they are usually conceptualized differently. That is, abuse is typically regarded as an act of commission (e.g., beating the child) whereas neglect is regarded as an act of omission or failure to provide some essential care (Kadushin, 1980; Polansky, Chalmers, Buttenwieser, & Williams, 1978; National Research Council, 1993).

Child neglect appears to be more prevalent (Eskin, 1980) and may actually be more harmful than abuse because it is often less conspicuous and, therefore, less apt to be reported (Polansky et al., 1978; Schwartz & Hirsh, 1982). Although definitions of neglect vary, child neglect is generally indicated when the caretaker cannot (or fails to) provide adequate food, clothing, medical care, education, or shelter. The child's shelter may be regarded as inadequate because of filth, the accumulation of trash, and the presence of decaying animals or other matter that could harbor disease and infestations of insects or vermin. Such neglect, often referred to as environmental neglect, represented more than one-fifth of all harms (both abuse and neglect) recently reported to the child welfare agency in Illinois (Figure 1).

It can be a difficult and sensitive matter for the state to make an official determination of environmental neglect. First, environmental conditions among households are apt to vary by degrees. Thus, it is only at some point along a hypothetical continuum that conditions are sufficiently bad to warrant state action. Second, impoverished families may be at particular risk for state intrusion for both legitimate and prejudicial reasons. The legacy of child welfare in this country includes periods in which the state has interceded in the family's affairs, and sometimes imposed punitive sanctions upon the parents, solely because the parents were poor (Giovannoni & Recerva, 1979). Indeed, even today subtle biases against poor families are evident for example, in a class action suit in which a federal district court has enjoined the state of Illinois from taking children into custody solely because of the poor physical conditions of the household when reasonable efforts could be made to improve those conditions (*Norman, Patterson, et al. v. Johnson*, 1990).

There may be no complete, technical solution to this problem. However, the problem could be alleviated if state authorities had objective criteria either to diagnose environmental neglect or at least to inform their judgment about whether or how severely it exists in particular cases. Similarly, such criteria could provide an objective basis for treatment agents who must establish reasonable goals for change and evaluate efforts to achieve them.

Some tools have been developed to assess the prevalence of safety hazards (Barone, Greene, & Lutzker, 1986; Tertinger, Greene, & Lutzker, 1984) and physically neglectful conditions in the home (Watson-Perczel, Lutzker, Greene, & McGimpsey, 1988). In the latter study an assessment protocol, the Checklist of Living Environments to Assess Neglect (CLEAN), was developed for purposes of evaluating the impact of treatment. To administer the CLEAN, individual rooms of the house are mapped into "item areas" (e.g., countertops, floor space between cabinets and living room, appliance surfaces). These item areas are then examined for (1) the presence of decaying organic matter, (2) obstructing accumulations of linen and clothing (e.g., in hallways), and (3) the presence of clutter (defined as items that are in unusual locations that the children's caretakers acknowledge as not the usual and preferred location for storing the item). CLEAN combines these three aspects of home cleanliness into a single index ranging from 0 to 100, reflecting progressively greater cleanliness. The reliability (interobserver agreement) of CLEAN has been established, and there is some evidence of its validity. Specifically, caseworkers have commented favorably on pre-post changes in two homes where environmental neglect was treated based on CLEAN (social validity). In addition, the households of a small number of families ($N = 4$) with no problem of environmental neglect were assessed and their CLEAN scores appeared to be in the range of the targeted families' posttreatment score (Watson-Perczel et al., 1986).

However, a more complete and formal use of the CLEAN would involve the development of standards or norms by which to compare and interpret the results from a particular household. That is, an acceptable range of cleanliness might be identified with normative data gathered from the homes of families from varied socioeconomic backgrounds. Accordingly, the purpose of this study was to gather and describe those normative data.

Method

Participants

Sixty-one families participated in this study. The families represented 6 groups from varied backgrounds with respect to socioeconomic status and child abuse/neglect history. All families had at least 1 child under 6 years of age living in the home. Some families were clients of Project 12-Ways.

Group 1: Low education and income/environmental neglect history. This group consisted of 10 families, clients of Project 12-Ways, for whom either an Illinois Department of Children and Family Services (DCFS) caseworker and/or a Project 12-Ways counselor identified home cleanliness or safety as an area in need of service. All families had low income (below $10,000 annually). In 5 of these families neither parent had a high school diploma; in 5, at least one parent had a high school diploma.

Group 2: Low education and income/abuse or neglect history but no environmental neglect. This group consisted of 10 families being served by Project 12-Ways for reasons other than environmental neglect. This group also had an annual income below $10,000. In 2 of these families neither parent in the home had a high school diploma; in 8 at least one parent had a high school diploma.

Recruitment procedures for Groups 1 and 2 (Project 12-Ways clients) were the same. Twenty-nine families being served at the time of the study had children under age 6. Nine were either unavailable or did not keep the appointments for the study.

The study was explained to the families eligible to participate by the staff member primarily responsible for serving the family. It was presented as a study done by Project 12-Ways in which participation was not a requirement for serving the family. The families who agreed to participate scheduled a time and date for the assessment.

Group 3: Low education and income/no abuse or neglect history. This group consisted of 11 families who, according to DCFS records, had no known history of child abuse and/or neglect. Otherwise, the selection criteria for this group were the same as for the Project 12-Ways groups, that is, low education (neither parent in the home had a college degree) and low income (below $10,000 annually).

Families were recruited during an outing of parents and children from a local Head Start. The experimenters approached about 40 parents and explained the study to them. Sixteen parents expressed interest. After a follow-up phone call 11 people agreed and scheduled a time for the assessment.

Group 4: High education and low income/no abuse or neglect history. This group consisted of 9 families who, according to DCFS records, had no known history of child abuse and/or neglect. These families were recruited from day-care centers operated by a university or in the university community for the families of its students and staff. All families had an annual income of less than $10,000. At least one parent in the home had a college degree and in 4 families, one or both parents were working on a graduate level degree.

Group 5: High education and income/no abuse or neglect history. This group consisted of 10 families who, according to DCFS records, had no known history of child abuse and/or neglect. At least one parent in the home had a graduate degree in a human service field and all families had an income over $30,000 annually.

Twenty potential participants were identified from among peers and colleagues in a university. They were contacted by mail and subsequently by telephone. Ten agreed to participate in the study for the assessment.

Group 6: State approved standard—foster families. This group consisted of 11 foster families licensed by the state to serve children under 6 years of age. This was the only selection criterion for this group. Their income varied from less than $10,000 to over $30,000 annually. Their education ranged from less than a high school diploma to a graduate-level degree.

In 5 of the 11 families, at least one parent in the home had a college degree. In 2 families at least one parent had some college experience. In 3 families at least one parent had a high school diploma. One family did not provide this information.

The group of foster parents was identified by obtaining a list of 40 homes from the child welfare agency. Twenty-six families declined to participate because of conflicts or because they simply were not interested in the study. Two families who initially agreed to participate failed to keep the appointments for the scheduled assessments. One family could not be contacted.

Table 2 provides demographic information pertaining to all groups.

Setting

The participants' homes in southern Illinois were the settings of the observations.

Assessment

Observational system. To administer the CLEAN, observers map individual rooms of the house into "item areas." For example, in the kitchen there may be several item areas such as countertop adjacent to sink, floor space between cabinets and living room, appliance surfaces, and so on. These item areas are then assessed along three dimensions: (1) the presence of organic matter in direct contact with the areas, (2) accumulations of clothing or linens, and (3) clutter, other than linen, composed of items which appear to be in unusual locations (e.g., a partial quart of oil on furniture) which the adult resident acknowledges is not the usual or preferred location for the item. A weighted point system is applied to each of these dimensions as outlined in Table 3.

The maximum score for an item area is 20 points. The CLEAN score for the room is derived by adding the scores for all item areas, dividing by the product of the number all areas assessed times 20 (Sum of All Item Areas 20 × Number of

Table 2. Social-Demographic Information Describing Participants

Family characteristic	Group					
	G_1	G_2	G_3	G_4	G_5	G_6
Children in the home						
Ave. no. children	2.6	2.3	1.7	1.8	1.9	2.3
Ave. age children	4.1	6.8	3.3	4.6	4.6	6.7
Adults in the home						
Ave. no. adults	1.7	1.8	1.1	1.7	2.0	2.3
Ave. age adults	30.9	31.4	25.9	29.6	33.6	44.3
Rooms in the home						
Ave. no. rooms	5.0	5.2	4.1	5.2	8.8	6.8
Type of housing—% of families living in						
Public housing	0	20	18.2	11.1	0	9.1
Trailer—rent	30	30	18.2	11.1	0	0
Trailer—own	20	10	9.1	77.8	0	0
Home/apt—rent	40	20	54.5	66.6	10	9.1
Home/apt—own	10	20	0	11.1	90	81.8
Income—% of families with income						
Under $5,000	40	20	45.5	11.1	0	0
$5,000–$10,000	60	70	54.5	88.9	0	27.3
$10,000–$20,000	0	10	0	0	0	27.3
$20,000–$30,000	0	0	0	0	0	36.3
Above $30,000	0	0	0	0	100	9.1
Educational level—% of parents with						
Some high school	33.3	25	0	0	0	0
High school diploma	58.3	66.6	64.3	0	0	52.4
Some college	8.3	8.3	35.7	18.8	5	19
College degree	0	0	0	56.2	20	23.8
Graduate school	0	0	0	25	75	4.8

Note: G_1: Low education and income/environmental neglect history
     G_2: Low education and income/abuse-neglect history but no environmental neglect
     G_3: Low education and income/no abuse-neglect history
     G_4: High education, low income/no abuse-neglect history
     G_5: High education and income/no abuse-neglect history
     G_6: Foster families

Items), and multiplying by 100 to yield a percentage score. An overall home cleanliness score is derived by averaging the scores from all rooms.

Observer training. Observers were Project 12-Ways staff who were trained by the experimenters. The staff studied and discussed the observation code, completed a quiz, and practiced scoring in a classroom set up to resemble a dining area and then in their own homes.

Staff who did not meet a criterion of 80% agreement were given specific feedback and were asked to read the package again and assess an additional house until the 80% criterion was met. Training took approximately 8 hours.

Application. At the time and date of the scheduled visit, two observers arrived at the family's home, reviewed the purpose of the study and obtained written consent. Participants were asked to identify areas in their home (e.g., specific

Table 3. Scoring of Item Areas Using CLEAN

Attribute of item area	Point value
Clean or dirty	10 or 0
Clothing/linen accumulation	
0 articles	5
1–5 articles	4
6–10 articles	3
11–15 articles	2
16–20 articles	1
>20 articles	0
Clutter	
0 items	5
1–5 items	4
6–10 items	3
11–15 items	2
16–20 items	1
>20 items	0
Total possible score for item area	20

cabinets) they did not want the observer to examine. The participants were invited to accompany the observers during the assessment or to continue with their own activities.

Data in the bathroom, kitchen, and living room were consistently available on all subjects. (Our experience has been that the bathroom and kitchen present greatest concerns for sanitation.)

Reliability. Reliability of cleanliness conditions was assessed throughout the study. Each occurrence of agreement or disagreement between the primary and secondary observer's recorded responses was calculated. Agreements were defined as agreement on the exact numerical range of "items not belonging" and "cloth/linens" and agreement on the "clean/dirty" condition. The percentage of agreement was calculated using the formula:

$$\frac{\text{Agreements}}{\text{Agreements} + \text{Disagreements}} \times 100$$

Reliability observations were taken for 44% of the home assessments. The results of the reliability calculations are shown in Table 4.

Results

Figure 3 presents mean composite cleanliness scores for each group of families in each of three rooms in their house (bathroom, kitchen, living room). A 6 (group) × 3 (room) analysis of variance with repeated measures (on the second factor) yielded a statistically significant main effect for group, $F(5,55) = 4.90$, $p <$

Table 4. Percentage Interobserver Agreement (Mean and Range)—
for Each Group by Room

Group	Room		
	Bathroom	Kitchen	Living room
Group 1			
Low education and income/environmental neglect history	94.6 (90–98.8)	88.1 (80.5–98.4)	91.2 (81.7–90.9)
Group 2			
Low education and income/abuse-neglect history but no environmental neglect	89.6 (82.3–98.5)	87.4 (68.3–98.7)	94.6 (91.8–99.1)
Group 3			
Low education and income/no abuse-neglect history	96.8 (91.1–100)	92.3 (86–99.4)	96.7 (93.4–99.4)
Group 4			
High education and low income/no abuse-neglect history	87.4 (72.9–100)	96.7 (91–100)	90.2 (87.7–92.7)
Group 5			
High education and income/no abuse-neglect history	92.6 (87.1–100)	94 (77.6–100)	97.3 (92.9–100)
Group 6			
Foster families	97.5 (91.4–100)	93.7 (87.5–99.6)	96.6 (92.5–100)

OOO9 and for room, F (2,110) = 31.43, p <.0001. Tukey tests indicated that the Project 12-Ways, Environmental Neglect Group was statistically different from all other groups (p = .05). The mean differences in cleanliness scores for all other groups were not statistically significant. The three rooms were statistically different from one another.

CLEAN scores averaged for all three rooms ranged from 69.16 in the Low Education and Income/Environmental Neglect History group, to 86.70 in the State approved standard: Foster Families group. Mean cleanliness scores in the Low Education and Income/Abuse or Neglect History (but not environmental neglect) group, the Low Education and Income Group/No Abuse or Neglect History group, the High Education/Low Income/No Abuse or Neglect History group and the High Education and Income/No Abuse or Neglect History group were 83.59, 86.43, 84.26, and 86.44, respectively. The ranges in room means were 77.53 (kitchen) to 89.66 (living room).

Figure 4 shows the percentage (cumulative) of families in the Project 12-Ways, Environmental Neglect Group versus all other groups combined whose composite cleanliness score fell at or below points along the cleanliness scale. From this distribution it is evident that the Environment Neglect Group distinguishes itself by lower scores and a greater percentage of families assessed at these lower levels of cleanliness.

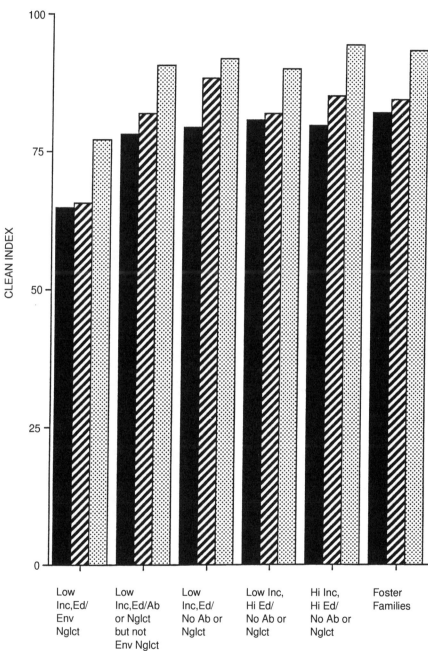

Figure 3. Mean CLEAN scores in each of three rooms in households of families with varied histories of neglect and varied incomes.

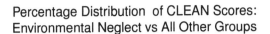

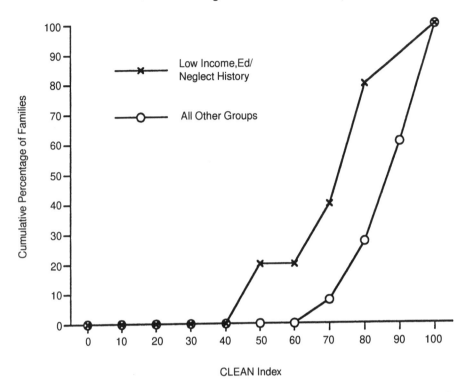

Figure 4. The cumulative percentage of families in each group whose households were assessed at or below the CLEAN index levels specified on the abscissa. The open circles represent households of families, including low income families, with no history of environmental neglect. The ×s represent households of low income families with a history of environmental neglect.

Discussion

The current study provides evidence for the discriminant validity of the CLEAN. That is, CLEAN was sensitive to the differences in cleanliness between homes of families with a history of environmental neglect and all other families from a broad range of educational backgrounds and economic conditions. Importantly, the latter group included families from a low socioeconomic background with a history of child abuse or neglect, but no environmental neglect specifically. This provides some assurance that the CLEAN does not discriminate solely on the basis of poverty (cf. Polansky et al., 1978).

The data confirmed our subjective impression that the households of families with an environmental neglect history had many more unrelated items in unusual locations (e.g., used automotive parts in the kitchen sink), rancid food products throughout the home, accumulated piles of clothing, linen and spent items (such as empty cans, bottles, broken toys, old newspapers) throughout the house. Moreover, these conditions seemed to be detected within a fairly narrow range of the

CLEAN index. That is, cases of severe environmental neglect appear at or below 70. Marginal conditions seemed prevalent at or just above 70.

The norms for the CLEAN serve a purpose comparable to the RDA. Specifically, the continuum of CLEAN scores derived from the homes of families with no history of environmental neglect provides the context for interpreting the results of a CLEAN assessment and making informed decisions in an individual case. That is, without the norms decision makers have no context or framework for interpreting a particular result (e.g., an index score of 60). However, it is evident from Figure 4 that no household in the normative sample scored at or below 60, but 20% of the households of the environmental neglect group did. As with the assessment of nutritional adequacy, our primary use of CLEAN norms and individual CLEAN assessments is to develop interventions to correct the situation. The norms provide the basis for establishing reasonable and achievable goals of such interventions.

FINAL REMARKS

It is not clear whether our efforts to establish quantitative continua for adequate parenting will be widely embraced. The general framework has been unquestionably helpful in our own clinical work and in establishing a credible presence in the child welfare system. We have found, for example, that our assessment of environmental neglect (i.e., CLEAN), interpreted in the context of its norms, is carefully considered in local juvenile court and other forums where decisions are made about the adequacy of parenting.

As mentioned, developing quantitative standards for other aspects of care, such as affection and the ongoing behavioral interactions between parents and children, may prove much more challenging. First, it is doubtful that any current assessment schemes capture the content of parenting outlined in Table 1. Second, if content-valid assessments could be developed, it is questionable whether normative data, gathered in a manner similar to the CLEAN, would provide an appropriate frame of reference for making judgments about parenting adequacy in an individual case. Consider parental affection. It is unlikely that normative data on simply the absolute level of parental affection would be useful without taking into consideration its context and timing. For example, two parents in two different families may deliver comparable levels of affection, but one may do so in a manner which actually reinforces maladaptive behavior of the children. Does this suggest that the behavior of the children should also be reflected in the norms?

Also, can there be valid norms for important parenting interactions given the infinite variety and continual changes in the composition and circumstances of families? For example, can the norms be relevant to a family if a child presents a challenge by virtue of a particular disability or behavior problem? Will this affect the nature of parenting that is minimally expected? Should the number of children in the family be considered in the norms? What about their ages, their genders? What about single- versus two-parent families, extended families, religious practices? If such variables are irrelevant to a judgment of the adequacy of parental affection or other interactions, there is no problem. However, if they are relevant, it is unlikely that their endless permutations can begin to be represented in any normative sample.

Such problems should not discourage research on strategies to develop quantitative frames of reference for assessing and improving the quality of parenting. There may be other tactics for dealing with these factors, some of which we are exploring in current research. In any case, it is important to remember that any empirical derivation of minimum parenting standards will be imperfect. However, if carefully constructed such standards are likely to be preferable to the common practice of judging parenting adequacy on the basis of psychological evaluations or the unsystematic and unreliable accounts of parenting that historically have filled case files and court records.

REFERENCES

Barone, V. J., Greene, B. F., & Lutzker, J. R. (1986). Home safety with families being treated for child abuse and neglect. *Behavior Modification, 10*(1), 93–114.

Eskin, M. (1980). *Child abuse and neglect: A literature review and selected bibliography.* Washington DC: National Institute of Justice.

Giovannoni, J. M., & Recerva, R. M. (1979). *Defining child abuse.* New York: Free Press.

Goldstein, S., Freud, A., Solnit, A. J. (1973). *Beyond the best interests of the child.* New York: Free Press.

Greene, B. F., Norman, K. R., Searle, M. S., Daniels, M., & Lubeck, R. C. (1995). Child abuse and neglect by parents with disabilities: A tale of two families. *Journal of Applied Behavior Analysis, 28,* 417–434.

Illinois Department of Children and Family Services (1985). *Child Welfare Services Practice Handbook.* Springfield, IL.

Illinois Department of Children and Family Services (1994). *Child abuse and neglect statistics: Annual Report—Fiscal Year 1994.* Springfield, IL.

Kadushin, A. (1980). *Child Welfare Services.* New York: Macmillan.

Kempe, C. H., Silverman, F. N., Steele, B., Droegemueller, W., & Silver, H. R. (1962). The battered child syndrome. *Journal of the American Medical Association, 181,* 107–112.

Lutzker, J. R. (1984). Project 12-Ways: Treating child abuse and neglect from an ecobehavioral perspective. In R. F. Dangel & R. A. Polster (Eds.), *Parent training: Foundations of research and practice.* New York: Guilford Press.

Mnookin, R. H. (1985). *In the interest of children.* New York: Freeman.

National Center for Child Abuse and Neglect. (1992, April). National Child Abuse and Neglect Data System, Working Paper 1, 1990 Summary Data. Component. Washington, DC: U.S. Department of Health and Human Services.

National Research Council. (1993). *Understanding child abuse and neglect.* Washington, DC: National Academy Press.

Norman, Patterson, et al. v. Johnson, 739 F. Supp. 1182 (N.D. Ill. 1990).

Patterson, G. R. (1982). *Coercive family processes.* Eugene, OR: Castalia.

Polansky, N. A., Chalmers, M. A., Buttenwieser, E., & Williams, P. (1978). Assessing adequacy of child caring: An urban scale. *Child Welfare,* 439–445.

Schwartz, A., & Hirsh, H. (1982). Child abuse and neglect: A survey of the law. *Medical Trial Technique Quarterly, 28,* 293–334.

Stein, T. J., Gambrill, E. D., & Wiltse, K. T. (1978). *Children in foster homes: Achieving continuity of care.* New York: Praeger.

Taylor, C. G., Norman, D. K., Murphy, J. M., Jellinek, M., Quinn, D., Poitrast, F. G., & Goshko, M. (1991). Diagnosed intellectual and emotional impairment among parents who seriously mistreat their children: Prevalence, type, and outcome in a court sample. *Child Abuse & Neglect, 15,* 389–401.

Tertinger, D. A., Greene, B. F., & Lutzker, J. R. (1984). Home safety: Development and validation of one component of an ecobehavioral treatment program for abused and neglected children. *Journal of Applied Behavior Analysis, 17,* 159–174.

Wahler, R.G. (1969). Oppositional children: A quest for parental reinforcement control. *Journal of Applied Behavior Analysis, 2,* 159–170.

Watson-Perczel, M., Lutzker, J. R., Greene, B. F., & McGimpsey, B. (1988). Assessment and modification of home cleanliness among families adjudicated for child neglect. *Behavior Modification, 12,* 57–81.

Part II

Assessment and Research

A frequent theme in this part is that assessments and research techniques in CAN have made some progress, but that more progress is necessary. For example, in their comprehensive chapter on assessment in CAN, Milner, Murphy, Valle, and Tolliver note that despite the number of assessment techniques currently available CAN, researchers and practitioners have few methods of clearly identifying risk and mitigating factors in CAN. In their chapter, these authors cover interviews, direct observation, personality measures, offender-specific measures, and risk assessments. Their overall conclusion is that risk assessment in the form of the Child Abuse Potential Inventory and direct assessment techniques currently offer the best assessment strattegies in CAN. Unfortunately, a child care worker is the least reliable predictor of further risk.

In his chapter on research, Ammerman reviews the work of the National Research Council and their recommendations about needed research and treatment in CAN. He calls for more work with males and better research designs and program evaluation. The latter problem is often noted by researchers contributing to this book.

Hansen, Warner-Rogers, and Hecht provide a review of factors that make treating CAN families difficult and suggest ways to produce more family cooperation and better treatment outcome. These authors describe the Family Interaction Skills Project (FISP), conducted by Hansen and his colleagues in West Virginia. The FISP is a multifaceted assessment and treatment program for families involved in CAN. Hansen and associates shed light on their successes and failures with FISP, which enabled them to make their recommendations based on their own applied research.

Chapter 7, by Kolko, provides additional insight into the pitfalls of trying to conduct applied research in CAN. As do so many authors in this volume, Kolko laments the overall dearth of good research techniques in the field, but also reviews the good research that is available and makes recommendations for improvements.

Finally, Webster-Stratton, like Hansen and colleagues, uses her own research to demonstrate how to conduct useful research in a related arena: families whose children are at risk for conduct disorder and who display violence. She describes a controlled study in which Head Start families received either the routine Head Start program or Head Start plus the PARTNERS parent training program, a comprehensive program that utilizes a number of features recommended by other contributors in this part for producing successful outcomes and conducting applied research with families. Of particular note in the PARTNERS parent training program were good attendance and very positive consumer validation, features often missing in working with CAN or high-risk families such as these.

Each of the chapters in this part emphasizes the need for continued empiricism in this field and the need to address variables/factors that mitigate against family cooperation in treatment services. Each makes suggestions that would create continued improvement in assessment, research, and treatment in CAN.

4

Assessment Issues in Child Abuse Evaluations

JOEL S. MILNER, WILLIAM D. MURPHY, LINDA A. VALLE, and RANDI M. TOLLIVER

Professionals have used a variety of techniques to evaluate offender characteristics thought to be related to child abuse. Current assessment approaches include the use of interviews, observations, general personality measures, offender-specific measures, and specialized risk assessment models. Offender evaluations are conducted for a variety of reasons, including screening for child abuse risk status, child abuse report confirmation, treatment planning, treatment evaluation, and prediction of reabuse. Unfortunately, as detailed here, supportive psychometric data are frequently lacking on the appropriateness of using available assessment techniques in various evaluation situations. Even when psychometric data exist, information is rarely available on the appropriateness of using different assessment techniques with demographically diverse populations.

Interview and observational techniques are universally used by child protective service providers and health professionals to assess parents. Consequently, this chapter begins with a description of these approaches and associated problems, including interviewer bias. Given the increasing use of general personality measures in child abuse assessment, particularly by psychologists (Straus, 1993), and the relatively recent development of offender-specific measures, this chapter focuses on some of the most frequently used general personality measures and specialized offender assessment techniques. In instances where multifactor scales exist, the review focuses on multifactor scales. In other instances, the review focuses on the measurement of specific constructs by single-factor measures. The review of assessment approaches concludes with a summary of recent work on the development of risk assessment models. In the discussion of each assessment method, when available, reliability and validity data are presented. To the extent

JOEL S. MILNER, LINDA A. VALLE, and RANDI M. TOLLIVER • Department of Psychology, Northern Illinois University, DeKalb, Illinois 60115.   **WILLIAM D. MURPHY** • Department of Psychiatry, University of Tennessee, Memphis, Tennessee 38105.

Handbook of Child Abuse Research and Treatment, edited by Lutzker. Plenum Press, New York, 1998.

possible, data are presented on the correct classification rates of offender status (sensitivity), the correct classification rates of nonoffender status (specificity), the misclassification rates of offender status (false negative classifications), and misclassification rates of nonoffender status (false positive classifications).

INTERVIEWS

Typically, child abuse interview procedures attempt to assess offender characteristics (risk factors) using a question and answer format. Structured interviews are preferred because they tend to generate more reliable data than unstructured interviews. In structured interviews, information is gathered through a planned process, in a systematic effort to ask questions about different domains of interest (i.e., cognitive/affective and behavioral factors). In some cases, structured interviews are very specific and assess individual characteristics, such as depression (Hamilton Rating Scale for Depression, Hamilton, 1986) and how parents view their children (e.g., Altemeier, O'Connor, Vietz, Sandler, & Sherrod, 1982; Kelly, 1983; Murphy, Orkow, & Nicola, 1985).

The validity of the information obtained from a structured interview depends upon a variety of factors (Milner, 1991d). General training in interviewing techniques and specific training in the evaluation of the characteristics of interest (e.g., depression, parental expectations) are needed. The interviewer must establish rapport with the client and must adhere to the recommended interview structure, which at times may be difficult because the interview process is interactive. One criticism of interview procedures is that they frequently have lower levels of reliability and validity than do objective tests. Nevertheless, the interview process has the advantage of allowing for idiographic assessment, in that the interviewer can deviate from the planned format to obtain personality data unique to the individual.

In child abuse assessment, there is a paucity of research on the relative predictive power of specific interviewing procedures in offender evaluations. However, for more than 50 years, evidence has existed indicating that the information gathered and the decisions made in the interview process can be contaminated by interviewer bias (e.g., Rice, 1929). In addition, interactionist theory posits that responses to child abuse case data are socially constructed and are affected by many factors, including the characteristics of the observer (Hawkins & Tiedeman, 1975). As anticipated, research findings suggest that many factors unrelated to the abuse event can impact child abuse evaluations and/or reporting decisions.

For example, personal characteristics of the evaluator/interviewer account for a significant part of the variance in child abuse evaluations. In a national sample, Nuttall and Jackson (1994) found that professionals (i.e., clinical social workers, pediatricians, psychiatrists, and psychologists) who had been sexually and/or physically abused as children were more likely to believe allegations of child sexual abuse. In terms of personal beliefs about the veracity of children's reports of sexual abuse, Kendall-Tackett and Watson (1991) found that professionals who believed that children do not lie about sexual abuse, compared to those who were neutral in their beliefs, were more likely to be convinced that child sexual abuse had occurred. With respect to personal acceptance of corporal punishment, Morris, Johnson, and Clasen (1985) reported that physicians who indicated a high tolerance for physical discipline were less likely to report child physical abuse.

Although data related to the impact of evaluator age on the assessment and reporting of child abuse appear to be highly variable (e.g., Beck, Ogloff, & Corbishley, 1994; Dukes & Kean, 1989; Morris et al., 1985; O'Toole, O'Toole, Webster, & Lucal, 1993), a substantial number of studies indicate that evaluator gender can impact the reaction to and interpretation of interview data. For example, Herzberger and Tennen (1985) reported that females were more likely than males to view harsh discipline as inappropriate. Hazzard and Rupp (1986) reported that women (professionals and students), compared to men, showed stronger emotional reactions (e.g., anger and sympathy) to child physical and sexual abuse. Wellman (1993) reported that female students displayed stronger "pro-social beliefs, attitudes, and emotional reactions to sexual abuse" (p. 539). Kendall-Tackett and Watson (1991) and Jackson and Nuttall (1993) reported that female, relative to male, professionals were more convinced that abuse had occurred when they evaluated vignettes describing possible child sexual abuse. Attias and Goodwin (1985) and Crenshaw, Lichtenberg, and Bartell (1993) reported that female, compared to male, professionals were more likely to report suspected child sexual abuse. In contrast, in a group consisting only of psychologists, Kalichman (1992) failed to find gender differences in attributions of responsibility, confidence that abuse had occurred, and the likelihood of reporting child physical and sexual abuse. Similarly, in a sample of nurses, O'Toole et al. (1993) failed to find gender differences in the recognition of child abuse and the likelihood of reporting child abuse. Thus, although gender effects are frequently reported, gender may selectively interact with other factors, such as professional affiliation, and study results appear to vary based on the type of dependent variable (emotional reaction, likelihood of reporting) under investigation.

Boat and Everson (1988) found that the profession of the evaluator was related to the type of information viewed as important. For example, in evaluating the likelihood of child sexual abuse, physicians, child protection workers, and mental health workers were more convinced by specific indicators (e.g., medical evidence, child's verbal description of abuse) than were law enforcement officers. Kendall-Tackett and Watson (1991) found that when general victim symptoms such as depression, aggression, and fear were present, law enforcement professionals, compared to mental health workers, were more convinced that abuse had occurred. In addition, the legal role assumed by a professional appears to impact their evaluation of case data. For example, Hartman, Karlson, and Hibbard (1994) reported that prosecuting attorneys, compared to defense attorneys, were more likely to evaluate sexual behavior between adults and children as sexual abuse.

The gender of the suspected offender and child victim have been shown to impact child abuse evaluations (e.g., Hampton & Newberger, 1985; O'Toole, Turbett, & Nalepka, 1983). With respect to offender gender, Kalichman (1992) found that fathers suspected of sexual abuse were viewed as more responsible than were fathers suspected of physical abuse. Furthermore, mothers were held more responsible in cases where the father was suspected of physical abuse. Wagner, Aucoin, and Johnson (1993) reported that psychologists attributed more responsibility to the offender when the offender in an adult–child sexual interaction was male. With respect to victim gender, Waterman and Foss-Goodman (1984) reported that sexually abused male children were held more responsible than were female children. Broussard and Wagner (1988) found that male undergraduate students attributed less responsibility to the offender when the sex abuse victim was male. Muller, Caldwell, and Hunter (1993), who asked students to evaluate physically abusive parent–child interactions, found that male children received greater blame than did female children and the victim gender effect was significantly greater when the offender was a male. Similarly, Dukes and Kean (1989) reported that daughters, compared to sons, were seen as more innocent in cases of physical abuse. These studies provide substantial support for the view that males are more likely to be blamed in abuse cases, especially by male evaluators.

Although the research findings indicating that some types of rater and interviewer bias in the evaluation of child abuse case data are relatively robust, evaluation bias does not always correlate in the anticipated manner with outcome events, such as the likelihood of reporting. For example, Dukes and Kean (1989) found that male victims of physical abuse cases were blamed to a greater degree than were female victims. However, the difference in the attribution of blame to male victims was not associated with the degree to which the parents' behavior was evaluated as abusive or with the likelihood that the rater would report the abuse incident. In addition, Horner, Guyer, and Kalter (1993) found that even when clinicians' estimates of likelihood of child sexual abuse by a father were low, the clinicians' recommendations to the court still tended to include limitations of father–child contacts.

What can be done to reduce interviewer bias in the interview process? Kendall-Tackett and Watson (1991) suggested that interviewers should be made aware of possible sources of bias, and such information should be included in interviewer training. Starr (1993) provides an excellent discussion of factors believed to affect the decision-making process. Guided by the work of Bazerman (1990), Starr describes a six-sequence decision-making process that can be used to guide child maltreatment decisions. The six steps include defining the problem, identifying the problem, weighing the criteria, generating solutions, comparing alternatives, and making the optimal decision. Interviewer biases can influence each of these decision-making steps, especially defining and identifying the problem and weighing the criteria. Starr points out that decisions usually are not made rationally, and that rationality is "bounded" because we lack the information necessary to complete each step of the decision-making sequence. He further states that professionals will probably never adhere to the six-step decision-making process and the ideal risk assessment technique will likely never be developed. Nevertheless, Starr believes that an understanding of the possible influences will minimize decision-making biases.

In a study of the decision-making process, Mandel, Lehman, and Yuille (1994) found that when "indeterminate" (ambiguous) child abuse and neglect information was presented in a vignette, almost 40% of a professional group with child maltreatment experience agreed with a decision to remove the child, whereas fewer than 20% strongly disagreed. Following additional analyses to determine the basis for the different professional decisions, Mandel and colleagues concluded that "the fewer unwarranted assumptions . . . professionals made, and the more they generated hypotheses and requested additional information," the less likely they were to agree that the child should be removed from the home (pp.

1058–1059), a decision viewed as appropriate given that the available information was indeterminate. Although the findings suggest topics for evaluator training, this investigation was an analogue study, and the results need to be replicated in field settings for different types of child maltreatment.

OBSERVATIONAL METHODS

Observational methods have been used in natural and laboratory settings. In each setting, observational techniques can be used to assess quantitative or qualitative aspects of the individual. The advantage of these techniques is that they provide direct observations of behavior rather than assessments of individual characteristics (e.g., attitudes and beliefs) assumed to be related to behavior. In natural settings (e.g., home), a parent is observed in daily activities and parent–child interactions. In structured situations, the individual is presented with a contrived situation and is asked to respond. A variety of situations have been used, such as providing an activity that requires parent–child interaction (e.g., parent–child puzzle completion task). The challenge is to develop situations that are realistic and that provide an opportunity to observe the behaviors of interest, such as the parent's disciplinary style. As was the case for interview procedures, observational methods often have modest reliability and validity. Even with rater/observer training and the specification of rating categories, observations depend on the subjective judgment of the rater, which, as previously noted, may be affected by a variety of rater characteristics.

An observational measure that examines primarily qualitative aspects of the parent's behavior (e.g., types of commands given to a child) as part of the parent–child interaction is the Interpersonal Behavior Construct Scale (Kogan, 1972; Kogan & Gordon, 1975). A coding system that examines primarily quantitative aspects of the parent's behavior as part of the analysis of the parent–child interaction is the Dyadic Parent–Child Interactional Coding System (Robinson & Eyberg, 1981). Another observational measure frequently used in child abuse research is the Home Observation for Measurement of the Environment (HOME, Caldwell & Bradley, 1978). About one-third of the HOME items are answered through parental interview and the remaining items are answered on the basis of home observations of the caregiver and the child. Modifying an existing technique, Wolfe, Sandler, and Kaufman (1981) developed a structured home observation of parenting practices measure that was used in a study of abusive parents. In a study of child abuse predictive factors, Rosenberg, Meyers, and Shackleton (1982) used a rating procedure that was completed in a hospital while the parent was observed undressing his or her child. Recently, Tuteur, Ewigman, Peterson, and Hosokawa (1995) used the Maternal Observational Matrix and the Mother–Child Interactional Scale to rate parent behavior (during a task) as abusive or nonabusive.

Although observational methods often show group differences, studies using observational methods to individually classify parents as abusive and nonabusive (e.g., on the basis of the type of parent behaviors observed in parent–child interactions) have yielded mixed results with respect to levels of sensitivity and specificity, ranging from chance to adequate levels (e.g., Deitrich-MacLean & Walden, 1988; Starr, 1987; Tuteur et al., 1995; Walden, Grisaff, & Deitrich-MacLean, 1990).

GENERAL PSYCHOLOGICAL ASSESSMENT

A variety of standardized personality measures have been used to assess child physical and sexual abusers (see Ammerman & Hersen, 1992; Hansen & MacMillan, 1990; Milner, 1991d; Straus, 1993, for reviews). In this section, we first describe some of the standardized measures that have been used to assess child physical abusers. Then, some of the personality measures that have been used to assess child sex offenders are described. In most cases, the different types of assessment devices are only briefly mentioned. However, in cases where substantial published data are available, more detailed discussions and critiques of the more commonly used standardized assessment approaches are provided.

Child Physical Abuse

In the study of child physical abuse, a large number of parent characteristics have been reported to be associated with physically abusive behavior (see Milner & Chilamkurti, 1991; Milner & Dopke, 1997; Starr, 1988, for reviews). Although there has been an increase in the number of adequately designed investigations with demographically matched comparison groups, few studies have demonstrated which factors are marker variables (often referred to as third variables that covary with but do not cause an event) and which are causal factors in child physical abuse. Even fewer data are available on the possible interactive effects of putative contributing and buffering factors. Research has also generally ignored the possibility that parental factors contributing to abuse may vary based on the developmental level of the child because different types of parenting skills are required at different developmental levels. Another problem is that the available studies on parental factors have been conducted primarily on physically abusive mothers.

Examples of abuse-related parent characteristics that have been assessed using standardized questionnaires include: life stress (e.g., Social Readjustment Scale, Holmes & Rahe, 1967), microstressors (e.g., Hassles and Uplifts Scale, Kanner, Coyne, Schaefer, & Lazarus, 1981), loneliness (e.g., the Revised UCLA Loneliness Scale, Russell, Peplau, & Cutrona, 1980), depression (e.g., Beck Depression Inventory, Beck, Ward, Mendelson, Mock, & Erbaugh, 1961), anxiety (e.g., State-Trait Anxiety Scale, Spielberger, Gorsuch, & Lushere, 1970), locus of control (e.g., Locus of Control Scales, Levenson, 1981; Parental Locus of Control Scales, Campis, Lyman, & Prentice-Dunn, 1986), parenting attitudes (e.g., Parent Attitude Research Inventory, Emmerich, 1969; Adult-Adolescent Parenting Inventory, Bavolek, 1984, 1989), conflict resolution techniques (Conflict Tactics Scale, Straus, 1979; Straus & Gelles, 1990) and alcohol use (Michigan Alcoholism Screening Test, Selzer, 1971). In addition, although the majority of physically abusive parents do not suffer from severe psychopathology, the Minnesota Multiphasic Personality Inventory (MMPI), a general measure of psychopathology, has shown some ability to distinguish between groups of child physical abusers and nonabusers (e.g., Gabinet, 1979; Paulson, Afifi, Chaleff, Thomason, & Liu, 1975; Paulson, Afifi, Thomason, & Chaleff, 1974). Although several MMPI profiles have been noted, no single abuser profile has been identified (e.g., Paulson et al., 1974).

Another standardized scale that has a substantial research base and appears to measure an important construct associated with problems in parenting and physically abusive behavior is the Parenting Stress Index (PSI, Abidin, 1995). The 120-item PSI is a self-report measure designed to assess three sources of stress: parent-related stress, child-related stress, and general life stress. The PSI provides a total stress score, a parent domain stress score, a child domain stress score, and a life stress score (which is said to be separate from the parent and child domains). PSI subscale scores (within the parent and child domains) are also available.

Abidin (1995) reported internal consistency estimates of .95, .93, and .89 for the PSI total stress scale, the parent domain scale, and the child domain scale, respectively. Internal consistency estimates for the parent and child domain subscales range from .55 to .80. Various estimates of the PSI temporal stability are available. Abidin (1995) reported 3-week test–retest reliabilities of .71 and .82 for the parent and child domain scores, respectively. For a 3-month interval, test–retest reliabilities of .69, .77, and .88 were reported for the parent, child, and total stress scores. For a 1-year interval, test–retest coefficients of .70, .55, and .65 were reported for the parent, child, and total stress scores, respectively. The internal consistency estimates are more than adequate for clinical use, and the test–retest reliabilities are adequate given that stress levels tend to be variable across time.

Although the PSI was not designed specifically as a child abuse measure, the questionnaire has been used to measure parent- and child-related stress in at-risk for physical abuse and physically abusive parents. For example, PSI scores, especially the Parent Domain Stress scores, correlate with child physical abuse potential (Holden & Banez, 1996; Milner, 1986a). In addition, several studies have reported that at-risk (Abidin, 1995) and physically abusive parents (Abidin, 1995; Mash, Johnston, & Kovitz, 1983), relative to comparison parents, earn higher PSI scores. In the PSI manual, Abidin (1995) cites several studies that indicate that PSI scores have shown pretreatment, posttreatment changes in program evaluation studies conducted with different problem parent groups.

Although the PSI has shown an ability to detect group differences between abusers and nonabusers, data are not available on the PSI individual classification rates (sensitivity and specificity) for child physical abusers and matched nonabusers. Furthermore, Abidin (1995) has indicated that the PSI scale scores are elevated for a variety of nonabusive parent groups experiencing child-related behavior problems. These data suggest that elevated PSI stress scores are not specific to physically abusive parents. Thus, the use of elevated PSI scores to indicate abuse may produce relatively high rates of false positive classification in some nonabusive parent groups.

Child Sexual Abuse

The child sexual abuse literature has described a number of offender and familial factors thought to be associated with the likelihood of child sexual abuse (see Hanson, Lipovsky, & Saunders, 1994; Milner, in press, for reviews). Examples of factors that have been assessed using standardized measures include assertiveness (e.g., Social Response Inventory, Keltner, Marshall, & Marshall, 1981), social anxiety (e.g., Social Avoidance and Distress Scale, Watson & Friend, 1969), self-esteem (e.g., Social Self-Esteem Inventory, Lawson, Marshall, & McGrath, 1979), sexual dysfunction (e.g., Derogatis Sexual Functioning Inventory, Derogatis & Meyer, 1979), sexual interest (e.g., Clarke Sexual History Questionnaire, Paitich,

Langevin, Freeman, Mann, & Handy, 1977), empathy (e.g., Hogan Empathy Scale, Hogan, 1969; Interpersonal Reactivity Index, Davis, 1983; Mehrabian and Epstein Empathy Scale, Mehrabian & Epstein, 1972) and family functioning (Family Environment Scale, Moos & Moos, 1986). Although mean scale score differences between offenders and nonoffenders are often found, substantial group overlap usually exists. In addition, the degree of false positive classifications of the measures is not known because studies often fail to include clinical comparison groups, who may exhibit characteristics (e.g., skill deficits) similar to those of sex offenders.

Initially, assessment of child sex offenders focused on either identifying psychological profiles that would characterize specific types of offenders or attempting to identify the "factor" having etiological significance in the development of deviant sexual behavior. Early studies used projective techniques to assess offenders (Derr, 1978; Hammer, 1955; Pascal & Herzberg, 1954). However, because of problems related to the samples tested and to the lack of standardized administration and scoring procedures, early projective studies added little to our understanding of offenders. Furthermore, due to the continued lack of controlled research supporting the utility of using projective techniques for offender assessment, there has been a shift toward the use of more objective measures. Unfortunately, except for studies using the MMPI, there are relatively few controlled studies on the appropriateness of using standardized instruments to assess the personality of the child sex offender (Levin & Stava, 1987; Murphy & Peters, 1992; Murphy, Rau, & Worley, 1994), and studies have not appeared on the utility of using the MMPI-2.

The use of the MMPI can be viewed as the application of a general psychological instrument (based on a general theory of psychopathology as the cause of sexual assault) to understand child sex offenders. On the surface, the MMPI would appear to offer an objective means of assessing sex offenders. In fact, many studies (Anderson & Kunce, 1979; Armentrout & Hauer, 1978; Erickson, Luxenburg, Walbek, & Seely, 1987; Hall, Maiuro, Vitaliano, & Proctor, 1986; Kalichman, 1991; Quinsey, Arnold, & Pruesse, 1980; Walters, 1987) suggest that sex offenders against children show a group mean MMPI profile consisting of elevations on Scale 4 (Psychopathic Deviance Scale) and Scale 8 (Schizophrenia Scale), with some studies also indicating elevations on Scale 2 (Depression), Scale 9 (Mania), and Scale 6 (Paranoia).

However, previous reviewers (Levin & Stava, 1987; Marshall & Hall, 1995; Murphy et al. 1994) have noted a number of problems with existing MMPI research. One problem is that group mean profiles are not highly reflective of the individual members of the group and thus can be misleading. Hall et al. (1986) reported that although their group of 406 offenders had a mean 4-8 MMPI profile, only 7% of the group actually displayed this profile and 7% of the individuals had normal profiles. In a group of 402 offenders, Erickson et al. (1987) reported that 14% of the group had the 4-8 profile, whereas 20% showed a normal profile. Out of the 45 possible 2-point MMPI codes, 43 2-point codes were observed.

Another problem in interpreting the MMPI literature is that the profiles observed in studies with offenders against children are not specific to this group. For example, Quinsey, Arnold, et al. (1980) found that the 4-8 MMPI profile observed in child sex abusers also occurred among rapists, murderers, arsonists, and property offenders seen in a forensic psychiatric setting. In the MMPI handbook, Dahlstrom, Welsh, and Dahlstrom (1972) also have indicated that a number of prison and psychiatric populations typically display a mean 4-8 MMPI profile.

In addition, MMPI elevation differences are not always found, especially between different types of offenders. For example, in a study of 28 child sex offenders, 35 rapists, and 75 nonsexual criminal comparisons in a military prison setting, Walters (1987) found no differences between child sex offenders and rapists. The only difference between child sex offenders and nonsexual criminals was that child sex offenders had slightly higher scores on Scale 5 (the Masculinity/Femininity scale). Yanagida and Ching (1993) found no differences between child sexual abuse perpetrators, child physical abuse perpetrators, and neglectful parents. There were also no differences between male and female perpetrators.

Child sexual abuse offenders also vary on factors such as level of denial, previous criminal history, relationship with the victim, and victim gender preference. A number of MMPI studies have attempted to investigate these factors. Degree of denial appears to have an impact on the type of MMPI profiles observed. For example, Lanyon and Lutz (1984) found that the typical 4-8 profile was found in offenders who admitted their offense, but normal profiles were found in offenders who denied their offense. Grossman and Cavanaugh (1990) reported that offenders who denied offenses or faced legal charges were more likely to minimize on the MMPI. Wasyliw, Grossman, and Haywood (1994) reported that 10 of 35 admitters exaggerated pathology, whereas only 2 of 37 nonadmitters exaggerated pathology. In an outpatient incest sample, Vaupel and Goeke (1994) compared admitters, nonadmitters, and a comparison group of outpatient psychiatric patients. Fifty-five percent of the admitters showed elevations above a T score of 70 on two or more MMPI scales and 70% of the comparison group showed elevations above 70 on at least two scales, but only 30% of the nonadmitters showed elevations on two or more scales. In addition, the mean profile of the nonadmitters showed no scales above 70, whereas the mean profile of the admitters was a 2-4 profile, and the mean profile of the psychiatric comparison group was a 2-4-8 profile.

In terms of previous criminal history, McCreary (1975) found a 4-8 MMPI profile in offenders with more than one previous criminal charge, whereas normal MMPI profiles were found in offenders with no previous convictions. The 4-8 profile has been found in child rapists and adult rapists, but not in nonviolent child molesters (Panton, 1978). Carroll and Fuller (1971) compared 50 nonviolent prisoners, 50 violent prisoners, and 50 sexual offenders. The sexual offenders differed from the nonviolent offenders on six MMPI scales, but were not different from the violent nonsex offenders. However, information regarding the composition of the sex offender group was not provided.

Evidence supporting the ability of the MMPI to distinguish between incestuous offenders and nonoffenders is mixed. Although some authors have reported elevated profiles (Kalichman, 1991), other authors have failed to find elevated MMPI profiles in incest offenders (Goeke & Boyer, 1993; Scott & Stone, 1986). Further complicating assessment, the degree of offender psychopathology may vary as a function of the nature of the relationship between the offender and victim and the age and gender of the victim (e.g., Groff & Hubble, 1984; Kalichman, 1991; Langevin, Paitich, Freeman, Mann, & Handy, 1978).

Because of the heterogeneity observed in MMPI profiles of offenders, there has been a move away from attempts to establish a single profile toward efforts to develop a range of profiles using cluster analytic methods. A variety of results have been reported. In four studies of outpatient samples, 8 (Duthie & McIvor, 1990), 6 (Kalichman & Henderson, 1991), 5 (Kalichman, Dwyer, Henderson, & Hoffman, 1992), and 10 profiles (Rau, Murphy, Worley, Haynes, & Flanagan, 1993) were identified. In an incarcerated group, 4 profile types were identified (Shealy, Kalichman, Henderson, Szymanowski, & McKee, 1991). Although each study found some reliable differences on various measures used to validate the profiles, the variability in study designs and samples makes it difficult to draw any firm conclusions about the reliability of specific profiles. The cluster analytic studies, however, do support the view that certain MMPI profiles may be associated with certain aspects of offending, such as degree of deviant sexual arousal (Rau et al., 1993), degree of general sexual deviation, and degree of distortions and justifications (Kalichman, Dwyer, et al., 1992; Rau et al., 1993). Unfortunately, existing MMPI profile data do not support the use of the MMPI as a screening device for differentiating child sex offenders from other deviant individuals and/or from general population individuals.

Summary

The review of the literature related to the use of general assessment measures with child physical and sexual abusers indicates that there is no one profile and no single characteristic that has been found consistently in these heterogeneous populations. For existing measures, sensitivity and specificity data are lacking or suggest inadequate classification rates. Nevertheless, the use of general assessment procedures may have some value in treatment planning. For example, extant standardized measures may identify significant areas of dysfunction in the offender and/or the offender's family that are in need of remediation. This application should not be confused with suggestions that these factors have some type of etiological significance or represent characteristics found in all child physical or sexual abusers.

SPECIALIZED OFFENDER ASSESSMENT TECHNIQUES

Two types of specialized assessment approaches have been used to evaluate child physical and sexual abusers: physiological assessments and self-report questionnaires. In this section, studies that have used physiological measures to assess child physical abusers and child sex offenders are reviewed. Then, we review the literature describing the two best known self-report measures that were originally designed for the purpose of screening and assessing physically abusive parents: the Michigan Screening Profile of Parenting (Helfer, Hoffmeister, & Schneider, 1978; Schneider, Helfer, & Pollock, 1972) and the Child Abuse Potential Inventory (Milner, 1986a, 1994). This review is followed by a description of the two most frequently used self-report child sex offender assessment devices: the Abel-Becker Cognition Scale (Abel et al., 1984) and the Multiphasic Sex Inventory (Nichols & Molinder, 1984).

Assessment of Physiological Reactivity

Physiological approaches have been used to assess both child physical and child sexual abusers. More specifically, autonomic nervous system measures, such as measures of heart rate, blood pressure, respiration, and skin conductance, have been used to assess child physical abusers, and measures of sexual arousal (penile tumescence) have been used to assess child sexual abusers. Although the research on the use of physiological measures to assess offenders indicates that these methods may have some utility, the procedures require special laboratory equipment and technical training that are not always available to practitioners. Relatively speaking, there is substantially less use of physiological methodology in the assessment of child physical abusers compared to child sexual abusers.

Child Physical Abuse

Seven studies have examined the psychophysiological reactivity of child physical abusers and at-risk individuals to child-related stimuli (Crowe & Zeskind, 1992; Disbrow, Doerr, & Caulfield, 1977; Friedrich, Tyler, & Clark, 1985; Frodi & Lamb, 1980; Pruitt & Erickson, 1985; Stasiewicz & Lisman, 1989; Wolfe, Fairbank, Kelly, & Bradlyn, 1983). A detailed review and critique of studies that investigated abusive parents is available elsewhere (McCanne & Milner, 1991). An underlying assumption of the studies is that child physical abusers and at-risk parents possess a hyperreactive trait (Knutson, 1978) or are hyperresponsive to child-related stimuli (Bauer & Twentyman, 1985). In the study with the most uniform findings, Frodi and Lamb (1980) reported that child physical abusers, compared to matched comparison parents, showed greater increases in heart rate and skin conductance in response to a crying infant video. Abusive parents were also physiologically reactive to a smiling infant video, whereas comparison parents did not show any change. In addition to the increased reactivity, abusive parents reported higher levels of negative affect in response to the infant videos.

Although the findings of studies on the psychophysiological reactivity of physically abusive and at-risk parents to child-related stimuli are mixed, all but one study (Stasiewicz & Lisman, 1989), which used undergraduate students who were assessed as at-risk for child abuse, have reported greater reactivity in abusive or at-risk individuals on at least some of the physiological measures used. In addition, a study of at-risk mothers' reactions to nonchild-related stressors provides additional support for the view that at-risk parents are hyperreactive. Casanova, Domanic, McCanne, and Milner (1992) examined the physiological reactivity of high- and low-risk mothers to four nonchild-related stimuli (a cold pressor, a film depicting industrial accidents, unsolvable anagrams, and a car horn) and found that high-risk mothers showed greater and more prolonged sympathetic activation to the two most stressful stimuli (i.e., cold pressor and film).

A limitation of studies that have investigated physiological responses to child-related and nonchild-related stimuli is that physically abusive and at-risk parents are assessed in laboratory settings and, even when reliable findings occur, questions of ecological validity remain. Also, data are lacking on the degree to which measures of physiological reactivity can be used to classify individual parents. However, an inspection of study results reveals that the degree of physiological reactivity is highly variable, especially within the physically abusive and at-risk parent groups. High variability on the psychophysiological measures suggests that, on an individual basis, physiological assessment may not adequately classify maltreating parents. In addition, nonabusive parents may show physiological reactivity that is unrelated to child abuse potential, which would result in false positive classifications. The usefulness of combining physiological data with other at-risk factors to classify individual parents as physically abusive and nonabusive needs additional study.

Child Sexual Abuse

As the MMPI is the most frequently studied standardized instrument in the sex offender area, assessment of sexual arousal via direct measurement of penile circumference or volume has been the most frequently investigated sex-offender-specific physiological methodology. Extended discussions of technical issues associated with this methodology, which are beyond the scope of this chapter, can be found elsewhere (e.g., Laws & Osborn, 1983; Murphy & Barbaree, 1994; O'Donohue & Letourneau, 1992). Data related to types of stimuli used in the assessment of sexual arousal can be found in Abel, Blanchard, and Barlow (1981).

In most instances, assessment of male sexual arousal involves the use of a circumferential type transducer, which is rather nonintrusive, to measure changes in penile circumference. Less often, a volumetric device, which encases the penis and is more intrusive, is used to measure total volume change. In assessing child molesters, two types of stimuli tend to be used: slides depicting males and females of various ages and audiotaped descriptions of sexual interactions between adults and children varying according to the level of aggression involved and the type of sexual behavior. At present, there appears to be a reduction in the use of slide stimuli because of ethical concerns regarding the use of slides of children. Although there is some variability across studies, stimuli traditionally are presented for approximately two minutes. Data produced by erectile measures are calculated in several ways, including millimeters of circumference change, percent of full erection, or as ipsative z scores. In addition, especially in classification studies, a deviant (pedophile) index is calculated by taking the ratio of deviant sexual arousal to nondeviant sexual arousal or by creating a difference score between deviant and nondeviant arousal.

Since the early work of Freund (1965, 1967a, 1967b), numerous studies of deviant arousal have demonstrated that extrafamilial child sex offenders can be reliably separated (on a group basis) from nonoffenders (e.g., Baxter, Marshall, Barbaree, Davidson, & Malcolm, 1984; Frenzel & Lang, 1989; Freund, Watson, & Dickey, 1991; Grossman, Cavanaugh, & Haywood, 1992; Lang, Black, Frenzel, & Checkley, 1988; Malcolm, Andrews, & Quinsey, 1993; Marshall, Barbaree, & Butt, 1988; Marshall, Barbaree, & Christophe, 1986; Murphy, Haynes, Stalgaitis, & Flanagan, 1986; Proulx, Cote, & Achille, 1993; Quinsey & Chaplin, 1988a; Quinsey, Chaplin, & Carrigan, 1979; Quinsey, Steinman, Bergersen, & Holmes, 1975). Only two studies failed to replicate these results (Hall, Proctor, & Nelson, 1988; Haywood, Grossman, & Cavanaugh, 1990). In both studies, however, participants showed extremely low levels of arousal, suggesting that individuals may have inhibited their arousal across stimuli. Hall et al. (1988) used participants who were actively involved in a long-term treatment program, and this may have affected the results. In addition, the audiotaped stimuli depicting children were twice as long as the stimuli depicting adults. Inadequate time for arousal to develop to the adult stimuli may have decreased discrimination between offenders and comparisons. Haywood et al. (1990) studied a heterogeneous group of offenders that included intrafamilial and extrafamilial child sex offenders, offenders against both male and female children, and a mixture of admitters and deniers; this may have contributed to the failure to replicate other studies.

The vast majority of studies on deviant arousal indicate that extrafamilial offenders can be discriminated from normals and other offender groups, but the research does not indicate similar discrimination success for incestuous offenders. Although Murphy (1990) and Abel, Becker, Murphy, and Flanagan (1981) found basically no arousal differences between a group of heterosexual incest offenders, a group of nonincestuous heterosexual pedophiles, and a mixed group of sexual deviates (e.g., rapists, voyeurs, homosexual pedophiles), most studies (Barbaree & Marshall, 1989; Grossman et al., 1992; Lang et al., 1988; Marshall et al., 1986; Murphy et al., 1986; Quinsey et al., 1979) report that incestuous offenders tend to respond more like nonoffenders than like extrafamilial sex offenders.

In examinations of aggressive sex offenders, Abel, Becker, et al. (1981) and Avery-Clark and Laws (1984), using a deviance index based on the ratio of arousal to aggressive sexual cues to arousal to nonaggressive sexual cues, were able to separate more aggressive pedophiles from less aggressive pedophiles. For example, Avery-Clark and Laws (1984) were able to correctly classify 92% of aggressive offenders and 70% of less aggressive offenders. Similarly, Marshall et al. (1986) found a positive relationship (.40) between degree of force in the offense and an aggression deviance index. Quinsey and Chaplin (1988a), however, found that a deviance index based on the difference between arousal to consenting adult stimuli and arousal to child coercive stimuli was significantly related to the offender's past history of victim damage, whereas a deviance index based on the difference between arousal to passively resisting child stimuli and arousal to child coercive stimuli was not. In addition, Lang et al. (1988) did not find significance (within groups) when comparing eight aggressive and eight nonaggressive pedophiles. Inspection of the data, however, suggests that the small sample size may have reduced the power of the analyses, as the trends were all in the predicted direction. Marshall et al. (1986), using a ratio of nonaggressive child sexual interactions and adult mutual interactions, found a substantial relationship (.66) with number of victims.

There is also evidence that arousal, primarily based on deviance indexes, is positively related to recidivism (e.g., Barbaree & Marshall, 1988; Malcolm et al., 1993; Quinsey, Chaplin, & Carrigan, 1980; Quinsey & Marshall, 1983; Quinsey, Rice, & Harris, 1995; Rice, Quinsey, & Harris, 1991). The only negative finding to date was reported by Hall et al. (1988). A recent meta-analysis of predictor variables of sex offender recidivism found a significant relationship (.32) between sexual preference for children measured physiologically and recidivism (Hanson & Bussiere, 1995). Albeit modest by some standards, in the prediction of criminal behavior this correlation is a relatively large association. For example, in the same meta-analyses, Hanson and Bussiere reported that recidivism correlated .20 and .14 with prior sexual offenses and prior nonsexual offenses, usually the best predictors of criminal recidivism.

Although group comparisons show reliable separation of extrafamilial offenders from nonoffenders, the ability to classify individuals based on erectile measures is more variable. In most of the classification studies, a deviance index with a specific cutoff score is used to classify individuals as either offenders or nonoffenders. Indices vary across studies, but generally are between .6 and 1.0. Abel, Becker, et al. (1981) and Murphy et al. (1986) report relatively high classification rates, all above 70%, although no normal participants were used. Similarly, Freund and Blanchard (1989) report extremely high classification rates (90%) for admitting offenders. In general, other studies have reported lower rates, ranging from 40% to 53%, of correct classification of child molesters, but in general fairly high rates (80% to 90%) of correct classification of normals (Barbaree & Marshall, 1989; Frenzel & Lang, 1989; Malcolm et al., 1993; Marshall et al., 1986). These studies suggest that many child sexual abusers do not, at least in the laboratory, display deviant sexual arousal patterns.

Barbaree and Marshall (1989) present data shedding light on the heterogeneity of patterns of sexual arousal in child molesters. Barbaree and Marshall found that individual judges could reliably sort arousal responses to slides depicting individuals of various ages into five profiles: an adult profile, a teen–adult profile, a nondiscriminating profile, a child profile, and a child–adult profile. Sixty-eight percent of the nonoffenders displayed the adult profile, and the remainder showed the teen–adult or nondiscriminating profiles. For incest cases, 40% showed an adult profile, 40% showed a nondiscriminating profile, and all but one of the remaining participants showed a teen–adult profile. The remaining incest offender showed a child–adult profile. For the extrafamilial offenders, 35% showed a child profile, and the rest were approximately equally divided among the other categories.

More recent data (e.g., Chaplin, Rice, & Harris, 1995; Harris, Rice, Quinsey, Chaplin, & Earls, 1992) suggest that part of the observed heterogeneity results from using procedures that do not maximize differences between offenders and nonoffenders. In a small group of intrafamilial and extrafamilial offenders against females, Chaplin et al. (1995) used stimuli that varied somewhat from traditional stimuli. Audiotapes, including stories told from the child's point of view and stories detailing significant child suffering, were used. Chaplin and colleagues reported 93% sensitivity and 100% specificity using one index, and 100% sensitivity and 100% specificity using a different index. In a reanalysis of a number of previous data sets, Harris et al. (1992) reported that discrimination between groups was enhanced when z-scores, rather than raw data, were used, when deviance indices were calculated using the differences in arousal between deviant and nondeviant stimuli, when the stimuli depicted brutal sexual coercion, and when pubescent-age stimuli were included in the determination of age preference. The Harris et al. data provide guidelines for improving discrimination.

Although the previous data would appear to provide some support for the use of physiological methods in child sex abuse assessment, there are additional problems. An important limitation is that research participants can intentionally alter responses in the laboratory (Abel, Barlow, Blanchard, & Mavissakalian, 1975; Laws & Holmen, 1978; Quinsey & Bergersen, 1976; Wydra, Marshall, Earls, & Barbaree, 1983). For example, in comparing admitting and nonadmitting offenders, Freund and Blanchard (1989) were able to correctly classify 90% of the admitters, but only 55% of the nonadmitters. Freund and Watson (1991) were able to correctly classify between 44% and 88% of the nonadmitting offenders, with better classification rates coming from offenders with male victims and with multiple victims. However, 14% to 28% of the patients were excluded for either low arousal or clear faking. Hall (1989) measured individuals' ability to inhibit sexual arousal in the laboratory by repeating the stimuli producing the highest level of arousal at the end of the assessment with specific instructions for individuals to inhibit their responses. Individuals who were able to inhibit displayed the lowest levels of arousal during the initial assessment.

Quinsey and Chaplin (1988b) describe a procedure developed to control faking behavior. Normal participants were tested under conditions where they were asked to fake an aggressive sexual interest under a normal testing condition and a condition where a semantic tracking test was employed. The semantic tracking test required participants to press a button on their right when sexual activity occurred and a button on their left when violence occurred. Participants could fake their responding under normal testing conditions, but not under the semantic tracking conditions. Proulx et al. (1993) replicated the study with pedophiles against male victims. In the first of two studies, a semantic tracking test was used with a group having no experience in the laboratory. In this case, the semantic tracking test did not appear to improve results and, in general, the group produced a deviant arousal pattern despite being assessed in a forensic situation. In the second study, including the semantic tracking test improved results with a group having experience in the laboratory. The group appeared to be less able to alter responses under the semantic tracking test. The Proulx et al. (1993) data suggest that as individuals become more familiar with laboratory assessment procedures, they may become more adept at altering physiological responding, thus raising concerns regarding the repeated assessment of arousal as a part of treatment evaluation.

Another limitation to the validity of arousal measures is the limited data on the impact of subject variables on sexual arousal. Data comparing different ethnic or cultural groups are generally lacking, and the primary data appear to be based on European-Americans. In addition, there are few data on the impact of such factors as anxiety and depression or other psychological states on sexual arousal and arousability. Data on socioeconomic status (SES) were presented by Barbaree and Marshall (1989), who found that individuals who displayed more classic child offender sexual arousal profiles were lower in SES than other profile groups. However, using a normal population sample, Murphy, Haynes, Coleman, and Flanagan (1985) found no relationship between arousal measures and income or education.

Finally, there are limited data on the reliability of arousal measures. Wormith (1985) reported a test–retest reliability of .53 for slide stimuli. Although this figure is relatively low, the nature of fluctuation of sexual arousal may make high test–retest reliability difficult to obtain. Quinsey and colleagues report relatively high levels of internal consistency (e.g., Harris et al., 1992), but most investigators do not report the temporal stability or internal consistency of arousal measures.

Researchers in the area of sex offender assessment have focused heavily on assessing sexual arousal. The data suggest that physiological measures do correctly identify offenders (especially extrafamilial child sexual abusers) beyond chance levels, and that sexual interest is related to other aspects of offending behavior, such as violence and recidivism. To date, no alternative approaches have sufficient data associated with them to replace arousal measures. However, as Peters and Murphy (1992) noted, there has been a disturbing trend in the sex offender field toward using arousal measures in criminal trials to show that some-one either fits or does not fit a sex offender profile. As the data related to classifi-cation rates clearly indicate, this is an inappropriate use of arousal measures because many known offenders do not show deviant arousal patterns. Thus, arousal measures cannot be used to state whether someone has or has not engaged in any specific sexual offense. In addition, the limitations related to individuals' ability to fake, lack of data on demographic factors, and limited reliability data, must be recognized.

Assessment Using Self-Report Measures

Child Physical Abuse

Michigan Screening Profile of Parenting (MSPP). The MSPP, which was de-veloped in the early 1970s (Schneider et al., 1972), is a 77-item self-report ques-tionnaire initially designed to screen for child "abuse and/or neglect" (Helfer et al., 1978). The MSPP has historical importance because it was the first published at-tempt to develop an objective screening scale specifically for child abuse. However, the stated purpose of the MSPP has changed since the measure was originally de-veloped. As a result of validity research, which indicated excessive levels of false positive classifications of general population and low-risk parents, the authors have appropriately modified the recommended use of the scale. The MSPP is now rec-ommended for the more general purpose of screening problems in parenting rather than for the specific purpose of child abuse and neglect screening.

The 77 MSPP items are divided into four sections, which ask about the re-spondent's demographic and social history, the respondent's childhood experi-ences and current relationships, the respondent's children, and the respondent's reactions to children (Helfer et al., 1978). The MSPP items assess four factors: Emo-tional Needs Met, Relationship with Parents, Expectations of Children, and Coping. The MSPP scoring is complex and requires computer analysis. According to the manual, the Emotional Needs Met (ENM) factor, which produces the fewest mis-classifications, is scored first to detect parents with problems in parenting. A sec-ond step in scoring involves a procedure called "convergence analysis," which is also used to screen parents as having problems in parenting. Convergence analysis appears to be a measure of inconsistent responding. Although other investigators have found that child physical abusers give inconsistent response patterns on self-report measures (Milner & Robertson, 1989), a problem with using inconsistent re-sponses to classify parents as child abusers is that nonabusive individuals with personal problems also often respond in an inconsistent manner on self-report questionnaires. Thus, using a measure of inconsistent responding to detect physi-cally abusive parents or parents with problems in parenting should be expected to result in high levels of false positive classifications.

Published MSPP classification rates for child physical abusers appear ade-quate; however, research reported by one of the test authors indicates that the MSPP scoring produces relatively high rates of false positive classifications, even in nurturing parent groups. Schneider (1982) reported that the mean MSPP sensitivity rate for six identified problem parent groups was 80%, indicating a 20% false negative classification rate. However, the mean MSPP specificity rate for five non-problem parent groups was 70%, indicating a 30% false positive classification rate for parents identified as low-risk for child abuse. Also important was the unexpected finding that the MSPP classified 60% of a group of general population parents as abusive. Since the MSPP identified the majority of general population parents as abusive, the authors suggested that the scale should be used to identify parents with problems in parenting rather than as a screen for child abuse. The authors have also indicated that the MSPP "is not a predictive instrument" and that it "is not a diagnostic test, and should not be used as such" (Helfer et al., 1978, p. 4).

MSPP construct validity data have been reported. As expected, MSPP scores were found to correlate with levels of family functioning (Siefert, Thompson, Ten-Bensel, & Hunt, 1983). Additional construct validity data has been sought by using the MSPP as a pretest, posttest measure in an effort to show that the scale is sensitive to treatment effects. However, in the two evaluation studies reported by one of the test authors, the MSPP scores increased rather than decreased following treatment (Schneider, 1982). The causes of these unexpected findings remain to be determined. It is not known whether the results were the result of treatment effects (e.g., an increased willingness of participants to admit problems), whether they were related to an inability of the MSPP to detect positive treatment changes, or whether the MSPP is accurately measuring negative treatment outcomes. Because the MSPP does not have a faking-good scale, it is not possible to determine whether the respondents were simply more honest during the posttreatment assessment. However, if participants' desire to distort their responses during the pretreatment assessment affected MSPP scores, this would indicate that the MSPP is susceptible to response distortion.

Child Abuse Potential (CAP) Inventory. The CAP Inventory is a 160-item questionnaire that is widely used as a child physical abuse screening device (Milner, 1986a, 1994). The CAP Inventory contains a physical abuse scale and six factor scales: distress, rigidity, unhappiness, problems with child and self, problems with family, and problems from others. The CAP Inventory also contains three validity scales: a lie scale, a random response scale, and an inconsistency scale. To detect response distortions, the validity scales are used to form three validity indexes: the faking-good index, the faking-bad index, and the random response index. Two special scales have been developed: the ego-strength scale (Milner, 1988) and the loneliness scale (Milner, 1990).

Information on the development, structure, reliability, and validity of the CAP Inventory are provided in a technical manual (Milner, 1986a), and details regarding scale score interpretation are provided in an interpretative manual (Milner, 1990). Reviews of the CAP Inventory are available (e.g., Hart, 1989; Kaufman & Walker, 1986; Melton, 1989). Although the applications and limitations of the CAP Inventory have been frequently discussed (e.g., Caldwell, Bogat, & Davidson, 1988; Melton, 1989; Melton & Limber, 1989; Milner, 1986a, 1986b, 1989b, 1989c, 1991a, 1991c, 1994), users have not always been attentive to the limitations of the CAP Inventory and misapplications have occurred, such as using the physical abuse scale to screen for child sexual abuse (Milner, 1989c).

Internal consistency and temporal stability estimates for the CAP Inventory scales have been reported in the technical manual (Milner, 1986a) and replicated in subsequent studies (e.g., Black et al., 1994; Burrell, Thompson & Sexton, 1992; Caliso & Milner, 1992; De Paul, Arruabarrena, & Milner, 1991; Kirkham, Schinke, Schilling, Meltzer, & Norelius, 1986; Merrill, Hervig, & Milner, 1996; Milner & Robertson, 1990; Pecnik & Ajdukovic, 1995). Split-half reliabilities for the abuse scale range from .96 to .98 and the KR-20 reliabilities range from .92 to .95 for general population ($n = 2,062$), at-risk ($n = 178$), neglectful ($n = 218$), and physically abusive ($n = 152$) groups (Milner, 1986a). Split-half reliabilities for the abuse scale range from .93 to .98 and KR-20 coefficients range from .85 to .96 for different gender, age, education, and ethnic groups (Milner, 1986a). General population test–retest reliabilities for the abuse scale for 1-day ($n = 125$), 1-week ($n = 162$), 1-month ($n = 112$), and 3-month ($n = 150$) intervals are .91, .90, .83, and .75, respectively (Milner, 1986a).

In addition to data indicating that the CAP abuse scale produces the expected group differences between child physical abusers and comparison groups (see Milner, 1986a, 1994 for reviews), individual classification rates have been reported. Initial abuse scale classification rates based on discriminant analysis indicated overall correct classification rates above 90% for physically abusive and matched comparison parents (Milner & Wimberley, 1980). However, in subsequent studies that used more diverse populations of abusive and matched comparison parents, classification rates in the mid-80% to low-90% range have been reported (e.g., Milner, Gold, & Wimberley, 1986; Milner & Robertson, 1989). Although these rates are encouraging, individual classification rates based on discriminant analysis provide the upper limits of correct classification because this procedure determines optimal item weights for each sample tested. To avoid this problem, several studies have determined abuse scale classification rates using the standard weighted item scoring procedure developed for field use (Milner, 1986a).

Before the removal of invalid protocols and using the 215-point cutoff score, Milner (1989a) reported that 73.8% of 110 child physical abusers and 99.1% of 110 matched comparison parents were correctly classified, producing an overall rate of 86.4%. A modestly higher overall rate of 88.5% was observed when the altarnate 166-point cutoff score, which was based on signal-detection theory, was used (Milner, 1986a). For valid protocols, the abuse scale correctly classified 81.4% of the physical abusers and 99.0% of the comparison parents, for an overall rate of 90.2%. Again, slightly higher overall rates of 92.2% were found when the 166-point cutoff score was used.

Using the standard scoring procedure, the 215-point cutoff score, and all protocols, Caliso and Milner (1992) found that the abuse scale correctly classified 87.7%, 73.3%, and 100% of child physical abusers with a childhood history of abuse, nonabusive comparison parents with a childhood history of abuse, and nonabusive comparison parents without a childhood history of abuse. Using the 166-point cutoff score and all protocols, the abuse scale classified 96.7%, 60.0%, and 83.3% of the child physical abusers with a childhood history of abuse, nonabusive comparison parents with a childhood history of abuse, and nonabusive comparison parents without a childhood history of abuse. Caliso and Milner did not report rates for valid protocols. However, Caliso and Milner did report data suggesting that classification rates of the nonabusive comparison parents with a childhood history of abuse might be improved through an examination of the rigidity and unhappiness factor scores as a follow-up to the initial abuse scale screening.

Data on the abuse scale specificity indicate 100% correct classification rates for groups of low-risk mothers (Lamphear, Stets, Whitaker, & Ross, 1985), nurturing mothers (Milner, 1986a, 1989a), and nurturing foster parents (Couron, 1981/1983). In a large sample study (n = 1,151) of the effects of medical stress on the abuse scale specificity, no distortions were found in the classification error rate (chance rate of 5%) in mothers with vaginal and C-section delivery, with and without complications (Milner, 1991b). However, a reduction in the abuse scale specificity (modest increase in error rate from chance) was observed when parents of children with certain types of injury (e.g., severe burns) and illness (e.g., gastric problems) were tested. These data indicate that the abuse scale specificity appears to be affected when a parent presents a child with a medical problem; however, some of the parents with elevated abuse scores may have been undetected cases of child abuse. Although the change in specificity was modest, research is needed on this issue because the abuse scale should discriminate between parents with an injured child who are abusive and those who are not.

Abuse scale classification rates have also been reported for maltreatment groups other than recently identified nontreated physical child abusers. For example, in a combined group of child physical abusers, child neglecters, and a group of comparison parents, Couron (1981/1982) reported an abuse scale classification rate of 72.6%. In addition, Holden, Willis, and Foltz (1989) reported abuse scale classification rates that were far below any other reported rates. When all protocols were used, a correct classification rate of 25% was found for a combined group of physically and sexually abusive parents who were referred from a treatment group. Using only valid protocols, Holden and associates found a classification rate of 28%. Classification data for the subgroup of child physical abusers were not reported. Furthermore, the meaningfulness of these data are difficult to interpret; child physical abusers who have received treatment should not be included in a group to determine concurrent classification rates of the abuse scale because treatment has been shown to lower abuse scores (e.g., Milner, 1986a).

To provide a stringent test of the abuse scale validity, Matthews (1984/1985) studied the abuse classification rates for "mildly" abusive and comparison parents. Moderate and severe physical abusers were excluded, and all comparison parents had children with emotional and behavioral problems. Both abusers and nonabusers were receiving treatment. Using a cutoff score developed from one-half of the study sample, Matthews reported a correct classification rate of 72.7%. Given that only mild abuse cases were included, that the comparison group had children with problems, that both groups were in treatment, and that a local sample cutoff was used, direct comparisons to other concurrent validity studies must be made with caution. However, existing data suggest that when groups other than untreated, recently identified child physical abusers are used, the abuse scale classification rates are lower. In addition, although abuse scores tend to be higher for child physical abusers, compared to other child maltreatment groups, research indicates an overlap in abuse scores across child maltreatment groups (e.g., Milner & Robertson, 1990).

Milner, Gold, Ayoub, and Jacewitz (1984) reported a prospective study in which an at-risk parent group (n = 200) was tested at the beginning of a prevention program and followed to determine subsequent child maltreatment. Forty-two parents were confirmed for later child maltreatment: 11 for physical child abuse, 15 for child neglect, and 16 for their children's failure-to-thrive. A significant relationship (Cramer's V = .34, omega squared = .32) was found between abuse scores and subsequent physical abuse. A significant, though modest, relationship was also found between abuse scores and later neglect. No significant relationship was observed between abuse scores and later occurrence of failure-to-thrive children. Milner and associates pointed out that although all parents who later were abusive earned abuse scores above the cutoff, the majority of parents, who earned elevated abuse scores did not become abusive. Because parents were tested during a pretreatment assessment, some of the parents may have had their abuse risk reduced by treatment (i.e., treatment successes), whereas others did not show change (i.e., treatment failures). Since posttreatment abuse scores were not collected, determining how many of the parents with elevated pretreatment abuse scores were actually treatment successes, instead of failures in abuse scale prediction of subsequent abuse, was not possible.

Extensive construct validity data for the CAP Inventory has been reported. In varying degrees, physiological studies have reported a relationship between elevated abuse scores and physiological reactivity to child-related and nonchild-related stimuli (Casanova et al., 1992; Crowe & Zeskind, 1992; Pruitt & Erickson, 1985). With only one exception (Haskett, Johnson, & Miller, 1994), abuse scores are correlated in the expected manner with the observation and receipt of abuse during childhood (Caliso & Milner, 1992; Crouch, Milner, & Caliso, 1995; Litty, Kowalski, & Minor, 1996; Mee, 1983; Merrill et al., 1996; Miller, Handal, Gilner, & Cross, 1991; Milner & Foody, 1994; Milner, Robertson, & Rogers, 1990). Elevated abuse scores are correlated with social isolation/lack of social support (Burge, 1982; Crouch et al., 1995; De Paul, Milner, & Mugica, 1995; Kirkham et al., 1986; Litty et al., 1996; Matthews, 1984/1985; McCurdy, 1995; Milner et al., 1990; Whissell, Lewko, Carriere, & Radford, 1990), and, with one exception (Kolko, Kazdin, Thomas, & Day, 1993), abuse scores have been correlated with negative family interactions (Arruabarrena & De Paul, 1992; Caliso & Milner, 1992; Lamphear et al., 1985; Mollerstrom, Patchner, & Milner, 1992; Nealer, 1992; Whissell et al., 1990).

Individuals with elevated CAP abuse scores report lower levels of self-esteem and ego-strength (Fulton, Murphy, & Anderson, 1991; McCurdy, 1995; Robertson & Milner, 1985; Robitaille, Jones, Gold, Robertson, & Milner, 1985; Whissell et al., 1990). Those with elevated abuse scores report more life stress and personal distress (Burge, 1982; Holden & Banez, 1996; Holden et al., 1989; Kolko et al., 1993; Mee, 1983; Milner, 1991b; Milner, Charlesworth, Gold, Gold, & Friesen, 1988). Studies have uniformly reported the expected relationship between elevated abuse scores and negative affect (Aragona, 1983; Arruabarrena & De Paul, 1992; De Paul & Rivero, 1992; Holden & Banez, 1996; Kirkham et al., 1986; Kolko et al., 1993; Matthews, 1984/1985; McCurdy, 1995; Milner et al., 1988; Milner, Halsey, & Fultz, 1995; Nealer, 1992; Robertson & Milner, 1985; Robitaille et al., 1985). Associations between drug use and elevated abuse scores have also been reported (Black et al., 1994; McCurdy, 1995; Merrill et al., 1996; Moss, Mezzich, Yao, Gavaler, & Martin, 1995).

With respect to knowledge of child development, one study failed to find the expected relationship (Osborne, Williams, Rappaport, & Tuma, 1986), whereas two studies reported a relationship between elevated abuse scores and lower levels of knowledge (Fulton et al., 1991; Whissell et al., 1990). Studies have reported the expected relationship between elevated abuse scores and negative evaluations of children's behavior (Aragona, 1983; Chilamkurti & Milner, 1993; Kolko et al., 1993) and inappropriate expectations for children's behavior (Chilamkurti & Milner, 1993; Oliva, Moreno, Palacios, & Saldana, 1995). Individuals with elevated abuse scores also make external attributions for their own behavior (Ellis & Milner, 1981; Stringer & La Greca, 1985) and are less likely to change their child-related attributions of responsibility after receiving mitigating information regarding the child's negative behavior (Milner & Foody, 1994). Data are mixed on the degree of relationship between elevated abuse scores and authoritarianism (Robitaille et al., 1985; Whissell et al., 1990) and infant attachment problems (Mee, 1983).

Perhaps most important for a scale that purports to measure abusive parenting, elevated CAP abuse scores have been shown to be related to problems in parent–child interactions (Aragona, 1983; Hann, 1989; Kolko et al., 1993; McCurdy, 1995; Schellenbach, Monroe, & Merluzzi, 1991), and individuals with elevated abuse scores are uniformly reported to use more harsh discipline techniques and less positive parenting practices (Aragona, 1983; Chilamkurti & Milner, 1993; McCurdy, 1995; Milner & Foody, 1994; Monroe & Schellenbach, 1989; Osborne et al., 1986; Schellenbach et al., 1991; Whissell et al., 1990). An interaction between abuse scores and stress also has been reported. As abuse scores increase, stress increases the degree to which parents are rejecting and punishing (Schellenbach et al., 1991).

Finally, the CAP abuse scale has been used successfully to evaluate a variety of secondary and tertiary prevention programs (e.g, Acton & During, 1992; Barth, 1989; Black et al., 1994; D'Agostino, Chapin, & Moore, 1984; Fulton et al., 1991; Mollerstrom, 1993; National Committee for the Prevention of Child Abuse, 1992; Thomasson et al., 1981; Wolfe, Edwards, Manion, & Koverola, 1988). Although the abuse scale appears to have sufficient sensitivity to detect treatment effects, additional information is needed on the relationship between the observed posttreatment and follow-up abuse scores and behavioral outcomes such as subsequent child abuse.

Child Sexual Abuse

In assessing and treating sex offenders, cognitive behavioral models have guided much of the research and many of the treatment approaches. Within this model, cognitive factors, specifically cognitive distortions, have been posited as one important factor that maintains the offender's behavior (Conte, 1985; Murphy, 1990). Cognitive distortions refer to minimizations and justifications that offenders use to excuse their behavior. Examples include such statements as "She didn't say no," "I was drinking," or "It was sex education." The Abel-Becker Cognition Scale (Abel et al., 1984) and the Justifications Scale and the Cognitive Distortion and Immaturity Scale of the Multiphasic Sex Inventory (Nichols & Molinder, 1984) have been used widely in research studies and clinical sites to evaluate cognitive distortions.

Abel-Becker Cognition Scale. The Abel-Becker Cognition Scale (Abel et al., 1984) was the first empirical scale designed to assess the cognitive distortions typically heard from child sexual abusers. The scale consists of 29 items rated from strongly agree to strongly disagree. Primary psychometric data came from a dissertation (Gore, 1988) and a subsequent publication from this dissertation (Abel et al., 1989), which reported an overall scale test–retest reliability over a 1-week to 3-week period of .76. Six factor analytic derived subscales have acceptable internal consistency (alphas = .59 to .84). The overall scale and six subscales differentiated a group of 240 child molesters from a group of 86 normal comparison males. There were no significant differences, however, between child molesters and a group of 48 mixed paraphiliacs. In addition, the mean difference between groups on each of the subscales was small, with substantial overlap between groups, suggesting that sensitivity and specificity rates might not be adequate. Further, Pithers (1990) failed to find any pretreatment differences on the scale between a group of 10 incarcerated child molesters and 10 rapists.

In support of the Abel-Becker Cognition Scale, Stermac and Segal (1989) found that the measure discriminated child molesters from a number of comparison groups including rapists, clinicians, lay persons, lawyers, and police. The amount of group overlap is unknown, however, because no means, standard deviations, or individual classification rates were presented. In another study, Hayashino, Wurtele, and Klebe (1995) found that extrafamilial offenders scored higher on cognitive distortions than did incest offenders, rapists, incarcerated nonsex offenders, and lay persons. Again, individual classification rates were not reported.

Limited data are available on the Abel-Becker Cognition Scale's relationship with other aspects of offending. Abel et al. (1989) reported that the six subscale factors accounted for 24% of the variance in the duration of child molestation and 11 % of the variance in the number of different categories of molestation in which the individual was involved (e.g., male vs. female victims, incest vs. nonincest, child vs. adolescent). The factors did not account for significant variance in the aggressiveness of the offenses or in the number of children molested. As noted by Horley and Quinsey (1994), the items on the scale are relatively obvious and raise concerns about social desirability influences. Although Stermac and Segal (1989) found no significant relationship (.25) between the Abel-Becker Cognition Scale and the Marlow-Crowne Social Desirability Scale, Haywood, Grossman, Kravitz, and Wasyliw (1994) reported significant correlations of .30 and .33 between the Cognition Scale and the F-K index and Obvious-Subtle Index from the MMPI.

The Abel-Becker Cognition Scale appears to have adequate reliability and initial validity data to support the view that the scale can separate offenders from nonoffenders. Data are needed, however, on individual classification rates (sensitivity and specificity) across a variety of offender and nonoffender groups. In addition, data are needed on the cognitive distortions used by incestuous and nonincestuous child sex offenders. For example, incest offenders may use a narrower range of cognitive distortions and, therefore, score lower on this scale than extrafamilial child sex offenders.

Multiphasic Sex Inventory. A second widely used specialized sex offender assessment instrument is the 300-item Multiphasic Sex Inventory (MSI, Nichols & Molinder, 1984). The MSI contains specific paraphilia subscales (child molestation, rape, and exhibitionism) along with subscales measuring sexual obsessions, social/sexual desirability, cognitive distortions and immaturity, justifications, sexual knowledge and beliefs, and sexual inadequacies. Also included are a Lie Scale and a Treatment Attitudes Scale. The MSI Child Molestation Scale measures the extent of child molestation by sampling specific behaviors, whereas the MSI Justifications Scale measures excuses used by the offender. The MSI Cognitive Distortions and Immaturity (CDI) Scale, however, is more complex and has been suggested to measure self-accountability and early childhood cognition. The CDI scale was specifically designed to measure the concept of victim stance, which appears to be a more characterological trait. Inspection of items suggests that although some appear to reflect the concept of victim stance, other items appear to measure denial of sexual feelings or cognitive distortions. This interpretation is supported by a factor analysis. Although the Justifications Scale items loaded on one factor, the CDI items showed moderate loadings on three factors, including a positive loading on a sexual fantasy factor and a dysfunctional/justifications factor and a negative loading on a normal factor (Simkins, Ward, Bowman, & Rinck, 1989).

Overall, the MSI has substantial face validity, is sex offender specific, and taps a variety of areas thought to be important in sex offender treatment. At present, however, psychometric data are limited and most of the available psychometric data are summarized in the test manual (Nichols & Molinder, 1984). Internal consistency of the MSI subscales is adequate (.58 to .92). In addition, the MSI has adequate temporal stability, with most subscale 3-month test–retest reliabilities falling between .8 and .9. Three-month test–retest reliability coefficients for the CDI and Justifications Scales of .71 and .78, respectively, have been reported in a sample of outpatient child molesters (Simkins et al., 1989). Internal consistencies for the CDI, Justifications, and Child Molestation Scales of .53, .82, and .90, respectively, were found in a group containing incarcerated and nonincarcerated child molesters and rapists (Kalichman, Henderson, Shealy, & Dwyer, 1992).

Validity data for the MSI are derived primarily from a comparison of 140 child molesters and 46 college students and a comparison of the 140 child molesters pretreatment to 54 child molesters posttreatment (Nichols & Molinder, 1984). The college student sample was younger than the pedophile sample and the samples may have differed in other ways. Also, it is not clear if the 54 child molesters tested posttreatment were part of the pretreatment group. The majority of MSI subscales separated child molesters from college students and rapists from college students. In addition, a number of subscale scores significantly decreased after treatment, although Nichols and Molinder (1984) have noted that posttreatment scores may increase as offenders become more honest about their past offending behavior.

Simkins (1993) reported significant CDI differences between sexually repressed and nonrepressed sex offenders. Intrafamilial groups also scored lower on the CDI than the extrafamilial or mixed offender groups and offenders with female victims scored lower than those with male victims or victims of both sexes (Simkins et al., 1989). The results on familial relationshp and victim sex, however, may have been confounded because the majority of intrafamilial victims are females. On the Justifications Scale, intrafamilial offenders, extrafamilial offenders, and a mixed group of offenders (with both intrafamilial and extrafamilial victims) did not show significant mean differences. Mean Justifications scores of groups of offenders with either male, female, or both male and female victims also did not differ. Beckett, Beech, Fisher, and Fordham (1994), however, found no differences on offenders' and nonoffenders' scores on either the CDI or Justifications Scale.

Although no data are provided, Beckett and colleagues suggested that extrafamilial, mixed offenders, and offenders with more victims appeared to have higher scores on the CDI.

Two reports by Kalichman (Kalichman, 1990; Kalichman, Szymanowski, McKee, Taylor, & Craig, 1989) found that offenders with the most extreme MMPI elevations had higher scores on the MSI Cognitive Distortions and Paraphilic scales, although rapists were the focus of investigation. Using a variety of offender groups, Kalichman, Henderson, et al. (1992) found associations between MMPI and MSI scales, but they also reported data indicating areas where the MMPI and MSI scales did not overlap. For example, although the CDI scale scores appeared to be related to overall psychopathology, the Justifications Scale scores appeared to be independent of general psychopathology. Kalichman, Henderson, et al. concluded that the MSI provides information beyond that gained from traditional personality assessment.

Evidence suggests the MSI scale scores are related to social desirability. Kalichman, Henderson, et al. (1992) reported significant correlations between the Marlow-Crowne Social Desirability Scale and the CDI, Child Molestation, and Justifications scales of $-.32$, $-.25$, and $-.17$, respectively. Haywood et al. (1994) found significant correlations of .76 and .77 between the CDI scale and the MMPI F-K and Obvious-Subtle indexes, respectively, and significant correlations of .39 and .44 between the Justifications Scale and the MMPI F-K and Obvious-Subtle indices, respectively. Although there were no significant differences between admitters and deniers on the CDI scale, both studies noted that offenders who denied offending scored significantly lower on the Justifications Scale than did offenders who admitted offenses. The Justifications Scale items may be problematic for deniers because the questions basically require the respondent to admit the offense in order to answer the questions. Abusers who are in denial tend to answer "no" to all questions, which may reflect denial of the offense rather than their cognitive processes.

Limited data exist on the relationship between the MSI scales and other components of offending. In a report from the Sex Offender Treatment and Evaluation Program in California (Marques, Nelson, West, & Day, 1994), no relationships were found between sexual recidivism and the CDI or Justifications Scales in a group of 116 offenders, which included both rapists and child molesters. The CDI, however, was marginally associated with new nonsexual violent offenses.

MSI scores appear to have some clinical utility for descriptive purposes, although the limited amount of validity data requires that MSI scores must be interpreted with caution. As the test developers have made clear, the MSI should not be used for screening general populations. In known offender groups, however, the MSI may provide useful information on the degree of offenders' minimization and cognitive distortions, which may be helpful in making treatment decisions.

SPECIALIZED RISK ASSESSMENT MODELS

Traditionally, risk assessment in Child Protective Services (CPS) relied heavily on worker expertise and agency policies and guidelines (Cicchinelli, 1995). In the past 15 years, however, specialized risk assessment models have been developed and implemented in CPS agencies in 42 states (Berkowitz, 1991) to increase the thoroughness and consistency of assessing the likelihood of future child maltreatment (English & Pecora, 1994). The specialized systems, compared to traditional CPS assessment methods, tend to be more systematic and structured in defining the criteria used to determine risk of abuse (Doueck, English, DePanfilis, & Moote, 1993).

Specialized risk assessment models differ from the assessment methods previously reviewed here by including, in addition to assessment of abuser characteristics, various case, child, and demographic variables. For example, demographic and case variables associated in the empirical literature with child physical abuse include low educational level, younger parents, being of female gender, low intelligence, larger families, younger children, and prior history of child abuse (see Milner & Chilamkurti, 1991; Milner & Dopke, 1997, for reviews). Demographic and case predictor variables associated with child sexual abuse include a nonbiological relationship with the victim, use of force in a previous offense, having male victims, prior criminal history, and being of male gender (e.g., Hall, 1988; Hall & Proctor, 1987; Rice, Quinsey, & Harris, 1991). Additional demographic variables associated with various types of child maltreatment include lower SES, unemployment, single marital status, a higher ratio of children to adults, frequent relocation, and short terms of residency (e.g., Coulton, Korbin, Su, & Chow, 1995).

Specialized risk assessment instruments used in different states vary in the way risk is defined (Berkowitz, 1991; Cicchinelli, 1995), in the degree of training provided in the use of the instruments (Cicchinelli, 1990; Pecora, 1991), and in the degree to which the instruments are incorporated into practice (Murphy-Berman, 1994; Pecora, 1991). Instruments also vary in the type and range of information obtained (Cicchinelli, 1990; English & Pecora, 1994; Murphy-Berman, 1994). For example, McDonald and Marks (1991) identified 88 variables assessed across 8 different risk assessment instruments. Variables most commonly assessed include primary caretaker and child characteristics, family characteristics, the nature of the maltreatment incident, and environmental factors (Berkowitz, 1991; Cicchinelli, 1990, 1995; McDonald & Marks, 1991; Palmer, 1990). Models are continually being revised as factors that are determined to be more or less relevant and predictive are added or deleted (Berkowitz, 1991; Doueck, English, et al., 1993). Instruments also differ in how the information is combined and used to guide decision making and risk determination (Cicchinelli, 1990; English & Pecora, 1994; Murphy-Berman, 1994). For example, Likert-type ratings for different risk items may be summed to arrive at a total risk rating, critical risk factors may simply be identified, or regression or path analytic models may be developed (Cicchinelli, 1990). The majority of instruments categorize cases by risk factors perceived to contribute to risk and in need of intervention, as well as by an overall risk level (English & Pecora, 1994).

Pecora (1991) has divided current risk assessment models into four categories. In the first category, matrix models, models are composed of 16 to 35 factors that are generally rated on scales representing low, moderate, and high levels of risk. The factors included are generally associated in the empirical literature with different types of child maltreatment and include parenting skills, child age, and the severity and frequency of maltreatment. The second category consists of empirical prediction models, which are based on public health and juvenile correction risk studies. Empirical prediction models generally are composed of a limited number of risk factors such as parenting skills, demonstrated to be predictive of child maltreatment. The third category of risk assessment models, the Child at Risk Field (CARF), developed by ACTION for Child Protection, rates 14 factors associated with child maltreatment according to perceived level or risk. The CARF is generally considered to be the most comprehensive model due to the breadth of areas assessed and putative applicability with different types of child maltreatment and across the life of a maltreatment case. A final category of risk assessment models consists of family assessment scales (e.g., Child Well-Being Scales, Magura & Moses, 1986), which are primarily used to assess child and family functioning as opposed to identifying risk of abuse.

A review of all the individual risk assessment models in use is beyond the scope of this chapter. However, the CARF system is presented here because a number of psychometric studies have been conducted (e.g., Doueck, Levine, & Bronson, 1993; Evans, Whiteside, & Cohen, 1992). The CARF system is not the most frequently used model. For example, surveys suggest that the CARF system has been implemented in from 4 (Berkowitz, 1991) to 10 states (Costello, 1990), whereas the Illinois Risk Assessment Model (CANTS) or a modified version of the Illinois model has been implemented in 15 states (Berkowitz, 1991). ACTION for Child Protection, however, provides training in the implementation of the CARF and controls modifications to the system across locations (Doueck, Levine, et al., 1993), suggesting that the CARF may be implemented in a more consistent manner and form across sites than are versions of the Illinois model.

The CARF consists of 14 open-ended questions organized around 5 elements (i.e., child, parent, family, maltreatment, and intervention). Information is rated on a risk scale ranging from 0 to 4. As mentioned previously, the CARF was designed to assess risk factors for all types of child maltreatment at various intervals from intake through case closure (Costello, 1990). Specific assessment phases include intake, initial assessment, safety determination, family assessment, case planning, case closure, supervisory review, and documentation of services. Materials used vary with the phase of assessment involved. For example, during intake, information gathered from the 14 questions is compared with a checklist of factors considered to pose a threat to the child, in order to identify the need for immediate intervention by CPS workers. During the initial assessment phase, additional qualifiers are included that measure the duration and pervasiveness of negative influences that may be contributing to risk of maltreatment and caretaker acknowledgement and control of these influences. A final risk score for the initial assessment, ranging from no likelihood to a high likelihood of maltreatment, is derived by combining the average ratings on the 14 risk factors and 4 qualifiers and dividing by two (Costello, 1990).

Information concerning the development of the CARF is provided by Doueck, English, et al. (1993). Group interrater reliability coefficients (Cronbach's Alpha) for the initial assessment risk scores for a nonindicated physical abuse/neglect case of .96 have been reported (Fluke et al., 1994). Interrater reliability coefficients for the elements ranged from .00 to .52. The 6-month assessment risk score coefficient was .98 for the same case, with element coefficients ranging from .00 to .64. For an indicated sexual abuse case, group interrater reliability coefficients for the initial assessment risk score and 6-month assessment risk score were .97 and 1.00, respectively. Interrater reliability coefficients for the elements for the sexual abuse case ranged from .06 to .56 at initial assessment and from .00 to .95 at the 6-month assessment. Internal consistency coefficients (Cronbach's Alpha) of the risk scores for the physical abuse and sexual abuse cases were .57 and .77, respectively, at initial assessment, and .72 and .75, respectively, at the 6-month assessment.

Risk ratings of 30 CPS case workers with hypothetical sexual abuse, physical abuse, and physical neglect cases were reported for a modified version of the initial assessment worksheet of the CARF (Doueck, English, et al., 1993). Internal consistency coefficients for the sexual abuse, physical abuse, and physical neglect cases of .77, .83, and .85, respectively, were reported. Internal consistency coefficients for the safety determination phase of the CARF were described as comparable. Interrater reliability coefficients using the same sample were .85, .76, and .79 for the hypothetical sexual abuse, physical abuse, and physical neglect cases, respectively.

Results of studies examining the validity of the CARF are less supportive. Using an unfounded physical abuse/neglect case and a founded sexual abuse case, Fluke et al. (1994) reported that 62.1% and 82.8% of the caseworkers in their sample ($n = 29$) determined the risk of future abuse or neglect to be very likely following initial assessment for the unfounded and founded cases, respectively. Doueck, Levine, et al. (1993) compared 89 cases evaluated with the CARF with 118 cases evaluated prior to implementation of the CARF over equal periods of time. Cases with higher CARF final risk ratings were more likely to remain open following initial investigation and were provided more services. A trend for cases with higher final risk ratings to have a subsequent report of recurrence was reported. More specifically, subsequent reports of child maltreatment occurred in 5% of the cases rated as low risk. No subsequent maltreatment reports, however, occurred in 72% of the cases rated as high risk using the CARF. Doueck, Levine, et al. noted that the study results may have been affected by the imperfect implementation of the CARF (e.g., completion of forms ranged from 80% to 100%). However, similar results were obtained by Sheets (1992), who reported a significant relationship between risk ratings obtained with the CARF and case decision making, but no relationship between recidivism and CARF initial assessment risk scores, CARF single elements, or CARF combinations of elements. Five CARF elements and two CARF forces derived through discriminant analyses were no better at predicting child maltreatment over a 9-month period than CARF overall risk ratings (Evans et al., 1992).

Despite a relationship between CARF risk ratings and caseworker decisions, two studies (Evans et al., 1992; Fluke et al., 1994) reported no differences between case decision making using the CARF and that using other comparison instruments (both reliable and unreliable). Doueck, Levine, et al. (1993) and Sheets (1996) have suggested that caseworkers may complete risk assessment instruments following an initial interview or later in the assessment process after important case decisions have already been made. The high correspondence between risk ratings and case decision making thus may result from completing the risk assessment instrument to correspond with the caseworker's decisions on substantiation and placement (Doueck, Levine, et al., 1993).

Although limited research has been generated on many specialized risk assessment models, problems with validity, particularly predictive validity, do not appear to be unique to the CARF (English & Pecora, 1994). One source of problems appears to result from the process used to develop many of the instruments. Often large numbers of variables are included that have been associated with maltreatment, in the empirical literature or in clinical experience, and these variables thus have high face validity (Johnson, 1991; Pecora, 1991; Wald & Woolverton, 1990). The variables included in different instruments, however, may have no causal relationships with abuse (i.e., marker variables) or may not be predictive of abuse. For example, Johnson (1991) compared an empirically validated risk assessment model with a face-validated risk assessment model and found the empirically derived model accurately predicted recurrence of abuse in 73.3% of cases, whereas the face-validated model accurately predicted abuse in 59% of the cases ($n = 120$). The face-validated instrument included 14 items, 3 of which were statistically related to reabuse, whereas the empirically derived model contained 5 items, all of which were related to abuse recurrence. At present, only two states (Alaska and Michigan) rely solely on predictive factors to determine risk status (Cicchinelli, 1995).

In addition, items derived from comparisons of maltreating and nonmaltreating parents in the general population may be less predictive of the likelihood of abuse recurrence than when only agency cases are used. The extent to which variables relevant to initial incidents of abuse are related to incidents of reabuse is not known (Pecora, 1991; Wald & Woolverton, 1990). In a similar vein, agencies often use the same model to determine risk for different types of maltreatment (e.g., sexual abuse, physical abuse, neglect). Research (e.g., Baird, 1988; English, Aubin, & Fine, 1993; McDonald, 1991) suggests that different risk factors may be associated with different types of abuse and with cases involving multiple types of child maltreatment. For example, English et al. (1993), using the Washington state risk matrix, found 8 factors associated with physical abuse and 12 factors associated with risk of neglect or combined physical abuse and neglect. Sexual abuse cases were excluded from the analyses.

McDonald (1991) and Murphy-Berman (1994) noted that the higher reliability coefficients reported for some models may result from the inclusion of easily observable and objective data, such as age and gender. As models include a greater proportion of more subjective, unobservable risk variables, such as parenting skills and social isolation, reliability coefficients tend to decline (Murphy-Berman, 1994). Including more objective variables in models may increase reliability; however, the inclusion of demographic variables in risk assessment models may result in increased numbers of false positives. Although demographic or case variables may statistically predict risk status, many variables (e.g., gender, severity of past incident, SES, caretaker's childhood history of abuse) are not responsive to intervention and therefore are useless for treatment planning. In addition, an individual identified as high risk on the basis of demographic and case variables will remain at risk despite intervention, and nonabusive individuals possessing the demographic characteristics will also tend to be classified as high risk. High percentages of false positives contribute to the low classification rates observed in many models. Pecora (1991) noted that correct classification rates for current specialized risk assessment models range from 15% to 83% and that no models have sufficiently high sensitivity and specificity for use as the sole determinant of risk status. The methods used to combine various risk factors in some models also may result in inaccurate estimates of risk by ignoring the intercorrelations and interactions between factors (Murphy-Berman, 1994; Wald & Woolverton, 1990).

A final problem involves the evaluation processes used with specialized risk assessment models. Increasingly, researchers have argued that the criterion measure for evaluating risk assessment instruments should be recurrence of maltreatment (e.g., Johnson, 1994) or risk of future harm to a child (e.g., Weld & Woolverton, 1990). Many instruments, however, are evaluated by comparing risk ratings to substantiation of reports, placement decisions (e.g., Doueck, Levine, et al., 1993), or caseworkers' ratings of risk (e.g., English et al., 1993; Fanshel, Finch, & Grundy, 1994). In a prospective longitudinal study involving 289 child maltreatment cases, however, Johnson (1994) reported a correlation of .00 between the clinical predictions of child welfare workers and recurrence of abuse. As noted previously, bias may affect maltreatment evaluations, report substantiation, and placement decisions. Correlations between these criteria and the risk ratings derived from a risk assessment model, however, are often assumed to be evidence of the model's validity.

CONCLUSIONS

Practitioners often have the need to assess child physical abuse and sexual abuse offenders for purposes of screening, report confirmation, treatment planning, treatment evaluation, and recidivism prediction. The present review of assessment approaches indicates that the amount of literature available to support these uses varies with the measure used and the desired assessment application. As suggested in guidelines developed by Monahan (1993), it is incumbent upon the test user to have adequate clinical and legal education before a child abuse assessment is conducted. This includes a knowledge of "basic concepts of risk assessment (e.g., predictor and criterion variables, true and false positive and negatives, decision rules, and base rates)" and an awareness of the "key findings in risk assessment research" (Monahan, 1993, p. 243), including a knowledge of the psychometric data on the various risk assessment approaches.

Although extant data suggest that some of the general personality measures and specialized child abuse measures may be appropriately used for screening, treatment planning, and program evaluations, other applications are not supported. For example, existing measures do not adequately differentiate subgroups of child abusers. In most cases where sensitivity and specificity data are reported, measures have substantial error rates (excessive false positive and/or false negative classifications). Given the presence of classification errors and the fact that no single offender profile has emerged for child physical or child sexual abuse, data from existing measures should not be used as conclusive evidence of abuse and should not be used in court proceedings as evidence that the individual has or has not abused a child. Ultimately, given that a great variety of assessment techniques and applications is possible, the test user is responsible for determining whether the reliability and validity data are sufficient for a particular application in a specific population (e.g., see guidelines in the Standards for Education and Psychological Testing, American Psychological Association, 1985).

ACKNOWLEDGMENTS

Preparation of this chapter was supported in part by National Institute of Mental Health Grant MH34252 to Joel S. Milner.

REFERENCES

Abel, G. G., Barlow, D. H., Blanchard, E. B., & Mavissakalian, M. (1975). Measurement of sexual arousal in male homosexuals: The effects of instructions and stimulus modality. *Archives of Sexual Behavior, 4,* 623–629.

Abel, G. G., Becker, J. V., Cunningham-Rathner, J., Rouleau, J. L., Kaplan, M., & Reich, J. (1984). *The treatment of child molesters.* Atlanta: Emory University Press.

Abel, G. G., Becker, J. V., Murphy, W. D., & Flanagan, B. (1981). Identifying dangerous child molesters. In R. B. Stuart (Ed.), *Violent behavior: Special learning approaches to prediction, management, and treatment* (pp. 116–137). New York: Brunner/Mazel.

Abel, G. G., Blanchard, E. B., & Barlow, D. H. (1981). Measurement of sexual arousal in several paraphilias: The effects of stimulus modality, instructional set and stimulus content on the objective. *Behaviour Research and Therapy, 19,* 25–33.

Abel, G. G., Gore, D. K., Holland, C. L., Camp, N., Becker, J. V., & Rathner, J. (1989). The measurement of the cognitive distortions of child molesters. *Annals of Sex Research, 2,* 135–152.

Abidin, R. R. (1995). *Parenting Stress Index—Manual* (3rd ed.). Odessa, FL: Psychological Assessment Resources.

Acton, R. G., & During, S. M. (1992). Preliminary results of aggression management training for aggressive parents. *Journal of Interpersonal Violence, 7,* 410–417.

Altemeier, W. A., O'Connor, S., Vietz, P. M., Sandler, H. M., & Sherrod, K. B. (1982). Antecedents of child abuse. *Journal of Pediatrics, 100,* 823–829.

American Psychological Association. (1985). *Standards for educational and psychological testing.* Washington, DC: Author.

Ammerman, R. T., & Hersen, M. (Eds.). (1992). *Assessment of family violence: A clinical and legal sourcebook.* New York: Wiley.

Anderson, W. P., & Kunce, J. T. (1979). Sex offenders: Three personality types. *Journal of Clinical Psychology, 35,* 671–676.

Aragona, J. A. (1983). Physical child abuse: An interactional analysis (Doctoral dissertation, University of South Florida, 1983). *Dissertation Abstracts International, 44,* 1225B.

Armentrout, J. A., & Hauer, A. L. (1978). MMPIs of rapists of adults, rapists of children, and non-rapist sex offenders. *Journal of Clinical Psychology, 34,* 330–332.

Arruabarrena, M. I., & De Paul, J. (1992). Validez convergente de la version espanola preliminar del Child Abuse Potential Inventory: Depresion y ajuste marital. *Child Abuse & Neglect, 16,* 119–126.

Attias, R., & Goodwin, J. (1985). Knowledge and management strategies in incest cases: A survey of physicians, psychologists, and family counselors. *Child Abuse & Neglect, 9,* 527–533.

Avery-Clark, C. A., & Laws, D. R. (1984). Differential erection response patterns of child sexual abusers to stimuli describing activities with children. *Behavior Therapy, 15,* 71–83.

Baird, C. (1988). Development of risk assessment indices for the Alaska Department of Health and Social Services. In T. Tatara (Ed.), *Validation research in CPS risk assessment: Three recent studies* (pp. 85–139). Occasional monograph series of APWA Social R&D Department, 2. Washington, DC: American Public Welfare Association.

Barbaree, H. E., & Marshall, W. L. (1988). Deviant sexual arousal, offense history, and demographic variables as predictors of reoffense among child molesters. *Behavioral Sciences and the Law, 6,* 267–280.

Barbaree, H. E., & Marshall, W. L. (1989). Erectile responses among heterosexual child molesters, father-daughter incest offenders and matched nonoffenders: Five distinct age preference profiles. *Canadian Journal of Behavioral Science, 21,* 70–82.

Barth, R. P. (1989). Evaluation of a task-centered child abuse prevention program. *Children and Youth Services Review, 11,* 117–131.

Bauer, W. D., & Twentyman, C. T. (1985). Abusing, neglectful, and comparison mothers' responses to child-related and non-child-related stressors. *Journal of Consulting and Clinical Psychology, 53,* 335–343.

Bavolek, S. J. (1984). *Adult-Adolescent Parenting Inventory (AAPI).* Eau Clair, WI: Family Development Resources.

Bavolek, S. J. (1989). Assessing and treating high-risk parenting attitudes. In J. T. Pardeck (Ed.), *Child abuse and neglect: Theory, research, and practice* (pp. 97–110). New York: Gordon & Breach.

Baxter, D. J., Marshall, W. L., Barbaree, H. E., Davidson, P. R., & Malcolm, P. B. (1984). Deviant sexual behavior: Differentiating sex offenders by criminal and personal history, psychometric measures, and sexual response. *Criminal Justice and Behavior, 11,* 477–501.

Bazerman, M. H. (1990). *Judgement in managerial decision making* (2nd ed.). New York: Wiley.

Beck, A. T., Ward, C. H., Mendelson, M., Mock, J., & Erbaugh, J. (1961). An inventory for measuring depression. *Archives of General Psychiatry, 4,* 561–571.

Beck, K. A., Ogloff, J. R. P., & Corbishley, A. (1994). Knowledge, compliance, and attitudes of teachers toward mandatory child abuse reporting in British Columbia. *Canadian Journal of Education, 19,* 15–29.

Beckett, R., Beech, A., Fisher, D., & Fordham, A. S. (1994). *Community-based treatment for sex offenders: An evaluation of seven treatment programmes.* (Home Office Occasional Paper). London: Home Office.

Berkowitz, S. (1991, December). *Key findings on definitions of risk to children and uses of risk assessment by state CPS agencies from the state survey component of the study of high risk child abuse and neglect groups.* Paper presented at the National Center on Child Abuse and Neglect Symposium on Risk Assessment, Washington, DC.

Black, M. M., Nair, P., Kight, C., Wachtel, R., Roby, P., & Schuler, M. (1994). Parenting and early development among children of drug-abusing women: Effects of home intervention. *Pediatrics, 94,* 440–448.

Boat, B. W., & Everson, M. D. (1988). Use of anatomical dolls among professionals in sexual abuse evaluations. *Child Abuse & Neglect 12,* 171–179.

Broussard, S. D., & Wagner, W. G. (1988). Child sexual abuse: Who is to blame? *Child Abuse & Neglect, 12,* 563–569.

Burge, E. B. (1982). Child abusive attitudes and life changes in an overseas military environment (Doctoral dissertation, United States International University, 1982). *Dissertation Abstracts International, 43,* 562A.

Burrell, B., Thompson, B., & Sexton, D. (1992). The measurement integrity of data collected using the Child Abuse Potential Inventory. *Educational and Psychological Measurement. 52,* 933–1001.

Caldwell, B. M., & Bradley, R. H. (1978). *Home Observation for Measurement of Environment.* Little Rock: University of Arkansas.

Caldwell, R. A., Bogat, G. A., & Davidson, W. S., II. (1988). The assessment of child abuse potential and the prevention of child abuse and neglect: A policy analysis. *American Journal of Community Psychology, 16,* 609–624.

Caliso, J. A., & Milner, J. S. (1992). Childhood history of abuse and child abuse screening. *Child Abuse & Neglect, 16,* 647–659.

Campis, L. K., Lyman, R. D., & Prentice-Dunn, S. (1986). The Parental Locus of Control Scale: Development and validation. *Journal of Clinical Child Psychology, 19,* 260–267.

Carroll, J. L., & Fuller, G. B. (1971). An MMPI comparison of three groups of criminals. *Journal of Clinical Psychology, 27,* 240–242.

Casanova, G. M., Domanic, J., McCanne, T. R., & Milner, J. S. (1992). Physiological responses to non-child-related stressors in mothers at risk for child abuse. *Child Abuse & Neglect, 16,* 31–44.

Chaplin, T. C., Rice, M. E., & Harris, G. T. (1995). Salient victim suffering and the sexual responses of child molesters. *Journal of Consulting and Clinical Psychology, 63,* 249–255.

Chilamkurti, C., & Milner, J. S. (1993). Perceptions and evaluations of child transgressions and disciplinary techniques in high- and low-risk mothers and their children. *Child Development, 64,* 1801–1814.

Cicchinelli, L. F. (1990). Risk assessment models: CPS agencies and future directions. In *CPS Risk Assessment Conference "From research to practice: Designing the future of child protective services"* (pp. 79–96). Washington, DC: American Public Welfare Association.

Cicchinelli, L. F. (1995). Risk assessment: Expectations and realities. *The APSAC Advisor, 8*(4), 3–8.

Conte, J. R. (1985). Clinical dimensions of adult sexual abuse of children. *Behavioral Sciences and the Law, 3,* 341–354.

Costello, T. (1990). Practice issues: Risk assessment and the CPS worker. In *CPS Risk Assessment Conference "From research to practice: Designing the future of child protective services"* (pp. 97–123). Washington, DC: American Public Welfare Association.

Coulton, C. J., Korbin, J. E., Su, M., & Chow, J. (1995). Community level factors and child maltreatment rates. *Child Development, 66,* 1262–1276.

Couron, B. L. (1982). Assessing parental potentials for child abuse in contrast to nurturing (Doctoral dissertation, United States International University, 1981). *Dissertation Abstracts International, 42*, 3412B.

Crenshaw, W. B., Lichtenberg, J. W., & Bartell, P. A. (1993). Mental health providers and child sexual abuse: A multivariate analysis of the decision to report. *Journal of Child Sexual Abuse, 2*(4), 19–42.

Crouch, J., Milner, J. S., & Caliso, J. A. (1995). Childhood physical abuse, perceived social support, and socio-emotional status in adulthood. *Violence and Victims, 10*, 273–283.

Crowe, H. P., & Zeskind, P. S. (1992). Psychophysiological and perceptual responses to infant cries varying in pitch: Comparison of adults with low and high scores on the Child Abuse Potential Inventory. *Child Abuse & Neglect, 16*, 19–29.

D'Agostino, P. A., Chapin, F., & Moore, J. B. (1984, September). *Rainbow Family Learning Center: Help for parents, haven for children.* Paper presented at the meeting of the Fifth International Congress on Child Abuse and Neglect, Montreal.

Dahlstrom, W. G., Welsh, G. S., & Dahlstrom, L. E. (1972). *An MMPI handbook: Volume 1: Clinical interpretation.* Minneapolis: University of Minnesota Press.

Davis, M. G. (1983). Measuring individual differences in empathy: Evidence for a multidimensional approach. *Journal of Personality and Social Psychology, 44*, 113–126.

Deitrich-MacLean, G., & Walden, T. (1988). Distinguishing teaching interactions of physically abusive from nonabusive parent-child dyads. *Child Abuse & Neglect, 12*, 469–479.

De Paul, J., Arruabarrena, I., & Milner, J. S. (1991). Validation de una version Espanola del Child Abuse Potential Inventory para su uso en Espana. *Child Abuse & Neglect. 15*, 495–504.

De Paul, J., Milner, J. S., & Mugica, F. (1995). Childhood physical abuse, perceived social support, and child abuse potential in a Basque sample. *Child Abuse & Neglect. 19*, 907–920.

De Paul, J., & Rivero, A. (1992). Version Espanola del Inventario Child Abuse Potential: Validez convergente y apoyo social. *Revista de Psicologia General y Aplicada, 45*, 49–54.

Derogatis, L. R., & Meyer, J. K. (1979). A psychological profile of the sexual dysfunctions. *Archives of Sexual Behavior, 8*, 201–223.

Derr, J. (1978). Using the Rorschach inkblot test in the assessment of parents charged with child abuse and neglect. *Projective Psychology, 23*, 29–31.

Disbrow, M. A., Doerr, H. O., & Caulfield, C. (1977). Measuring the components of parents' potential for child abuse and neglect. *Child Abuse & Neglect, 1*, 279–296.

Doueck, H. J., English, D. J., DePanfilis, D., & Moote, G. T. (1993). Decision-making in child protective services: A comparison of selected risk-assessment systems. *Child Welfare, 72*, 441–452.

Doueck, H. J., Levine, M., & Bronson, D. E. (1993). Risk assessment in child protective services: An evaluation of the Child at Risk Field System. *Journal of Interpersonal Violence, 8*, 446–467.

Dukes, R. L., & Kean, R. B. (1989). An experimental study of gender and situation in the perception and reportage of child abuse. *Child Abuse & Neglect, 13*, 351–360.

Duthie, B., & McIvor, D. L. (1990). A new system for cluster-coding child molester MMPI profile types. *Criminal Justice and Behavior 17*, 199–214.

Ellis, R. H., & Milner, J. S. (1981). Child abuse and locus of control. *Psychological Reports, 48*, 507–510.

Emmerich, W. (1969). The parental role: A functional-cognitive approach. *Monographs of the Society for Research in Child Development, 34* (8, Serial No. 132).

English, D. J., Aubin, S. W., & Fine, D. (1993). Evaluation of conformance between individual risk factors and overall level of risk. In T. Tatara (Ed.), *Sixth National Roundtable on CPS Risk Assessment* (pp. 235–260). Washington, DC: American Public Welfare Association.

English, D. J., & Pecora, P. J. (1994). Risk assessment as a practice method in child protective services. *Child Welfare, 73*, 451–473.

Erickson, W. D., Luxenburg, M. G., Walbek, N. H., & Seely, R. K. (1987). Frequency of MMPI two-point code types among sex offenders. *Journal of Consulting and Clinical Psychology, 55*, 566–570.

Evans, J., Whiteside, D., & Cohen, M. (1992). Evaluation results of the pilot of the Child-at-Risk Field. In T. Tatara (Ed.), *Fifth National Roundtable on CPS Risk Assessment* (pp. 37–53). Washington, DC: American Public Welfare Association.

Fanshel, D., Finch, S. J., & Grundy, J. F. (1994). Testing the measurement properties of risk assessment instruments in child protective services. *Child Abuse & Neglect, 12*, 1073–1084.

Fluke, J. D., Wells, S., England, P., Walsh, W., English, D., Johnson, W., Gamble, T., & Woods, L. (1994). Evaluation of the Pennsylvania approach to risk assessment: Summary of the results for project objectives 1, 2, and 4. In T. Tatara (Ed.), *Seventh National Roundtable on CPS Risk Assessment* (pp. 115–170). Washington, DC: American Public Welfare Association.

Frenzel, R. R., & Lang, R. A. (1989). Identifying sexual preferences in intrafamilial and extrafamilial child sexual abusers. *Annals of Sex Research, 2*, 255–275.

Freund, K. (1965). Diagnosing heterosexual pedophilia by means of a test for sexual interest. *Behaviour Research and Therapy, 3*, 229–234.

Freund, K. (1967a). Diagnosing homo- or heterosexuality and erotic age-preference by means of a psychophysiological test. *Behaviour Research and Therapy, 5*, 209–228.

Freund, K. (1967b). Erotic preference in pedophilia. *Behaviour Research and Therapy, 5,*. 339–348.

Freund, K., & Blanchard, R. (1989). Phallometric diagnosis of pedophilia. *Journal of Consulting and Clinical Psychology, 57*, 100–105.

Freund, K, & Watson, R. J. (1991). Assessment of the sensitivity and specificity of a phallometric test: An update of phallometric diagnosis of pedophilia. *Psycholoyical Assessment, 3*, 254–260.

Freund, K., Watson, R. J., & Dickey, R. (1991). Sex offenses against female children perpetrated by men who are not pedophiles *The Journal of Sex Research, 28*, 409–423.

Friedrich, W. N., Tyler, J. D., & Clark, J. A. (1985). Personality and psychophysiological variables in abusive, neglectful, and low-income control mothers. *Journal of Nervous and Mental Disease, 173*, 449–460.

Frodi, A. M., & Lamb, M. E. (1980). Child abusers' responses to infant smiles and cries. *Child Development, 51*, 238–241.

Fulton, A. M., Murphy, K. R., & Anderson, S. L. (1991). Increasing adolescent mothers' knowledge of child development: An intervention program. *Adolescence, 26*, 73–81.

Gabinet, L. (1979). MMPI profiles of high-risk and outpatient mothers. *Child Abuse & Neglect, 3*, 373–379.

Goeke, J. M., & Boyer, M. C. (1993). The failure to construct an MMPI-based incest perpetrator scale. *International Journal of Offender Therapy and Comparative Criminology, 37*, 271–277.

Gore, D. K. (1988). *Cognitive distortions of child molesters and the cognition scale: Reliability. validity, treatment effects, and prediction of recidivism.* Unpublished doctoral dissertation, Georgia State University, Atlanta.

Groff, M. G., & Hubble, L. M. (1984). A comparison of father–daughter and stepfather–stepdaughter incest. *Criminal Justice and Behavior, 11*, 461–475.

Grossman, L. S., & Cavanaugh, J. L. (1990). Psychopathology and denial in alleged sex offenders. *The Journal of Nervous and Mental Diseases, 178*, 739–744.

Grossman, L. S., Cavanaugh, J. L., & Haywood, T. W. (1992). Deviant sexual responsiveness on penile plethysmography using visual stimuli: Alleged child molesters vs. normal control subjects. *The Journal of Nervous and Mental Diseases, 180*, 207–208.

Hall, G. C. N. (1988). Criminal behavior as a function of clinical and actuarial variables in a sexual offender population. *Journal of Consulting and Clinical Psychology, 56*, 773–775.

Hall, G. C. N. (1989). Sexual arousal and arousability in a sexual offender population. *Journal of Abnormal Psychology, 98*, 145–149.

Hall, G. C.. N., Maiuro, R. D., Vitaliano, P. P., & Proctor, W. D. (1986). The utility of the MMPI with men who have sexually assaulted children. *Journal of Consulting and Clinical Psychology, 54*, 493–496.

Hall, G. C. N., & Proctor, W. C. (1987). Criminological predictors of recidivism in a sexual offender population. *Journal of Consulting and Clinical Psychology, 55*, 111–112.

Hall, G. C. N., Proctor, W. C., & Nelson, G. M. (1988). The validity of physiological measures of pedophilic sexual arousal in a sexual offender population. *Journal of Consulting and Clinical Psychology, 56*, 118–122.

Hamilton, M. (1986). The Hamilton Rating Scale for Depression. In N. Sartorius & T. A. Ban (Eds.), *Assessment of depression* (pp. 143–152). Berlin: Springer-Verlag.

Hammer, E. F. (1955). A comparison of H-T-P's of rapists and pedophiles. *Journal of Projective Techniques, 18*, 346–354.

Hampton, R. L., & Newberger, E. H. (1985). Child abuse incidence and reporting by hospitals: Significance of severity, class, and race. *American Journal of Public Health, 75*, 56–60.

Hann, D. M. (1989). A systems conceptualization of the quality of mother–infant interaction. *Infant Behavior and Development, 12*, 251–263.

Hansen, D. J., & MacMillan, V. M. (1990). Behavioral assessment of child-abusive and neglectful families: Recent developments and current issues. *Behavior Modification 14*, 225–278.

Hanson, R. F., Lipovsky, J. A., & Saunders, B. E. (1994). Characteristics of fathers in incest families. *Journal of Interpersonal Violence, 9*, 155–169.

Hanson, R. K., & Bussiere, M. (1995, September). *Predictors of sexual offender recidivism.* Paper presented at the NOTA Conference, Cambridge, England.

Harris, G., T., Rice, M. E., Quinsey, V. L., Chaplin, T. C., & Earls, C. (1992). Maximizing the discriminant validity of phallometric assessment data. *Psychological Assessment, 4*, 502–511.

Hart, A. N. (1989). Review of the Child Abuse Potential Inventory, Form IV. In J. C. Conoley & J. J. Kramer (Eds.). *The tenth mental measurements yearbook* (pp. 152–153). Lincoln, NE: Buros Institute of Mental Measurement.

Hartman, G. L., Karlson, H., & Hibbard, R. A. (1994). Attorney attitudes regarding behaviors associated with child sexual abuse. *Child Abuse & Neglect, 18*, 657–662.

Haskett, M. E., Johnson, C. A., & Miller, J. W. (1994). Individual differences in risk of child abuse by adolescent mothers: Assessment in the perinatal period. *Journal of Child Psychology and Psychiatry and Allied Disciplines, 35*, 461–476.

Hawkins, R., & Tiedeman, G. (1975). *The creation of deviance: Interpersonal and organizational determinants,* Columbus, OH: Merrill.

Hayashino, D. S., Wurtele, S. K., & Klebe, K. J. (1995). Child molesters: An examination of cognitive factors. *Journal of Interpersonal Violence, 10*, 106–116.

Haywood, T. W., Grossman, L. S., & Cavanaugh, J. L. (1990). Subjective versus objective measurements of deviant sexual arousal in clinical evaluations of alleged child molesters. *Psychological Assessment, 2*, 269–275.

Haywood, T. W., Grossman, L. S., Kravitz, H. M., & Wasyliw, O. E. (1994). Profiling psychological distortion in alleged child molesters. *Psychological Reports, 75*, 915–927.

Hazzard, A., & Rupp, G. (1986). A note on the knowledge and attitudes of professional groups toward child abuse. *Journal of Community Psychology, 14*, 219–223.

Helfer, R. E., Hoffmeister, J. K., & Schneider, C. J. (1978). *MSPP: A manual for the use of the Michigan Screening Profile of Parenting.* Boulder, CO: Express Press.

Herzberger, S. D., & Tennen, H. (1985). "Snips and snails and puppy dog tails": Gender of agent, recipient, and observer as determinants of perceptions of discipline. *Sex Roles, 12*, 853–865.

Hogan, R. (1969). Development of an empathy scale. *Journal of Consulting and Clinical Psychology, 33*, 307–316.

Holden, E. W., & Banez, G. A. (1996). Child abuse potential and parenting stress within maltreating families. *Journal of Family Violence, 11*, 1–12.

Holden, E. W., Willis, D. J., & Foltz, L. (1989). Child abuse potential and parenting stress: Relationships in maltreating parents. *Psychological Assessment, 1*, 64–67.

Holmes, T. H., & Rahe, R. H. (1967). The social readjustment scale. *Journal of Psychosomatic Research, 11*, 213–218.

Horley, J., & Quinsey,V. L. (1994). Assessing the cognitions of child molesters: Use of the semantic differential with incarcerated offenders. *The Journal of Sex Research, 31*, 171–178.

Horner, T. M., Guyer, M. J., & Kalter, N. M. (1993). Clinical expertise and the assessment of child sexual abuse. *Journal of the American Academy of Child and Adolescent Psychiatry, 32*, 925–931.

Jackson, H., & Nuttall, R. (1993). Clinician responses to sexual abuse allegations. *Child Abuse & Neglect, 17*, 127–143.

Johnson, W. (1991). Accuracy, efficiency, and research standards for risk assessment systems. In T. Tatara (Ed.), *Fourth National Roundtable on CPS Risk Assessment* (pp. 145–159). Washington, DC: American Public Welfare Association.

Johnson, W. (1994). Maltreatment reference as a criterion for validating risk assessment. In T. Tatara (Ed.), *Seventh National Roundtable on CPS Risk Assessment* (pp. 173–182). Washington, DC: American Public Welfare Association.

Kalichman, S. C. (1990). Affective and personality characteristics of MMPI profile subgroups of incarcerated rapists. *Archives of Sexual Behavior, 19*, 443–459.

Kalichman, S. C. (1991). Psychopathology and personality characteristics of criminal sexual offenders as a function of victim age. *Archives of Sexual Behavior, 20*, 187–197.

Kalichman, S. C. (1992). Clinicians' attributions of responsibility for sexual and physical child abuse: An investigation of case-specific influences. *Journal of Child Sexual Abuse, 1*(2), 33–46.

Kalichman, S. C., Dwyer, M., Henderson, M. C., & Hoffman, L. (1992). Psychological and sexual functioning among outpatient sexual offenders against children: A Minnesota Multiphasic Personality

Inventory (MMPI) cluster analytic study. *Journal of Psychopathology and Behavioral Assessment, 14,* 259–276.

Kalichman, S. C., & Henderson, M. (1991). MMPI profile subtypes of nonincarcerated child molesters: A cross-validation study. *Criminal Justice and Behavior, 18,* 379–396.

Kalichman, S. C., Henderson, M. C., Shealy, L. S., & Dwyer, M. (1992). Psychometric properties of the Multiphasic Sex Inventory in assessing sex offenders. *Criminal Justice and Behavior, 19,* 384–396.

Kalichman, S. C., Szymanowski, D., McKee, J., Taylor, J., & Craig, M. (1989). Cluster analytically derived MMPI profile subgroups of incarcerated adult rapists. *Journal of Clinical Psychology, 45,* 149–155.

Kanner, A. D., Coyne, J. C., Schaefer, C., & Lazarus, R. S. (1981). Comparison of two modes of stress measurement: Daily hassles and uplifts versus major events. *Journal of Behavioral Medicine, 4,* 1–39.

Kaufman, K. L., & Walker, C. E., (1986). The Child Abuse Potential Inventory. In D. J. Keyser & R. C. Sweetland (Eds.), *Test critiques* (Vol. 5, pp. 55–64). Kansas City, MO: Test Corporation of America.

Kelly, J. (1983). *Treating child-abusive families.* New York: Plenum Press.

Keltner, A. A., Marshall, P. G., & Marshall, W. L. (1981). The description of assertiveness in a prison population. *Corrective and Social Psychiatry, 27,* 41–47.

Kendall-Tackett, K. A., & Watson, M. W. (1991). Factors that influence professionals' perceptions of behavioral indicators of child sexual abuse. *Journal of Interpersonal Violence, 6,* 385–395.

Kirkham, M. A., Schinke, S. P., Schilling, R. F., Meltzer, N. J., & Norelius, K. L. (1986). Cognitive-behavioral skills, social supports, and child abuse potential among mothers of handicapped children. *Journal of Family Violence, 1,* 235–245.

Knutson, J. G. (1978). Child abuse as an area of aggression research. *Journal of Pediatric Psychiatry, 3,* 20–27.

Kogan, K. L. (1972). Specificity and stability of mother–child interactional styles. *Child Psychiatry and Human Development, 2,* 160–168.

Kogan, K. L., & Gordon, B. M. (1975). Interpersonal behavior constructs: A revised approach to defining dyadic interactional styles. *Psychological Reports, 36,* 835–846.

Kolko, D. J., Kazdin, A. E., Thomas, A. M., & Day, B. (1993). Heightened child physical abuse potential: Child, parent, and family dysfunction. *Journal of Interpersonal Violence, 8,* 169–192.

Lamphear, V. S., Stets, J. P., Whitaker, P., & Ross, A. O. (1985, August). *Maladjustment in at-risk for physical child abuse and behavior problem children: Differences in family environment and marital discord.* Paper presented at the meeting of the American Psychological Association, Los Angeles.

Lang, R. A., Black, E. L., Frenzel, R. R., & Checkley, K. L. (1988). Aggression and erotic attraction toward children in incestuous and pedophilic men. *Annals of Sex Research, 1,* 417–441.

Langevin, R., Paitich, D., Freeman, R., Mann, K., & Handy, L. (1978). Personality characteristics and sexual anomalies in males. *Canadian Journal of Behavioral Science, 10,* 222–238.

Lanyon, R. I., & Lutz, R. W. (1984). MMPI discrimination of defensive and nondefensive felony sex offenders. *Journal of Consulting and Clinical Psychology, 52,* 841–843.

Laws, D. R., & Holmen, M. L. (1978). Sexual response faking by pedophiles. *Criminal Justice and Behavior, 5,* 343–356.

Laws, D. R., & Osborn, C. A. (1983). How to build and operate a behavioral laboratory to evaluate and treat sexual deviance. In J. G. Greer & I. R. Stuart (Eds.), *The sexual aggressor: Current perspectives on treatment* (pp. 293–335). New York: Van Nostrand Reinhold.

Lawson, J. S., Marshall, W. L., & McGrath, P. (1979). The Social Self-Esteem Inventory. *Education and Psychological Measurement, 39,* 803–811.

Levenson, H. (1981). Differentiating among externality, powerful others and chance. In H. M. Lefcourt (Ed.), *Research with the locus of control construct* (pp. 15–63). New York: Academic Press.

Levin, S. M., & Stava, L. (1987). Personality characteristics of sex offenders: A review. *Archives of Sexual Behavior, 16,* 57–79.

Litty, C. G., Kowalski, R., & Minor, S. (1996). Moderating effects of physical child abuse and perceived social support on potential to abuse. *Child Abuse & Neglect, 20,* 305–314.

Magura, S., & Moses, B. S. (1986). *Outcome measures for child welfare services: Theory and applications.* Washington, DC: Child Welfare League of America.

Malcolm, P. B., Andrews, D. A., & Quinsey, V. L. (1993). Discriminant and predictive validity of phallometrically measured sexual age and gender preference. *Journal of Interpersonal Violence, 8,* 486–501.

Mandel, D. R., Lehman, D. R., & Yuille, J. C. (1994). Should this child be removed from home? Hypothesis generation and information seeking as predictors of case decisions. *Child Abuse & Neglect, 18*, 1051–1062.

Marques, J., Nelson, C., West, M. A., Day, D. M. (1994). The relationship between treatment goals and recidivism among child molesters. *Behaviour Research and Therapy, 32*, 577–588.

Marshall, W. L., Barbaree, H. E., & Butt, J. (1988). Sexual offenders against male children: Sexual preferences. *Behaviour Research and Therapy, 26*, 383–391.

Marshall, W. L., Barbaree, H. E., & Christophe, D. (1986). Sexual offenders against female children: Sexual preferences for age of victims and type of behavior. *Canadian Journal of Behavioral Science, 18*, 424–439.

Marshall, W. L., & Hall, G. C. N. (1995). The value of the MMPI in deciding forensic issues in accused sexual offenders. *Sexual Abuse: A Journal of Research and Treatment, 7*, 205–219.

Mash, E. J., Johnston, C., & Kovitz, K. (1983). A comparison of the mother–child interactions of physically abused and non-abused children during play and task situations. *Journal of Clinical Child Psychology, 12*, 337–346.

Matthews, R. D. (1985). Screening and identification of child abusing parents through self-report inventories (Doctoral dissertation, Florida Institute of Technology, 1984). *Dissertation Abstracts International, 46*, 650B.

McCanne, T. R., & Milner, J. S. (1991). Physiological reactivity of physically abusive and at-risk subjects to child-related stimuli. In J. S. Milner (Ed.), *Neuropsychology of aggression* (pp. 147–166). Norwell, MA: Kluwer Academic.

McCreary, C. P. (1975). Personality differences among child molesters. *Journal of Personality Assessment, 39*, 591–593.

McCurdy, K. (1995). Risk assessment in child abuse prevention programs. *Social Work Research, 19*(2), 77–87.

McDonald, T. P. (1991). Recurrence of maltreatment in relation to assessed risks. In T. Tatara (Ed.), *Fourth National Roundtable on CPS Risk Assessment* (pp. 59–73). Washington, DC: American Public Welfare Association.

McDonald, T, & Marks, J. (1991). A review of risk factors assessed in child protective services. *Social Service Review, 65*, 112–132.

Mee, J. (1983). *The relationship between stress and the potential for child abuse*. Unpublished thesis, Macquarie University, New South Wales, Australia.

Mehrabian, A., & Epstein, N. (1972). A measure of emotional empathy. *Journal of Personality, 40*, 525–543.

Melton, G. B. (1989). Review of the Child Abuse Potential Inventory, Form IV. In J. C. Conoley, & J. J. Kramer (Eds.), *The tenth mental measurements yearbook* (pp. 153–155). Lincoln, NE: Buros Institute of Mental Measurements.

Melton, G. B., & Limber, S. (1989). Psychologists' involvement in cases of child maltreatment: Limits of role and expertise. *American Psychologist, 44*, 1225–1233.

Merrill, L. L., Hervig, L. K., & Milner, J. S. (1996). Childhood parenting experiences, intimate partner conflict resolution, and adult risk for child physical abuse. *Child Abuse & Neglect, 20*, 1049–1065.

Miller, T. R., Handal, P. J., Gilner, F. H., & Cross, J. F. (1991). The relationship of abuse and witnessing violence on the Child Abuse Potential Inventory with Black adolescents. *Journal of Family Violence, 6*, 351–363.

Milner, J. S. (1986a). *The Child Abuse Potential Inventory: Manual* (2nd ed.). Webster, NC: Psytec.

Milner, J. S. (1986b). Assessing child maltreatment: The role of testing. *Journal of Sociology and Social Welfare, 13*, 64–76.

Milner, J. S. (1988). An ego-strength scale for the Child Abuse Potential Inventory. *Journal of Family Violence, 3*, 151–162.

Milner, J. S. (1989a). Additional cross-validation of the Child Abuse Potential Inventory. *Psychological Assessment, 1*, 219–223.

Milner, J. S. (1989b). Applications and limitations of the Child Abuse Potential Inventory. In J. T. Pardeck (Ed.), *Child abuse and neglect: Theory, research and practice* (pp. 83–95). London: Gordon and Breach Science Publishers.

Milner, J. S. (1989c). Applications of the Child Abuse Potential Inventory. *Journal of Clinical Psychology, 45*, 450–454.

Milner, J. S. (1990). *An interpretive manual for the Child Abuse Potential Inventory*. Webster, NC: Psytec.

Milner, J. S. (1991a). Additional issues in child abuse assessment. *American Psychologist, 46,* 80–81.

Milner, J. S. (1991b). Medical conditions and the Child Abuse Potential Inventory specificity. *Psychological Assessment, 3,* 208–212.

Milner, J. S. (1991c). Physical child abuse perpetrator screening and evaluation. *Criminal Justice and Behavior, 18,* 47–63.

Milner, J. S. (1991d). Measuring parental personality characteristics and psychopathology in child maltreatment research. In R. H. Starr & D. A. Wolfe (Eds.), *The effects of child abuse and neglect: Issues and research* (pp. 164–185). New York: Guilford Press.

Milner, J. S. (1994). Assessing physical child abuse risk: The Child Abuse Potential Inventory. *Clinical Psychology Review, 14,* 547–583.

Milner, J. S. (in press). Individual and family characteristics associated with intrafamilial child physical and sexual abuse. In P. K. Trickett & C. Schellenbach, *Violence against children in the family and the community.* Washington, DC: American Psychological Association.

Milner, J. S., Charlesworth, J. R., Gold, R. G., Gold, S. R., & Friesen, M. R. (1988). Convergent validity of the Child Abuse Potential Inventory. *Journal of Clinical Psychology, 44,* 281–285.

Milner, J. S., & Chilamkurti, C. (1991). Physical child abuse perpetrator characteristics: A review of the literature. *Journal of Interpersonal Violence, 6,* 345–366.

Milner, J. S., & Dopke, C. A. (1997). Child physical abuse: Review of offender characteristics. In D. A. Wolfe, R. J. McMahon, & R. deV. Peters (Eds.), *Child abuse: New directions in prevention and treatment across the life span* (pp. 25–52). Thousand Oaks, CA: Sage Publications.

Milner, J. S., & Foody, R. (1994). The impact of mitigating information on attributions for positive and negative child behavior by adults at low- and high-risk for child abusive behavior. *Journal of Social and Clinical Psychology, 13,* 335–351.

Milner, J. S., Gold, R. G., Ayoub, C. A., & Jacewitz, M. M. (1984). Predictive validity of the Child Abuse Potential Inventory. *Journal of Consulting and Clinical Psychology, 52,* 879–884.

Milner, J. S., Gold, R. G., & Wimberley, R. C. (1986). Prediction and explanation of child abuse: Cross-validation of the Child Abuse Potential Inventory. *Journal of Consulting and Clinical Psychology, 54,* 865–866.

Milner, J. S., Halsey, L., & Fultz, J. (1995). Empathic responsiveness and affective reactivity to infant stimuli in high- and low-risk for physical child abuse mothers. *Child Abuse & Neglect, 19,* 767–780.

Milner, J. S., & Robertson, K. R. (1989). Inconsistent response patterns and the prediction of child maltreatment. *Child Abuse & Neglect, 13,* 59–64.

Milner, J. S., & Robertson, K. R. (1990). Comparison of physical child abusers, intrafamilial sexual child abusers, and child neglecters. *Journal of Interpersonal Violence, 5,* 37–48.

Milner, J. S., Robertson, K. R., & Rogers, D. L. (1990). Childhood history of abuse and adult child abuse potential. *Journal of Family Violence, 5,* 15–34.

Milner, J. S., & Wimberley, R. C. (1980). Prediction and explanation of child abuse. *Journal of Clinical Psychology, 36,* 875–884.

Mollerstrom, W. W. (1993, January). *U.S. Air Force Family Advocacy Program research initiative.* Paper presented at the seventh annual meeting of the San Diego Conference on Responding to Child Maltreatment, San Diego.

Mollerstrom, W. W., Patchner, M. A., & Milner, J. S. (1992). Family functioning and child abuse potential. *Journal of Clinical Psychology, 48,* 445–454.

Monahan, J. (1993). Limiting therapist exposure to Tarasoff liability: Guidelines for risk containment. *American Psychologist, 48,* 242–250.

Monroe, L. D., & Schellenbach, C. J. (1989). Relationship of Child Abuse Potential Inventory scores to parental responses: A construct validity study. *Child & Family Behavior Therapy, 11,* 39–58.

Moos, R. H., & Moos, B. S. (1986). *Family Environment Scale manual.* Palo Alto, CA: Consulting Psychologists Press.

Morris, J. L., Johnson, C. F., & Clasen, M. (1985). To report or not report: Physicians' attitudes toward discipline and child abuse. *American Journal of Diseases of Children, 139,* 194–197.

Moss, H. B., Mezzich, A., Yao, J. K., Gavaler, J., & Martin, C. S. (1995). Aggressivity among sons of substance-abusing fathers: Association with psychiatric disorder in the father and son, parental personality, pubertal development, and socioeconomic status. *American Journal of Drug and Alcohol Abuse, 21,* 195–208.

Muller, R. T., Caldwell, R. A., & Hunter, J. E. (1993). Child provocativeness and gender as factors contributing to the blaming of victims of physical child abuse. *Child Abuse & Neglect, 17,* 249–260.

Murphy, S., Orkow, B., & Nicola, R. M. (1985). Prenatal prediction of child abuse and neglect: A prospective study. *Child Abuse & Neglect, 9,* 225–235.

Murphy, W. D. (1990). Assessment and modification of cognitive distortions in sex offenders. In W. L. Marshall, D. R. Laws, & H. E. Barbaree (Eds.), *Handbook of sexual assault: Issues, theories, and treatment of the offender* (pp. 331–342). New York: Plenum Press.

Murphy, W. D., & Barbaree, H. E. (1994). *Assessments of sexual offenders by measures of erectile response: Psychometric properties and decision making,* Brandon, VT: Safer Society Press.

Murphy, W. D., Haynes, M. R., Coleman, E. M., & Flanagan, B. (1985). Sexual responding of 'nonrapists' to aggressive sexual themes: Normative data. *Journal of Psychopathology and Behavioral Assessment, 7,* 37–47.

Murphy, W. D., Haynes, M. R., Stalgaitis, S. J., & Flanagan, B. (1986). Differential sexual responding among four groups of sexual offenders against children. *Journal of Psychopathology and Behavioral Assessment, 8,* 339–353.

Murphy, W. D., & Peters, J. M. (1992). Profiling child sexual abusers: Psychological considerations. *Criminal Justice and Behavior, 19,* 24–37.

Murphy, W. D., Rau, T. J., & Worley, P. J. (1994). The perils and pitfalls of profiling child sex abusers. *APSAC Advisor, 7*(3–4), 28–29.

Murphy-Berman, V. (1994). A conceptual framework for thinking about risk assessment and case management in child protective services. *Child Abuse & Neglect, 18,* 193–201.

National Committee for Prevention of Child Abuse. (1992). *Evaluation of the William Penn Foundation child abuse prevention initiative.* Chicago: Author.

Nealer, J. B. (1992). A multivariate study of intergenerational transmission of child abuse (Doctoral dissertation, Ohio State University, 1992). *Dissertation Abstracts International, 53,* 1848A.

Nichols, H. R., & Molinder, I. (1984). *Multiphasic Sex Inventory.* Tacoma, WA: Authors.

Nuttall, R., & Jackson, H. (1994). Personal history of childhood abuse among clinicians. *Child Abuse & Neglect, 18,* 455–472.

O'Donohue, W., & Letourneau, E. (1992). The psychometric properties of the penile tumescence assessment of child molesters. *Journal of Psychopathology and Behavioral Assessment, 14,* 123–174.

Oliva, A., Moreno, M. C., Palacios, J., & Saldana, D. (1995). Ideas sobre la infancia y predisposicion hacia el maltrato infantil. *Infancia y Aprendizaje, 71,* 111–124.

Osborne, Y. H., Williams, H. S., Rappaport, N. B., & Tuma, J. M. (1986, March). *Potential child abusers: Deficits in childrearing knowledge and parental attitudes.* Paper presented at the meeting of the Southeastern Psychological Association, Atlanta.

O'Toole, A. W., O'Toole, R., Webster, S., & Lucal, B. (1993). Nurses' responses to child abuse: A factorial survey. *Journal of Interpersonal Violence, 9,* 194–206.

O'Toole, R., Turbett, P., & Nalepka, C. (1983). Theories, professional knowledge, and diagnosis of child abuse. In D. Finkelhor, R. J. Gelles, G. T. Hotaling, & M. A. Straus (Eds.), *The dark side of families: Current family violence research* (pp. 349–362). Beverly Hills, CA: Sage.

Paitich, D., Langevin, R., Freeman, R., Mann, K., & Handy, L. (1977). The Clarke SHQ: A clinical sex history questionnaire for males. *Archives of Sexual Behavior, 6,* 421–436.

Palmer, M. (1990). Multi-state analysis of risk assessment systems—Findings and implications for practice. In *CPS Risk Assessment Conference "From research to practice: Designing the future of child protective services"* (pp. 71–78). Washington, DC: American Public Welfare Association.

Panton, J. H. (1978). Personality differences appearing between rapists of adults, rapists of children, and non-violent sexual molesters of female children. *Research Communications in Psychology, Psychiatry, and Behavior, 3,* 385–393.

Pascal, G. R., & Herzberg, F. I. (1954). The detection of deviant sexual practice from performance on the Rorschach test. *Journal of Projective Techniques, 16,* 366–373.

Paulson, M. J., Afifi, A. A., Chaleff, A., Thomason, M. L., & Liu, V. Y. (1975). An MMPI scale for identifying "at-risk" abusive parents. *Journal of Clinical Child Psychology,* 422–24.

Paulson, M. J., Afifi, A. A., Thomason, M. L., & Chaleff, A. (1974). The MMPI: A descriptive measure of psychopathology in abusive parents. *Journal of Clinical Psychology, 30,* 387–390.

Pecnik, N., & Ajdukovic, M. (1995). The Child Abuse Potential Inventory: Cross validation in Croatia. *Psychological Reports, 76,* 979–985.

Pecora, P. J. (1991). Investigating allegations of child maltreatment: The strengths and limitations of current risk assessment systems. *Child and Youth Services, 15,* 73–92.

Peters, J. M., & Murphy, W. D. (1992). Profiling child sexual abusers: Legal considerations. *Criminal Justice and Behavior, 19,* 38–53.

Pithers, W. D. (1990). Relapse prevention with sexual aggressors: A method for maintaining therapeutic gain and enhancing external supervision. In W. L. Marshall, D. R. Laws, & H. E. Barbaree (Eds.), *Handbook of sexual assault: Issues, theories and treatment of the offender* (pp. 343–361). New York: Plenum Press.

Proulx, J., Cote, G., & Achille, P. A. (1993). Prevention of voluntary control of penile response in homosexual pedophiles during phallometric testing. *The Journal of Sex Research, 30,* 140–147.

Pruitt, D. L., & Erickson, M. T. (1985). The Child Abuse Potential Inventory: A study of concurrent validity. *Journal of Clinical Psychology, 41,* 104–111.

Quinsey, V. L., Arnold, L. S., & Pruesse, M. G. (1980). MMPI profiles of men referred for a pretrial psychiatric assessment as a function of offense type. *Journal of Clinical Psychology, 36,* 410–417.

Quinsey, V. L., & Bergersen, S. G. (1976). Instructional control of penile circumference in assessments of sexual preference. *Behavior Therapy, 7,* 489–493.

Quinsey, V. L., & Chaplin, T. C. (1988a). Penile responses of child molesters and normals to descriptions of encounters with children involving sex and violence. *Journal of Interpersonal Violence, 3,* 259–274.

Quinsey, V. L., & Chaplin, T. C. (1988b). Preventing faking in phallometric assessments of sexual preference. In R. A. Prentky & V. L. Quinsey (Eds.), *Human sexual aggression: Current perspectives* (Vol. 528, pp. 49–58). New York: Annals of the New York Academy of Sciences.

Quinsey, V. L., Chaplin, T. C., & Carrigan, W. F. (1979). Sexual preferences among incestuous and nonincestuous child molesters. *Behavior Therapy, 10,* 562–565.

Quinsey, V. L., Chaplin, T. C., & Carrigan, W. F. (1980). Biofeedback and signaled punishment in the modification of inappropriate sexual age preferences. *Behavior Therapy, 11,* 567–576.

Quinsey, V. L., & Marshall, W. L. (1983). Procedures for reducing inappropriate sexual arousal:·An evaluation review. In J. G. Greer & I. R. Stuart (Eds.), *The sexual aggressor: Current perspectives on treatment* (pp. 267–289). New York: Van Nostrand Reinhold.

Quinsey, V. L., Rice, M. E., Harris, G. T. (1995). Actuarial prediction of sexual recidivism. *Journal of Interpersonal Violence, 10,* 85–105.

Quinsey, V. L., Steinman, C. M., Bergersen, S. G., & Holmes, T. F. (1975). Penile circumference, skin conductance, and ranking responses of child molesters and 'normals' to sexual and nonsexual visual stimuli. *Behavior Therapy, 6,* 213–219.

Rau, T. J., Murphy, W. D., Worley, P. J., Haynes, M. R., & Flanagan, B. (1993, November). *History of physical and sexual abuse in adult sexual abusers: Psychometric comparisons*. Paper presented at the 12th Annual Research and Treatment Conference of the Association of the Treatment of Sexual Abusers, Boston.

Rice, M. E., Quinsey, V. L., & Harris, G. T. (1991). Sexual recidivism among child molesters released from a maximum security psychiatric institution. *Journal of Consulting and Clinical Psychology, 59,* 381–386.

Rice, S. A. (1929). Contagious bias in the interview. *American Journal of Sociology, 35,* 420–423.

Robertson, K. R., & Milner, J. S. (1985). Convergent and discriminant validity of the Child Abuse Potential Inventory. *Journal of Personality Assessment, 49,* 86–88.

Robinson, E. A., & Eyberg, S. M. (1981). The dyadic parent-child interactional coding system: Standardization and validation. *Journal of Consulting and Clinical Psychology, 49,* 245–250.

Robitaille, J., Jones, E., Gold, R. G., Robertson, K. R., & Miner, J. S. (1985). Child abuse potential and authoritarianism. *Journal of Clinical Psychology, 41,* 839–843.

Rosenberg, N. M., Meyers, S., & Shackleton, N. (1982). The Revised UCLA Loneliness Scale: Concurrent and discriminant validity evidence. *Journal of Personality and Social Psychology, 39,* 472–480.

Russell, D., Peplau, L. A., & Cutrona, C. E. (1980). The Revised UCLA Loneliness Scale: Concurrent and discriminant validity evidence. *Journal of Personality and Social Psychology, 39,* 472–480.

Schellenbach, C. J., Monroe, L. D., & Merluzzi, T. V. (1991). The impact of stress on cognitive components of child abuse potential. *Journal of Family Violence, 6,* 61–80.

Schneider, C. J. (1982). The Michigan Screening Profile of Parenting. In R. H. Starr, Jr. (Ed.), *Child abuse prevention: Policy implications* (pp. 157–174). Cambridge, MA: Ballinger.

Schneider, C. J., Helfer, R. E., & Pollock, C. (1972). The predictive questionnaire: A preliminary report. In C. H. Kempe & R. E. Helfer (Eds.), *Helping the battered child and his family* (pp. 271–282). Philadelphia: Lippincott.

Scott, R. L., & Stone, D. A. (1986). MMPI profile constellations in incest families. *Journal of Consulting and Clinical Psychology, 54,* 364–368.

Selzer, M. L. (1971). The Michigan Alcoholism Screening Test: The quest for a new diagnostic instrument. *American Journal of Psychiatry, 127,* 89–94.

Shealy, L., Kalichman, S. C., Henderson, M. C., Szymanowski, D., & McKee, G. (1991). MMPI profile subtypes of incarcerated sex offenders against children. *Violence and Victims, 6,* 201–212.

Sheets, D. A. (1992). Implications of research for the designs and implementation of the Texas Risk Assessment Model. In T. Tatara (Ed.), *Fifth National Roundtable on CPS Risk Assessment* (pp. 169–186). Washington, DC: American Public Welfare Association.

Sheets, D. A. (1996). Caseworkers, computers, and risk assessment: A promising partnership. *APSAC Advisor, 9*(1), 7–12.

Siefert, K., Thompson, T., Ten-Bensel, R. W., & Hunt, C. (1983). Perinatal stress: A study of factors linked to the risk of parent problems. *Health and Social Work, 8,* 107–121.

Simkins, L. (1993). Characteristics of sexually repressed child molesters. *Journal of Interpersonal Violence, 8,* 3–17.

Simkins, L., Ward, W., Bowman, S., & Rinck, C. M. (1989). The Multiphasic Sex Inventory as a predictor of treatment response in child sexual abusers. *Annals of Sex Research, 2,* 205–226.

Spielberger, C. D., Gorsuch, R., & Lushere, R. (1970). *Manual for the State-Trait Anxiety Scale.* Palo Alto, CA: Consulting Psychologists Press.

Starr, R. H. Jr. (1987). Clinical judgement of abuse-proneness based on parent–child interactions. *Child Abuse & Neglect, 11,* 87–92.

Starr, R. H., Jr. (1988). Physical abuse of children. In in. B. Van Hasselt, R. L. Morrison, & A. S. Bellack (Eds.), *Handbook of family violence* (pp. 119–155). New York: Plenum Press.

Starr, R. H., Jr. (1993). Cognitive factors underlying worker decision bias. In T. Tatara (Ed.), *Sixth national roundtable on CPS risk assessment: Summary of highlights* (pp. 195–212). Washington: American Public Welfare Association.

Stasiewicz, P. R., & Lisman, S. A. (1989). Effects of infant cries on alcohol consumption in college males at risk for child abuse. *Child Abuse & Neglect, 13,* 463–470.

Stermac, L. E., & Segal, Z. V. (1989). Adult sexual contact with children: An examination of cognitive factors. *Behavior Therapy, 20,* 573–584.

Straus, M. A. (1979). Measuring intrafamilial conflict and violence: The Conflict Tactics (CT) Scale. *Journal of Marriage and the Family, 41,* 75–88.

Straus, M. A. (1993). *Measurement instruments in child abuse research.* Unpublished manuscript, University of New Hampshire, Durham.

Straus, M. A., & Gelles, R. J. (Eds.). (1990). *Physical violence in American families.* New Brunswick, NJ: Transaction.

Stringer, S. A., & La Greca, A. M. (1985). Correlates of child abuse potential. *Journal of Abnormal Child Psychology, 13,* 217–226.

Thomasson, E., Berkovitz, T., Minor, S., Cassle, G., McCord, D., & Miner, J. S. (1981). Evaluation of a family life education program for rural "high risk" families: A research note. *Journal of Community Psychology, 9,* 246–249.

Tuteur, J. M., Ewigman, B. E., Peterson, L., Hosokawa, M. C. (1995). The Maternal Observation Matrix and the Mother-Child Interactional Scale: Brief observational screening instruments for physically abusive mothers. *Journal of Clinical Child Psychology, 24,* 55–66.

Vaupel, S. G., & Goeke, J. M. (1994). Incest perpetrator MMPI profiles and the variable of offense admission status. *International Journal of Offender Therapy and Comparative Criminology, 38,* 69–77.

Wagner, W. G., Aucoin, R., & Johnson, J. T. (1993). Psychologists' attitudes concerning child sexual abuse: The impact of sex of perpetrator, sex of victim, age of victim, and victim response. *Journal of Child Sexual Abuse, 2*(2), 61–74.

Wald, M. S., & Woolverton, M. (1990). Risk assessment: The emperor's new clothes? *Child Welfare, 69,* 483–511.

Walden, T. A., Grisaff, D., & Deitrich-MacLean, G. (1990). Observing interactions of abusive and nonabusive dyads: Information extracted by accurate and inaccurate judges. *Journal of Abnormal Child Psychology, 18,* 241–254.

Walters, G. D. (1987). Child sex offenders and rapists in a military prison setting. *International Journal of Offender Therapy and Comparative Criminology, 31,* 261–269.

Wasyliw, O. E., Grossman, L. S., & Haywood, T. W. (1994). Denial of hostility and psychopathology among alleged child molesters. *Journal of Personality Assessment, 63,* 185–190.

Waterman, C. K., & Foss-Goodman, D. (1984). Child molesting: Variables relating to attribution of fault to victims, offenders, and nonparticipating parents. *Journal of Sex Research, 20,* 329–349.

Watson, D., & Friend, R. (1969). Measurement of social-evaluation anxiety. *Journal of Consulting and Clinical Psychology, 33,* 448–457.

Wellman, M. M. (1993). Child sexual abuse and gender differences: Attitudes and prevalence. *Child Abuse & Neglect, 17,* 539–547.

Whissell, C., Lewko, J., Carriere, R., & Radford, J. (1990). Test scores and sociodemographic information as predictors of child abuse potential scores in young female adults. *Journal of Social Behavior and Personality, 5,* 199–208.

Wolfe, D. A., Edwards, B., Manion, I., & Koverola, C. (1988). Early interventions for parents at risk for child abuse and neglect: A preliminary investigation. *Journal of Consulting and Clinical Psychology, 56,* 40–47.

Wolfe, D.A., Fairbank, J. A., Kelly, J. A., & Bradlyn, A. S. (1983). Child abusive parents' physiological responses to stressful and nonstressful behavior in children. *Behavioral Assessment, 5,* 363–371.

Wolfe, D. A., Sandler, J., & Kaufman, K. (1981). A competency-based parent training program for abusive parents. *Journal of Consulting and Clinical Psychology, 49,* 633–640.

Wormith, J. S. (1985). *Some physiological and cognitive aspects of assessing deviant sexual arousal.* (Report No. 1985-26.) Ottawa: Ministry of the Solicitor General of Canada.

Wydra, A., Marshall, W. L., Earls, C. M., & Barbaree, H. E. (1983). Identification of cues and control of sexual arousal by rapists. *Behaviour Research and Therapy, 21,* 469–476.

Yanagida, E. H., & Ching, J. W. J. (1993). MMPI profiles of child abusers. *Journal of Clinical Psychology, 49,* 569–576.

5

Methodological Issues in Child Maltreatment Research

ROBERT T. AMMERMAN

INTRODUCTION

In 1993, the National Research Council (Panel on Research on Child Abuse and Neglect) published the findings and recommendations of a distinguished group of established researchers in child maltreatment. The purpose of this document was to summarize and integrate extant research findings, and to establish goals and suggestions for future scientific study of the abuse and neglect of children. Among other things, the Panel lamented the significant methodological shortcomings that characterized the empirical literature up to that point: "The research literature in the field of child maltreatment is immense . . . Despite this quantity of literature, researchers generally agree that the quality of research on child maltreatment is relatively weak in comparison to health and social science research studies in areas such as family systems and child development" (p. 45). Indeed, they pointed out that research on child abuse and neglect was largely "undervalued," and that limited resources allocated to empirical investigations, coupled with the comparatively nascent development both theoretically and methodologically in the child maltreatment field, conspired to limit both the quantity and quality of empirical work in this area. Despite this caveat, a considerable body of work has accrued in the past 35 years, and we now know more about the causes, consequences, and treatment of child abuse and neglect than we ever have before. Considerable work awaits researchers in this area, however, offering both substantial challenges and potential rewards in terms of understanding and preventing maltreatment of children.

Table 1 presents the specific priorities for future research recommended by the Panel on Research on Child Abuse and Neglect (National Research Council, 1993). What is most striking about this list of priorities is the emphasis on fundamental

ROBERT T. AMMERMAN • MCP ♦ Hahnemann School of Medicine, Allegheny University of the Health Sciences, Pittsburgh, Pennsylvania 15212.

Handbook of Child Abuse Research and Treatment, edited by Lutzker. Plenum Press, New York, 1998.

Table 1. Research Priorities Recommended by the Panel on Research on
Child Abuse and Neglect, National Research Council (1993)

Priority 1

A consensus on research definitions needs to be established for each form of child abuse and neglect.

Priority 2

Reliable and valid clinical-diagnostic and research instruments for the measurement of child maltreatment are needed to operationalize the definitions discussed under Research Priority 1.

Priority 3

Epidemiologic studies on the incidence and prevalence of child abuse and neglect should be encouraged, as well as the inclusion of research questions about child maltreatment in other national surveys.

Priority 4

Research that examines the processes by which individual, family, community, and social factors interact will improve understanding of the causes of child maltreatment and should be supported.

Priority 5

Research that clarifies the common and divergent pathways in the etiologies of different forms of child maltreatment for diverse populations is essential to improve the quality of future prevention and intervention efforts.

Priority 6

Research that assesses the outcomes of specific and combined types of maltreatment should be supported.

Priority 7

Research is needed to clarify the effects of the many forms of child victimization that often occur in the social context of child maltreatment. The consequences of child maltreatment may be significantly influenced by a combination of risk factors that have not been well described or understood.

Priority 8

Studies of similarities and differences in the etiologies and consequences of various forms of maltreatment across various cultural and ethnic groups are necessary.

Priority 9

High-quality evaluation studies of existing program and service interventions are needed to develop criteria and instrumentation that can help identify promising developments in the delivery of treatment and prevention services.

Priority 10

Research on the operation of the existing child protection and child welfare systems is urgently needed. Factors that influence different aspects of case handling decisions and the delivery and use of individual and family services require attention. The strengths and limitations of alternatives to existing institutional arrangements need to be described and evaluated.

Priority 11

Research on existing state data service systems should be conducted to improve the quality of child maltreatment research information as well as to foster improved service interventions.

Priority 12

The role of the media in reinforcing or questioning social norms relevant to child maltreatment needs further study.

Priority 13

Federal agencies concerned with child maltreatment research need to formulate a national research plan and provide leadership for child maltreatment research.

Priority 14

Governmental leadership is needed to sustain and improve the capabilities of the available pool of researchers who can contribute to studies of child maltreatment. National leadership is also required to foster the integration of research from related fields that offer significant insights into the causes, consequences, treatment, and prevention of child maltreatment.

Table 1. (*Continued*)

Priority 15
  Recognizing that fiscal pressures and budgetary deficits diminish prospects for significant increases in research budgets generally, special efforts are required to find new funds for research on child abuse and neglect and to encourage research collaboration and data collection in related fields.

Priority 16
  Research is needed to identify organizational innovations that can improve the process by which child maltreatment findings are disseminated to practitioners and policy makers. The role of state agencies in supporting, disseminating, and utilizing empirical research deserves particular attention.

Priority 17
  Researchers should design methods, procedures, and resources that can resolve ethical problems associated with recruitment of research subjects: informed consent, privacy, confidentiality, and autonomy, assignment of experimental and control research participants, and debriefing.

Source: Adapted from National Research Council. (1993). *Understanding child abuse and neglect*. Washington, DC: National Academy Press. Reprinted with permission.

aspects of conducting research in this area (e.g., Priority 1: definition, Priority 2: instrumentation). It is evident that a firm foundation in the field has yet to form. To their credit, the Panel has admirably sifted through a sizable and diverse literature and established meaningful, worthwhile, and largely achievable goals. At the same time, this document underscores the need for a higher standard of research in child abuse and neglect, one that will ensure continued accumulation of useful, relevant, and clinically applicable knowledge. Admittedly, this is no easy task. Child maltreatment is an enormously complicated problem with many logistic and practical barriers to conducting controlled, methodologically rigorous research. Overcoming these obstacles, at least in part, is essential to the advancement of scientific work in this area.

Why is research in child maltreatment so important? The Panel on Research on Child Abuse and Neglect (National Research Council, 1993) cited five reasons why research was critical to understanding and ameliorating child maltreatment: (1) research can provide a scientific basis for identifying solutions to a broad range of individual and social disorders; (2) research can provide insight and understanding that can benefit abused and neglected children and their families; (3) research can lead to cost savings in areas affected by child maltreatment, such as mental health, criminology, and foster care; (4) research findings can guide legal and other organizational decisions involving children and families; and (5) research on the causes of maltreatment can directly inform the design and implementation of prevention efforts.

The purpose of this chapter is to explore some of the more salient difficulties in conducting research on child abuse and neglect. At the outset, it is imperative to point out that child maltreatment is a very complicated phenomenon, and that many of the shortcominngs in the field arise from the difficulties inherent in systematically studying it. This is a relatively new field, and growing pains are to be expected. At the same time, it is essential that we take stock of achievements, acknowledge shortcomings, and map out a future for research in child abuse and neglect. Moreover, because methodological challenges and weaknesses abound in child maltreatment, it is equally important that we be frank and direct in confronting the limitations of findings in the field.

What follows is a discussion of some of the major pitfalls in conducting research and interpreting findings in child abuse and neglect, as well as suggestions for improving the quality of empirical work in this area. It is not meant to be a "how to" treatise on experimental methodology and design; many references (e.g., Kazdin, 1992) exist to guide social and behavioral scientists in this endeavor. Also, it is not meant to cover the entire universe of research issues in the field, issues that vary considerably depending on the questions asked and populations studied. Rather, the overarching objective of this chapter is to assist in the recognition of common impediments to controlled research in child abuse and neglect, and to contribute to the enhancement of the quality of empirical work on this topic.

DEFINITION

Reliably and operationally defining child maltreatment research has been elusive. Indeed, difficulties in arriving at clear and widely accepted definitions have undermined the research endeavor as a whole, given the primary importance of definition in developing a firm scientific base of understanding. The National Research Council (1993) plainly lays out some of the impediments to arriving at universally accepted definitions of abuse and neglect. First, there is a lack of a societal consensus regarding inadequate and inappropriate parenting. Moreover, different cultures have diverse standards for optimal parenting skills and values. To further complicate the picture, as Garbarino (1990) points out, societal views on parenting (and its deviant forms) are in a state of flux, changing over time and in response to cultural movements and shifting mores. Second, there has been confusion about whether to define maltreatment based on specific parent behaviors or child outcome. A third, and related, problem is the role of perpetrators' intent to harm in defining child maltreatment. And fourth, definitions of maltreatment are used for different purposes in disparate settings and systems (e.g., child protection, legal, clinical), and there is an inherent conflict between these groups that precludes arriving at a widely accepted view as to what constitutes maltreatment. Of course, because abuse and neglect are typically private acts, and thus hidden from public scrutiny, definitions are also reliant on indirect indicators (e.g., self-report) or intermittently occurring outcomes (e.g., injury), thereby further preventing accurate and consistent identification.

Although there tends to be agreement about the most severe forms of maltreatment, other aspects of deviant caregiving (e.g., psychological and emotional abuse), which may also be deleterious to the child's development and well-being, are debated among clinicians, researchers, and other professionals (see Giovannini, 1989). Although researchers have relied primarily on categorical definitions of maltreatment (e.g., abused vs. nonabused), others (Zuravin, 1991) have argued for more fine-grained distinctions between forms of inadequate parenting. Because we have little idea about what parenting abilities and skills are required for positive outcomes in children, however, we are stymied when trying to decide how to define and categorize parenting approaches that constitute maltreatment. We are in no position, then, to determine whether molecular indices (e.g., how many times a week the child was hit with a paddle) are preferable to more broadly based categorizations (e.g., child abuse suspected by a child protective service agency).

From a research perspective, it is imperative that definitions be reliable and replicable. Therefore, molecular approaches to definition and measurement are desirable. The Conflict Tactics Scale (Straus, 1979), and the lengthier but comprehensive Child Abuse and Neglect Interview Schedule (Ammerman, Hersen, & Van Hasselt, 1987), are useful tools for this purpose. Gathering and reporting highly specific data also facilitates communication among researchers and comparability between studies. Finally, more global categorizations can be derived from such data, using empirical methods (e.g., confirmatory factor analysis, cluster analysis) rather than subjective and potentially biased methods. The Panel on Research on Child Abuse and Neglect (National Research Council, 1993) recommends that multidisciplinary panels of experts be formed with the goal of arriving at standard definitions of maltreatment. Although this is a worthwhile endeavor with several benefits, it is difficult to arrive at consensus definitions if we do not yet know what to measure. Until a more coherent theoretical conceptualization of maltreatment emerges, researchers should (1) clearly articulate the definitions of maltreatment used in their investigations, (2) measure molecular aspects of the phenomena studied, and (3) routinely report these data in articles to enhance communication among members of the scientific and clinical communities.

SUBJECT SAMPLING

Just as there has been confusion and disagreement about what constitutes child abuse and neglect, research with maltreated children and their families has relied on a variety of sampling strategies to choose subjects. There is no one location where maltreated children and perpetrators reside or receive services and, as a result, many different settings have provided subject populations. Variability in the types of settings where recruitment occurs leads to questions about whether selected samples are representative of abused and neglected children in general. Scrutiny of sampling methods reveals that biases and error in sample selection decrease the generaizability of findings to other populations of maltreated children and their families (see Widom, 1988). Issues related to the settings in which subjects are recruited and methods of sampling will each be considered in turn.

Sampling Sources

Abuse and neglect are so widespread that there are few places where maltreated children (or individuals with a history of maltreatment) are not found. Although much research has been conducted with children and families who are involved with child protective service agencies (the largest setting for maltreated children), a significant amount of research (if not the major part) has been carried out with other samples in which maltreatment is thought to be found at a high rate. Illustrative settings include hospital emergency rooms, criminal courts, psychiatric clinics, shelters for battered women, inpatient hospital units, self-help organizations, schools, residential treatment settings, colleges, and group homes, to name a few. There is nothing inherently wrong with investigating maltreatment in subjects recruited from diverse settings. Indeed, depending on the questions asked, a specific population may be required (e.g., are conduct-disordered children referred for clinical evaluation more likely to have histories of abuse than other types of psychiatrically disordered children?). The unique characteristics of a population, however, limits comparisons between populations.

Child protective service agencies offer a prime example of how recruitment setting influences sampling and ultimately biases research results. In 1993, almost 3 million children were involved in reports of maltreatment to child protective service agencies in the United States, reports most of which were substantiated (c.f., Curtis, Boyd, Liepold, & Petit, 1995). It is generally believed that the actual number of maltreated children is larger than this figure, given that the private nature of abuse and neglect and the often temporary or absent physical effects of maltreatment result in a significant portion of children not coming to the attention of authorities. Thus, child protective service agencies are at the center of the simultaneous overreporting (as indicated by unsubstantiated cases) and underreporting (as indicated by the number of cases that are undiscovered) of child maltreatment. Therefore, subjects recruited from this setting are not representative of abused and neglected children as a whole, but, rather, they reflect only those children and families who have been identified. The processes of identification are variable from state to state, where laws and risk assessment approaches differ. They also vary within child protective service agencies, where an individual caseworker's style, training, and caseload all contribute to differences in identification and substantiation. In fact, in some urban settings, where child abuse and neglect reports are rising and agency resources are shrinking, there is pressure to focus almost exclusively on the most severe reports of maltreatment. Clearly, the types of children served in urban settings will differ from those in locations where caseloads are more manageable and less severe forms of maltreatment are more likely to be represented.

What other factors contribute to decreasing the representativeness of samples recruited from child protective service agencies? There is a skewed representation of poor children and families in these settings. A causal link between poverty and maltreatment is compelling (Gelles, 1992), but even when this is taken into account, it is probable that a disproportionate number of poor children, relative to the general population, are found in child protective service agencies. In addition, parents who are difficult, cognitively limited, or socially unskilled are more likely to have problems working with service providers in general, making it more likely that they will be referred for investigation. In summary, it is clear that subjects recruited from child protective service agencies are not representative of abused and neglected children as a whole, and caution is necessary in interpreting findings from these populations and comparing results to those of other groups.

Other settings have their own unique filters that bias the type of child and family identified. Emergency rooms will have children who have suffered physical injury as a result of maltreatment. Self-help groups will select potentially abusive parents who are motivated to change their behavior. Families recruited through criminal courts may reflect particularly severe forms of maltreatment or concurrent involvement in illegal activities (such as substance abuse). Psychiatric clinics have children with behavioral and emotional problems and tend not to have children who may be more resilient in adverse environments. College students who report histories of maltreatment have at least demonstrated the cognitive abilities and resourcefulness to graduate from high school and enroll in college, in sharp contrast to the educational underachievement characteristic of many maltreated youth. Furthermore, the unique features of children and families recruited from different settings may conceal possibly more significant differences between groups. For example, whereas psychiatric disorder may emerge as a result of maltreatment, it may also reflect a genetic vulnerability to the disorder. Parents who are motivated to seek out self-help groups probably differ from their peers who do not seek out such assistance on a variety of dimensions, including personality, coping skills, and resourcefulness.

In sum, there is no setting from which subjects are recruited that is fully representative of abused and neglected children and perpetrators. Each has inherent "gates" that influence entrance into these settings, and the resulting biases affect the type, meaning, and generalizability of research findings. In the child maltreatment field, it is often the case that settings are selected because of convenience (e.g., college students are readily available and may be compelled to participate in research, host organizations are cooperative or facilitative, some agencies are easier to work with than others). When there is a mismatch between the research questions asked and the recruitment setting used, both the internal and external validity of the research suffers, and subsequent findings are of restricted heuristic value.

Sampling Methods

Once a setting has been selected, a method of recruitment must be determined. Here, too, potential problems and difficulties exist. Ideally, a random selection of subjects will be made from a sufficiently large pool of subjects to prevent systematic biases in subject selection. Unfortunately, this is very difficult in child maltreatment research, and as a result it is an unrealized ideal in the majority of studies. Most scientific investigations of child maltreatment ask intrusive questions and deal with sensitive areas. Families may not want to undergo such an assessment, or they may be concerned about the potential consequences of divulging information that may prompt the investigator to make a report to child protective services. For example, much has been written about whether a significant number of families refuse to participate in family violence research because of these concerns. Some researchers have suggested the use of a Certificate of Confidentiality, which purportedly limits the reporting obligations should additional abuse and neglect be discovered (cf., Socolar, Runyan, & Amaya-Jackson, 1995). However, it is not clear whether this approach can stand up in a court of law; it has been argued that the ethical obligation to protect the child supersedes the research desire to collect and keep confidential information that is both accurate and complete. Because child maltreatment is in the forefront of public discussion and media attention, both as a societal problem and as a focus of controversy (e.g., false memory syndrome, spurious allegations of abuse, use of facilitated communication to identify abused children who are nonverbal and those who have developmental disabilities), most potential subjects know that harsh corporal punishment is looked down upon (at least officially), and that the consequences of admitting to "losing control" are potentially devastating. Thus, a certain number of subjects are likely to decline to participate in or may withdraw prematurely from research because of the perceived risks of doing so. This may be especially true for subjects already in contact with child protective systems, where they have already experienced legal involvement with their children. A related concern, of course, is that subjects will participate in research but will provide socially desirable and inaccurate information about parameters of interest to the researcher so as to avoid triggering a report of child abuse.

Of course, subjects turn down participation in research for other reasons. Some have neither the time nor the interest. Others may lead especially disorganized or chaotic lives, and are unable to make arrangements to visit a clinic or laboratory (or even to be available for a home visit). Low remunerations are likely to attract less participation than higher subject payments (Capaldi & Patteon, 1987). Longitudinal and treatment outcome studies suffer from attrition and dropouts. It is evident, therefore, that virtually all studies will encounter individuals who decline or fail to participate. These numbers are likely to be higher in clinical research than in studies with "captive" populations (e.g., college students). It is unknown how these "lost" subjects affect study findings. Some researchers contrast participants with nonparticipants on demographic variables to demonstrate that the groups are equivalent. However, such comparisons are rarely conducted on the variables of greatest interest (e.g., disciplinary practices, psychiatric disorder, IQ), and these are almost always unavailable to investigators.

These factors undermine a random sampling strategy, yet most subjects are not selected randomly. Rather, they are selected based on convenience. Whether it is a class of college students, the clinic where one works, the school where one consults, or the shelter that is willing to cooperate in a research study, each is a unique sampling site with limited applicability to the population as a whole.

Comments

The inherent difficulties in conducting rigorous, well-controlled research in child maltreatment are most evident in the identification and recruitment process. Carefully conceived hypotheses are often compromised by barriers to sampling, thereby threatening both internal and external validity. Unfortunately, few studies in applied clinical research in general, and child maltreatment in particular, escape some or many of the sampling problems just described. What, then, is to be done to enhance the quality of research in this area? First, at least some problems can be avoided by careful planning prior to conducting investigations. For example, it is well documented that sizable monetary remunerations reduce the chance of attrition in longitudinal research with at-risk families (Capaldi & Patterson, 1987). Second, attention must be paid to matching the research question to the appropriate sample and selection strategy. And third, it is critical that researchers report, *in detail*, the sampling methods used and the problems encountered along the way. Difficulties experienced should be revisited in discussion sections of research articles to highlight limitations of study findings. Providing such information will facilitate comparison between studies and assist reviewers (especially those who conduct meta-analyses) in extracting patterns of findings and conclusions from the literature as a whole.

MEASUREMENT AND DESIGN

The child maltreatment literature has been plagued by a variety of measurement problems. Adherence to basic psychometric principles of reliability, validity, and standardization has been inconsistent. Measurement of overt behaviors is still relatively rare in research on child maltreatment, although this is explained by the fact that aspects of abuse and neglect are difficult to measure directly, and logistic barriers interfere with such assessment approaches. Like much of the research on children and families, there is an overreliance on reports from mothers (Fantuzzo & Twentyman, 1986), despite considerable evidence that such reports are skewed and biased in child maltreatment populations (Reid, Kavanangh, & Baldwin, 1987). It is rare for child maltreatment researchers to report the reliabilities of measures administered in their samples, although this is becoming standard practice in the child development literature as a whole. Given the negative and pejorative connotations of abuse and neglect, it is likely that some aspects of subject reporting are susceptible to socially desirable response patterns. Yet, only a few measures have lie scales, and researchers rarely assess response biases. Inattention to psychometric issues has contributed to the general impression that the child maltreatment literature is weak, and future studies must focus on these critical areas.

Experimental design has been another topic of concern in the scientific study of child maltreatment. There is a preponderance of retrospective research designs in this area, characterized by the lack of experimental control, proneness to error and bias, and inability to establish causative relationships. Longitudinal designs are still relatively rare, despite their importance in developing and testing causal models, and in studying the processes of maladaptive development and family functioning. Significant advances in the field await the application of these more rigorous and potentially informative design strategies.

DATA ANALYTIC STRATEGIES

The National Research Council (1993) is quite explicit in its recommendations regarding data analysis: "Research using multivariate models and etiological theories that integrate ecological, transactional, and developmental factors will improve our understanding of the causes of child maltreatment. . . . Rather than focusing on specific factors . . . the interactions of variables at multiple ecological levels should be examined (p. 140). Complex, multidetermined phenomena such as child abuse and neglect necessitate multivariate data analytic strategies. Whereas the dominant theoretical formulations (e.g., ecological model) readily acknowledge the intricate interplay among etiologic variables in bringing about and maintaining child maltreatment, the sophistication of statistical procedures used to analyze data has lagged behind.

There are several reasons for the relatively slow progress in the use of more advanced statistical approaches to child abuse and neglect. First, it has been only recently that more than one perspective (e.g., individual, community) has been represented in research in this area. As different levels of functioning and different systems have been assessed and integrated, the need for multivariate approaches has become evident. Second, longitudinal studies (which typically require multivariate approaches) have been infrequent in child maltreatment. As these designs are used more often, multivariate methods of analysis will be more widely utilized. Finally, large sample sizes are typically required for multivariate analyses, yet they are relatively rare in child maltreatment research. In addition, significant amounts of missing data are common problems in clinical research in general, further undermining sample size and decreasing statistical power. In sum, the field is in need of more research that (1) uses measures that collect data from many levels (e.g., individual, family, community), (2) is longitudinal, and (3) has larger sample sizes.

Complex relationships can be elucidated only by using data analytic strategies that are capable of describing and examining such associations. For example, Baron and Kenny (1986) describe the identification of mediating and moderating variables; both types abound in the intricacies of child maltreatment. Moderator variables affect the strength or direction of the relationship between an independent or predictor variable and a dependent or criterion variable. Mediator variables, on the other hand, account for the strength of association between two variables. Both types of variables are identified upon systematic application of multiple regression analyses. Of course, this kind of approach requires a theory-driven conceptualization of the interrelationships among variables measured, rather than an exploratory, atheoretical data analytic strategy.

Structural equation modeling (SEM) has also been underutilized in child maltreatment research. SEM permits testing of causal models using nonexperimental data (see Hoyle, 1995). Specifically, SEM uses exploratory factor analysis and simultaneous multiple regression to test the goodness of fit between obtained data and prior hypotheses regarding the interrelationships among specific constructs. There are several advantages of SEM over more traditional statistical approaches. First, it allows the testing of causal models using correlational data. The results confirm or disconfirm the utility of the model, thus evaluating the validity of hypothesized links between constructs. Second, exploratory factor analysis is used to derive latent constructs, which reflect common variances among two or more similar variables and minimize potentially confounding measurement error. And third, SEM delineates the interrelationships among variables simultaneously, thereby making it an ideal procedure for identifyinng factors that mediate the relationships among other factors. These attributes are especially useful in child maltreatment research, which has (1) a frequent lack of a priori theoretical formulations in the conducting of data analyses, (2) significant problems with measurement error, and (3) a need for the development of unified constructs independent of specific measurement devices. Once again, SEM requires large sample sizes and is most often applied to longitudinal data sets, which are relatively rare in the child maltreatment field. SEM and other multivariate strategies (e.g., linear growth modeling) have the potential, however, to greatly enhance our understanding of child abuse and neglect and assist in the development of more effective preventive and treatment interventions.

INTERVENTION EVALUATION

Although the child maltreatment literature has burgeoned in the past two decades, empirical investigation of intervention outcome has lagged behind the rest of the field. As a result, most of our interventions (either prevention or treatment) have not been subjected to controlled clinical trials, and replication of studies is all but absent. Of course, this is due, in part, to the relative nascence of the field as a whole. In addition, the same barriers to controlled research that undermine assessment and etiology studies also occur in outcome investigations. In some cases, these are magnified (e.g., problems in conducting multiple assessments over a long period of time). Clearly, there is a great need to evaluate interventions so as to more effectively allocate resources and maximize the child's recovery and the family's rehabilitation.

The need for outcome studies is even more acute when one considers that most examinations of intervention effectiveness in clinical settings are disappointing, suggesting that the long-term benefits of treatment are quite limited (e.g., Cohn & Daro, 1987). Yet the few controlled research studies on treatment outcome (the majority of which are single-case) demonstrate that treatment, particularly cognitive–behavioral intervention, is successful, at least in the short run (e.g., see Kolko, 1996). (There are exceptions to these positive findings—see Ammerman, Hersen, & Lubetsky, 1996.) What accounts for this discrepancy?

Clues can be found in the child clinical psychology literature. Recent meta-analyses have documented the effectiveness of psychotherapy with children. For example, Weisz, Weiss, Alicke, and Klotz (1987) examined 105 outcome studies of psychological intervention with children ages 4 to 18 years. They found a mean effect size of 0.79 for treatment versus control comparison. Behavior therapy was found to be more effective than other forms of treatment, and children were more likely to improve when compared with adolescents. Moreover, a recent meta-analysis (Serketich & Dumas, 1996) of parent training interventions (the most frequently used intervention for child-abusing parents) concluded that "the average child whose parents participated in BPT (*Behavioral Parent Training*) was better adjusted after treatment than approximately 80% of children whose parents did not" (p. 179).

Yet, although laboratory findings are quite positive (as in the child maltreatment literature), treatment outcome in clinic settings is markedly inferior (also as in the child maltreatment literature; Weisz, Donenberg, Han, & Weiss, 1995). Weisz and associates explored 10 reasons that were hypothesized to account for the divergence of outcome in these two settings. They reported that research treatment of children differed from interventions carried out in the clinical setting in that clinic samples were more psychopathologically disturbed, research settings had superior resources, and behavior therapy (which has been found to be more effective overall) is more likely to be used in research rather than clinic settings. Although this investigation did not look at the child maltreatment literature, it is likely that the findings are applicable and relevant. Abused and neglected children and their families typically exhibit many problems that require many services involving several agencies that often have limited resources. In contrast, research studies often exclude the most severely disturbed families, have considerably more resources at their disposal, and are able to devote the time and effort required to optimize treatment outcome.

In addition, because of the high proportion of single-case research studies in the child maltreatment literature, there may be a skewed representation of treatment successes relative to failures. The reason for this is that single-case studies are designed to demonstrate the functional relationship between manipulations in interventions and subsequent changes in behavior. While negative results in group outcome studies are often difficult to publish in professional journals (yet critical for evaluating psychotherapy outcome—see Mohr, 1995), it is all but impossible to have failed single-case results disseminated in these forums. As a result, the extant empirical literature may provide an overly optimistic and distorted picture about the effectiveness of our interventions.

It is apparent, then, that significantly more research on treatment outcome with abused and neglected children and their families is needed. Moreover, the gap between research and clinic interventions needs to be narrowed. This can be accomplished in two ways. First, more rigorous empirical designs should be applied to program evaluations of existing services in the clinic and community. And second, research programs should recruit participants who reflect the many problems and the more severe disorders that are common among maltreated children and their families. Through such changes, the research literature will be made more relevant to clinicians, and more comprehensive and controlled evaluation of clinic programs can be conducted.

There is also a need, of course, for improvement in the quality of intervention outcome research in child maltreatment. Indeed, there is a unique opportunity to take advantage of what has been learned in the psychosocial treatment literature as a whole, and to apply it to the emergent child maltreatment field. To this end, Kazdin (1990) outlined 10 issues, needs, and areas that should be addressed in conducting treatment outcome research with children and families: (1) increased evaluation of clinical samples, (2) consideration of diagnostic comorbidity, (3) evaluation of underresearched treatment modalities, (4) evaluation of combined interventions, (5) outcome measurement of both symptom reduction and increased psychosocial functioning, (6) consideration of clinical versus statistical significance, (7) use of psychometrically strong and appropriate assessment measures, (8) monitoring of treatment integrity, (9) longer and more frequent posttreatment follow-up assessments, and (10) consideration of statistical power to detect differences between two or more treatments.

In the following sections, potential problem areas and strategies to enhance research quality in treatment outcome in child abuse and neglect are discussed.

INTERVENTION INTEGRITY

In the clinic setting, interventions are individually tailored to meet the needs of clients. This approach is essential in the treatment of children and families in general, and in child maltreatment in particular, given the great variability in strengths and needs displayed by abused and neglected children and their families. Although some leeway exists in providing treatment in research outcome studies, clinicians in research programs must adhere to a standardized protocol in order to maintain internal validity. Preserving integrity of research treatment protocols (i.e., ensuring that the treatment is being carried out consistently and accurately) has received much attention in the treatment outcome literature as a whole, but it is all but absent from the child maltreatment literature. Assessing adherence to treatment protocols provides assurance that the intervention (and not extraneous and confounding variables) is responsible for beneficial changes in functioning, and also facilitates replication of results in future studies.

The most common way of enhancing intervention integrity is to prepare, in advance, a comprehensive and concise treatment manual. Manuals should be clear and should permit replication of the intervention approach. Independent validity checks can confirm whether or not the protocol is being followed. Videotaped or audiotaped sessions, or written transcripts of sessions, can be systematically reviewed in a standardized way to determine fidelity to the protocol. While these procedures are time-consuming and labor intensive, they have become standard in other treatment literatures, and adoption of such practices will significantly elevate the quality of outcome research in child maltreatment.

Assessment

Intervention outcome research requires a comprehensive assessment battery. This is especially true in the case of child maltreatment, given that variables which may be primary targets for change (e.g., use of harsh disciplinary practices) may be difficult or impossible to observe and measure directly. As a result, assessment strategies focus primarily on indirect indices of child and family functioning, indices that are hypothesized to change in response to the intervention being evaluated. Assessment batteries, then, ideally consist of several analog and self and other report measures which describe and quantify the type and severity of the problems targeted for change as a function of treatment. Finally, assessment of intervention outcome requires some additional measures. These include process variables (e.g., resistance) and consumer satisfaction.

Design Considerations

Issues in experimental design in intervention outcome research have spawned several recent articles (e.g., VadenBos, 1996). Under the best of circumstances, evaluation of treatment effectiveness is an arduous undertaking, fraught with potential confounds and threats to empirical rigor. Not surprisingly, these problems are compounded in child maltreatment research. There are five major impediments to well-controlled outcome studies in child abuse and neglect, particularly studies involving groups: (1) random sampling, (2) random assignment, (3) concurrent interventions, (4) control groups, and (5) therapist effects.

As previously noted, random sampling from a population is essential to maximize generalizability to the population as a whole. It is rare, however, in the child maltreatment literature to be able to sample randomly from a setting, for the reasons noted in the section on subject selection. As a result, it is likely that systematic biases will exist in subject selection, thereby imposing limitations to study results at the outset. Assuming that such biases have been minimized, random assignment to groups is the sine qua non of valid treatment outcome studies.

A problem unique to the child maltreatment field is the fact that families who have been identified as abusive and/or neglectful typically receive many services. Often these interventions are mandated. As a result, researchers may be working with children and families who are being served concurrently by other providers.

Illustrative programs include substance abuse treatment, respite programs, and transportation assistance, among others. It is possible that improvement in family functioning over time is attributable, at least in part, to support services provided independent of the intervention being evaluated. In some instances, researchers will be the sole providers of treatment. Alternatively, researchers may work with families who do not require such extensive support, although in these instances such families are probably functioning at a higher level than those typically served by child protective service agencies. Careful documentation and reporting of simultaneously received services is an essential feature of dissemination of intervention outcome research.

A related concern is selection of control groups. Both ethical and legal considerations preclude the use of "no treatment" control groups. The latter might endanger the safety of the child, prolong suffering, and "no treatment" is untenable if child protective service agencies mandate intervention. Control groups, then, are typically receiving some form of intervention. Ideally, the intervention provided in the control group will be under the direction of the researcher. For example, Cohen and Mannarino (1996) evaluated a cognitive–behavioral treatment for sexually abused children. In that study, the control group consisted of children who received nondirective supportive therapy, an intervention involving providing empathy, encouraging expression of feelings, and providing a safe, therapeutic environment in sessions. This is both a viable treatment alternative and one that does not contain the core features of cognitive–behavior therapy that are thought to be critical to success. Unfortunately, such control groups have not been widely used in the research on child maltreatment intervention. More typical are comparisons between the treatment under consideration and interventions received in the community (e.g., Ammerman et al., 1996; Lutzker, 1990), which are usually beyond the control of the investigator.

SUMMARY

Child abuse and neglect has become an overwhelming societal problem, and it has been a daunting task for researchers to study, describe, and understand it. At the outset, research in the behavioral and social sciences is fraught with methodological and measurement problems. These are magnified dramatically in child maltreatment (cf. Herrenkohl, 1990). Yet tremendous advances have been made in the past two decades. We now have a clearer picture of the causes of maltreatment, and are in a better position to design effective prevention and treatment programs. The next generation of child maltreatment research, however, must address the formidable barriers that impede progress in the field. At the very least, a more open dialogue among researchers is needed as to the problems encountered and the explication of the limitations of findings. In addition, standardized procedures for gathering and reporting data, particularly as they pertain to defining and describing maltreatment, are needed. Finally, enhancements in research design, measurement, sampling strategies, data analysis, and intervention outcome studies are required to move the field forward. The inevitable evolution of research in child maltreatment toward greater sophistication and rigor will, no doubt, lead to improved understanding and more effective clinical interventions for abused and neglected children and their families.

ACKNOWLEDGMENT

This chapter was written with support from Grants Nos. H133A40007 and H133G-100008 from the National Institute on Disabilities and Rehabilitation Research, U.S. Department of Education. The opinions expressed herein are solely those of the author, and no official endorsement by the U.S. Department of Education should be inferred.

REFERENCES

Ammerman, R. T., Hersen, M., & Van Hasselt, V. B. (1987). *Child Abuse and Neglect Interview Schedule*. Unpublished instrument, Western Pennsylvania School for Blind Children, Pittsburgh.

Ammerman, R. T., Hersen, M., & Lubetsky, M. J. (1996, November). Difficulties in implementing interventions in chronic child maltreatment. In J. R. Lutzker (Chairperson), *Child abuse and neglect: The cutting edge*. Symposium conducted at the annual convention of the Association for Advancement of Behavior Therapy, New York.

Baron, R. M., & Kenny, D. A. (1986). The moderator-mediator variable distinction in social psychological research: Conceptual, strategic, and statistical considerations. *Journal of Personality and Social Psychology, 51*, 1173–1182.

Capaldi, D., & Patterson, G. R. (1987). An approach to the problem of recruitment and retention rates for longitudinal research. *Behavioral Assessment, 9*, 169–178.

Cohen, J. A., & Mannarino, A. P. (1996). A treatment outcome study for sexually abused preschool children: Initial findings. *Journal of the American Academy of Child and Adolescent Psychiatry, 35*, 42–50.

Cohn, A. E., & Daro, D. (1987). Is treatment too late: What ten years of evaluative research tell us. Special Issue: Child abuse and neglect. *Child Abuse & Neglect, 11*, 433–442.

Curtis, P. A., Boyd, J. D., Liepold, M., & Petit, M. (1995). *Child abuse and neglect: A look at the states*. Washington, DC: Child Welfare League of America.

Fantuzzo, J. W., & Twentyman, C. T. (1986). Child abuse and psychotherapy research: Merging social concerns and empirical investigation. *Professional Psychology: Research and Practice, 17*, 375–380.

Garbarino, J. (1990). Future directions. In R. T. Ammerman & M. Hersen (Eds.), *Children at risk: An evaluation of factors contributing to child abuse and neglect* (pp. 291–298). New York: Plenum Press.

Gelles, R. J. (1992). Poverty and violence toward children. *Behavioral Scientist, 35*, 258–274.

Giovannoni, J. (1989). Definitional issues in child maltreatment. In D. Cicchetti & V. Carlson (Eds.), *Child maltreatment: Theory and research on the causes and consequences of child abuse and neglect* (pp. 3–37). New York: Cambridge University Press.

Herrenkohl, R. C. (1990). Research directions related to child abuse and neglect. In R. T. Ammerman & M. Hersen (Eds.), *Children at risk: An evaluation of factors contributing to child abuse and neglect* (pp. 85–108). New York: Plenum Press.

Hoyle, R. H. (1995). *Structural equation modeling: Concepts, issues, and applications*. Thousand Oaks, CA: Sage.

Kazlin, A. E. (1990). Psychotherapy for children and adolescents. *Annual Review of Psychology, 41*, 21–54.

Kadin, A. E. (Ed.). (1992). *Methodological issues and strategies in clinical research*. Washington, DC: American Psychological Association.

Kolko, D. J. (1996). Child physical abuse. In J. Briere, L. Berliner, J. A. Bulkley, C. Jenny, & T. Reid (Eds.), *The APSAC handbook on child maltreatment* (pp. 21–50). Thousand Oaks, CA: Sage.

Lutzker, J. R. (1990). Project 12-ways: Treating child abuse and neglect from an ecobehavioral perspective. In R. F. Dangel & R. F. Polster (Eds.), *Parent training: Foundations of research and practice* (pp. 260–291). New York: Guilford Press.

Mohr, D. C. (1995). Negative outcome in psychotherapy: A critical review. *Clinical Psychology: Science and Practice, 2*, 1–27.

National Research Council. (1993). *Understanding child abuse and neglect*. Washington, DC: National Academy Press.

Reid, J. B., Kavanagh, K., & Baldwin, D. V. (1987). Abusive parent's perceptions of child problem behaviors: An example of parental bias. *Journal of Abnormal Child Psychology, 15*, 457–466.

Serketich, W. J., & Dumas, J. E. (1996). The effectiveness of behavioral parent training to modify anti-social behavior in children: A meta-analysis. *Behavior Therapy, 27,* 171–186.

Socolar, R. R. S., Runyan, D. K., & Amaya-Jackson, L. (1995). Methodological and ethical issues related to studying child maltreatment. *Journal of Family Issues, 16,* 565–586.

Straus, M. A. (1979). Measuring family conflict and violence: The Conflict Tactics Scales. *Journal of Marriage and the Family, 41,* 75–88.

VandenBos, G. R. (1996). Guest editor. Special issue: Outcome assessment of psychotherapy. *American Psychologist, 51,* 1005–1079.

Weisz, J. R, Weiss, B., Alicke, M. D., & Klotz, M. L. (1987). Effectiveness of psychotherapy with children and adolescents: A meta analysis for clinicians. *Journal of Consulting and Clinical Psychology, 55,* 542–549.

Weisz, J., Donenberg, G., Han, S., & Weiss, B. (1995). Bridging the gap between the lab and the clinic in child and adolescent psychotherapy. *Journal of Consulting and Clinical Psychology, 63,* 688–701.

Widom, C. S. (1988). Sampling biases and implications for child abuse research. *American Journal of Orthopsychiatry, 58,* 260–270.

Zuravin, S. J. (1991). Research definitions of child physical abuse and neglect: Current problems. In R. Starr & D. Wolfe (Eds.), *The effects of child abuse and neglect: Issues and research.* New York: Guilford Press.

6

Implementing and Evaluating an Individualized Behavioral Intervention Program for Maltreating Families
Clinical and Research Issues

DAVID J. HANSEN, JODY E. WARNER-ROGERS, and DEBRA B. HECHT

Child abuse and neglect is a multidimensional problem that requires comprehensive, individualized treatment. The multiproblem nature of maltreating families presents many assessment and treatment difficulties for clinicians and researchers. A variety of factors contribute to difficulties in treating these families, including (1) the presence of multiple stressors and limited financial, personal, and social resources within the family for coping with stressors, (2) the often coercive nature of the referral and the possibility that participation in services may be involuntary or under duress, (3) the fact that abusive behavior cannot be readily observed, and (4) the need for many different interventions to treat several target areas (Azar & Wolfe, 1989; Hansen & Warner, 1992, 1994; Wolfe, 1988). Abusive and neglectful families are a very heterogeneous group for which individualized intervention approaches are needed.

Physical abuse and neglect may be seen as the result of complex maladaptive interactions and/or lack of essential caretaking behaviors that are influenced by parental skill or knowledge deficits and other stress factors (Hansen, Conaway, & Christopher, 1990; Hansen & Warner, 1992; Kelly, 1983). Parental skill deficits may be found in areas such as child management and parent–child interaction, anger

DAVID J. HANSEN and DEBRA B. HECHT • Department of Psychology, University of Nebraska, Lincoln, Nebraska 68588.   JODY E. WARNER-ROGERS • MRC Child Psychiatry Unit, London SE5 8AF, England.

Handbook of Child Abuse Research and Treatment, edited by Lutzker. Plenum Press, New York, 1998.

and stress control for child-related and nonchild-related stressors, or problem solving for familial or other stressors. Maltreating parents may also have unrealistic expectations and distorted judgments of child behavior. In addition, a lack of motivation (e.g., related to personal values, cultural standards) may interfere with adequate parenting behavior.

Research on the use of particular treatment approaches (e.g., parent training) with individual or small groups of maltreating parents has suggested that behavioral procedures may be effective for improving family functioning and reducing recurrence of maltreatment (e.g., Crimmins, Bradlyn, St. Lawrence, & Kelly, 1984; Scott, Baer, Christoff, & Kelly, 1984; Wolfe, Edwards, Manion, & Koverola, 1988). However, the multiplicity of problems characteristic of maltreating families, in combination with the need for individualized and comprehensive intervention, has made the evaluation of the effectiveness of such treatment procedures very difficult. In their review of 21 intervention studies, Wolfe and Wekerle (1993) highlight some of the difficulties, including a relative paucity of well-designed studies (e.g., adequate control groups, proper randomization procedures, establishment of sufficient statistical power) and a lack of long-term follow-up to assess recidivism.

A notable exception to the relatively narrow focus of the treatment research is Project 12-Ways, a multifaceted behavioral treatment program for abusive and neglectful parents (cf. Lutzker, 1984; Lutzker, Wesch, & Rice, 1984; Wesch & Lutzker, 1991). These evaluations have indicated that families receiving Project 12-Ways services showed generally lower recidivism rates and less frequent removal of children from the home than those who had not received such services. Unfortunately, little is known about the characteristics and effectiveness of the many other agencies and programs nationwide that utilize behavioral interventions to treat maltreating families.

Given the massive amount of societal, clinical, and research attention to child abuse and neglect in recent decades, there is a relative dearth of empirical evidence on how to provide effective and comprehensive treatment for these multi-problem families. The problem lies partially in the fact that research designs are so incredibly difficult to implement under the circumstances (e.g., heterogeneous population, multiple problems and stressors, multiple etiological and maintaining factors, inability to randomly assign subjects to control or comparison conditions).

Published treatment projects, whether they are individual subject or group design, must often sacrifice external validity (generalizability) for internal validity (e.g., focus on only one intervention approach such as parent training). It also seems that when maltreating families are presented or described in treatment research, the multidimensional nature of their problems and the multidimensional nature of their treatment are not addressed (e.g., involvement of other agencies, crisis and problem-solving interventions to address problems that are not the focus of the study).

This chapter discusses the clinical and research issues that arise when evaluating the effectiveness of an individualized behavioral intervention program for maltreating families. Specifically, we describe the Family Interaction Skills Project (FISP) at West Virginia University, a behavioral program located within a university-based clinic, which specialized in the assessment and treatment of physically abusive and neglectful families. An overview of FISP is provided, including client and therapist characteristics, assessment and treatment procedures, practical issues that arose in implementing services, research design issues, and evidence for the effectiveness of FISP.

OVERVIEW OF THE FAMILY INTERACTION SKILLS PROJECT

The Quin Curtis Center for Psychological Training, Research, and Service is a clinic operated by the Department of Psychology of West Virginia University. The Family Interaction Skills Project for physically abusive and neglectful families was one of the specialized projects in the Curtis Center. Funded by a grant from the West Virginia Department of Health and Human Resources, FISP provided free services to maltreating parents referred by Child Protective Services workers. All families were referred by Child Protective Services workers.

During the initial years of FISP, the Curtis Center was housed in space provided by the local community mental health center. In the final years of the project, the Curtis Center opened new space in the psychology department on the university's main campus. One-way glass and videotaping equipment were available in the center for purposes of clinical supervision and training as well as for clinical observation and assessment.

The program was conducted by a clinical psychology faculty member and students of the psychology department. The graduate students who served as therapists were in the child clinical track of the department's doctoral program in clinical psychology. Direct assessment and treatment services were provided primarily by these therapists. Each year a graduate student was selected to serve in the role as services coordinator. Undergraduate clinical assistants served a variety of functions: scoring assessments, observation and data collection in home or schools, summarizng data, participating in sessions, and interacting with children while the therapist(s) worked with the parent(s). Many families were served by two co-therapists. Two staff members generally attended home sessions.

All therapists were supervised by the faculty member who served as project director. Therapists and the project director supervised the clinical assistants. Individual and group supervision were provided. Inexperienced therapists and students were trained via readings, discussions, presentations, and by working closely with an experienced therapist. "Vertical team" opportunities were available, whereby less experienced graduate students gained experience by working with advanced graduate students.

Clinical assessment and treatment services were provided for physically abusive and/or neglectful parents and their children. Parents and children participated in an individualized comprehensive assessment procedure designed to assess potential factors related to abuse or neglect. These factors included psychopathology, child-management skills deficits, child behavior problems, parent–child interaction deficits, insufficient knowledge about child development and behavior, stress- and anger-control deficits, and problem-solving skills deficits for coping with family stressors and other risk factors.

A variety of treatment procedures were available and treatment programs were structured to meet the needs of the participants as indicated by the assessment results. Treatments included parenting-skills training, problem-solving skills training, stress-management or anger-control training, and interventions to improve personal cleanliness or safety (e.g., from sexual abuse), home-cleanliness or safety, and nutrition. Length of treatment was based on client needs and was variable. Treatment was conducted with individual families, usually in their own home (approximately 85% of sessions were conducted within the home). The provision of services in the natural environment, as opposed to the artificial nature of clinic settings, is important for enhancing the effectiveness, generalization, and maintenance of treatment (Wolfe & Wekerle, 1993).

Periodic summary and progress reports were made to the referral source (Child Protective Services). Frequent phone contacts were made between FISP staff, especially the services coordinator, and the Child Protective Services staff. FISP staff regularly participated in court hearings regarding placement and custody of children. This type of affordable, comprehensive, individualized clinical services was in short supply in the region. The flexibility to hold sessions in the home or at the school and to schedule several sessions or contacts per week if needed were also unique aspects of the program.

ASSESSMENT PROCEDURES

The initial assessment for each family was tailored to address the specific referral issues. In general, domains targeted for assessment in FISP included (1) history and risk of abuse and neglect, (2) parental psychopathology and substance abuse, (3) knowledge and expectations regarding child development and behavior, (4) child behavior problems, (5) child management and parent–child interaction skills, (6) stress and anger control deficits, (7) problem-solving and coping skills deficits, (8) adaptive social contacts and social support, and (9) marital/relationship problems. Additional target areas for neglectful families included home cleanliness, home safety, and other dimensions related to the facilitation of optimal child development (e.g., child nutrition, intellectual stimulation). These assessment procedures are briefly described below. See Hansen and MacMillan (1990) and Hansen and Warner (1992) for more detailed reviews.

Throughout the assessment process, a functional analytic perspective, essential for conducting a thorough treatment-relevant assessment (Hansen & MacMillan, 1990; Hansen & Warner, 1992), was adopted. Potential antecedents of maltreatment, including child misbehaviors, conflict between parents, unrealistic expectations or lack of knowledge regarding child development and behavior, substance abuse, and other stressors or interaction problems were identified. The role of potential positive consequences for maltreatment was examined. For example, maltreating behavior may function to remove an aversive event such as noncompliance or tantrumming. It may bring praise or approval to the maltreating parent from others who perceive the actions as appropriate child-rearing practices. The absence of negative consequences may also contribute to continued maltreatment (Hansen & Warner, 1992).

Clinical interviewing was a critical component of the assessment process; it provides an essential procedure for identifying circumstances around maltreatment, assessing risk, and identifying targets for intervention, Interviews with a variety of individuals, including parents, children, and caseworkers, were generally needed. Although not a standardized or structured interview, Wolfe's (1988) Parent Interview and Assessment Guide is helpful for identification of general problem areas and assessment of parental responses to child-rearing demands.

Use of Existing Measures

A variety of widely used measures were helpful in assessment of the families seen through FISP. The majority of measures discussed, with a few exceptions, have known psychometric properties that support their use. Following the initial assessment, many devices were used repeatedly throughout treatment for the purposes of evaluating behavior change.

Measures commonly employed to address parental psychopathology were the Symptom-Checklist-90–Revised (SCL-90-R; Derogatis, 1983) and the Minnesota Multiphasic Personality Inventory–2 (MMPI-2; Butcher, Dahlstrom, Graham, Tellegen, & Kaemmer, 1989). The 90-item SCL-90-R was particularly useful, given its relative brevity and the breadth of symptoms covered (Somatization, Obsessive–Compulsive, Interpersonal Sensitivity, Depression, Anxiety, Hostility, Phobic Anxiety, Paranoid Ideation, Psychoticism, and global indices).

A widely researched measure for detection of at-risk status is Milner's (1986) Child Abuse Potential (CAP) Inventory. The Abuse Potential Scale of the CAP Inventory can be divided into six factor scales: Distress, Rigidity, Unhappiness, Problems with Child and Self, Problems with Family, and Problems from Others. Distortion indexes of Fake-Good, Fake-Bad, and Random Responding are derived from the validity scales of Lie, Random Response, and Inconsistency. The CAP Inventory is careful in screening, as it can detect individuals who exhibit characteristics associated with difficulties in the parent–child relationship, as well as many risk factors that can increase the likelihood that abuse will occur (Milner, 1994); however, because of the possibility of misclassification, it is not intended to be used in isolation for identification of abuse potential.

Parental knowledge and expectations about child development and behavior is a particularly difficult area to assess because normative levels and timing of child behaviors are so varied. Fortunately, a few measures are available to evaluate general parental belief and attitudes. The Parent Opinion Questionnaire (Azar & Rohrbeck, 1986) assesses the appropriateness of expectations related to a variety of child behaviors. In addition to the total score, six subscales are scored: Self-Care, Family Responsibility and Care of Siblings, Help and Affection to Parents, Leaving Children Alone, Proper Behavior and Feelings, and Punishment. The Family Belief Inventory (Roehling & Robin, 1986) is a useful measure of adherence to unreasonable belief in parent–adolescent conflict situations. For parents, the belief measured are ruination, perfectionism, approval, obedience, self-blame, and malicious intent. For adolescents, the beliefs are ruination, unfairness, autonomy, and approval.

A variety of procedures were used for assessing child management and parent–child interaction skills. Parent-report measures of child behavior problems were commonly used. Two of the most useful were the Child Behavior Checklist (CBCL; Achenbach, 1991) and the Eyberg Child Behavior Inventory (ECBI; Eyberg & Ross, 1978). The CBCL consists primarily of ratings of 118 items describing specific behavior problems. In addition, several questions are included to evaluate the child's social strengths. Behavior Problem scales of the CBCL vary according to the age and sex of the child, but may include Schizoid or Anxious, Depressed,

Uncommunicative, Obsessive–Compulsive, Somatic Complaints, Social Withdrawal, Ineffective, Aggressive, and Delinquent. Social Competence scales include Activities, Social, and School. The ECBI (Eyberg & Ross, 1978) is brief and can be repeated readily to monitor changes in child behavior. Thirty-six behavior problems are rated on a 7-point scale for frequency (or intensity). Parents are also asked to indicate which behaviors they consider a problem.

A measure developed to assess parental knowledge about child management is the Knowledge of Behavioral Principles as Applied to Children (KBPAC; O'Dell, Tarler-Benlolo, & Flynn, 1979). The KBPAC was occasionally useful, but the advanced reading level required for the 50-item multiple-choice measure precluded the ability of many clients to complete the measure independently.

Direct observations of parent–child interactions and parenting behavior are essential for a complete assessment. FISP staff found videotaping to be a practical, informative, and integral part of assessment, especially given the portability and availability of video recording equipment. Parent–child interactions were often observed in unstructured play situations using the Child's Game procedure (Forehand & McMahon, 1981). A parent was instructed to play with his or her child, allowing the child to structure the activity. The interactions were generally observed for approximately 10 minutes and ended with the parent asking the child to put away the toys. Target behaviors included parent descriptions, imitations, praise statements, questions, and commands. Child and parent responses to questions and commands (e.g., compliance) were also recorded. More complex direct observation instruments, such as the Dyadic Parent–Child Interaction Coding System (DPICS; Eyberg & Robinson, 1981), were also useful for assessing the quality and content of parent–child interactions. The DPICS assesses a variety of positive and negative behaviors. The frequency of 14 parent behaviors (e.g., direct or indirect commands, descriptive or reflective statements, positive or negative physical behavior) and 10 child behaviors (e.g., cry, yell, destructive, compliance, noncompliance) are coded.

General measures of stress were helpful in examining recent stressful experiences of maltreating families. Such measures included the Life Experiences Survey (Sarason, Johnson, & Siegel, 1978), which assesses occurrence and impact of major life events, and the Hassles Scale (Kanner, Coyne, Schaefer, & Lazarus, 1981), which assesses occurrence and impact of minor, commonly occurring stressors. Both of these measures were often included in a FISP assessment protocol in order to gather information on stressors outside the parent–child relationship that may impact parenting ability.

For the purposes of evaluating stressors associated specifically with parenting, the Parenting Stress Index (Abidin, 1986) was used. This measure was developed for assessing dysfunctional parent–child relationships and stress associated with parenting. The Child Domain scales are Adaptability, Acceptability, Demandingness, Mood, Distractibility/Hyperactivity, and Reinforces Parent. The Parent Domain scales are Parent Health, Depression, Attachment, Restrictions of Role, Sense of Competence, Social Isolation, and Relationship with Spouse. Life Stress is an optional scale.

The Issues Checklist (Robin & Foster, 1989) was useful for assessment of anger related to parent–adolescent conflict in maltreating families. It is a self-report measure of conflict issues and intensity of anger during interactions about these issues. Examples include telephone calls, doing homework, cursing, lying, and sex.

The presence and quality of social contacts and social support were assessed through interview and self-monitoring. Availability and use of the various types of social support, such as guidance and advising, emotional support, socializing, tangible assistance, self-disclosure, and support related to child problems (e.g., advice on how to handle tantrums, emotional support for handling child-related stressors) were evaluated. Wahler's (1980) Community Interaction Checklist was useful for evaluation of social contacts for some clients.

When both parents were present in the home, the quality of their partnership was assessed. Self-report measures commonly used in the assessment of marital problems included the Dyadic Adjustment Scale (DAS; Spanier, 1976) and the Marital Adjustment Scale (MAS; Locke & Wallace, 1959). The DAS, which is similar to the MAS, is a brief questionnaire using primarily Likert-style rating scales to assess the quality of dyadic relationships. The DAS yields a standard score that represents the degree of dissatisfaction in the relationship, which can be compared to distressed and nondistressed norms.

The Conflict Tactics Scale (Straus, 1979), a brief measure designed to assess individual responses to situations involving conflict within the family, was used for some families to assess conflict resolution tactics between parents and children or between spouses. It was administered in interview or questionnaire fashion. Items assess a wide range of tactics, from "discussed the issue calmly" to "kicked, bit, or hit with a fist" and the subscales are Reasoning, Verbal Hostility, and Physical Aggression.

Psychophysiological measures were not used in FISP, but research has suggested that they may be useful (e.g., Wolfe, Fairbank, Kelly, & Bradlyn, 1983). Physiological measurements of arousal may be taken during exposure to audio- or video-recorded stimuli (e.g., child deviant behavior) or in vivo exposure to deviant child behavior (Hansen & MacMillan, 1990). Research suggests that use of imagery enhanced by audio-recorded descriptions of child-related problems may facilitate measurement of anger and arousal (Hansen & MacMillan, 1990).

Additional measures were useful for families at risk for neglect. Neglectful parents may fail to meet several important needs of their children, including safety, cleanliness, health and nutrition, and education. Methods of assessment included interview, direct observation during home visits, and behavioral monitoring by parents, children, and teachers (Hansen & Warner, 1992). Lutzker and his colleagues developed two very useful observational rating systems for identifying and monitoring problems in the home. The Checklist for Living Environments to Assess Neglect (CLEAN; Watson-Perczel, Lutzker, Greene, & McGimpsey, 1988) is designed to assess home cleanliness. Item areas in targeted places (e.g., sink, counter) are rated for cleanliness according to three dimensions: presence of dirt or organic matter, number of clothes or linens in contact with the item area, and number of nonclothing items or other nonorganic matter in contact with the item area.

The Home Accident Prevention Inventory (HAPI; Tertinger, Greene, & Lutzker, 1984) was developed to assess the safety of home environments of families identified as abusive or neglectful. The HAPI assess hazards in five categories of home items: fire and electrical hazards, suffocation by ingested object, suffocation by mechanical objects, firearms, and solid and liquid poisons. The total number of hazardous items, as well as the type and number of categories under which these hazardous items are organized, can be identified.

Development of Measures

In addition to use of the available standardized measures just noted, FISP staff also developed standardized procedures for assessing parental problem-solving skills, as well as anger and arousal specifically related to child behavior. These target areas were seen as important in the overall assessment, but there were no appropriate measures available.

It is hypothesized that inability to solve problems related to parenting and other aspects of daily living results in frustration or inability to cope and leads to problematic parental behavior such as physical abuse or neglect (Hansen et al., 1995). The Parental Problem-Solving Measure (PPSM) (Hansen, Pallotta, Tishelman, Conaway, & MacMillan, 1989; Hansen, Pallotta, Christopher, Conaway, & Lundquist, 1995) assesses problem-solving skills for child-related as well as nonchild-related areas. Problem situations for the PPSM are classified into one of five problem areas: (1) child behavior and child management, (2) anger and stress control, (3) finances, (4) child care resources, and (5) interpersonal problems. Responses are rated for the number of solutions generated and the effectiveness of each chosen solution. An initial 25-item measure was shown to have good interrater reliability and internal consistency and to discriminate abusive and neglectful from nonmaltreating parents (Hansen et al., 1989). To save time in administration, it was reduced to 15 items in subsequent research (Smith, Conaway, Smith, & Hansen, 1988). The most recent study of the 15-item PPSM (Hansen et al., 1995) demonstrated the interrater reliability, internal consistency, and temporal stability of the PPSM and its five subscales (child behavior, interpersonal, anger/stress, financial, and child care problems). Support was also found for the convergent and discriminant validity of the measure. The problem-solving scales had moderate relationships with each other and with a measure of intellectual functioning. Scores on the PPSM were not significantly related to a measure of socially desirable response style. The PPSM also differentiated maltreating from nonmaltreating parents.

Anger specifically related to child behavior is sometimes an assessment priority with abusive parents (Hansen & Warner, 1992). The Parental Anger Inventory (PAI; previously known as the MacMillan-Olson-Hansen Anger Control Scale) (DeRoma & Hansen, 1994; MacMillan, Olson, & Hansen, 1988) was developed to assess anger experienced by maltreating parents in response to child misbehavior and other child-related situations. The development of the PAI was conducted in a number of phases to select items and demonstrate the reliability and validity of the scale (DeRoma & Hansen, 1994; MacMillan, Olson, & Hansen, 1988). Parents rate 50 child-related situations (e.g., child refuses to go to bed, child throws food) as problematic or nonproblematic and rate the degree of anger evoked by each situation. High item-total, split-half, and test–retest correlations support the internal consistency and temporal stability of the measure. Moderate correlations with other measures of child problems and with global stress also represent a psychometric strength of this measure. Comparison data based on a normative sample of 166 parents facilitates the utility of this measure for evaluation purposes (DeRoma & Hansen, 1994).

Situations in which discipline is attempted represent high risk for physical abuse and should be an assessment priority. Because directly observing actual discipline is often difficult, an assessment utilizing an adult actor to present deviant child behavior was developed for the FISP treatment project (MacMillan, Olson, & Hansen, 1991). The Home Simulation Assessment (HSA) measures parent ability to apply child management skills in realistic problem situations that may occur in the home. Parents are provided with instructions about tasks (e.g., dry the dishes) and asked to do their best to prompt the actor to complete the tasks. "Deviant" scripted behaviors are exhibited by the actor. A high-deviance segment of the HSA can be utilized to examine anger and stress responses to child behaviors. The high-deviance assessment uses an additional actor and increases the frequency of deviant actor behaviors. Parent self-report ratings of stress, anger, and anxiousness are also collected.

At times, as with all clinical services, it was useful to construct measures to address target behaviors of interest. Development of such client-specific measures was useful when there were no existing measures available. For example, in the treatment of a multiply distressed abusive and neglectful mother (described in more detail later), MacMillan, Guevremont, and Hansen (1988) created a self-report stress and anxiety measure that was completed two or three times per week by the client during audiotaped telephone interviews. The client was not able to read, so items had to be read to her. The items were generated based on her description of what she felt like when things were not going well for her (e.g., anxious, light-headed, headache). The client was asked, (1) How anxious did you feel? (2) How dizzy or light-headed did you feel? (3) Did you have a headache? (4) How much did you enjoy the day? and (5) How would you rate the overall day? Items were rated on a Likert-type scale ranging from *not at all* (1) to *very much* (5). For the same client, a measure of her affective state during sessions was created to further evaluate her progress. During the first 10 minutes of each session, she was asked to describe events occurring in the past week. Her description was audiotaped and scored as positive/neutral or negative using a 10-second whole interval recording system. Positive/neutral affect was defined as verbal or nonverbal client behaviors that were positive or neutral, such as laughing and talking about pleasant or routine activities. Negative affect was defined as verbal or nonverbal behaviors that were negative, such as crying, sighing, cursing, and expressing frustration, anger, or hopelessness.

In other cases, measures were as simple as recording toothbrushing by each child in a family (when dental hygiene was a serious concern) and recording praise statements made by the mother while the family was playing a game (Doepke, Watson-Perczel, & Hansen, 1988). Self-report procedures, such as monitoring of responses associated with arousing events, were also useful. For instance, a parent may be instructed to record a description of each incident that led to feelings of anger, frustration, or tension, the manner in which he or she dealt with the problem, the way it was resolved, and the feelings he or she had afterward (Hansen & Warner, 1992).

TREATMENT PROCEDURES AND EVALUATION

Traditional group design studies are extraordinarily complex in work with maltreating families. Researchers are dealing with a heterogeneous population. The families are experiencing multiple problems and stressors. A variety of etiological factors may have precipitated the maltreatment and may be different from the factors that maintain the abuse. Furthermore, researchers cannot randomly assign subjects to control or comparison conditions. The lack of a comprehensive theory of the causes and consequences of maltreatment makes it difficult to develop treatments. In addition, treatment groups and procedures for maltreatment often form in response to community needs and the focus is on providing services to families in crisis, not on empirical control and evaluation

Despite these difficulties, the evaluation of treatment efficacy obviously is important. The resources allocated to address child maltreatment are limited, making it imperative that funds are directed to the most efficacious treatments. Thus, documentation and empirical evaluation of treatment outcome should be a critical component of any treatment program. We have found that two methods, a program evaluation approach (cf. Posavac & Carey, 1992) and single-subject designs (cf. Barlow & Hersen, 1984), were particularly valuable for understanding and evaluating our treatment efforts.

In the following sections, the nature of the treatments provided and realistic and practical procedures for evaluation are described in the context of presenting several projects that evaluated aspects of FISP. This approach represents our adaptation of the research literature into a treatment program, and in return, our contributions to the literature.

Program-Evaluation Approach

Program evaluation approaches can be useful in providing a broader perspective about a project, including its clients, procedures, and impact. In conducting such program evaluation research, the size and characteristics of a target population are determined and the impact of a treatment program on this target group is assessed. Additionally, the specific program elements or resources expended are identified such that a cost-benefit analysis of the program can be made. Program evaluations can be based primarily on archival-type examination of clinical records; this highlights one of the many reasons why detailed, consistent record keeping throughout assessment and treatment is paramount.

There were three program evaluation projects designed to describe and evaluate specific dimensions of FISP. The first project focused on description of FISP, in terms of staff, clients, and services provided, as well as global measures of outcome. The second project addressed treatment adherence within FISP. The third focused on evaluating social validity. Unlike the individual subject design strategies (described in the next section), these projects did not provide detailed information relevant to the treatment of individuals (e.g., the modification or extension of interventions with a particular family), but, rather, outlined the main components of our project, its services, and their effectiveness.

Program Description and Evaluation

Unfortunately, little is known about the characteristics and effectiveness of the many agencies and programs nationwide which utilize behavioral interventions to treat maltreating families. To address this gap in the literature, Malinosky-Rummell, Eli, Warner, Ujcich, Carr, and Hansen (1991) conducted an archival program evaluation project to describe and evaluate FISP services.

The subjects in this evaluation were 45 physically abusive and neglectful parents and two additional maltreated children (who came to treatment without parents). Of the parents, 32 were mothers and 13 were fathers. Collectively, these parents had a total of 90 children (with an average of 2.59 per family) who also received services from FISP.

Independent measures included demographic and descriptive data regarding parents (e.g., age, gender, education, income, number of children, marital status, occupation, and history of maltreatment) and their children (e.g., age, gender, grade, placement, and custody status). Data on the following treatment variables were collected: whether the subjects were court-ordered for services, whether the spouse was also participating in treatment, and the type of treatment (e.g., parent training, home cleanliness, marital therapy). Data regarding the average and total number of therapists per client were also recorded.

A variety of dependent outcome measures were also examined: number of sessions conducted in the home, clinic, and school; court hearings (including those scheduled with the therapist present and those in which FISP recommendations were followed); type of termination; child placement and custody status at the end of treatment; and recidivism (including reports of maltreatment while in treatment as well as re-referral to CPS or to FISP for treatment).

A checklist was developed to record the variables of interest from the client charts. A separate information sheet was completed regarding demographic data on all therapists involved in FISP, including their year in graduate school, gender, age, degree, and years as a project therapist. Data collection involved reviewing client files and transcribing the necessary information onto the checklist. Good interrater reliability was demonstrated by having 29% of the files coded separately by an undergraduate research assistant

Of the 20 therapists who had worked for the project at the time of this evaluation, 75% were female. The average age of the therapists was 25.58 years ($SD = 2.28$) and they had an average of 3.13 years of graduate-level education ($SD = 1.55$). Therapists worked an average of 2.25 years on the project ($SD = 1.07$). The average number of therapists working for FISP per year was 7.50 ($SD = 1.52$). The average number of therapists working with each client was 1.70 ($SD = .46$). Therapists consulted with CPS in all cases, and often consulted with other community agencies as well, such as the court system, schools, and other psychological service agencies.

The children served by FISP during the time frame of the evaluation ranged in age from 0 to 17 (mean = 7.50, $SD = 4.55$), were predominantly white (92%), and the majority were male (58%). The parents ranged in age from 20 to 61 years (mean = 34.38, $SD = 9.10$), with a mean of 10.38 years of education ($SD = 1.45$); all were white, and the majority were female (69%). Parents were primarily married, unemployed caretakers with an average annual income of $9,371 ($SD = $5,595$). The primary reason for referral was physical abuse (60.8%), with neglect being the second most common referral issue (49%). The majority of clients had a documented history of physical abuse and/or neglect (physical abuse, 19.6%; neglect, 23.5%; both physical abuse and neglect, 29.4%); 29.4% also had a documented history of sex abuse within the family. More than half of the clients (56.6%) had a spouse or significant other involved in treatment. Only 5.7% of the clients had a spouse or partner who did not participate in treatment.

Most of the sessions (62%) were scheduled in the client's home. Clients spent an average of 11.39 months in treatment ($SD = 11.73$). Parent training in child-management and problem-solving skills served as the primary interventions in 81.1% and 71.7% of the cases, respectively. Additional treatment targets included hygiene (30.2%), safety and self-protection skills (30.2%), financial issues and budgeting skills (28.3%), school problems (28.3%), school placement issues (22.6%), home cleanliness (20.8%), marital problems (18.9%), nutrition (17.0%), prenatal care (11.3%), medical problems (7.5%), anger control (7.5%), and social skills training (1.9%). Several clients (13.2%) were referred to other agencies for additional services (e.g., for financial assistance). On the average clients attended 61.7% of scheduled home visits compared to 34.5% of sessions scheduled in the clinic.

Court orders for treatment existed for 22.6% of FISP clients. Of the 23 court hearings scheduled for all clients, FISP staff participated in all but one hearing. Furthermore, the court followed FISP recommendations in 73.9% of the cases.

With regard to recurrence of maltreatment, physical abuse was reported in 22.6% of the cases and neglect was reported in 3.8% of the cases during the course of treatment. Thirty-six percent of the clients dropped out of treatment against therapist recommendations. At the beginning of treatment, 22% of the children were in CPS custody and 18% were placed out of the home, compared to 18% and 19%, respectively, at the end of treatment. Twenty-one percent of the cases were later reopened by CPS, and 23% were re-referred to FISP for treatment.

The number of therapists at the time the case was opened (which was generally 1 or 2), significantly predicted 44.9% of the variance in total sessions attended and 65% of the variance in home visits attended. This increased effectiveness of having more than one therapist working with the family suggests that the costs of increased resources per family may be outweighed by the benefits of increased client participation in treatment. The number of children in the family significantly predicted 44.1% of the variance in physical abuse reported during treatment, suggesting that therapists working with maltreating parents of large numbers of children should recognize the potential for recurrent physical abuse, and should alter their assessment and treatment approaches accordingly. Based on the findings of this initial program evaluation, the influence of other factors that may play a role in treatment adherence was explored in a subsequent program evaluation study.

Treatment Adherence Evaluation

Session attendance, an essential component in clinical interventions, is believed to be poor with maltreating families; however, few studies have investigated the session attendance of maltreating families. Poor rates of session attendance have been indicated in FISP research (e.g., Malinosky-Rummell et al., 1991) and other research, including surveys of professionals (Hansen & Warner, 1994).

Warner, Malinosky-Rummell, Ellis, and Hansen (1990) examined client demographic characteristics and treatment variables of 31 maltreating parents in order to identity features associated with session attendance. All of the clients were white, and they averaged 33.4 years in age with 10.13 years of education. Seventy-five percent were female.

Comparisons were made to a group of 16 subjects without a history of maltreatment who were seeking services at the same outpatient treatment facility. These families sought outpatient treatment for a variety of issues involving their children. None of these subjects had a history of documented maltreatment. All clients were white and 94% were female. Their ages and years of education were unavailable.

Independent measures included the following client demographic variables: race, sex, age, education, employment status, number and age of children. Treatment variables, including court-ordering of services, removal of children from the home, and location of treatment (i.e., home versus clinic) were also examined. Demographic and treatment variables were examined in relation to the percentage of sessions attended by the client, calculated by dividing the number of sessions attended by the number of sessions scheduled.

A checklist was developed to record variables of interest from client charts in the maltreating group. Data collection involved reviewing client files. Every available file from FISP was used. Files from the nonmaltreating families seen through the general services program of the clinic were reviewed and were eliminated if the client had a history of maltreatment or was being seen for treatment which did not involve her or his children. In cases where general service files were eliminated, another file was selected randomly as a replacement. All sessions with general services clients were based in the clinic.

The mean percentage of sessions attended by the nonmaltreating clients was 82.1% ($SD = 15.7$). The mean percentage of sessions attended by maltreating clients, regardless of session site, was 67.4% ($SD = 22.4$), significantly lower than the rate for nonmaltreating clients. However, an interesting finding emerged when the influence of session site was examined for the maltreating group. The mean percentage of sessions attended in the home was 71.6% ($SD = 23.1$), which was not significantly different from the attendance of nonmaltreating families. The mean for clinic sessions was 61.8% ($SD = 30.2$), significantly lower than the rate for nonmaltreating families.

Examination of various demographic variables in the maltreating group provided valuable insight into factors associated with good session attendance. Level of education proved to be an influential variable related to session attendance for the maltreating group. FISP clients with more education (more than 11.5 years of school) had a significantly higher mean attendance rate of 77.5% ($SD = 20.0$) than the 61.1% rate ($SD = 22.3$) of less educated clients (who had less than 11.5 years of school). Younger clients (under 32 years old) had a significantly higher attendance rate (75.5%; $SD = 18.5$) than did clients over 32 years old (58.8%; $SD = 23.7$). This finding is in contrast to other studies, which have suggested that younger clients are more likely to be noncompliant, even if the services are court-ordered (e.g., Butler, Radia & Magnatta, 1994). However, our definition of "younger client" (i.e., less than 32 years of age), which was determined based on the average age of our clients (33.4 years), was slightly higher than that used in other studies (e.g., the mean age of "younger client" in the Butler et al. study was 27 years).

Interestingly, employment status (employed vs. unemployed), number of children (less than or equal to 2 vs. more than 2), court involvement (court order vs. no court order), and children removed from home (yes or no) were not significantly related to attendance. Multiple regression analyses revealed a four-variable model which significantly accounted for 30.6% of the variance: having sessions in the clinic, number of children, being married, and parental age demonstrated a negative relationship with attendance.

Court involvement was not as influential as initially expected. Court involvement was, however, positively related to clinic attendance. Perhaps the added effort required on the part of the client to attend sessions outside their homes can most effectively be elicited in the context of legal ramifications.

Social Validity Evaluation

An essential feature of intervention programs that has received little attention in the treatment of abuse and neglect is the social validity of the goals, procedures, and effects of intervention (Kazdin, 1977). Social validity can be examined from the perspective of the clients served, as well as from that of the other professionals in the community who collaborate with and benefit from the services provided by the treatment program. Clients may be more likely to adhere to—and subsequently benefit from—those aspects of an intervention they find most socially valid. Information on those features of the program that the other professionals in the community find most and least socially valid can contribute to the establishment of the most optimal multidisciplinary service provision, as services can be tailored to maximize their usefulness to the other professionals involved. A study of the social validity of FISP services was conducted by Warner, Ujcich, Ellis, Malinosky-Rummell, and Hansen (1992).

At the time of this evaluation there had been 25 FISP therapists. Like all FISP clients, parents and children participated in a comprehensive individualized behavioral assessment. Intervention programs were structured to meet the needs of the participants as indicated by the assessment results. Areas targeted for intervention included training to improve parenting skills (81.1% of clients), problem solving (71.9%), hygiene (30.2%), home safety (30.2%), budgeting/finances (28.3%), school problems (28.3%), and home cleanliness (20.8%). The length of treatment was based on client participation and needs (mean length of treatment was 11.39 months). The majority (61.9%) of sessions were held in the home, with the remainder in the clinic or in a school. As part of providing services to the families, therapists from FISP often worked collaboratively with professionals from other disciplines, such as CPS workers, judges, lawyers, and school counselors.

Although a total of 58 clients had been served by FISP at this time, not every client was available or eligible for participation. Clients who terminated with FISP prior to two years earlier were not asked to participate, as it was believed that the length of time since their contact with the project might affect their ability to provide an accurate evaluation of the services they received. Several of the eligible clients (15.5%) had moved out of the area, and several others (8.6%) could not be located. One eligible client declined to participate and one had died. A total of 15 clients participated in this study (25.9% of the total number of clients served by FISP). Ten of the fifteen participants were female. Other demographic characteristics (e.g., age, education, race, income) were also representative of FISP clientele.

The second group of subjects were eleven professionals in the community who had significant contact with the therapists and clients from FISP. Eight of the professionals (72.7%) were CPS workers. The other professionals included one judge, one prosecuting attorney, and one school counselor. The number of cases that they had collaborated on with FISP therapists ranged from 5 to 35 cases. Data from the professionals in the community were collected via a mail survey.

Data were collected on the social validity of three general areas: (1) usefulness of the formats of intervention; (2) usefulness of the skills involved in the intervention; and (3) overall satisfaction with the program, therapists, and goals and effectiveness of treatment.

A Social Validation Questionnaire (SVQ), based on a measure by Forehand and McMahon (1981), was developed for the study. Separate forms were created for clients (SVQ-C) and professionals (SVQ-P). A therapist involved with the family approached the parent and discussed the purpose of the study. If the parent expressed a desire to participate, the therapist provided the parent with a copy of the SVQ-C and an envelope. The parent was instructed to complete the SVQ-C and place it in the envelope. The therapist either waited or picked up the sealed envelope at a later date. If a parent had difficulty reading or comprehending the material in the questionnaire, a clinical aide or therapist reviewed the SVQ-C with them.

Parents rated all formats of intervention as useful to very useful, including therapist talking about a new skill, therapist demonstrating a new skill, practicing a skill with the therapist, homework assignments, and written materials. Practicing a skill with a therapist and receiving written material regarding skills were rated as most useful. Interestingly, practicing a skill with a child was the least useful.

The percentage of clients who worked on specific target areas and the ratings of the usefulness of the skills they learned in those areas were assessed. Paying attention to child's good behavior, rewarding good behavior, giving good commands, and learning time-out were the most common, with 85 to 95% of clients reporting that they received them. Interventions targeting more basic needs, such as home safety and cleanliness, nutrition, and personal hygiene, were rated by parents as most useful. Specific child management skills, especially time-out, were rated as less useful.

Client ratings of satisfaction with overall treatment and therapists were very positive. The goals established for treatment, the procedures used, the effectiveness of new skills, and therapist interest and concern for family were rated very positively. Therapist ability to teach new skills, preparation for sessions, and the overall rating for the therapists were lower, but still indicated satisfaction.

Professionals indicated that they were very satisfied overall with the services provided by FISP. More specifically, interagency collaboration and communication, FISP therapist involvement in court hearings, and the helpfulness of FISP reports were viewed as the most useful. Professionals also found the services provided by FISP to the clients to be very socially valid. The mean ratings were reduced somewhat by the lower ratings provided by the one school professional. Her slightly lower ratings might reflect the different goals held by the school system (e.g., homework completion, parent participation in school activities) as opposed to those held by the legal and social services agencies (e.g., safe home, children's basic needs met).

Overall, clients and professionals were very satisfied with the services provided by FISP. Clients generally indicated that they would recommend the project to a friend and believed that their therapists were interested in and concerned about their family. Lower satisfaction ratings for the format of treatment may have implications for treatment adherence and generalization. For example, one could speculate that parents who do not find it useful to "practice a new skill with a child" during a session may be less likely to utilize that skill outside of session. Subsequently, views of treatment effectiveness may be affected. If parents do not consistently use new skills, the potential for change in the target areas could be compromised, making the treatment appear less effective.

Behaviorally oriented parent training is often a major component in the treatment of maltreating families. Parents in this study rated the usefulness of one "critical" child management skill, time-out, as "neutral." Comments written on the questionnaires by the clients revealed that parents found time-out a difficult technique to implement. Therapists working with maltreating parents should be aware that time-out may not be viewed favorably by this population and attempt to address specific difficulties clients may have with implementing this potentially effective, nonphysical discipline technique. Research with maltreating parents (e.g., Kelley, Grace, & Elliott, 1990), as well as nonmaltreating parents (e.g., Frentz & Kelley, 1986; Heffer & Kelley, 1987), suggests that as practitioners we must be sensitive to the varying acceptability of behavioral treatment procedures such as time-out.

The results suggest that clients view certain formats and interventions as more useful than others. These views may affect treatment adherence and subsequent treatment effectiveness. Therapists may benefit from assessing the social validity of their interventions throughout therapy to determine potential areas of dissatisfaction and modify the formats and interventions as much as possible to meet the client's needs and treatment goals.

Examples of Single-Subject Designs

Individual subject designs were frequently used to evaluate the effectiveness of intervention procedures. Designs such as multiple-baselines across subjects or behaviors and A-B-A type designs replicated across clients were useful, practical, and efficient ways to evaluate the impact of our efforts. Clinically, all of our work had characteristics of individual subject designs, including evaluation prior, during, and after treatment, repeated measurement, and attempts to obtain objective and behavioral measures.

Parent-Training for High-Demand Situations

Available evidence suggests that many parents do not apply to new settings or problems the skills acquired during treatment (MacMillan, Olson, & Hansen, 1991). The results of poor generalization of parenting skills to the home is particularly critical for abusive populations given that the goal is to prevent the reemergence of abusive behavior. A reason for poor generalization of parenting skill use from the clinic to the home is that clinic training may not routinely involve skill training in realistic, stressful situations. Parenting skills may be mastered only during low-demand clinic assessments, and may not be rehearsed in high-demand situations which are more representative of the parent's natural environment.

Because directly observing parent performance in home or clinic discipline contexts is often difficult, utilization of analogue situations (e.g., adult actors) to present deviant child behavior can be helpful for assessment as well as intervention practice. Assessment of abusive parents in high-demand child-management situations is particularly important, given the connection between parental discipline efforts and physically abusive behavior (MacMillan et al., 1991).

MacMillan et al. (1991) examined the utility of a parent-training program which included training to facilitate generalization to high-demand child-management situations, and employed structured analogue assessments of parent discipline performance in high-demand situations. A single-subject A-B-B+C design (baseline, parent training, parent training plus generalization training) was used to evaluate the effects of intervention with three physically abusive parents. The use of parenting skills was observed during free-play assessments with the parent and child (in clinic and home) and two home-simulation assessments (low- and high-deviance) with clinical assistants enacting scripted child behaviors. Results supported the effectiveness of the parent-training package and the usefulness of the low- and high-demand home-simulation assessments. One client in particular demonstrated differences in performance between low- versus high-demand situations. Because the parent reported higher levels of assessment-evoked stress, anger, and anxiousness relative to other subjects, it is reasonable to expect her performance to evidence greater impairment, particularly in high-demand situations. Her performance improved in response to high-demand generalization training, while the other two achieved similar benefits from the standard parent-training components. The results suggest that a standard parent-training program can successfully improve parent performance in both low- and high-demand simulations of natural child-management situations. For some parents, specialized generalization training may further improve performance in high-demand situations.

Other Parent-Training Interventions

Other projects have been conducted to evaluate parent-training interventions. For example, in one project, videotape recordings of in-clinic and in-home parent–child interactions were used to provide feedback as well as to enhance the parents' relationship, especially as it related to child management (MacMillan, Olson, & Hansen, 1987). An abusive mother and her husband were prompted to identify appropriate and positive self and spouse behaviors in videotaped as well as live interactions of their own family. Results suggested that training in the detection of the targeted parent behaviors was associated with increases in their occurrence.

Illiteracy is not an uncommon problem in low-income, maltreating families. Combined with economic and familial stressors, illiteracy can make it difficult to develop or implement measures through which parents will monitor their own and their children's behavior. In a case study with an illiterate maltreating mother, Christopher, Malinosky-Rummell, and Hansen (1990), monitored the effectiveness of parent training using multiple repeated measures procedures, including (1) in-home observations of unprompted maternal praise; (2) observations of maternal and child behaviors during the Child's Game and Clean-Up procedures (Forehand & McMahon, 1981); (3) weekly reading of the Eyberg Child Behavior Inventory (ECBI; Eyberg & Ross, 1978) by the therapist with recording of oral responses of the parent. Eventually, a paper-and-pencil measure to chart implementation of a token/point system was implemented using symbols recognized by the parent. In addition, a posttreatment Parent Consumer Satisfaction Questionnaire (Forehand & McMahon, 1981) was read to the parent. ECBI scores demonstrated a substantial decrease in child behavior problems for the targeted child following intervention. This decrease coincided with an increase in unprompted maternal praise of the children, and increases in praise and attend statements. The mother's responses on the Parent Consumer Satisfaction Questionnaire indicated that she felt the target child's behavior had greatly improved, and she enjoyed the treatment program as well. At four-month follow-up, the mother not only demonstrated maintenance of her in-session praise and skill with the target child, she also demonstrated generalization of parenting skills (i.e., praise and attend statements) with her other child. The measures were efficient (i.e., brief), provided a variety of sources of information to evaluate progress, and were effectively used with a mother who was unable to read.

Problem-Solving Training

Problem-solving training provides a promising means for enhancing appropriate parental judgment with respect to child-care responsibilities and for increasing parental competence to deal effectively with daily stressors. A problem-solving intervention was evaluated with a multiply distressed, abusive and neglectful mother (MacMillan, Guevremont, & Hansen, 1988). Problem-solving skills were trained sequentially in a multiple-baseline across-skills design (i.e., training in generation of alternative solutions followed by training in effective solution planning). Training focused on improving judgments related to child-care problems and managing daily stress. Problem-solving training resulted in a substantial increase in generation of alternative solutions and in the quality of plans to implement solutions on both training and generalization vignettes.

Social insularity, negative affect, and self-reported stress, which appeared to compromise child-care abilities, were reduced as a result of problem-solving training. The daughter was returned to the mother's custody after training. Follow-up data indicated that the mother maintained most of the treatment gains for the five months following intervention. In addition, there was no evidence or report of maltreatment 21 months after the daughter's return to the home.

The improvement across the various outcome measures (i.e., social contacts, affect, anxiety/stress) with the acquisition of problem-solving skills was important and striking. Several factors may account for the success of the intervention. First, significant psychopathology, anger control problems, or disturbances in parent–child attachment was not evidenced on comprehensive screening. Second, the problem vignettes used for training were tailored to "real life" problems encountered by the mother rather than intuitively generated vignettes. Third, because the mother was of borderline intellectual functioning, training was extremely concrete, and modeling and rehearsal were extensively employed. Fourth, approximately half of the training sessions were conducted in the mother's home to enhance the likelihood of generalization. Finally, problem solving was designed specifically to enhance the mother's judgment and ability to deal successfully with multiple stressors.

Involving Children as Behavior Change Agents

It is often difficult to implement behavior change programs with maltreating parents. Common obstacles to treatment implementation are parental lack of skills and resources, noncompliance with treatment strategies, and a myriad of other problems (e.g., financial, interpersonal). Even when parental compliance to treatment suggestions within a clinic setting is achieved, competing contingencies may prevent generalization of treatment effect to home environments. Research and clinical literature on interventions with maltreating parents has emphasized the need to overcome obstacles to generalization and maintenance (Azar & Wolfe, 1989; Lundquist & Hansen, Chapter 19, this volume). Doepke et al (1988) demonstrated the use of children as behavior change agents to enhance generalization of treatment effects in a maltreating home. Subjects were a single mother and her five children (ages 2, 5, 7, 9, and 11). The mother had limited intellectual ability along with limited financial and social resources. She was referred and identified as abusive and neglectful by CPS. A severe and chronic lack of routine dental hygiene, identified as an area of neglect by both the children's schoolteachers and the CPS caseworker, was targeted for intervention. Prior to treatment, one child had extensive dental work for tooth decay and infection. An increase in positive maternal attention for appropriate child behavior was identified as the second goal. The design consisted of baseline, treatment, and maintenance phases for dental hygiene, and baseline and treatment phases for praise, with periodic measures of generalization. Treatment abruptly ended when the family moved. Contact was reinstated 10 months later, which allowed for one follow-up assessment of positive attention.

After initial intervention (i.e., direct instruction, modeling, rehearsal feedback, and prompting) with the mother failed, the children were incorporated into the procedures. Through the use of weekly individual and group contingencies, such as special treats or privileges, the older two children were taught to self-record toothbrushing by placing a check on a daily chart, and subsequently to remind their mother to deliver the stickers and remind the younger children to brush their teeth.

The mother was cooperative with initial attempts to teach her to praise appropriate child behavior, but there was little retention. The children were then included in the behavior change plan. Through the use of a structured "praise game" taught to the children and mother, in which the participants earned points for the frequency of praise statements, the children were utilized to model and prompt the use of appropriate praise statements. Daily practice in the "praise game" continued throughout the treatment phase, and the participants were taught to self-record frequency of praise statements during the game. Reliability of self-recording was assessed weekly. In addition, three months after the initiation of the praise game, a praise chart with four "praise statements" was posted on the refrigerator. The children were allowed to initial the chart on a daily basis if their mother used designated statements to praise behavior. Individual and group contingencies were used to teach the children to prompt their mother in the use of these statements. The frequency of the mother's praise statements, both within the context of the game and in other natural home sessions, was assessed.

Daily charts indicated that the rate of toothbrushing rapidly increased for each child, from zero to an average of two times daily. During the intervention, the children required no special dental attention. Daily practice of the "praise game" resulted in a significant increase in mother's praise statements both within the context of the game and in other natural home situations. Parent report and direct observation indicated improvement in the children's compliance and behavior.

PRACTICAL ISSUES IN IMPLEMENTATION AND EVALUATION OF SERVICES

A variety of practical details learned during the implementation and evalua- tion of FISP should be noted, as they may be applicable to other treatment pro- grams dealing with abusive and neglectful families. For example, coordination with other agencies (e.g., CPS, schools) is essential for providing informed, com- prehensive, and multidisciplinary services. In addition, the likelihood of duplica- tion of services to a family (e.g., child seen by school psychologist and FISP for behavioral problems) is decreased when services across agencies and profes- sionals are well coordinated. Prompt initial contact with the relevant CPS worker, followed by regular contact by phone or periodic written updates, facilitates com- munication. It is also helpful to clarify the goals of all parties (i.e., therapist, client, CPS workers) and to discuss with the client the therapist's distinction from and re- lationship with CPS.

Conducting sessions in the home can enhance session attendance (Warner et al., 1990) and program effectiveness (Wolfe & Wekerle, 1993). However, sending therapists into the homes of families who have a history of abuse can present a personal safety risk, especially for those programs like FISP, which are located in rural communities where houses may be in isolated areas with few if any neigh- bors. Having therapists work in pairs appears not only to increase the likelihood that clients will attend sessions (e.g., Malinosky-Rummell et al., 1991) but also in- creases personal safety. Furthermore, in FISP the initial home visit was not con- ducted until the therapist had discussed the case at length with a professional from the referring agency who was familiar with the family and home environ- ment and who identified any potential safety risks (e.g., no telephone in the home, a parent with a history of verbal or physical aggression toward professionals). In cases where safety was a concern, initial visits were scheduled in the clinic until a therapeutic relationship was established. Home visits were then arranged if and when the therapist and program director felt that the safety of FISP staff would not be compromised. It is also useful to have a centrally located logbook in which all home visits are recorded combined with a "safety check-in system," such that someone is always aware of the location of all home visits and when the therapist is expected to return. A mobile telephone, although an expensive acquisition, may be a worthwhile investment for treatment teams.

Aside from safety concerns, there are a variety of obstacles to providing ser- vices to this population, such as clients' lack of transportation to clinics and lim- ited financial resources and motivation. It is helpful if the presence of such issues can be identified early, ideally in the initial assessment phase, and addressed as quickly as possible. Efforts to decrease the influence of factors that can hinder treatment may help build client rapport and increase motivation. For example, by arranging to see clients in their home, the therapist has acknowledged the issue (e.g., lack of transportation, inconvenience of making the trip with children, prohibitive costs of public transportation) and increased the likelihood that the client will attend the sessions.

Attention has recently been directed toward the acceptability of treatment procedures to parents receiving treatment (e.g., Hansen & Warner, 1994; Kelley, Grace, & Elliott, 1990). Research is needed that examines the acceptability of various treatment procedures for maltreating parents and the conditions that may make procedures more or less acceptable. The more acceptable clients find the treatment, the more likely they may be to practice, use, and subsequently benefit from new skills. Program evaluation of FISP services suggests that maltreating parents may not view some of the more traditional child management techniques (e.g., time-out) very positively. Such views may affect client motivation to use the techniques.

Another potential obstacle to treatment is the fact that maltreating parents often do not identify themselves as having a problem and are usually not self-referred for evaluation or treatment (Kelly, 1983; Wolfe, 1988). It is not surprising, then, that recent research indicates that session attendance and homework completion are problems with maltreating families (e.g., Hansen & Warner, 1994; Warner et al., 1990). The variety of behaviors that comprise treatment adherence can be classified into three primary areas: (1) attendance, whether it is the home, clinic, or elsewhere; (2) participation with the session—the most complicated and least understood aspect of adherence; and (3) completion of assignments to be carried out outside of the session—that is, "homework." Session attendance includes not only coming to appointments but also arriving on time. Within-session adherence responses include talking about relevant topics, following session goals and procedures, and practicing new skills within the session. Adherence to homework assignments encompasses a wide variety of responses, such as accurately collecting data, self-monitoring, practicing skills, and otherwise implementing the treatment programs.

Professionals must be sensitive to the variety of factors that may contribute to noncompliance, such as inadequate instructions and rationale, lack of skills or motivation to perform the assignment, and competing contingencies that may reinforce noncompliance or punish compliance (Hansen & Warner, 1992; Lundquist & Hansen, Chapter 19, this volume). Use of strategies to improve attendance, as well as participation within and after the session (e.g., homework), are essential and should begin in the early phases of contact. Antecedent prompting strategies include attendance policies, additional stimuli (e.g., reminders), written commitments, and training in tasks assigned. Consequent strategies include reinforcement (e.g., praise), tangibles (e.g., clothing, movie tickets, money), and attention to nonadherence responses (e.g., open discussion). Combined antecedent and consequent strategies include contingency contracting and involving children in assignments to be carried out in the home. Results on the effectiveness of court orders, which may or may not specify positive (e.g., return of the child to the home) or negative (e.g., removal of the child from the home) consequences for participation in assessment or therapy, have been inconclusive. Effectiveness of other procedures to enhance compliance has not been empirically tested with maltreating families (Hansen & Warner, 1992, 1994).

Therapists who work with physically abusive and neglectful families can expect to have interactions with the legal system. These interactions can be with the local child protective services agency, law enforcement officials, lawyers, or the judicial system (Hansen & Warner, 1992). There are generally two areas of legal involvement regarding child maltreatment. The first, the protection of children, is typically addressed through civil procedures. The second, criminal prosecution of the child abuser, occurs when the abuse is severe. When working with a family, it is important for practitioners to confine their part in the legal process to either investigator, evaluator, or therapist (Melton & Limber, 1989). Attempting more than one role may result in a conflict of interest or require a breach of confidentiality that could be detrimental to the therapeutic relationship (Hansen & Warner, 1992). Clinicians working with maltreating families should have a working knowledge of and cooperative relationship with the local court and child protective services system and should be prepared to participate in the judicial process. The active involvement of FISP staff in court hearings and the high percentage of FISP recommendations followed by the courts emphasizes the effectiveness that these systems attributed to FISP.

The evaluation of FISP highlighted several recommendations for therapists working with maltreating families: (1) conduct regular home visits; (2) work in therapist pairs; (3) plan to provide a broad range of therapeutic interventions, including training in child-management skills, problem-solving skills, hygiene, safety, and financial issues, as well as school intervention; (4) consider using children as agents of behavioral change; (5) collaborate and communicate frequently with legal and child protective systems; and (6) be prepared to make recommendations regarding child custody and to provide court reports and/or testimony about this information (Malinosky-Rummell et al., 1991). Actively addressing issues such as treatment adherence, generalization, and social (functional) validity are also critical for successful intervention.

CONCLUSION

Child abuse and neglect is a complex, multidimensional problem that requires comprehensive individualized treatment. Thus, research on the effectiveness of such intervention approaches can be very difficult. The present chapter described the approach taken by one of many treatment programs in the United States. Efforts were made to use a scientist-practitioner approach: assessment and treatment procedures were based on the available empirical literature; attempts were made to develop and evaluate assessment procedures to fill gaps that existed in the pool of available measures; treatment approaches were evaluated by therapists using a variety of measures; program evaluation and single-subject procedures were used to examine the effectiveness of the approaches used. We learned much from our effort.

The FISP clients were primarily white, unemployed, low-income, female caretakers who had not graduated from high school. The clients had an average of more than two young children, and the majority of clients had a spouse or significant other involved in treatment as well. The clients presented with multiple problems, including physical abuse and neglect, as well as sexual abuse. The therapists serving these clients were typically M.A. level female clinical psychology graduate students in their mid-20s. Primary intervention strategies included parent training in child-management skills and problem-solving training. Other focuses of treatment included hygiene, safety, financial issues, school problems, home cleanliness, marital problems, and more. Active consultation with other agencies, such as school systems, legal systems, child protective services, and other mental health facilities, also comprised a substantial part of treatment activity. The wide range of interventions used highlights the extensive expertise needed to treat these families.

The available research literature on the evaluation of the treatment of maltreating families often fails to address the complexity and comprehensiveness of the existing intervention programs. We have attempted to illustrate this through a description of a treatment program for physically abusive and neglectful families. Use of existing measures and the development of standardized and client-specific measures were essential for providing and evaluating clinical services. We found that two methods, a program evaluation approach and individual subject designs, were particularly valuable for understanding and evaluating our treatment efforts. The procedures and projects described in this chapter provide a variety of support for the effectiveness of the individualized behavior intervention program and elucidate the difficulties associated with treating these families.

ACKNOWLEDGMENTS

The authors wish to acknowledge the efforts of the many therapists who participated in the project, with special thanks to Virginia MacMillan DeRoma, Jeanette Smith Christopher, James Ellis, Robin Malinosky-Rummell, Ralph Olson, and Kim Ujcich. We also wish to acknowledge the efforts of the Child Protective Services workers who facilitated our efforts, especially Vicki Lemine, and the many families who participated and let us into their homes and lives.

REFERENCES

Abidin, R. R (1986). *Parenting Stress Index* (2nd ed.). Charlottesville, VA: Pediatric Psychology Press.

Achenbach, T. M. (1991). *Manual for the Child Behavior Checklist/4-18 and 1991 Profile.* Burlington, VT: University of Vermont.

Azar, S. T., & Rohrbeck, C. A (1986). Child abuse and unrealistic expectations: Further validation of the Parent Opinion Questionnaire. *Journal of Consulting and Clinical Psychology, 54,* 867–868.

Azar, S. T., & Wolfe, D. A (1989). Child abuse and neglect. In E. J. Mash & R. Barkley (Eds.), *Treatment of childhood disorders* (pp. 451–489). New York: Guilford Press.

Barlow, D. H., & Hersen, M. (1984). *Single case experimental designs: Strategies for studying behavior change* (2nd ed.). New York: Pergamon.

Butcher, J. N., Dahlstrom, W. G., Graham, J. R, Tellegen, A, & Kaemmer, B. (1989). *Minnesota Multiphasic Personality Inventory–2 (MMPI-2): Manual for administration and scoring.* Minneapolis: University of Minnesota Press.

Butler, S. M., Radia, N., & Magnatta, M. (1994). Maternal compliance to court-ordered assessment in cases of child maltreatment. *Child Abuse & Neglect, 18,* 203–210.

Christopher, J. S., Malinosky-Rummell, R., and Hansen, D. J. (1990, November). *Monitoring effectiveness of parent training: A case example with an illiterate maltreating mother.* Presented at the meeting of the Association for the Advancement of Behavior Therapy, San Francisco.

Crimmins, D. B., Bradlyn, A. S., St Lawrence, J. S., & Kelly, J. A. (1984). A training technique for improving the parent–child interaction skills of an abusive-neglectful mother. *Child Abuse & Neglect, 8,* 533–539

Derogatis, L. R. (1983). *SCL-90-R: Administration, scoring, and procedures manual–II.* Towson, MD: Clinical Psychometric Research.

DeRoma, V. M., & Hansen, D. J. (1994, November). *Development of the Parental Anger Inventory.* Presented at the meeting of the Association for the Advancement of Behavior Therapy, San Diego, CA.

Doepke, K. J., Watson-Perczel, M., & Hansen, D. J. (1988, November). *Modification of an abusive and neglectful home environment: Children as behavior change agents.* Presented at the meeting of the Association for the Advancement of Behavior Therapy, New York.

Eyberg, S. M., & Robinson, E. A. (1981). *Dyadic Parent–Child Interaction Coding System: A manual* (Ms. No. 2582). San Rafael, CA: Social and Behavioral Sciences Documents, Select Press.

Eyberg, S. M., & Ross, A. W. (1978). Assessment of child behavior problems: The validation of a new inventory. *Journal of Clinical Child Psychology, 7,* 113–116.

Forehand, R., & McMahon, R. (1981). *Helping the noncompliant child: A clinician's guide to parent training.* New York: Guilford Press.

Frentz, C., & Kelley, M. L. (1986). Parents' acceptance of reductive treatment methods: The influence of problem severity and perception of child behavior. *Behavior Therapy, 17,* 75–81.

Hansen, D. J., Conaway, L. P., & Christopher, J. S. (1990). Victims of child physical abuse. In R. T. Ammerman & M. Hersen (Eds.), *Treatment of family violence: A sourcebook* (pp. 17–49). New York: Wiley.

Hansen, D. J., & MacMillan, V. M. (1990). Behavioral assessment of child abusive and neglectful families: Recent developments and current issues. *Behavior Modification, 14,* 255–278.

Hansen, D. J., Pallotta, G. M., Christopher, J. S., Conaway, R. L., & Lundquist, L. M. (1995). The Parental Problem-Solving Measure: Further evaluation with maltreating and nonmaltreating parents. *Journal of Family Violence, 10,* 319–336.

Hansen, D. J., Pallotta, G. M., Tishelman, A. C., Conaway, L. P., & MacMillan, V. M. (1989). Parental problem-solving skills and child behavior problems: A comparison of physically abusive, neglectful, clinic, and community families. *Journal of Family Violence, 4,* 353–368.

Hansen, D. J., & Warner, J. E. (1992). Child physical abuse and neglect. In R. T. Ammerman & M. Hersen (Eds.), *Assessment of family violence: A clinical and legal sourcebook* (pp. 123–147). New York: Wiley.

Hansen, D. J., & Warner, J. E. (1994). Treatment adherence of maltreating families: A survey of professionals regarding prevalence and enhancement strategies. *Journal of Family Violence, 9,* 1–19.

Heffer, R., & Kelley, M. L. (1987). Mother's acceptance of behavioral interventions for children: The influence of parent race and income. *Behavior Therapy, 18,* 153–163.

Kanner, A. D., Coyne, J., Schaefer, C., & Lazarus, R. S. (1981). Comparison of two modes of stress measurement: Daily hassles and uplifts versus major events. *Journal of Behavioral Medicine, 4,* 1–39.

Kazdin, A. E. (1977). Assessing the clinical or applied importance of behavior change through social validation. *Behavior Modification, 1,* 427–452.

Kelley, M. L., Grace, N., & Elliott, S. N. (1990). Acceptability of positive and punitive discipline methods: Comparisons among abusive, potentially abusive, and nonabusive parents. *Child Abuse & Neglect, 14,* 219–226.

Kelly, J. A (1983). *Treating child-abusive families:Intervention based on skills-training principles.* New York: Plenum Press.

Locke, H. J., & Wallace, K. M. (1959). Short marital adjustment and prediction tests: Their reliability and validity. *Journal of Marriage and Family Living, 21,* 251–255.

Lutzker, J. R. (1984). Project 12-Ways: Treating child abuse and neglect from an ecobehavioral perspective. In R. F. Dangel and R. A. Polster (Eds.), *Parent training* (pp. 260–297). New York: Guilford Press.

Lutzker, J. R., Wesch, D., & Rice, J. M. (1984). A review of Project 12-Ways: An ecobehavioral approach to the treatment and prevention of child abuse and neglect. *Advances in Behavior Research and Therapy, 6,* 63–74.

MacMillan, V. M., Guevremont, D. C., & Hansen, D. J. (1988). Problem-solving training with a multiply distressed abusive and neglectful mother: Effects on social insularity, negative affect, and stress. *Journal of Family Violence, 3,* 313–326.

MacMillan, V. M., Olson, R. L., & Hansen, D. J. (1987). *Facilitating the maintenance of relationship building skills in a parent training program for a physically abusive mother and her husband.* Presented at the Rivendell Conference of Clinical Practitioners, Memphis, TN.

MacMillan, V. M., Olson, R. L., & Hansen, D. J. (1988). *The development of an anger inventory for use with maltreating parents.* Presented at the meeting of the Association for the Advancement of Behavior Therapy, New York.

MacMillan, V. M., Olson, R. L., & Hansen, D. J. (1991). Low and high deviance analogue assessment of parent-training with physically abusive parents. *Journal of Family Violence, 6,* 279–301.

Malinosky-Rummell, R, Ellis, J. T., Warner, J. E., Ujcich, K., Carr, R. E., & Hansen, D. J. (1991, November). *Individualized behavioral intervention for physically abusive and neglectful families: An evaluation of the Family Interaction Skills Project.* Presented at the meeting of the Association for the Advancement of Behavior Therapy, New York.

Melton, G. B., & Limber, S. (1989). Psychologists' involvement in cases of child maltreatment. *American Psychologist, 44,* 1225–1233.

Milner, J. S. (1986). *The Child Abuse Potential Inventory: Manual* (2nd ed.). Webster, NC: PSYTEC.

Milner, J. S. (1994). Assessing physical child abuse risk: The Child Abuse Potential Inventory. *Clinical Psychology Review, 14,* 547–583

O'Dell, S. L., Tarler-Benlolo, L., & Flynn, J. M. (1979). An instrument to measure knowledge of behavioral principles as applied to children. *Journal of Behavior Therapy and Experimental Psychiatry, 10,* 29–34.

Posavac, E. J., & Carey, R. G. (1992). *Program evaluation: Methods and case studies* (4th ed.). Englewood Cliffs, NJ: Prentice Hall.

Robin, A. L, & Foster, S. L. (1989). *Negotiating parent-adolescent conflict: A behavioral-family systems approach.* New York: Guilford Press.

Roehling, P. V., & Robin, A. L. (1986). Development and validation of the Family Beliefs Inventory: A measure of unrealistic beliefs among parents and adolescents. *Journal of Consulting and Clinical Psychology, 54,* 693–697.

Sarason, I. G., Johnson, J. H., Siegel, J. M. (1978). Assessing the impact of life change: Development of the Life Experiences Survey. *Journal of Consulting and Clinical Psychology, 46,* 932–946.

Scott, W. O., Baer, G., Christoff, K. A., & Kelly, J. A. (1984). The use of skills training procedures in the treatment of a child-abusive parent. *Journal of Behavioral Therapy and Experimental Psychiatry, 15,* 329–336.

Smith, J. M., Conaway, R. L., Smith, G. M., & Hansen, D. J. (1988, November). Evaluation of a problem-solving measure for use with physically abusive and neglectful parents. Present at the meeting of the Association for the Advancement of Behavior Therapy, New York

Spanier, G. B. (1976). Measuring dyadic adjustment: New scales for assessing the quality of marriage and similar dyads. *Journal of Marriage and the Family, 38,* 15–28.

Straus, M. A. (1979). Measuring intrafamily conflict and violence: The Conflict Tactics (CT) Scales. *Journal of Marriage and the Family, 41,* 75–88.

Tertinger, D. A, Greene, B. F., & Lutzker, J. R. (1984). Home safety: Development and validation of one component of an ecobehavioral treatment for abused and neglected children. *Journal of Applied Behavior Analysis, 2,* 159–174.

Wahler, R. (1980). The insular mother: Her problems in parent child treatment. *Journal of Applied Behavior Analysis, 13,* 207–219.

Warner, J. E., Malinosky-Rummell, R., Ellis, J. T., & Hansen, D. J. (1990, November). *An examination of demographic and treatment variables associated with session attendance of maltreating families.* Presented at the annual conference of the Association for the Advancement of Behavior Therapy, San Francisco.

Warner, J. E., Ujcich, K, Ellis, J. T., Malinosky-Rummell, R, & Hansen, D. J. (1992). *Social validity of an individualized behavioral intervention program for physically abusive and neglectful families: Further evaluation of the Family Interaction Skills Project.* Presented at the meeting of the Association for the Advancement of Behavior Therapy, Boston.

Watson-Perczel, M., Lutaker, J. R., Greene, B. F., & McGimpsey, B. J. (1988). Assessment and modification of home cleanliness among families adjudicated for child neglect. *Behavior Modification, 12,* 57–81.

Wesch, D., & Lutzker, J. R. (1991). A comprehensive 5-year evaluation of Project 12-Ways: An ecobehavioral program for treating and preventing child abuse and neglect. *Journal of Family Violence, 6,* 17–35.

Wolfe, D. A. (1988). Child abuse and neglect. In E. J. Mash & L. G. Terdal (Eds.), *Behavioral assessment of childhood disorders* (2nd ed., pp. 627–669). New York: Guilford Press.

Wolfe, D. A., Edwards, B. E., Manion, I., & Koverola, C. (1988). Early intervention for parents at risk for child abuse and neglect: A preliminary investigation. *Journal of Consulting and Clinical Psychology, 56,* 40–47.

Wolfe, D. A., Fairbank, J. A., Kelly, J. A., & Bradlyn, A. S. (1983). Child abusive parents' physiological responses to stressful and non-stressful behavior in children. *Behavioral Assessment, 5,* 363–371.

Wolfe, D. A. & Wekerle, C. (1993). Treatment strategies for child physical abuse and neglect: A critical progress report. *Clinical Psychology Review, 13,* 473–500.

7

Integration of Research and Treatment

DAVID KOLKO

This chapter seeks to promote the integration of research and treatment practices in the area of child abuse and neglect. By encouraging this conceptual and practical rapprochement, it is hoped that the knowledge base in the area of child maltreatment can be expanded and made more relevant. A primary objective is to describe areas that may benefit from further empirical attention in clinical practice. As background, I will summarize recent literature describing or evaluating interventions and programs in the areas of sexual abuse, physical abuse, various forms of neglect, psychological maltreatment, and exposure to family violence. Of course, there may be considerable overlap among these subtypes. Certainly, progress is needed in further articulating clinical and therapeutic characteristics and the context in which treatment occurs. There are several excellent sources for gaining a more comprehensive perspective on the treatment outcome literature and details of relevant studies along with insightful recommendations for future work in each area (see Becker et al., 1995; Finkelhor & Berliner, 1995; Lutzker & Campbell, 1994; Oates & Bross, 1995; Wolfe, 1994).

Across all forms of child maltreatment, there is increasing attention to understanding the developmental sequelae of child abuse and identifying areas requiring further attention. As reviewed by Finkelhor (1995), developmental concepts have been applied to a traumatagenic model of child sexual abuse, highlighting the importance of understanding the developmental context of both the risks for and the effects of victimization. The first concerns the study of variables that increase a child's risk for abuse and neglect and the second reflects the developmental impact of increased risk for abuse and neglect. Finkelhor (1995) provides a nice summary of the manifestations of the effects of abuse at different developmental stages and their implications for both research and treatment in the area. The developmental approach is important to keep in mind as primary findings regarding treatment are

DAVID KOLKO • University of Pittsburgh Medical Center, Western Psychiatric Institute and Clinic, Pittsburgh, Pennsylvania 15213.

Handbook of Child Abuse Research and Treatment, edited by Lutzker. Plenum Press, New York, 1998.

interpreted and directions for future work discussed. Recent research findings regarding the evaluation and outcome of treatment first will be reviewed.

PRIMARY RESEARCH FINDINGS

Overview of Status of Treatment Research

Several reviews in different areas have documented research studies on treatment or intervention in the area of child sexual abuse (Beutler, Williams, & Zetzer, 1994; Finkelhor & Berliner, 1995) and child physical abuse (Kolko, 1996b; Oates & Bross, 1995; Wolfe, 1994), with a few recent reviews dealing with neglect (DePanfilis, 1996; Gaudin, 1993; Gaudin, Wodarski, Arkinson, & Avery, 1991) and exposure to violence (Peled & Edleson, 1995). Work in the area of child sexual and physical abuse has emphasized child and parent applications, respectively, though much more empirical work has been done in the area of child sexual abuse. Treatment of sexual abuse has been directed toward such diverse problems as hypersexuality and sexual behavior problems, fear, anxiety, and depression, dysfunctional attributions, and social or interpersonal difficulties. With the exception of sexual behavior, many of the same difficulties have been targeted during treatment of these other forms of maltreatment. The long-term effects of sexual abuse and physical abuse, in particular, support the need for intervention and follow-up (cf., Green, 1993; Malinosky-Rummell & Hansen, 1993).

It is important to bear in mind that the empirical literature examining treatment is quite limited in that many treatment outcome studies are not controlled or carefully conducted experiments. Although most studies have reported quasi-experimental designs, a few have used experimental designs. Clearly, most reports are descriptive in nature and may include attention to certain methodologic or empirical characteristics (e.g., pre/post measures, comparison or control group, follow-up, random assignment). Still, several findings have been described regarding child treatment of child sexual abuse victims and parent treatment in the area of physical abuse. Studies also have varied in several parameters, including the age ranges of the clients (children vs. adolescents), type of treatment approach (cognitive-behavioral treatment, or CBT, vs. psychoeducation), and format of treatment (group vs. individual therapy), among other treatment characteristics.

Individual Child Treatment

Given children's diverse needs and characteristics, existing direct services for children have varied along a continuum of care ranging from minimal outpatient visits to intensive treatment in different contexts. For example, individual child therapy in sexual abuse has been directed toward minimizing symptoms in multiple areas, such as traumatic stress, dissociation and anger, depression and anxiety, and sexual concerns (Lanktree & Briere, 1995). Level of improvement in these domains has actually varied with time, the latter symptoms requiring more extensive treatment (one year) before improvements were realized. Other forms of individual treatment also report improvements in children's behavior problems (Sullivan, Scanlan, Brookhouser, & Schulte, 1992).

Individual treatment research in physical abuse has been limited to studies of specific behavioral and social learning procedures directed toward improving the preschool physically abused child's peer relations and social adjustment using peer social initiation techniques designed to encourage social overtures to peers (Fantuzzo, Stovall, Schachtel, Goins, & Hall, 1987). This intervention has been found superior to adult initiations in improving the children's social adjustment and peer initiations (Davis & Fantuzzo, 1989; Fantuzzo, Jurecic, Stovall, Hightower, & Goins, 1988), although both interventions were somewhat limited in overall efficacy. Interestingly, withdrawn children responded better to peer sessions, whereas aggressive children showed an increase in negative behavior in response to peers (Davis & Fantuzzo, 1989; Fantuzzo et al., 1987, 1988). These studies would be enhanced by having follow-up assessments of program maintenance and an evaluation of the impact on recidivism. Greater attention to the child's developmental competence seems warranted (Wolfe, Edwards, Manion, & Koverola, 1988).

Group Treatment

Group therapy studies are common in the area of sexual abuse (Sinclair, Larzclere, Paine, Jones, Graham, & Jones, 1995), but have not been done in the area of physical abuse. With sexually abused children, group discussions of abusive experiences, support, and suggestions regarding prevention and protection appear to be effective in reducing behavior problem severity (e.g., conduct problems, attention problems/immaturity, anxiety, withdrawal) and both the overall intensity and range of problem behavior, relative to controls (McGain & McKinzey, 1995). The improvements found in externalizing problems, especially aggression, are notable, but are qualified by the absence of repeated measures analyses. In another experimental study (Berliner & Saunders, 1995), structured CBT groups have resulted in several gains (e.g., amelioration of anxiety, fear, depression, traumatic effects, sexual behavior, internalizing symptoms), but were not improved by the addition of a brief stress inoculation and gradual exposure component designed to minimize fear and anxiety. The rigor of this study deserves mention (e.g., monitoring of treatment integrity), but it is possible that most patients' levels of fear and anxiety were not substantial prior to treatment.

Studies of individual or group child treatment are rare in other areas (e.g., neglect, exposure) where such services often are incorporated in multicomponent or multimodal studies. An exception is the work by Jaffe and colleagues (Jaffe, Wilson, & Wolfe, 1986, 1988; Jaffe, Wolfe, & Wilson, 1990) showing that witnessing children may be likely to learn that violence is an appropriate form of conflict resolution, among other studies suggesting the adverse impact of exposure (Fantuzzo et al., 1991). Jaffe et al. (1988) described the initial use and benefit of a group program (the Child Witnesses of Wife Abuse [CWWA]) that combines psychoeducation about spouse abuse and cognitive–behavioral exercises designed to teach prosocial conflict resolution and appropriate attitudes about wife abuse. Indeed, they documented pre/post improvements showing that children had a better understanding of the dynamics of wife abuse and showed improvements in safety skill development and an increase in positive impressions of their parents following group training. However supportive, these findings are limited by the absence of a control or comparison group, and of symptom measures. As reported by Peled and Edleson (1995), other changes following training have been found in the content of participants' responses to semistructured interviews (e.g., feelings or thoughts about the group, special experiences, changes noticed, home influences), among other areas targeted by the group, such as definitions of violence, expression of feelings, sharing of personal experiences, self-esteem.

A more recent experimental evaluation of the CWWA program with preadolescents showed greater improvements in attitudes about and responses to anger situations, and a sense of responsibility for parents and the violence that occurred in their homes in treated vs. control children (Wagar & Rodway, 1995). Of course, such results did not include ratings of child behavior or parent/family functioning, or a follow-up assessment of the maintenance of treatment gains. Other skills training components suggested to enhance program outcome could be easily included in this program (e.g., social skills).

Other Child Treatment Programs

In the area of physical abuse, treatments directed toward children have been described as part of day and residential treatment programs incorporating multiple therapeutic activities (e.g., learning) and modalities (e.g., family counseling). For example, intensive group-based treatment and developmental programming, with other family services, has been associated with several improvements (e.g., perceived cognitive competence, peer acceptance, maternal acceptance, and developmental scores on standardized measures), relative to a control group (Culp, Little, Letts, & Lawrence, 1991). A similar program, Kempe Early Education Project Serving Abused Families (KEEPSAFE), that incorporates a therapeutic preschool and home visitation for young sexually or physically abused children has found improvements in general intellectual functioning and receptive language by discharge one year later (Oates, Gray, Schweitzer, Kempe, & Harmon, 1995), with several children entering regular classrooms. Other programs for young maltreated children and their families incorporate multiple services for children (developmental milieu), parents (individual therapy), and families (Ghuman, 1993). Programs to address the problem of neglect generally target parental behavior and functioning, and, thus, infrequently describe the role of child-directed treatment strategies (see Wolfe, 1994).

Individual and Group Parent Training-Treatment

In physical abuse, parent training in positive/nonviolent child management practices, anger-control skills, or stress management techniques is one of the most common and effective treatment approaches (see National Academy of Sciences, 1993; Wolfe & Wekerle, 1993). Programs that combine these elements report improvements in both parent (e.g., child abuse potential, parental depression) and child (e.g., behavior problems) targets (Wolfe et al., 1988). Other cognitive–behavioral applications for parents conducted in a group format have reported positive outcomes in terms of anger management, communication, and problem-solving skills (Acton & During, 1992; Nurius, Lovell, & Edgar, 1988; Whiteman, Fanshel, &

Grundy, 1987), although these studies suffer from certain methodological limitations, such as the lack of a comparison group.

A related short-term group for parents of sexually abused children focused on encouraging disclosure and understanding of guilt and anger in the context of a supportive environment and providing educational information regarding parenting effectiveness and behavior modification (Winton, 1990). After participating in the group, parents reported reductions in certain child dysfunctional behaviors (e.g., fear, neurotic behavior, sexual behavior), but not in externalizing or social competence problems or in level of parenting stress. Parents' subjective ratings suggested that they learned coping skills and became more confident as parents. The possible confound due to providing parallel treatment for the children and the absence of a comparison group suggest the need for more rigorous evaluation of the impact of group treatment with parents.

Parallel Child and Parent Treatment

In one of the few clinical trials with sexually abused preschoolers, Cohen and Mannarino (1996) found that cases randomly assigned to individual child and parent cognitive–behavioral therapy (CBT; see Cohen & Mannarino, 1993) had fewer problems on measures of internalizing symptoms, home problems, and sexual behavior problems at posttreatment, with no differences in externalizing symptoms or social competence, than those assigned to nondirective-supportive treatment (NST).

Fewer cases were removed from treatment in CBT (0) than NST (6). The study is noteworthy for several positive features, such as the use of a therapist crossover design, report of client satisfaction with both protocols, inclusion of parents and children in parallel treatment, and application of abuse-specific measures. It also clearly shows that younger children, like their parents, can profit from CBT and learn self-management skills.

Novel applications in sexual abuse have also examined CBT with nonoffending mothers and their abused preschool children (Stauffer & Deblinger, 1996), where changes in parent practices and child sexual behavior have been found after services and have been maintained by 3-month follow-up. There was a high level of satisfaction with the helpfulness of treatment (95%), but also a high level of dropout (44%).

A related study evaluated the short-term treatment of physically abused, school-aged children and their offending parents/families (Kolko, 1996). This study compared the outcome of 55 cases who were randomly assigned to individual child and parent cognitive–behavioral therapy (CBT) or family therapy (FT) with those who received routine community services (RCS). Measures of child, parent, and family dysfunction and adjustment were both collected from participants and supplemented with official social service records to evaluate the efficacy of treatment through one-year follow-up. Relative to RCS, CBT and FT were associated with improvements in child-to-parent violence and child externalizing behavior, parental distress and abuse risk, and family conflict and cohesion. All three conditions reported several improvements across time (e.g., child depression, parent management). One parent participant each in CBT and FT and three in RCS had engaged in another incident of physical maltreatment by the end of follow-up. No differences between CBT and FT were observed on consumer satisfaction or maltreatment risk ratings at termination. Such provide additional support for the continued development and evaluation of individual and family treatments involving child victims of physical abuse.

Multimodal Family Treatment

In sexual abuse, multimodal treatment in one agency (individual, group, parent/family work) has had an impact on aggression and social behavior, sexualized behavior, and maternal and family functioning, but not on depression or self-esteem (Friedrich, Luecke, Beilke, & Place, 1992). Other forms of family treatment have been evaluated in recent experimental comparisons with sexually abused children. Family/network meetings dealing with multiple issues (e.g., communication, protection, marital problems) with or without child/family groups (e.g., information on social development, self-protection, secrecy, parental response) have been found similarly effective on standardized measures of child outcomes (e.g., children's health and behavior, child depression, self-concept), but not on children's reports of their own behavior or self-concept, or on teachers' reports of symptoms. Clinicians' ratings following treatment reflected comparable percentages of cases classified with good, moderately good, or little or no improvement. However, clinicians' ratings revealed some superiority for the combined condition on several treatment aims (e.g., child sharing painful feelings and having more positive self-concept, family perception of child's needs). A high percentage of children saw group work as a positive experience (71%) and as helpful in preventing further abuse (78%). Although the inclusion of offenders in services is a new practice, the absence of outcome data (i.e., means) for primary measures or treatment integrity measures precludes clear interpretation of the findings.

In-Home, Family-Based Services—Ecological, Contextual, and Multisystemic

Several interventions directed at the more global or contextual risk factors associated with abuse have been evaluated, though most do not include experimental designs or measures. In-home, family-based services, such as Homebuilders, have reported improvements in family functioning (e.g., problem behaviors, communication skills), but without comparison data in some cases (Amundson, 1989; Whittaker, Kinney, Tracy, & Booth, 1990). Indeed, some comparison data do not favor family preservation services over routine services in reducing child placements following the termination of services (Nelson, 1990).

Brunk, Henggeler, and Whelan (1987) applied a multisystemic approach to target problems in various systems affecting the family using services; this approach emphasizes skills training in parent–child interaction, and parental control strategies. Improvements were found in these domains and other areas (child behavior) relative to parent training. In another treatment outcome study, family casework using behavioral techniques (modeling, reinforcement) and play therapy was conducted to alter individual behavior and family interactions (Nicol et al., 1988). These findings, however, were somewhat qualified by the absence of clear targets for certain conditions (Nicol et al., 1988), follow-up information (Brunk et al., 1987; Nicol et al., 1988), and minimal treatment conditions (Brunk et al., 1987). Improvements were reported in family coercion, but not in positive behavior. Subsequent evidence suggests that improvements in family functioning are sometimes difficult to achieve with more violent families (Ayoub, Willett, & Robinson, 1992; Willett, Ayoub, & Robinson, 1991).

The Project 12-Ways program (Lutzker, 1990) has documented multiple gains in various areas (e.g., interactions, child management training, social support, assertion training, job training, home safety, and finances training) following individualized home-based services using various skills training methods with families in abuse or neglect. Improvements in parent-identified goals and reduced reabuse rates relative to comparison cases have been reported (Lutzker & Rice, 1987), but maintenance of reduced rates has not always been found (Wesch & Lutzker, 1991). Lutzker and Campbell (1994) nicely articulate the collective evidence supporting the use of structured assessment and training procedures to modify individualized concerns related to abuse or neglect (e.g., environmental hazards, child illnesses). Recent applications of Project 12-Ways highlight the variability in family outcomes following training. One case in which multiple targets reflecting diverse parenting skills and a few child behaviors (e.g., positive and negative response, play) responded well to specialized in-home training, but another case was only minimally successful (Greene, Norman, Searle, Daniels, & Lubeck, 1995). A significant asset of this approach is the use of objective behavior measures designed to facilitate training and evaluation.

An extension of this program, Project SafeCare, provides specific services to families with young children (birth to age 5) adjudicated or at-risk for abuse or neglect (e.g., health and physical care, safety and accident prevention, parent–child relationships). Initial reports have evaluated the efficacy of using videotaped training or in-home counselors to identify and modify environmental and health-related risks (Taub, Kessler, & Lutzker, 1995) and to promote positive parent–child interactions (Bigelow, Kessler, & Lutzker, 1995). These programs are noteworthy for their content validity based on questionnaires sent to and completed by experts, the simplified checklist format of specific parental behaviors, and the use of training routines that promote behavioral competence. A strong emphasis of the program is its evaluation of the observations of both child (e.g., smiling, verbal, imitations) and parent behavior (e.g., looking, touch, play) that are likely to enhance the quality of family interactions. Home visiting programs may help to target children's development and parental functioning and competencies (see Wasik & Roberts, 1994; Wolfe, 1994).

Intervention studies in the area of neglect (e.g., DePanfilis, 1996) emphasize primarily the role of parental functioning and involvement (e.g., Gaudin, 1993; Gaudin et al., 1991). In one of the few family-based intervention studies, Gaudin and colleagues (1991) found that case management and advocacy services (mobilization of informal social networks) was more effective than traditional casework on specific (parenting attitudes) and global (worker ratings) measures, although there was a high attrition rate. Such work has suggested the importance of using only a few primary providers who work with the family over a long period of time. Only a few of these programs seemed to offer specific services to children, primarily through therapeutic day care, with some services available in multiservice models (e.g., support groups, behavioral skills training), similar to Project 12-Ways (Crittenden, 1996). Day-care programs that include several child and parent services report improvements for most child participants upon discharge (Stehno, 1984; Miller & Whittaker, 1988).

Comments and Critique

A few conclusions seem warranted based on this brief review. It is clear that these treatment programs have different theoretical approaches and therapeutic foci, and incorporate diverse content. Many studies, though, emphasize training in cognitive–behavioral skills or techniques (e.g., Berliner & Saunders, 1995; Cohen & Mannarino, 1996). Moreover, the cases targeted both across and within treatment programs vary widely in age and developmental status, which may influence the degree of improvement achieved by each child. Finally, studies vary by format (individual, group, family), although few direct comparisons of different treatments have been conducted. The findings reported in recent experimental studies support those of prior reports in documenting clinical improvements following treatment and, in some cases, in follow-up.

Studies that compare alternative treatments in sexual abuse have revealed fewer group differences beyond the effects of group CBT (Berliner & Saunders, 1995) or family/network meetings alone (Hyde et al., 1995). Besides some evidence for treatment differences in the area of physical abuse and neglect (Brunk et al., 1987; Wolfe et al., 1988), few such studies have been conducted in these and other areas. Most programs have been directed toward preschoolers (Culp, Heide, & Richardson, 1987; Culp et al., 1991; Davis & Fantuzzo, 1989; Fantuzzo et al., 1988). Studies of services provided directly to older children and adolescents are needed to determine if the programs minimize the effects of maltreatment or risk for another incident (Finkelhor & Berliner, 1995; Kolko, 1996a; Oates & Bross, 1995; Wolfe, 1994). In the other areas, there is little recent literature on the impact of treatment specifically on child victims of neglect or exposure to family violence, or on adult offenders; this precludes any summary of findings and implications on the role of treatment for each participant. Further development of research needed on the treatment of child abuse and neglect is discussed in the following section.

CLINICAL CONSIDERATIONS

Comprehensive Psychosocial/Clinical Evaluation

There is increased recognition of the need to conduct an adequate clinical evaluation in this area. Given much diversity in the symptom pictures of abused children and their parents, an effort should be made to conduct a careful, comprehensive, intake evaluation that incorporates multiple domains of functioning (e.g., behavior, social), informants (e.g., child, parent, siblings), and methods (e.g., interviews, checklists, observations). Various aspects of child and parent functioning, or competence (e.g., child symptoms, parental mood state), and the family environment (e.g., caretaking routines, stimulation, activities), including areas of personal and family resources (Azar & Wolfe, 1989), deserve evaluation because of their relationship to abuse or neglect. Several innovative and specialized assessment measures are available (Hansen & MacMillan, 1990). Helpful guidelines for conducting a clinical evaluation of relevant symptoms and disorders can be found in Chaffin, Bonner, Worley & Lawson (1996).

The evaluation has implications for the types of therapeutic problems that need to be pursued at different levels (e.g., child, parent, family). Problems such as excessive child misbehavior, heightened parental anger, and/or family stress may place the child at increased risk for reabuse, interfere with successful social adjustment, and/or increase personal distress. Certainly, interventions aimed at both promoting a prosocial repertoire and minimizing the psychological sequelae of abusive behavior can be selected only if each family's idiosyncratic characteristics and relational style are considered in this formulation (Graziano & Mills, 1992).

Because diverse forms of maladjustment have been documented among abused children and their families, a understanding of the child's and family's strengths is an important therapeutic prerequisite. Issues for consideration in a comprehensive clinical evaluation include the nature and extent of the child's level of adjustment, social support and family functioning, and potential resources or compensatory skills (Azar & Wolfe, 1989; Kolko, 1996a).

Goals and Targets

Even with the accumulation of clinical data, the development of a constructive formulation of the case and the identification of realistic, individualized goals remains a complicated task. One primary consideration in articulating these goals is how to balance the child's needs with those of the family, and how strongly to focus on individuals or on the family system. Although children's needs and vulnerabilities are often addressed in initial evaluations of risk status, they seem to receive less follow-up attention once service options are reviewed. In fact, it may seem at times that greater attention is paid to goals related to the containment (prevention) of reabuse than to treatment of the sequelae of abuse and improving the quality of life (Baglow, 1992). The initial emphasis on containment and protection is understandable, but adequate intervention services that focus on environmental risk factors and psychological reactions to abusive caretaking are equally important (Graziano & Mills, 1992). Potential targets for child-focused intervention include health promotion, social and developmental stimulation, behavior management, and education (cf., Mannarino & Cohen, 1990). Potential targets for parents include parent management skill; individual counseling for problems with anger, drug abuse, depression, and self-control; developmental knowledge; and social support. Regardless of the specific nature of the goals selected, there should be a balance between the focus on negative or deviant behavior and that on personal competencies or strengths. This dual focus seems justified, given findings that implicate both behavioral deficiencies and excesses.

Participants, Settings, and System Linkages

Among the other parameters of treatment to be considered are the potential participants and the settings in which services are to be delivered. There is minimal evidence regarding the relative advantages of certain treatment formats and the impact of having different individuals included in treatment. Whereas some studies have targeted either children or parents, several have targeted children and parents in parallel services (e.g., Cohen & Manarino, 1996; Kolko, 1996b) or the entire family in coordinated services (Brunk et al., 1987; Hyde, Bentovin, & Monck, 1995; Lutzker, 1990). These considerations may influence greatly the types of services and approaches selected for use and their likelihood of success.

In addition, one must appreciate the relationship between treatment and other aspects of the systemic response to an individual case. For example, the nature of the integration of the mental health service with the overall range of services (e.g., legal/criminal, social services) is often difficult to describe or evaluate. The role of case management services and accountability are two issues that could be emphasized in this context. Issues include system obstacles or conflicts, the relationship between court mandate and treatment participation, and the level of communication among all systems. Finally, one would hope that these developments occur in the context of a well-coordinated service system that can efficiently and sensitively help children and their families to make contact with and profit from therapeutic resources. As outlined by Baglow (1992), a cooperative framework is needed to facilitate cross-agency collaboration in the identification of case management priorities, and the prevention of casework breakdown (e.g., therapy vs. containment, monitoring of intervention).

OPPORTUNITIES FOR CLINICAL–RESEARCH INTEGRATION

Models

In the sexual abuse area, conceptual and therapeutic models have provided clinical guidelines for the treatment of child and adult victims that integrate treatment stages incorporating the concepts of trauma, treatment, and recovery (Lebowitz, Harvey, & Herman, 1993). Clinical strategies associated with these concepts are being developed to provide abuse-specific treatments and they deserve both elaboration and empirical examination. This is illustrated by the work of Cohen and Mannarino (1993) whose cognitive–behavioral approach to the parallel individual treatment of preschool sexual abuse victims and their parents targets both the symptoms commonly observed in these participants and relevant clinical issues for children (e.g., safety, assertion, ambivalence) and parents (attributions, support, child management). Group treatment models have also generated specific techniques to enhance cohesion, coping, expression, and support (Zaidi & Gutierrez-Kovner, 1995) and the integration of skills training (e.g., relaxation, social skills), psychotherapy (e.g., feeling recognition, peer relations), and education (e.g., sexuality, self-protection) with sexual abuse victims (Lindon & Nourse, 1994). Documentation of the usefulness of these methods is necessary to facilitate their judicious application.

Developments in family therapy also require greater technical and applied evaluation (Roesler, Savin, & Grozs, 1993), especially in terms of its hypothesized advantages for discussing traumatic experiences and conducting systemic work incorporating offenders (Greenspun, 1994). Indeed, other approaches have integrated specific procedures based on the effects of sexual abuse in children (e.g., attachment, behavioral and emotional regulation, self-concept) at the individual (e.g., play treatment), group (e.g., didactics), and family level (e.g., goal attainment) (Friedrich, 1996; see p.116), with methods to enhance the process of treatment with adolescents and their families (Chaffin et al., 1996).

In contrast, few models have been proposed to guide treatment in other areas. For example, interventions for physical abuse based on the social-situational model have generally emphasized parent training in the use of nonviolent disciplinary skills, anger control and stress management, and contingency management (Azar & Siegel, 1990; Kolko, 1996a; Wolfe & Wekerle, 1993) and other concurrent clinical or support services (e.g., self-help groups, child development information). Such interventions may both promote a prosocial repertoire and minimize the psychological sequelae of abusive behavior. Given the complexities inherent in most cases of abuse, it is suggested that parent-directed methods to eliminate abusive behavior be supplemented with evaluation, education, treatment, and follow-up of abused children to promote their social-psychological development (Graziano & Mills, 1992). Recent work using Parent-Child Interaction Training (PCIT) has been advocated for clinical application in the treatment of physical abuse (Urquiza & Bodiford-McNeil, 1996). PCIT may help parents develop more positive relationships with their children and learn appropriate parenting techniques through ongoing coaching efforts during observed interactions in various stages in the treatment process (e.g., assessment, training of behavioral play and discipline skills, booster sessions).

The ecological model is an alternative approach that views physical abuse from a systemic perspective and seeks to address various child (e.g., feelings), parent (e.g., poor empathy, physical punishment) and/or family issues (e.g., role reversal), emphasizing the interrelationships among individual, family, and social support factors (e.g., family communication, extra familial contacts; Belsky, 1993). Multisystemic Therapy (Henggeler & Borduin, 1990) is one approach that can address several targets in different domains by providing individualized, family-based services conducted in the home and community. Recent empirical studies support the efficacy of such applications with various adolescent offender populations (Henggeler, 1994).

Models used to guide treatment applications with neglectful families have been based on social learning and behavioral principles (Lutzker & Campbell, 1994), and the role of social support and social network development (DePanfilis, 1996; Gaudin, 1993a, b). These models generally speak to the need to target multiple aspects of the family environment in an effort to enhance child, parent, and family functioning (see Oates et al., 1995; Wasik & Roberts, 1994). Far less work has been conducted in the area of psychological maltreatment or neglect, although some conceptualizations have been developed (e.g., Brassard, Germain, & Hart, 1987; Erickson, 1988). Unfortunately, few reports of treatment studies have been made based on either of these approaches or on any other conceptual framework.

Bullying in school (American Psychological Association [APA], 1993; Farrington, 1993; Olweus (1993a,b) and ritual abuse (Faller, 1994) are among some of the other less well studied and understood forms of victimization for which children may receive intervention services. Efforts to minimize the extent and severity of bullying have been made successfully by using a school-based program that incorporates complementary modalities (e.g., teaching training, classroom management). Specialized intervention models or treatments for ritualistic abuse have not yet been reported and, as a consequence, formal outcome studies have yet to appear in this area (see Kelley, 1996).

Methods for Evaluation

Empirical Case Evaluation and Replication

The greater use of empirical designs that permit clearer understanding of the effects of a intervention is important. Evaluation studies that address issues of internal and external validity, and experimental control, and that are prospective in format, are clearly needed. In general, experimental and statistical methods are needed to increase confidence in our conclusions and to rule out alternative, more parsimonious explanations of outcome. If the role of a child or parent treatment/ intervention is to be carefully evaluated, studies should use such features as multiple measures, informants, and methods (multitrait-multimethod); multivariate analyses; repeated measures; control or comparison groups; and/or formal follow-up evaluations (e.g., Berliner & Saunders, 1995; Cohen & Mannarino, 1996). Evidence of this nature would encourage an understanding of the key ingredients of intervention with this population. Several helpful sources identify issues for consideration in psychotherapy trials and outcome studies (see Beutler, 1993; Kazdin, 1993; Pilkonis, 1993).

At the same time, the demands incurred in designing, conducting, and completing an experimental study of treatment often exceed available resources, especially those present in agency or private practitioner settings. Short of implementing something as complex as a clinical trial, data collection from several individual cases treated and assessed in a standardized manner may prove helpful. The clinical replication series, for example, is useful in evaluating the effectiveness and limitations of a given treatment when pre/post information can be obtained on several cases receiving the treatment (see Kazdin, 1993). A set of accumulated cases possessing such data will highlight the overall efficacy of a intervention approach and variations found in individual cases.

There is little information about the comparative effectiveness of treatments that differ in format, such as the manner in which children are integrated into intervention (e.g., individual child, separate child and parent training, family therapy), clinical site (community systems vs. home vs. clinic), single vs. multicomponent interventions, and the timing or sequence of intervention components (e.g., how interventions are tailored to children's developmental stages). Different interventions should be studied in order to elaborate on findings showing that certain outcomes are associated with specific parent training methods (e.g., improved problem solving and/or parent–child relationships with family-directed therapy; Brunk et al., 1987). Other methodologic and clinical advances are needed to evaluate the impact of intervention on family functioning (e.g., Willet et al., 1991).

Systematic and Ongoing Assessment of Treatment Progress

Kazdin (1993) has advocated the routine and ongoing assessment of individual cases as a means to develop more definitive observations regarding treatment course and outcome. Systematic assessment of client response may permit operationalization of treatment goals, enhance information-gathering, provide more opportunities to examine change and improve client care, and facilitate accurate decision making. Obtained throughout treatment, such information may help practitioners better understand a client's response to treatment and identify the presence of clinical obstacles to improvement. Such "clinical course" measures have the potential to flag, early in treatment, threats to a child's welfare or deteriorating family conditions that may require alternative interventions and child protection/safety plans. Systematic evaluation in clinical practice has been useful in determining differences among violent families in their response to preventive intervention based on monthly therapists' ratings of family functioning (Ayoub, Willett, & Robinson, 1992; Willett et al., 1991) and differences among physically abusive families based on weekly child and parent ratings (Kolko, 1996b). Families characterized by problems of violence and high levels of distressed parenting were least likely to improve during intervention compared to other families and actually showed consistently negative changes that reflected a deterioration in functioning.

Measurement and Assessment

Abuse History and Status

Progress has been made in documenting the functional context and parameters of abusive interactions (e.g., frequency, severity, chronicity, situational context) (see Barnett, Manly, & Cicchetti, 1993). Delineation of the reliability and validity of structured case record measures and interviews deserves greater clinical attention to evaluate the overall utility of these coding systems. For example, clinical practitioners could evaluate the accuracy of judgments of cases perceived to be at "low" vs. "high" risk of reabuse, especially among those cases that receive rapid closure following intake. Other instruments, such as the Abuse Dimensions Inventory (ADI; Chaffin, Wherry, Newlin, Crutchfield, & Dykman, 1997), Brief Assessment of Traumatic Events (BATE; Lipovsky, 1992), and Survey of Exposure to Community Violence (Richters & Saltzman, 1990) seem to capture helpful descriptive characteristics of an abusive experience, but merit further clinical and empirical testing. Regardless of the instrument used, development of operational criteria would encourage depiction of the severity of the sample and permit cross-study comparisons.

Clinical Symptoms/Status

One of the primary directions for evaluation efforts is the need to enhance the assessment/measurement process by selecting measures with a clear tie to the constructs of interest. When these issues are addressed, measures should possess population sensitivity (clear tie to unique features of sample, including developmental level) and/or therapeutic specificity (clear tie to treatment procedures), be psychometrically sound, and permit replication across studies (e.g., Trauma Symptom Checklist for Children [TSC-C]; Briere, 1996). The scope of assessment and followup could be expanded to include more information on the effects of treatment on child and family functioning (e.g., suicidality, aggression, peer relations), and development of psychiatric disorders, re-abuse rates, and family integrity.

For example, measures can be suggested for the following areas that represent common domains of clinical assessment: (1) aggression/antisocial behavior: Child Behavior Checklist (CBCL), Interview for Antisocial Behavior (IAB; Kazdin & Esveldt-Dawson, 1986), and Parent Daily Report (PDR; Chamberlain & Reid, 1987); (2) family violence: Conflict Tactics Scales (CTS; Straus, 1990); (3) attributions and distortions: Children's Negative Cognitive Error Questionnaire (CNCEQ; Leitenberg et al., 1986), and Parent Opinion Questionnaire (POQ; Azar et al., 1984); (4) Stress and Anger: Parenting Stress Inventory (PSI, Form 5; Abidin, 1983); (5) Risk for child abuse and maltreatment: Child Abuse Potential Inventory (CAPI; Milner, 1986) and Caseworker Ratings of Maltreatment Risk Status (Wolfe et al., 1988); (6) treatment utility/acceptability: Goal Attainment Scaling (GAS; Brunk et al., 1987), Treatment Evaluation Inventory (TEI; Kazdin et al., 1987), Child Evaluation Inventory (CEI; Kazdin et al., 1987), and Consumer Satisfaction Questionnaire (see Kolko, 1995). Other suggestions for clinical assessment measures in this area can be found elsewhere (Rittner & Wodarski, 1995).

Adjustment and Functional Impairment

Measures to document the cognitive-behavioral skills (competencies) targeted by training and prosocial or adaptive behaviors that may facilitate coping are also needed to evaluate the overall effects of treatment, as reflected in the following domains: (1) child behavior management and disciplinary skills: Knowledge of Behavioral Principles as Applied to Children (KOBPAC; O'Dell, Tarler-Benlolo, & Flinn, 1979), Child Rearing Interview (CRI; Stouthamer-Loeber & Loeber, 1985), and Parent Behavior Inventory—Child Version (PBI; Crook, Raskin, & Elliot, 1981); (2) parent–child interaction: Structured Clinical Observation System (SCOS; Budd, Riner, & Brockman, 1983), and (3) child/family functioning and adjustment: Home Environment Questionnaire (HEQ; Laing & Sines, 1982).

Service Delivery and Treatment Integrity

There are other forms of intervention in which examination is of clinical relevance because of their potential impact on both short- and long-term outcome. An interesting survey by Berliner and Conte (1995) interviewed child victims and their parents regarding the effects of disclosure and intervention. The study reported several important findings: (1) children most often told their mothers about the abuse (48%) and said it is good to tell (97%); (2) children's perceptions of professional treatment were generally positive; (3) adverse family experiences were associated with the perceived level of distress experienced by the child as rated by parents; (4) children saw as helpful counselors who showed understanding, concern, and sincerity. These findings suggest that children are influenced by the ways in which they are evaluated and treated, and that they benefit from the professional contacts they receive in the aftermath of abuse. Such findings are in accord with evidence showing that children who testified once in juvenile court have shown symptom improvements relative to those who have not testified (Runyart, Everson, Edelsohn, Hunter, & Coulter, 1988). Runyan et al. (1988) also found that children who are placed outside the home may show higher levels of distress initially than those who remain in the home, but they may later exhibit compara-ble levels of improvement.

Few studies have reported information about treatment integrity, attrition and treatment removal, but virtually all devote at least some attention to enhanc-ing engagement with the child. Treatment integrity has been established for cer-tain CBT protocols for sexual abused (Cohen & Mannarino, 1996) and physically abused children (Kolko, 1996b), but deserves greater consideration in future re-search because of its potential impact on clinical outcome. For those studies re-porting other details, low levels of attrition and removal have been found with sexual abuse (22%; Cohen & Mannarino, 1996), physical abuse (23%; Kolko, 1996b), and exposed children (10%; Wagar & Rodway, 1995), which may account for somewhat heightened consumer satisfaction. Engagement strategies have been incorporated in some studies to promote peer cohesion in group therapy (Sinclair et al., 1995; Stauffer & Deblinger, 1996) and to enhance rapport and the thera-peutic relationship during individual or family therapy (Brunk et al., 1987; Wolfe et al., 1988). Just how these methods work and which ones work best would be of clinical import.

Monitoring of Treatment Course and Response

Families recommended for services following investigation may struggle as much in handling the investigation experience as they do the sequelae of the abuse incident, although the reactions to both experiences may be exacerbated by the lack of a supportive process of referral for intervention. The presence of vari-ous problems at the individual and family level, not to mention social insularity and limited resources, may minimize the potential to participate actively in treat-ment and benefit from intervention. This may encourage the use of methods to monitor the family's initial reaction and response to treatment.

Clinical (high-risk) indicators. One of the few comparisons of initial re-sponse to alternative interventions that included children as participants during treatment was recently reported by Kolko (1996b). Weekly reports of high-risk in-dicators were obtained from physically abused, school-aged children and their parents or guardians who were randomly assigned to Individual Child and Parent Cognitive–Behavioral Treatment (CBT) or Family Therapy (FT). The measures, consisting of parental anger and physical discipline/force, and family problems, were obtained each weekly session in order to monitor the course of treatment. These reports showed moderate stability over time and parent–child correspon-dence. The overall levels of parental anger and physical discipline/force were found to be lower in CBT than FT families, though each group showed a reduction on these items from the early to late treatment sessions. Equally important, be-tween 20% and 23% of all children and their parents independently reported high levels of physical discipline/force during the early and late phases of treatment, although few incidents seemed to result in injuries, and an even higher percentage of cases reported heightened parental anger and family problems. Early treatment reports from both sets of informants predicted late period reports, but only parent reports were related to validity measures.

These findings suggest some benefit to routine monitoring of clinical course during intervention, especially in the identification of cases at risk of re-abuse, and the need to be prepared to respond to incidents of physical punishment. The study is limited by the small number of self-report items used to reflect high-risk behavior in the home. However, by identifying families exhibiting high levels of coercive behavior, treatment course data may help in understanding the heterogeneity of abusive families, document the need for individualized interventions (Ayoub et al., 1992; Willett et al., 1991), assist in targeting contextual problems and guide decisions about the level of protection afforded to children or priorities for additional services (Daro, 1993; Toth & Cicchetti, 1993), or identify predictors of poor prognosis. Repeated assessment of high-risk clinical indicators of child and family dysfunction may help to monitor the immediate effects of, and receptivity to, intervention with physically abusive families (Ayoub et al., 1992; Kazdin, 1993). As few studies have described treatment course in physical abuse or other areas, further development of clinical measures of parent–child adjustment that can efficiently document therapeutic response seems warranted.

Adherence and treatment process. Across all types of intervention studies, problems with engagement, compliance, and dropout have been reported among abusive or neglectful families (Cohn & Daro, 1987). Lower rates of clinic attendance have been found in maltreating than nonmaltreating families; this may be influenced by certain procedures (e.g., court ordering of treatment, child removal) (Warner, Malinosky-Rummell, Ellis, & Hansen, 1990). Malinosky-Rummell et al. (1991), for example, also reported a 38% no-show rate at home, a 66% clinic no-show rate, and a 36% dropout rate among 45 families. Physical abuse was noted during treatment in 23% of the cases and case reopening by child protective services (CPS) workers occurred in 21% of the cases. In the general literature, high rates of recidivism during treatment (about one-third; Cohn & Daro, 1987) and after treatment (30–47%; Daro, 1988) have been reported. These and other obstacles to successful resolution of family conflict provide a significant challenge for resolution to both researchers and to the practitioners.

Efforts to enhance treatment adherence are especially relevant given the low rates of attendance found in maltreating families. In their survey of professionals, Hansen and Warner (1994) report average rates of attendance and homework completion of 84% and 64%, respectively, and several predictors of good attendance (e.g., educational level of parent, experience treating maltreatment, home site) and completion (e.g., education and low age of parent, home site). Certain procedures were reported to be the most effective in improving attendance (e.g., praise, tangible rewards), while in-session practice worked best to improve homework completion. These and other suggestions for enhancing participation lend themselves to clinical testing (e.g., rapid establishment of the first contact, conducting certain sessions in the family's home, showing sensitivity to the child's developmental level and sociocultural background). Attention to therapeutic process is also important, but rarely evaluated. For example, evidence indicating that maltreated adolescents who failed to develop positive therapeutic alliances with their therapists tended to show poorest outcome in a hospitalized sample should encourage more formal assessment of initial treatment relationships (Eltz, Shirk, & Sarlin,

1995). Certainly, greater attention to treatment participation should enhance both acquisition and program maintenance.

Maintenance and Follow-up

Once clients complete treatment and are discharged, the assessment of follow-up becomes an important concern. Maintenance of treatment gains has been reported for internalizing symptoms, avoidance, dissociation, and/or sexual behavior in some sexually abused children (Hack, Osachuk, & De Luca, 1994; Lanktree & Briere, 1995; Stauffer & Deblinger, 1996) and for child behavior problems in physically abused children (Wolfe et al., 1988). However, other program evaluation findings highlight the continuity of child and family problems following services (Daro, 1988). Indeed, some intervention studies have shown limited evidence for maintenance of gains (e.g., Lutzker, 1990; Wolfe et al., 1988). The majority of treatment studies do not examine the maintenance of improvements at follow-up (Finkelhor & Berliner, 1995; Kolko, 1996b).

Much work still needs to be done to promote the development and application of psychosocial interventions directed at multiple risk factors for abuse (National Academy of Sciences, 1993). Whether treated children continue to experience improvements in the issues at referral and other clinical symptoms cannot be determined at this point. Such data are necessary to document the relationship between treatment outcome and both follow-up status and recidivism. Modest rates of recidivism have been reported by follow-up studies of maltreated children and youth referred to a inpatient assessment program (Levy, Markovic, Chaudhry, Ahart, & Torres, 1995) or the court (16%; Jellinek et al., 1995), highlighting the importance of tracking children and using assessment information to guide treatment and placement decisions. Thus, collection of follow-up information is an important aspect of evaluating the impact of services. Additional attention should be paid to the collection of follow-up reports and official child abuse records, use of repeated measures analyses and appropriate statistical tests, and extension of alternative treatment procedures. Comparative outcome studies that report follow-up information are clearly needed to identify the influence of treatment well after treatment has ended, both on measures of clinical status and adjustment, and on risk for re-abuse (e.g., Fantuzzo et al., 1988). Follow-up services may be a necessary extension of intervention. An examination of therapeutic methods, then, should help promote greater stability of improvements (e.g., "check-ups," service calls). This consideration gains importance given that the greatest risk of recidivism probably occurs during the first two years following program discharge (Levy et al., 1995).

SUMMARY

This chapter has identified several areas of clinical interest and involvement in working with abusive and neglectful families that deserve further empirical attention. In general, much more work should be directed toward understanding the impact and role of treatment with children who have been exposed to physical or psychological maltreatment, domestic or family violence, and neglect, and offenders of the latter three categories of maltreatment, given the dearth of studies in these areas. The clinical benefits and limitations of alternative interventions could be evaluated using existing assessments, and examining treatment process and course, including patient–therapist relationships and treatment credibility, clinical outcomes relating to child adjustment, and risk for re-abuse. Various services make up a continuum of care ranging from minimal outpatient visits to intensive treatment in different contexts or settings (community vs. home vs. clinic). These include abuse-specific vs. general treatment programs, skills training and experiential methods, individual vs. family therapy approaches, and special parallel or combined programs for children and their parents/families (Cohen & Mannarino, 1996; Hyde et al., 1995; Kolko, 1996b). Treatment approaches would benefit from information regarding the relative impact of treating the sequelae of abuse (e.g., psychological reactions to an abusive experience) and targeting environmental risk factors (e.g., dysfunctional caretaking or family interactions) (Grazianno & Mills, 1992).

Even with the broad array of measures reported in the literature, it is important to consider collecting information from both children and parents, as well as other sources such as teachers, clinicians, or archival records (Cohen & Mannarino, 1996; Hyde et al., 1995; Jaffe et al., 1988; Kolko, 1996b; Sinclair et al., 1995). The development of new measures related to the sequelae of abuse and neglect seems warranted, especially those that reflect the child's perception of the abusive experience. Outcome measures or measures that evaluate the targets of intervention may help to identify children's adjustment in its developmental context (e.g., medical status, social and developmental stimulation, behavior management, and education (see Mannarino & Cohen, 1990). Measures of service delivery and consumer satisfaction are likewise important in order to document client impressions of abuse-specific services (Cohen & Mannarino, 1996; Friedrich et al., 1992; Hyde et al., 1995; Stauffer & Deblinger, 1996).

Related to these issues, more progress is needed in evaluating how treatment obstacles and parameters may influence process and course (e.g., cognitive limitations, chronic stress, substance abuse, family discord, limited financial and social resources, resistance/poor motivation, coercion, frequent attrition, positive orientation to treatment). High rates of recidivism are common both during (about one-third; Cohn & Daro, 1987) and after treatment (30–47%; Daro, 1988), suggesting the importance of monitoring and modifying high-risk behaviors during treatment related to sexual abuse (Cohen & Mannarino, 1996) and physical abuse (Kolko, 1996a). Certain variables have been found to moderate the impact of sexual abuse (e.g., sex of victim, and that of perpetrator, relationship to victim, support following incident, parental depression); these and other variables, such as parental functioning in cases of physical abuse (Haskett, Myers, Pirrello, & Dombalis, 1995) may affect children's subsequent adjustment, and they deserve empirical study. Moreover, client reactions to and progress during treatment may influence service participation and impact. Studies are needed to determine how these variables mediate therapeutic efficacy. The integration of research methods in the development and extension of clinical intervention is a necessary step toward enhancing both the delivery and the effectiveness of treatment services to victims and offenders in child abuse and neglect.

REFERENCES

Abidin, R. R. (1983). *Parenting stress index.* Odessa, FL: Psychological Assessment Resources.

Acton, R. G., & During, S. M. (1992). Preliminary results of aggression management training for aggressive parents. *Journal of Interpersonal Violence, 7,* 410–417.

American Psychological Association. (1993). *Violence and youth: Psychology's response. Vol. I: Summary of the American Psychological Association Commission on Violence and Youth.* Washington, DC: America Psychological Association.

Amundson, M. J. (1989). Family crisis care: A home-based intervention program for child abuse. *Issues in Mental Health Nursing, 10,* 285–296.

Ayoub, C., Willett, J. B., & Robinson, D. S. (1992). Families at risk of child maltreatment: Entry-level characteristics and growth in family functioning during treatment. *Child Abuse & Neglect, 16,* 495–511.

Azar, S. T., Robinson, D. R., Hekimian, E., & Twentyman, C. T. (1984). Unrealistic expectations and problem-solving ability in maltreating and comparison mothers. *Journal of Consulting and Clinical Psychology, 52,* 687–691.

Azar, S. T., & Siegel, B. R. (1990). Behavioral treatment of child abuse. A developmental perspective. *Behavior Modification, 14,* 279–300.

Azar, S. T., & Wolfe, D. A. (1989). Child abuse and neglect. In E. J. Marsh & R. A. Barkley (Eds.), *Treatment of childhood disorders* (pp.451–493). New York: Guilford Press.

Baglow, L. J. (1992). A multidimensional model for treatment of child abuse: A framework for cooperation. *Child Abuse & Neglect, 14,* 387–395.

Bassard, M. R, Germain, R, & Hart, S. N. (Eds.). (1987). *Psychological maltreatment of children and youth.* Elmsford, NY: Pergamon.

Barnett, D., Manly, J. T., & Cicchetti, D., (1993). Defining child maltreatment: The interface between policy and research. In D. Cicchetti & S. L. Toth (Eds.), *Child abuse, child development, and social policy* (pp. 7–74). Norwood, NJ: Ablex.

Becker, J. V., Alpert, J. L., Bigfoot, D. S., Bonner, B. L., Geddie, L. F., Henggeler, S. W., & Kaufman, K. L., (1995). *Journal of Clinical Child Psychology.*

Belsky, J. (1993). Etiology of child maltreatment: A developmental–ecological analysis. *Psychological Bulletin, 114,* 413–434.

Berliner, L., & Conte, J. R. (1995). The effects of disclosure and intervention on sexually abused children. *Child Abuse & Neglect, 19,* 371–384.

Berliner, L., & Saunders, B. (1995). *Grantee Status Report National Center on Child Abuse and Neglect.* Washington, DC.

Beutler, L. E. (1993). Designing outcome studies: Treatment of adult victims of child sexual abuse. *Journal of Interpersonal Violence, 8,* 402–414.

Beutler, L. E., Wllliams, R. E., & Zetzer, H. A. (1994). Efficacy of treatment for victims of child sexual abuse. *Sexual Abuse of Children, 4,* 156–175.

Bigelow, K. M., Kessler, M. L., & Lutzker, J. R. (1995, June). Improving the parent–child relationship in abusive and neglectful families. In M. L. Kessler (Chair), *Treating Physical Abuse and Neglect: Four Approaches.* Symposium conducted at the 3rd Annual American Professional Society on the Abuse of Children Colloquium, Tucson, Arizona.

Briere, J. (1996). *Trauma Symptom Checklist for Children.* Psychological Assessment Resources, Inc. Professional Manual.

Brunk, M, Henggeler, S. W., & Whelan, J. P. (1987). Comparison of multisystemic therapy and parent training in the brief treatment of child abuse and neglect. *Journal of Consulting and Clinical Psychology, 55,* 171–178.

Budd, K. S., Riner, L. S., & Brockman, M. P. (1983). A structured observation system for clinical evaluation of parent training. *Behavioral Assessment, 5,* 373–393.

Chaffin, M., Bonner, B. L., Worley, K. B., & Lawson, L. (1996). Treating abused adolescents. In J. Briere, L. Berliner, J. A. Bulkey, C. Jenny, & T. Reid (Eds), *The APSAC handbook on child maltreatment* (pp. 119–139). Thousand Oaks, CA: Sage.

Chaffin, M., Wherry, J., Newlin, C., Crutchfield, A., & Dykman, R. (1997). The abuse dimension inventory: Initial data on a research measure of abuse severity. *Journal of Interpersonal Violence, 12,* 569–589.

Chamberlain, P., & Reid, J. B. (1987). Parent observation and report of child symptoms. *Behavioral Assessment, 9,* 97–100.

Cohen, J. A., & Mannarino, A. P. (1993). A treatment model for sexually abused preschoolers. *Journal of Interpersonal Violence,* 8, 115–131.

Cohen, J. A., & Mannarino, A. P. (1996). A treatment outcome study for sexually abused preschool children: Initial findings. *Journal of the American Academy of Child and Adolescent Psychiatry, 35,* 42–50.

Cohn, A. H., & Daro, D. (1987). Is treatment too late: What ten years of evaluative research tell us. *Child Abuse & Neglect, 11,* 433–442.

Crittenden, P. M. (1996). Research on maltreating families: Implications for intervention. In J. Briere, L. Berliner, J. A. Bulkey, C. Jenny, & T. Reid (Eds.), *The APSAC handbook on child maltreatment* (pp. 158–174). Thousand Oaks, CA: Sage.

Crook, T., Raskin, A., & Elliot, J. (1981). Parent–child relationships and adult depression. *Child Development, 52,* 950–957.

Culp, R. E., Heide, J., & Richardson, M. T. (1987). Maltreated children's developmental scores: Treatment versus nontreatment. *Child Abuse & Neglect, 11,* 29–34.

Culp, R. E., Little, V., Letts, D., Lawrence, H. (1991). Maltreated children's self-concept: Effects of a comprehensive treatment program. *American Journal of Orthopsychiatiy, 61,* 114–121.

Daro, D. (1993). Child maltreatment research: Implications for program design. In D. Cicchetti, & S. L. Toth (Eds.), *Child abuse, child development, and social policy* (pp. 331–367). Norwood, NJ: Ablex.

Daro, D. (1988). *Confronting child abuse: Research for effective program design.* New York: Free Press.

Davis, S., & Fantuzzo, J. W. (1989). The effects of adult and peer social initiations on social behavior of withdrawn and aggressive maltreated preschool children. *Journal of Family Violence, 4,* 227–248.

DePanfilis, D. (1996). Social isolation of neglectful families: A review of social support assessment and intervention models. *Child Maltreatment, 1,* 37–52.

Eltz, M. J., Shirk, S. R, & Sarlin, N. (1995). Alliance formation and treatment outcome among maltreated adolescents. *Child Abuse & Neglect, 19,* 419–431.

Erickson, M. F. (1988, March). *School psychology in preschool settings.* Paper presented at the meeting of the National Association of School Psychologists, Chicago.

Faller, K. C. (1994). Ritual abuse: A review of research. *APSAC Advisor, 7,* 19–27.

Fantuzzo, J. W., DePaola, L. M., Lambert, L., Martino, T., Anderson, G., & Sutton, S. (1991). Effects of interparental violence on the psychological adjustment and competencies of young children. *Journal of Consulting and Clinical Psychology, 59,* 258–265.

Fantuzzo, J. W., Jurecic, L., Stovall, A., Hightower, A. D., & Goins, C. (1988). Effects of adult and peer social initiations on the social behavior of withdrawn, maltreated preschool children. *Journal of Consulting and ClinicalPsychology, 56,* 34–39.

Fantuzzo, J. W., Stovall, A., Schachtel, D., Coins, C., & Hall, R. (1987). The effects of peer social initiations on the social behavior of withdrawn maltreated preschool children. *Journal of Behavior Therapy and Experimental Psychiatry, 18,* 357–363.

Farrington, D. P. (1993). Understanding and preventing bullying. In M. Tonry (Ed.), *Crime and justice: A review of research* (pp. 381–458). Chicago: University of Chicago Press.

Finkelhor, D. (1995). The victimization of children: A developmental perspective. *American Journal of Orthopsychiatry, 65,* 177–193.

Finkelhor, D., & Berliner, L. (1995). Research on the treatment of sexually abused children: A review and recommendations. *Journal of the American Academy of Child and Adolescent Psychiatry, 34,* 1408–1423.

Friedrich, W. N. (1996). An integrated model of psychotherapy for abused children. In J. Briere, L. Berliner, J. A. Bulkey, C. Jenny, & T. Reid (Eds.), *The APSAC handbook on child maltreatment* (pp. 104–118). Thousand Oaks, CA: Sage.

Friedrich, W. N., Luecke, W. J., Beilke, R. L., & Place, V. (1992). Psychotherapy outcome of sexually abused boys: An agency study. *Journal of Interpersonal Violence, 7,* 396–409.

Gaudin, J. (1993). Effective intervention with neglectful families. *Criminal Justice and Behavior, 20,* 66–89.

Gaudin, J. M., Jr., Wodarski, J. S., Arkinson, M. K., & Avery, L. S. (1991). Remedying child neglect: Effectiveness of social network interventions. *Journal of Applied Social Sciences, 15,* 97–123.

Ghuman, J. K. (1993). An integrated model for intervention with infants, preschool children and their maltreating parents. *Infant Mental Health Journal, 14,* 147–157.

Graziano, A. M., & Mills, J. R (1992). Treatment for abused children: When is a partial solution acceptable? *Child Abuse & Neglect, 16,* 217–228.

Green, A. H. (1993). Child sexual abuse: Immediate and long-term effects and intervention. *Journal of the American Academy of Child and Adolescent Psychiatry, 32,* 890–902.

Greene, B. F., Norman, K. R., Searle, M. S., Daniels, M., & Lubeck, R. C. (1995). Child abuse and neglect by parents with disabilities: A tale of two families. *Journal of Applied Behavior Analysis, 28,* 417–434.

Greenspun, W. S. (1994). Internal and interpersonal: The family transition of father–daughter incest. *Journal of Child Sexual Abuse, 3,* 1–14.

Hack, T. F., Osachuk, T. A., & De Luca, R. V. (1994). Group treatment of sexually abused preadolescent boys. *Families in Society: The Journal of Contemporary Human Services, 75,* 217–224.

Hansen, D. J., & MacMillan, V. M. (1990). Behavioral assessment of child-abusive and neglectful families: Recent developments and current issues. *Behavior Modification, 14,* 255–278.

Hansen, D. J., & Warner, J. E. (1994). Treatment adherence of maltreating families: A survey of professionals regarding prevalence and enhancement strategies. *Journal of Family Violence, 9,* 1–19.

Haskett, M. E., Myers, L. W., Pirrello, V. E., & Dombalis, A. O. (1995). Parenting styles as a mediating link between parental emotional health and adjustment of maltreated children. *Behavior Therapy, 26,* 625–642.

Henggeler, S. W. (1994). A consensus: Introduction to the APA Task Force report on innovative models of treatment and service delivery for children, adolescents, and their families. *Journal of Clinical Child Psychology, 23,* 3–6.

Henggeler, S. W., & Borduin, C. M. (1990). *Family therapy and beyond: A multisystemic approach to treating behavior problems of children and adolescents.* Pacific Grove, CA: Brooks/Cole.

Hyde, C., Bentovin, A., & Monck, E. (1995). Some clinical and methodological implications of a treatment outcome study of sexually abused children. *Child Abuse & Neglect, 19,* 1387–1399.

Jaffe, P., Wilson, S., & Wolfe, D. A. (1986). Promoting changes in attitudes and understanding of conflict resolution among child witnesses of family violence. *Canadian Journal of Behavioral Science, 18,* 357–366.

Jaffe, P., Wilson, S., & Wolfe, D. A. (1988). Specific assessment and intervention strategies for children exposed to wife battering: Preliminary empirical investigation. *Canadian Journal of Community Mental Health, 7,* 157–163.

Jaffe, P., Wolfe, D. A., & Wilson, S. (1990). *Children of battered women.* Newbury Park, CA: Sage.

Jellinek, M. S., Little, M., Benedict, K., Murphy, J. M., Pagano, M., Poitrast, F., & Quinn, D. (1995). Placement outcomes of 206 severely maltreated children in the Boston juvenile court system: A 7.5-year follow-up study. *Child Abuse & Neglect, 19,* 1051–1064.

Kazdin, A. E. (1993). Evaluation in clinical practice: Clinically sensitive and systematic methods of treatment delivery. *Behavior Therapy, 24,* 11–45.

Kazdin, A. E., & Esveldt-Dawson, K. (1986). The Interview for Antisocial Behavior: Psychometric characteristics and concurrent validity with child psychiatric inpatients. *Journal of Psychopathology and Behavioral Assessment, 8,* 289–303.

Kazdin, A. E., Esveldt-Dawson, K., French, N. H., & Unis, A. S. (1987). Problem-solving skills training and relationship therapy in the treatment of antisocial child behavior. *Journal of Consulting and Clinical Psychology, 55,* 76–85.

Kelley, S. J. (1996). Ritualistic abuse of children. In J. Briere, L. Berliner, J. A. Bulkley, C. Jenny, & T. Reid (Eds.), *APSAC Handbook of child maltreatment,* (pp. 90–99). Thousand Oaks, CA: Sage.

Kolko, D. J. (1995). Multimodal partial/day treatment of child antisocial behavior: Description and multilevel program evaluation. *Continuum: Developments in Ambulatory Health Care, 2,* 3–24.

Kolko, D. J. (1996a). Clinical monitoring of treatment course in child physical abuse: Child and parent reports. *Child Abuse & Neglect, 20,* 23–43.

Kolko, D. J. (1996b). Child physical abuse. In J. Briere, L. Berliner, J. A. Bulkley, C. Jenny, & T. Reid (Eds.), *APSAC Handbook of child maltreatment,* (pp. 21–50). Thousand Oaks, CA: Sage.

Laing, J. A., & Sines, J. O. (1982). The home environment questionnaire: An instrument of assessing several behaviorally relevant dimensions of children's environment. *Journal of Pediatric Psychology, 7,* 425–449.

Lanktree, C. B., & Briere, J. (1995). Outcome of therapy for sexually abused children: A repeated measures study. *Child Abuse & Neglect, 19,* 1145–1155.

Lebowitz, L., Harvey, M. R., & Herman, J. L. (1993). A stage-by-dimension model of recovery from sexual trauma. *Journal of Interpersonal Violence, 8,* 378–391.

Levy, H. B., Markovic, J., Chaudhry, U., Ahart, S., & Torres, H. (1995). Reabuse rates in a sample of children followed 5 years after discharge from a child abuse inpatient assessment program. *Child Abuse & Neglect, 19,* 1363–1377.

Lindon, J., & Nourse, C. A. (1994). A multi-dimensions model of group work for adolescent girls who have been sexually abused. *Child Abuse & Neglect, 18,* 341–348.

Lipovsky, J. A. (1992). Brief Assessment of Traumatic Events (BATE). Unpublished instrument. Charleston: Medical University of South Carolina.

Lutzker, J. R. (1990). Project 12-Ways: Treating child abuse and neglect from an ecobehavioral perspective. In R. F. Dangel & R. F. Polster (Eds.), *Parent training: Foundations of research and practice.* New York: Guilford Press.

Lutzker, J. R., & Campbell, R V. (1994). *Ecobehavioral family interventions in developmental disabilities.* Pacific Groves, CA: Brooks Cole.

Lutzker, J. R., & Rice, J. M. (1987). Using recidivism data to evaluate Project 12-Ways: An ecobehavioral approach to the treatment and prevention of child abuse and neglect. *Journal of Family Violence, 2,* 283–289.

Malgady, R. G., Rogler, L. H., & Costantino, G. (1990). Hero/heroine modeling for Puerto Rican adolescents: A preventive mental health intervention. *Journal of Consulting and Clinical Psychology, 58,* 469–474.

Malinosky-Rummell, R., Ellis, J. T., Warner, J. E., Ujcich, K., Carr, R. E., & Hansen, D. J. (1991, November). *Individualized behavioral intervention for physically abusive and neglectful families: An evaluation of the family interaction skills project.* Paper presented at the 25th Annual Conference of the Association for the Advancement of Behavior Therapy, New York, NY.

Malinosky-Rummell, R., & Hansen, D. J. (1993). Long-term consequences of child physical abuse. *Psychological Bulletin, 114,* 68–79.

Mannario, A. P., & Cohen, J. A. (1990). Treating the abused child. In R. T. Ammerman & M. Hersen (Eds.), *Children at Risk: An Evaluation of Factors Contributing To Child Abuse and Neglect* (pp. 249–266). New York: Plenum Press.

McGain, B., & McKinzey, R. K. (1995). The efficacy of group treatment in sexually abused girls. *Child Abuse & Neglect, 19,* 1157–1169.

Miller, J. L., & Whittaker, J. K. (1988). Social services and social support: Blended programs for families at risk of child maltreatment. *Child Welfare, 67,* 161–174.

Milner, J. S. (1986). *The Child Abuse Potential Inventory: Manual* (2nd ed.). Webster, NC: Psytec Corporation.

National Academy of Sciences (1993). *Understanding child abuse and neglect.* Washington, DC: National Academy Press.

Nelson, K. (1990, Fall). How do we know that family-based services are effective? *The Prevention Report, 1–3.* University of Iowa: National Resource Center on Family Based Services.

Nicol, A. R., Smith, J., Kay, B., Hall, D., Barlow, J., & Williams, B. (1988). A focused casework approach to the treatment of child abuse: A controlled comparison. *Journal of Child Pyschology and Psychiatry, 29,* 703–711.

Nurius, P. S., Lovell, M., & Edgar, M. (1988). Self-appraisals of abusive parents. *Journal of Interpersonal Violence, 3,* 458–467.

Oates, R. K., & Bross, D. C. (1995). What have we learned about treating child physical abuse? A literature review of the last decade. *Child Abuse & Neglect, 19,* 463–473.

Oates, R. K., Gray, J., Schweitzer, L., Kempe, R. S., & Harmon, R. J. (1995). A therapeutic preschool for abused children: The Keepsake Project. *Child Abuse & Neglect, 19,* 1379–1386.

O'Dell, S. L., Tarler-Benlolo, L., & Flynn, J. M. (1979). An instrument to measure knowledge of behavioral principles as applied to children. *Journal of Behavior Therapy and Experimental Psychiatry, 10,* 29–34.

Olweus, D. (1993a). Bully/victim problems among schoolchildren: Long-term consequences and an effective intervention program. In S. Hodgins (Ed.), *Mental disorder and crime* (pp. 317–349). Newbury Park, CA: Sage.

Olweus, D. (1993b). *Bullying at school: What we know and what we can do.* Cambridge, MA: Blackwell.

Peled, E. & Edleson, J. L. (1995). Process and outcome in small groups for children of battered women. In E. Peled, P. G. Jaffe, & J. L. Edelson (Eds.), *Ending the cycle of violence: Community responses to children of battered women* (pp. 77–96). Thousand Oaks, CA: Sage.

Pilkonis, P. A. (1993). Studying the effects of treatment in victims of childhood sexual abuse. *Journal of Interpersonal Violence, 8,* 392–401.

Richters, J. E., & Saltzman, W. (1990). *Survey of children's exposure to community violence: Parent report.* Rockville, MD: National Institute of Mental Health.

Rittner, B., & Wodarski, J. S. (1995). Clinical assessment instruments in the treatment of child abuse and neglect. *Early Child Development and Care, 106,* 43–58.

Roesler, T. A., Savin, D., & Grozs, C. (1993). Family therapy of extrafamilial sexual abuse. *Journal of the American Academy of Child and Adolescent Psychiatry, 32,* 967–970.

Runyan, D. K., Everson, M D., Edelsohn, G. A., Hunter, W. M., Coulter, M. L. (1988). Impact of legal intervention on sexually abused children. *Journal of Pediatrics, 113,* 647–653.

Sinclair, J. J., Larzclere, R. E., Paine, M., Jones, P., Graham, K., & Jones, M. (1995). Outcome of group treatment for sexually abused adolescent females living in a group home setting. *Journal of Interpersonal Violence 10,* 533–542.

Stauffer, L. B., & Deblinger, E. (1996). Cognitive behavioral groups for nonoffending mothers and their young sexually abused children: A preliminary treatment outcome study. *Child Maltreatment, 1,* 65–76.

Stehno, S. (1984, August). *The care and treatment program, Seattle Day Nursery.* Notes from presentation to the American Psychological Association Convention,

Steinberg, R, & Sunkenberg, M. (1994). A group intervention model for sexual abuse: Treatment and education in an inpatient child psychiatric setting. *Journal of Child and Adolescent Group Therapy, 4,* 61–73.

Stouthammer-Loeber, M., & Loeber, R. (1985). Child Rearing Practices—pilot version. Unpublished instrument, Pittsburgh Youth Study, University of Pittsburgh, Western Psychiatric Institute and Clinic, Pittsburgh, PA.

Straus, M. A. (1990). Measuring intra family conflict and violence: The Conflicts Tactics (CT) Scales. In M. A. Straus & R. J. Gelles (Eds.), *Physical violence in American families. Risk factors and adaptations to violence in 8,145 families* (pp. 29–47). New Brunswick, NJ: Transaction.

Taub, H. B., Kessler, M. L., & Lutzker, J. R (1995, June). Teaching neglectful families to identify and address environmental and health-related risks. In M. L. Kessler (Chair), *Treating Physical Abuse and Neglect: Four Approaches.* Symposium conducted at the Third Annual APSAC Colloquim, Tucson, Arizona.

Toth, S. L., & Cicchetti, D. (1993). Child maltreatment: Where do we go from here in our treatment of victims? In D. Cicchetti & S. L. Toth (Eds.), *Child abuse, child development, and social policy* (pp. 399–437). Norwood, NJ: Ablex.

Urquiza, A. J., & Bodiford-McNeil, C. (1996). Parent-child interaction therapy: An intensive dyadic intervention for physically abusive families. *Child Maltreatment, 1,* 134–144.

Wagar, J. M., & Rodway, M. R (1995). An evaluation of a group treatment approach for children who have witnessed wife abuse. *Journal of Family Violence, 10,* 295–306.

Warner, J. D., Malinosky-Rummell, R, Ellis, J. T., & Hansen, D. J. (1990). *An examination of demographic and treatment variables associated with session attendance of maltreating families.* Paper presented at the 24th Annual Conference of the Association for the Advancement of Behavior Therapy, San Francisco.

Wasik, B. H., & Roberts, R. N. (1994). Survey of home visiting programs for abused and neglected children and their families. *Child Abuse & Neglect, 18,* 271–283.

Wesch, D., & Lutzker, J. R. (1991). A comprehensive 5-year evaluation of Project 12-Ways: An ecobehavioral program for treating and preventing child abuse and neglect. *Journal of Family Violence, 6,* 17–35.

Whiteman, M., Fanshel, D., & Grundy, J. F. (1987, November–December). Cognitive–behavioral interventions aimed at anger of parents at risk of child abuse. *Social Work,* 469–474.

Whittaker, J., Kinney, J., Tracy, E. M., & Booth, C. (Eds.). (1990). *Reaching high risk families: Intensive family preservation in human services.* New York: Aldine de Guyter.

Willett, J. B., Ayoub, C. C., & Robinson, D. (1991). Using growth modeling to examine systematic differences in growth: An example of change in the functioning of families at risk of maladaptive parenting, child abuse, or neglect. *Journal of Consulting and Clinical Psychology, 59,* 38–47.

Winton, M. A. (1990). An evaluation of a support group for parents who have a sexually abused child. *Child Abuse & Neglect, 14,* 397–405.

Wolfe, D. A. (1994). The role of intervention and treatment services in the prevention of child abuse and neglect. In G. B. Melton & F. D. Barry (Eds.), *Protecting children from child abuse and neglect: Foundations for a new national strategy* (pp. 224–303). New York: Guilford Press.

Wolfe, D., Edwards, B., Manion, I., & Koverola, C. (1988). Early intervention for parents at risk for child abuse and neglect: A preliminary report. *Journal of Consulting & Clinical Psychology, 56,* 40–47.

Wolfe, D. A., & Wekerle, C. (1993). Treatment strategies for child physical abuse and neglect: A critical progress report. *Clinical Psychology Review, 13,* 473–500.

Zaidi, L. Y., & Gutierrez-Kovner, V. M. (1995). Group treatment of sexually abused latency-age girls. *Journal of Interpersonal Violence, 10,* 215–227.

8

Parent Training with Low-Income Families

Promoting Parental Engagement through a Collaborative Approach

CAROLYN WEBSTER-STRATTON

Children from certain types of families are at particularly high risk for developing conduct disorders (CD): namely, families characterized by factors such as low income, low educational level, high levels of stress, single-parent status, lack of support, and a history of ongoing depression, criminal activity, substance abuse, or psychiatric illness (Farrington, 1992). Children whose parents' discipline approaches are inconsistent and erratic and who are physically abusive, highly critical, or lacking in warmth (Patterson, Capaldi, & Bank, 1991; Patterson, Stouthammer-Loeber, 1984; Reid, Taplin, & Loeber, 1981) are also at high risk for conduct disorder, as are children whose parents are disengaged from their children's school experiences and provide little instruction for prosocial behavior (for review, see Webster-Stratton, 1990). Moreover, the risk of a child developing conduct disorders seems to increase exponentially with the child's exposure to each additional risk factor (Coie et al., 1993; Rutter, 1980).

Head Start is a federally funded preschool program available to children whose parents are receiving welfare. This group of economically disadvantaged preschool children may be characterized as having increased risk for developing conduct disorders because so many risk factors are present at higher than average rates in this population. In a recent study of more than 500 Head Start families in the Seattle area, we found that over 74% of the sample had four or more of the risk factors noted above (Webster-Stratton, 1995). Approximately 42% of the mothers were in the high range for harsh, critical discipline as measured by independent observers.

CAROLYN WEBSTER-STRATTON • Parenting Clinic, Family & Child Nursing, University of Washington, Seattle, Washington 98105-4631.

Handbook of Child Abuse Research and Treatment, edited by Lutzker. Plenum Press, New York, 1998.

Consistent with what might have been predicted from these findings, 35% of the children were above the established cutoff point for conduct problems, falling in the clinical range according to the Achenbach Child Behavior Checklist (Achenbach & Edelbrock, 1991). Other larger scale investigations have also indicated that economically deprived children are at increased risk for mental health problems (Belle, 1990; Goldberg, Roghmann, McInerny, & Burke, 1984). Goldberg and colleagues (1984) demonstrated that children receiving Medicaid benefits had almost twice as many behavior problems when compared with children from more advantaged environments. Unfortunately, reports indicate that fewer than 66% of disadvantaged children who are in need ever receive services (Saxe, Cross, & Silverman, Batchelor, & Dougherty, 1987) and only 20% receive adequate treatment.

While not all the risk factors for conduct disorders are amenable to intervention (e.g., economic status or parental history of substance abuse), risk factors such as lack of parenting skills, lack of support networks, and lack of school involvement are; to reverse these risk factors is to build up protective factors which may help buffer some of the adverse effects of poverty and its accompanying stressors. The potential for addressing these factors through parent training programs suggests that parent training would be a highly useful intervention with Head Start families. However, despite Head Start's founding philosophy of strong parent involvement (Zigler & Styfco, 1993), there have been few studies examining the benefits of adding a comprehensive parent training intervention to Head Start's child-focused program.

INTERVENTION WITH LOW-INCOME FAMILIES

The parent training literature has suggested that parent training is less effective with disadvantaged parents—particularly low-income single mothers—who have been described by Wahler (1980) as "insular" and "multiply entrapped." It also has been reported that recruitment rates for parent training interventions with low-income families of children with conduct problems are low, especially if there is an evaluation component (Spoth & Redmond, 1995). This population has often been reported to be the most likely to drop out of treatment (Bernal, 1984; Eyberg & Johnson, 1974), and more likely to relapse or to fail to make clinically significant improvements following treatment or to maintain treatment effects over time (Dumas & Wahler, 1983). Such families have been described as unmotivated, resistant, unreliable, disengaged, chaotic, in denial, disorganized, uncaring, dysfunctional, and unlikely candidates for this kind of treatment—in short, unreachable. However, these families might well describe traditional clinic-based programs as "unreachable." Clinical programs may be too far away from home, too expensive, insensitive, distant, inflexible in terms of scheduling and content, foreign in terms of language (literally or figuratively), blaming or critical of their lifestyle. A cost-benefit analysis would, in all likelihood, reveal that the costs to these clients of receiving treatment far outweigh the potential benefits—even though they do genuinely want to do what is best for their children. Perhaps this population has been "unreachable" not because of their own characteristics, but because of the characteristics of the interventions they have been offered.

The paradox is that while on the one hand we decry the lack of efficacy of therapy (i.e., parent training) with economically disadvantaged families, we also maintain the belief that if we could just do *more therapy* focusing more broadly (i.e., on family dysfunction and parental psychopathology), we would be more effective. But the problem may not lie in the focus of the therapy (i.e., parenting skills vs. family dynamics), but, rather, in the therapeutic model or approach—namely, a traditional clinic-based model of parent training. Before abandoning parent training as an intervention with this population, we should examine alternative models of parenting.

PARTNERS PARENT TRAINING

Recently we conducted a randomized study wherein we examined the effectiveness of an established theory-based parent training program (PARTNERS) as a selective prevention intervention (Medicine, 1994) with a sample of 210 Head Start parents and their 4-year-old children. The programs proven effectiveness as a clinical intervention for young children with identified conduct problems suggested its potential as a community-based, early prevention program designed to enhance family protective factors by strengthening parenting competence, fostering parents' involvement in children's Head Start preschool experiences, and promoting social support networks. Eight Head Start centers were randomly assigned to two conditions: (1) an experimental condition in which parents participated in the parent training program (PARTNERS) as well as in the Head Start program, or (2) a control condition in which parents participated only in the regular center-based Head Start program (controls). Baseline assessments for all eight centers included teacher and parent reports of child behavior as well as interviews and independent observations of parent–child interactions in the home and child behavior in the classroom. Home interviews lasted 2–3 hours and were carried out by warm, friendly women who had extensive experience working with parents. In some cases the interviewers were Head Start mothers who had shown natural leadership and caring interpersonal qualities. These interviews were followed by the home observations; observers asked parents to do what they would normally do and to try to ignore their presence. Post assessments at the end of the school year included parent and teacher reports as well as independent observations in the home. Evaluation of parental engagement included attendance, dropout rate, consumer satisfaction, and percentage improvement in observable parenting behaviors.

Approximately 65% of the total enrollees in the four Head Start centers participated in the study. Of those assigned to the PARTNERS group, 88% attended more than two-thirds of the sessions. Only 12% attended fewer than four sessions or dropped out after attending the first session. Results of home observations by independent raters indicated that PARTNERS mothers made significantly fewer critical remarks, used less physically negative discipline, and were more positive, appropriate, and consistent in their discipline style when compared with control mothers. PARTNERS mothers perceived their family service workers as more supportive than did control mothers; furthermore, teachers reported that PARTNERS mothers were more involved in their children's education than control mothers. In turn, PARTNERS children were observed at home to exhibit significantly fewer negative behaviors, less noncompliance, more positive affect, and more prosocial behaviors than control children. Consumer satisfaction with the program was high, with 89% reporting "positive" to "very positive" overall satisfaction, 91% reporting they expected positive results, and 95% saying they would "highly recommend" the program to others. More than 85% of the parents in the intervention condition wanted the program to be longer and to continue into the kindergarten year.

In a second analysis we sought to determine the clinical significance of the intervention (Schmaling & Jacobson, 1987) and the particular characteristics of the families from the intervention condition who did not respond to the intervention. This question was of interest not only for the sake of evaluating our intervention, but also in light of the current debate regarding this population. Results indicated that for PARTNERS mothers, 71% showed a 30% reduction in critical statements, whereas 29% were categorized as nonresponders. Of the mothers who were nonresponders, 40% reported a history of drug abuse as compared with 17% of mothers categorized as responders. There was a trend ($p < .06$) for mother psychiatric illness also to differentiate responders from nonresponders. Responses to the program were not affected by educational level, minority status, depression level, number of negative life events, amount of support or history of physical or sexual abuse.

In contrast to what the literature has reported about parent training programs for disadvantaged families, the short-term results of this prevention program suggest that the intervention was successful in engaging at least two-thirds of the families, as evidenced by the high level of recruitment, low parent dropout rate, high percentage of families who made clinically significant improvements, and high consumer satisfaction with training methods and content. Why did this program succeed where others have failed? Because the content of this program is similar to many others, we hypothesize that it was other aspects of the intervention—our training model, our methods, our leadership style, or specific strategies—that contributed to the high level of parental engagement. To look at it a little differently, rather than characteristics of the families being the reason for the failure of previous interventions with low-income parents, we hypothesize that interventions with this population (or any population) may fail when they lack certain critical intervention characteristics that enable a family to remain engaged in a parent training program and thereby benefit from it.

The remainder of this chapter will focus on a closer examination of what we consider to be the critical features of the PARTNERS program by which we promoted parental engagement with this intervention program for this low-income group of families. More details regarding the research results of the intervention can be found elsewhere (Webster-Stratton, 1995).

Initial Steps to Promote Parental Engagement

Involving School Personnel and Parents in Planning

In launching the program, one key to attracting parents was the participation of administrators, teachers, and Head Start staff who were committed to the program's goals and methods. Because the actual staff (teachers and family service workers) at the Head Start centers were employed by school districts (although administered by Head Start), we felt that all levels of administrative support would be essential to the ultimate success of the project.

We began by developing an advisory steering committee consisting of Head Start administrators, parent policy council representatives, teachers, family service workers, and parents. This committee's function was to provide advice concerning recruitment of families, assessment procedures, and relevant content for the intervention. The committee also assisted in the important job of informing and soliciting input from the principals and superintendents of the five school districts where the Head Start centers were located. Shared participation in the process of designing the recruitment, training and evaluation strategies would, we believed, lead to shared ownership of the program and a commitment to its eventual success.

The advisory committee conducted a series of focus groups with the separate groups of teachers, family service workers, and parents in order to define and prioritize their needs and goals, as well as to develop a recruitment plan, select sites for the intervention, and agree upon a schedule and time line. In the first year, we conducted a pilot parent group to evaluate the program's relevance and acceptability to parents. This was followed by a series of workshops in which we presented the pilot group's findings and showed how the PARTNERS program meshed with their administrative and family goals and needs. Teachers and family service workers participated in mock parent groups so as to become familiar with the program content, process, and methods. As a result, they were able to serve as knowledgeable and enthusiastic recruiters for the program among Head Start parents.

We chose to train the family service workers within the Head Start organization to be the parent group trainers because of their ongoing involvement with families in the preschool setting during the week. About 30% of them had social work degrees and the others had baccalaureate degrees in psychology or some other helping profession. Some of them had been Head Start parents themselves and had firsthand knowledge of what it is like to live on welfare. Since we felt it was important for the group trainers to be as similar as possible to the parents in their cultural and linguistic background, in the second year of the project we selected representative parents to be trained as co-trainers to work alongside the family service workers. We felt that if parents perceived the group trainers and co-leaders as similar to themselves, their engagement with the program would be enhanced.

Encouraging Every Parent's Participation

The next step was to advertise the parenting program to *all* of the parents enrolled in the Head Start centers that had been randomly chosen for the intervention trial. We began this process in the spring when parents first indicated an interest in Head Start. The family service workers and teachers described Head Start as a program not just for children, but also for parents. The PARTNERS program was described as part of the Head Start curriculum, and flyers were handed out describing the content of PARTNERS. In the fall when families actually enrolled in Head Start, further discussion of the parenting program took place during orientation meetings. Parents who had participated in the pilot parent group attended these meetings and told parents about their positive experiences with the PARTNERS program. They also called parents who were reluctant to sign up and told them of their own initial reluctance, reiterating the program's possible benefits.

The program was offered in the centers as a "universal" intervention (i.e., offered to all parents) because we felt that singling out parents on the basis of either their increased risk factors or their child's negative behaviors would have a stigmatizing effect and therefore result in a low turnout. Although our ultimate goal was to reduce conduct problems, we advertised the program in terms of school success, for our focus groups had indicated that the majority of parents were interested in learning ways to promote their children's academic success.

Accessibility and Feasibility of Intervention

Quality child care is essential in order for parents to be able to attend parent training. In this case, child care was provided during the sessions for all children of participating parents (not just the Head Start child), organized largely by Head Start teachers and parents who had been trained in our program. This was perceived as an added bonus of participating in the program because it gave parents a much-appreciated break from child care. Where needed, we also provided families with transportation to and from parent groups.

Our goal was to offer the program in highly accessible locations (i.e., as close as possible to where the parents were living and working) at convenient times. Many of the Head Start centers did not have enough space to accommodate both a parent training group and the accompanying child care for 10 to 40 children at a time. We ended up holding sessions in schools, churches, and housing units.

Incentives

In addition to appealing to parents' intrinsic motives, we also offered some tangible benefits for participating in the program. Because baseline assessments involved a considerable time commitment from parents—a 2- to 3-hour home interview and completion of many questionnaires—we offered a $30 payment (often in the form of a voucher at a large department store) for completion of baseline assessments. In addition, if parents completed post-assessments at the end of the year and had attended at least two-thirds of the sessions, we paid them an additional $70. For each session missed, $10 was deducted from the final amount. Initially, we used raffles and lotteries as motivators, but we stopped these when feedback from parents indicated they felt it devalued their commitment to the goals of the program. Instead, we substituted periodic surprise celebrations of parents' efforts as a group and for individuals mastering a particularly difficult skill.

Food at group meetings was an additional incentive—and not only as refreshment or a snack. For many parents it made the difference between attending or not attending an evening group. For example, if a mother was picking up children from day care at 5 P.M., she could not feed them and herself and make it to a 6 P.M. meeting. By offering dinner at the meeting, we enabled them to come directly to the meeting. Furthermore, husbands and partners were more likely to attend when dinner was available. Thus offering dinner amounted to making the intervention more feasible for these parents. Well-balanced dinners were offered to parents as well as to their children. Parents participated in planning menus for groups and, in some groups, a different parent took responsibility each week for purchasing the food for the subsequent session (with funds provided). This rotation of responsibility resulted in a pleasant variety in the type of food provided. Afternoon sessions included substantial snacks of fruit, vegetables, and desserts.

At the end of the year we asked parents what motivated them to participate in the program in the first place. Approximately 80% of the parents said they attended because they wanted "to learn more about parenting"; 26% of these were concerned about particular behavior problems in their children and 17% said they felt "out of control as a parent." Of the total group, 22% said they participated specifically because they wanted to make new friends with other parents. Only 9.4% said they signed up because of the financial incentive. Of the parents, 95.8% said they would have participated even if they had not been given the financial incentives.

Training Model

Parent Training as Collaborative

There are many competing parent intervention models, each with different sets of assumptions about the cause of family problems, the role of the therapist and the nature of the relationship between parent and therapist, and the level of responsibility assumed by the parent and the therapist. In many—perhaps most—parent training programs, the model is *hierarchical:* The trainer's role is that of an expert who is responsible for uncovering and interpreting past experiences and family dynamics to the family. In such a model the parent's role is that of a relatively passive recipient of the trainer's knowledge and advice. In other models, parents are to blame for their children's behavior; misbehavior is evidence that the parent is unable to display effective parent skills and the trainer's role is to diagnose and repair the parent's deficit.

Our training model for working with families is collaborative. In a collaborative relationship, the trainer does not set him- or herself up as an "expert" dispensing advice to parents about how they should parent more effectively. With a root meaning of "to labor together," collaboration implies a reciprocal relationship based on utilizing equally the trainer's and the parent's knowledge, strengths, and perspectives. A collaborative model of parent training is non-blaming and non-hierarchical.

As professionals, we have considerable expertise in our fields. Does the collaborative trainer have to renounce this expertise? Hardly. The collaborative training model acknowledges that expertise is not the sole property of the therapist or trainer: The parents function as experts concerning their child, their particular family, and their community, and the trainer functions as expert concerning child development, family dynamics in general, behavior management principles, and so on. The collaborative trainer labors with parents by actively soliciting their ideas and feelings, understanding their cultural context, and involving them in the therapeutic process by inviting them to share their experiences, discuss their ideas, and engage in problem solving. Collaboration implies that parents actively participate in setting goals and the intervention agenda. It also implies that parents evaluate each session and the trainer is responsible for adapting the intervention so that it meets the families' needs.

Another aspect of the collaborative trainer's labor is working with parents to adapt concepts and skills to the particular circumstances of those parents and the particular temperament of their child. For example, a parent who lives in a one-room trailer will not have an empty room for time-out and will have difficulty even finding a suitable spot to put a time-out chair. A parent living in an apartment, where walls usually are not soundproofed, will be acutely sensitive to the possible reactions of neighbors when she or he tries to ignore the screaming child; with good reason, that parent may resist using the ignore technique. These parents may raise objections—apparently unrelated from the therapists' point of view—to the use of time-out or ignoring. In traditional (hierarchical) therapy, these would be seen as instances of resistance, and the therapist/trainer would try to overcome the parents' resistance. In contrast, the collaborative therapist/trainer would operate from the assumption that the parent had legitimate grounds for resisting this aspect of the training, would attempt to understand the living situation and other circumstances of each family, and would involve the parents in problem solving to adapt the concepts to their particular situation. To take another example, a highly active, impulsive child will not be able to sit quietly and play attentively with his parents for long periods of time. Such children will also have more difficulty sitting in time-out than will less active children. As another example, some children are not particularly responsive to tangible reward programs. The trainer needs to be sensitive to these differences in child temperament so that she or he can begin to collaborate with parents in defining the approaches that will work for them and their child.

A noncollaborative approach is didactic and nonparticipative—the trainer lectures, the parents listen. The noncollaborative trainer presents principles and skills to parents in terms of "prescriptions" for successful ways of dealing with their children. Homework assignments are rigid, given without regard for the particular circumstances of an individual family. We reject this approach because, for one thing, it is unsuccessful: It is likely to lead to higher attrition rates and poor long-term maintenance. Furthermore, it is ethically dubious to impose goals on parents which may not be congruent with their goals, values, and lifestyles and which are not adapted to the temperament of their child. This is particularly important when there are cultural or class differences between the trainer and the group; assumptions arising from the trainer's own background or training simply may not apply. The collaborative model implies that, insofar as possible, the trainer stimulates the parents to generate solutions based on their experience with their child, and based on their family's cultural, class, and individual background. When parents come up with solutions they view as appropriate, the trainer can then reinforce and expand on these ideas.

A collaborative style of trainership is demonstrated by open communication patterns within the group and the trainer's attitude of acceptance toward all the families in the program. By building a relationship based not on authority but on rapport with the group, the trainer creates a climate of trust, making the group a safe place for parents to reveal their problems and to risk new approaches. The collaborative leader is a careful listener. She or he uses open-ended questions when exploring issues, for they are more likely to generate discussion and collaboration, and she or he encourages debate and alternative viewpoints, treating all viewpoints with respect. The trainer's empathic understanding is conveyed by the extent to which she or he actively reaches out to the parents, elicits their ideas, and attempts to understand rather than analyze (see Webster-Stratton & Herbert, 1994, for a more comprehensive discussion of collaborative model).

Parent Training as Empowerment

This partnership between parents and group trainer has the effect of giving back dignity, respect and self-control to parents who, because of their problems, including poverty, may be in a vulnerable time of low self-confidence and intense feelings of guilt and self-blame (Spitzer, Webster-Stratton, & Hollinsworth, 1991). It is our hypothesis that a collaborative approach is more likely to increase parents' confidence and perceived self-efficacy than all other therapeutic approaches. The essential goal of collaborative intervention is to empower parents so that they feel confident about their parenting skills and about their ability to respond to new situations that may arise when the therapist is not there to help them. Bandura (1977) has called this strategy strengthening the client's "efficacy expectations"— that is, parents' conviction that they can successfully change their own and their child's behaviors. Bandura (1982, 1989) has suggested that self-efficacy is the mediating variable between knowledge and behavior. Therefore, parents with high self-efficacy will tend to persist at tasks until they succeed. The literature also indicates that people who have determined their own priorities and goals are more likely to persist in the face of difficulties and less likely to show debilitating effects of stress (e.g., Dweck, 1975; Seligman, 1975).

Moreover, this model is likely to increase parents' engagement in the intervention. Research (Backeland & Lundwall, 1975; Janis & Mann, 1977; Meichenbaum & Turk, 1987) suggests that the collaborative process has the multiple advantages of reducing attrition rates, increasing motivation and commitment, reducing resistance, increasing temporal and situational generalization, and giving parents and the therapist a joint stake in the outcome of the intervention. On the other hand, controlling or hierarchical modes of therapy, in which the trainer analyzes, interprets, and makes decisions *for* parents without incorporating their input, may result in a low level of commitment, dependency, low self-efficacy, and increased resistance (Janis & Mann, 1977; Patterson & Forgatch, 1985), as well as resentment of professionals. In fact, if parents are not given appropriate ways to participate, they may see no alternative but to drop out or resist the intervention as a means of asserting their control over the therapeutic process.

In short, the net result of collaborative parent training is to empower parents by strengthening their knowledge and skill base, their self-confidence, and their autonomy, instead of perpetuating a sense of inadequacy and creating dependence on the therapist or trainer. There is a further reason for this model: Because we want parents to adopt a participative, collaborative, empowering approach with their own children, it is important to use this approach with the parents in the program—that is, to model with them the relationship style we wish them to use with their children. This form of training leads to greater internalization of learning in children (and very likely adults) (Herbert, 1987).

Parent Training Groups as Support Systems

It is debatable whether there are clearly differentiated criteria for choosing between one-on-one intervention and group training. Our own research with clinic families has shown that group training utilizing videotape modeling is at least as therapeutically effective as one-on-one intervention and certainly more cost-effective (Webster-Stratton, 1984, 1985b). But aside from the obvious economic benefits, there is another benefit to the group format: greater parental engagement with the program, a particularly compelling benefit in the case of low-income single mothers, who have been reported by Wahler (1980) and others to be "insular"—that is, socially isolated, with little support and few friendships. "Insular" parents frequently report feeling criticized and otherwise rejected in their relationships with relatives, professionals, case workers, spouses, and girl- or boyfriends. Parent groups can become an empowering environment for these parents, decreasing their insularity and giving them new sources of support.

Many of the parents in our studies initially were reluctant to participate in groups, preferring the privacy of individual counseling. However, after completion of the training, 87.7% reported that group discussion was a very useful training method—ranking second to books in terms of effectiveness as a training method. After having had a successful group experience, many parents were for the first time willing to consider serving on PTA boards or participating in other school and community-related group functions.

In the parent group, parents learned how to collaborate in problem solving, how to express their appreciation for each other, and how to cheer each other's successes in tackling difficult problems. They also learned to share their feelings of guilt, anger and depression, as well as experiences that involve mistakes on their part or misbehaviors from their children. These discussions served as a powerful source of support. Through this sharing of feelings and experiences, commonality was discovered. Feelings of isolation decreased, and parents were empowered by the knowledge that they are not alone in their problems and that many of their problems are normal. And this sense of group support and kinship increased parents' engagement with the program. For instance, the following comments were made in one of our groups:

> FATHER: You know when this program is finished, I will always think about this group in spirit.
> MOTHER: This group is all sharing—it's people who aren't judging me, who are also taking risks and saying, "Have you tried this?" or "Have you considered you might be off track?"

One of the ways we helped our groups become support systems was by assigning everyone a parent "buddy" in the second session. Buddies were asked to call each other during the week to share how the homework assignment (e.g., praising, limit setting) was going. Parents were initially hesitant about making these calls, but as they experienced the sense of support they received from these phone conversations, they expressed a desire to continue them. Frequently, fathers voiced that this was the first time they had ever talked to another father about parenting. This assignment was carried out four times during the program, with different "buddies" each time.

Building Parent Support outside the Group

Parents often reported conflicts with partners and grandparents over how to handle the child's problems, resulting in stressed relationships and stressed individuals. Therefore, in addition to building the support system within the parent group, the program also emphasized building support within the family and home life. The program encouraged every parent to have a spouse, partner, close friend, or family member (such as a grandparent) in the program with them to provide mutual support. (Our own follow-up studies as well as others' have indicated that the greatest likelihood of relapse occurs in families in which only one person was involved in the intervention [Herbert, 1987; Webster-Stratton, 1985c]). During parent groups, partners were helped to define ways they could support each other when one was feeling discouraged, tired, or unable to cope.

Frequently, the energy required to care for children, coupled with financial constraints, leaves parents feeling exhausted, too tired to make plans to spend time with each other or with adult friends, let alone interact with them. Yet time away from the child with a partner or a friend can help parents feel supported and energized. It helps them gain perspective so they are better able to cope with parenting. Wahler's (1980) research has indicated that single mothers who have contact with other people outside the home fare much better in their parenting than do mothers without such contacts, while maternal insularity or social isolation results in the probability of intervention failure (Dumas & Wahler, 1983). In our group, sometimes parents almost seemed to have forgotten their identity as individuals other than as parents. One of the home assignments was to do some self-care activity so that parents learned how to take "caring moments" in which they do something nice for themselves. Emphasis was placed on inexpensive activities such as taking a walk or a hot bath, reading a book, listening to music, meeting a friend for coffee, and so forth. Paradoxically, the result of spending some time away in self-care activities was often a feeling of support and understanding from one's partner or the other adult who made it possible.

Training Content

There is a rather large body of literature describing the content of parent training programs. Commonly taught behavior management strategies such as time-out, praise, effective limit setting, differential attention, response cost, and so on, along with the behavioral principles that underlie them, have been described in detail in many parent training programs (e.g., Barkely, 1987; Forehand & McMahon, 1981; Patterson, 1982; Webster-Stratton, 1992a). The behavioral content of the PARTNERS program was presented under the following eight topics, which provided the focus for the eight weekly sessions: (1) How to Play with Your Child, (2) How to Help Your Child Learn, (3) Effective Praise and Encouragement, (4) How to Motivate Your Child, (5) Effective Limit Setting, (6) How to Follow Through with Limits and Rules, (7) Handling Common Misbehaviors, and (8) Problem Solving. These topics were selected based on information from parents and teachers as well as our own beliefs about which behavioral strategies were most important for the 4-year-old child.

The behavioral components of the program were intertwined with cognitive components, because several studies have shown that parents who learn the principles underlying the behavioral strategies are better able to generalize strategies to new situations and are more satisfied with their program (McMahon & Forehand, 1984; Glogower & Sloop, 1976). Consequently, we felt parental engagement would be enhanced by what we called *principle training* in which we sought to help parents determine which principle was operative in a given situation or might be used to influence a particular child behavior. For example, the modeling principle was important for parents to grasp so that they could understand why modeling a particular behavior (e.g., respect, self-control) would have long-term benefits for them in improving their child's behavior. Or, to take another example, a parent might come to the group with questions about her child's refusal to get dressed in the morning; the trainer would ask the parent to think about what principle might be operating to maintain the child's dawdling and refusal to dress (i.e., attention). In addition, parents were helped to *conceptualize the strategies* they had learned. For example, the trainer might say, "Now you have learned to praise your child and ignore misbehavior and you know how to do it, but what makes it hard to do at dinner time?" or "What are the times of the day or situations when you find it most difficult to stay positive?" Once these difficult situations or circumstances were identified, the group would discuss strategies the parent might use to minimize the impact of the situation on their parenting.

Group leaders also attempted to explain the rationale for particular behavioral strategies in terms of parents' stated goals. For example, when providing the rationale for doing child-directed play, the trainer would explain how this approach fosters the child's self-esteem, social competence, and success in school, at the same time decreasing the child's need to obtain control over parents through negative behaviors. In this example, the rationale was important not only because parents might not immediately have seen the connection between playing with their children more and helping their child be successful in school, but also because this rationale established a strong link between this new element in the training and the parents' original reason for agreeing to participate (i.e., to promote their child's academic success). Without this rationale, parents might not be motivated to do the play sessions. To take another example:

> FATHER: He hit her and hurt her. I have talked to him over and over about how he's making other children feel bad. I get so frustrated with him. He doesn't seem to have any guilt.
>
> TRAINER: It *is* frustrating. But it looks like you're doing a nice of job of beginning to help him understand the perspective of others in a situation. You know, the development of empathy in children—that is, the ability of a child to understand another person's point of view—takes years. Not until adulthood is this aspect of development fully matured. Young children are at the very beginning steps of gaining this ability. The paradox of this is that one of the best ways you can help your son learn to be sensitive to the feelings of others is for you to model your understanding of him. Children need to feel understood and valued by their parents before they can value others.

In this example, the trainer restates or echoes the parent's frustration with his son, shows empathy about it, reinforces the parent's efforts to promote empathy, brings up the behavioral principle of modeling, and explains some points of child development. In doing so, the trainer is collaborating with the parent's goal, yet suggesting a new method for pursuing this goal.

In the interest of promoting engagement (as well as for therapeutic reasons), it was also important to explore parents' affective responses to the training in general and to particular strategies they were learning. Trainers would acknowledge in the groups that some parents might be feeling resentful, critical, angry, and hopeless about their relationships with their children, their life situation, and their ability to alter the future. When these feelings are acknowledged, they lose some of their power to disrupt the parent's engagement with the training. The trainer was then able to help parents learn how to recognize and cope with feelings that might prevent them from engaging with their children. Discussing distressing thoughts in a parent group is also very reassuring for parents because it helps to "normalize" thoughts which they may previously have considered abnormal or crazy. As parents discover that other parents have the same kinds of "crazy" thoughts and reactions, they stop blaming themselves.

Many low-income parents experience quite understandable feelings of powerlessness, which are sometimes expressed in terms of feeling victimized by their children or by fate—"Why me?" The feeling of helplessness typically is accompanied by intense anger and a fear of losing control of themselves when trying to discipline their children. Parents' anger toward their children is likely to cause them to blame themselves and to then feel depressed in reaction to their guilt. Furthermore, they feel depressed about their interactions with their children, seeing themselves as causal factors in their children's problems. More than 50% of the parents in our Head Start study were in the clinical range for depression on the CES-D inventory (Rodloff, 1977).

As with the behavioral component, the affective dimension of parents' experience was addressed through a cognitive approach. Parents were helped to understand the factors—family dynamics, past experiences, the legacy of their families of origin, current life stressors, and so on—that might be disrupting their parenting. The parent program addressed parents' depression by focusing on helping them stop their spiraling negative self-talk and, more generally, to modify their negative thoughts. We tried to help them learn how to give themselves a psychological "pat on the back." Parents were encouraged to look at their strengths and think about how effectively they handled a difficult situation. We asked them to express their positive feelings about their relationship with their child and to remember good times before this stressful period. We taught parents to actively formulate positive statements about themselves such as, "I had a good day today with Billy; I handled that situation well," or, "I was able to stay in control; that was good." For example, a parent might say, "It's all my fault, I'm a terrible parent. This is more than I can cope with; everything's out of control." The trainer would then help the parent learn how to stop this kind of powerless, self-defeating train of thought and to substitute calmer, coping self-statements such as, "Stop worrying. These thoughts are not helping me. I'm doing the best I can. He's just testing my limits. All parents get discouraged at times. I'm going to be able to cope with this."

Parents were asked to keep records of their thoughts in response to extremely stressful situations with their children at home. We then invited them to share some of this record with the group. As the group discussed these thoughts, unrealistic expectations and irrational beliefs were challenged and became modified through discussion. These strategies are in accordance with the cognitive restructuring strategies described by Beck (1979). The process of learning to recognize angry, helpless, self-critical, blaming, catastrophizing thoughts, and to substitute more adaptive and positive thoughts, empowers parents by showing them they can cope with their thought patterns as well as their behaviors.

Training Methods

Videotape Modeling

Verbal training methods such as lectures and written handouts about parenting are inexpensive and can be widely disseminated; however, such methods have been shown to be relatively ineffective for changing actual parenting behaviors. In particular, those parents with a poor educational background show low satisfaction and poor engagement with such verbal training methods, perhaps because of associated low reading abilities or because they are not verbal learners (Chilman, 1973). Performance training approaches such as videotape feedback, role play and rehearsal, on the other hand, have been shown to be very effective for improving parenting behaviors. Our own research indicated that therapist-led group discussion based on videotape modeling was superior to therapist-led group discussion without videotapes. Even self-administered videotape modeling resulted in significant changes in parenting skills and fewer dropouts when compared to group discussion without videotape (Webster-Stratton, Kolpacoff, & Hollinsworth, 1988; Webster-Stratton, Hollinsworth, & Kolpacoff, 1989). Regardless of educational background, families showed more significant improvements if they were trained by videotape modeling rather than methods using no videotapes (Webster-Stratton, 1984).

The PARTNERS program relied heavily on videotape modeling. The series of videotape programs shows parents of different sexes, ages, cultures, socioeconomic backgrounds, and temperament styles interacting with their children in natural situations—during mealtime, getting children dressed in the morning, toilet training, handling child disobedience, playing together, and so forth. The 130 vignettes include scenes in which parents are "doing it right" and "doing it wrong." The intent in showing negative as well as positive examples was to demystify the notion that there is "perfect parenting" and to illustrate how parents can learn from their mistakes (Webster-Stratton, 1992b).

The videotapes were designed to be used in a collaborative way—as a catalyst for group discussion and problem solving, not as a device that renders the parents passive observers. After a videotape vignette was shown, the trainer would pause the tape to give parents a chance to react and discuss what they had observed. The trainer often would ask open-ended questions such as, "Do you think that was the best way to handle that situation?" or, "How would you feel if your child did that?" The goal was to have parents become actively engaged in problem solving and sharing ideas about the vignette. Trainers would also facilitate learning by asking the parents how the concepts illustrated in the vignettes applied or did not apply to their own situations. For example, a mother made the following comment after watching a few of the play vignettes:

> MOTHER: I don't have any toys at home. I can't afford toys like those shown on the tapes—I'm living on a welfare check.
> TRAINER: You know, even if you had the money it is not important to have fancy toys. In fact, some of the best toys for children are things like pots and pans, empty cereal boxes, dry macaroni and string. Why don't we brainstorm some ideas for inexpensive things you could use to play with your child at home?

Role-Playing and Rehearsal

Role-playing and modeling of newly acquired behaviors are one of the most common components of parent training programs; they have been shown to be quite effective in producing behavioral changes (Eisler, Hersen, & Agras, 1973; Twentyman & McFall, 1975). Role-play helps to evoke sequences in behavior, enabling parents to anticipate situations more clearly. However, some parents may feel reluctant to participate in role-playing, particularly if they feel inadequate regarding their own behavior as parents. Use of this method can lead to disengagement with therapy, and even dropout, if it is not handled well.

The PARTNERS program included two to three suggested role-plays for each session. Besides presenting a clear rationale for the role-play, the trainer would often do the first role-play in order to reduce parents' self-consciousness and anxiety. If the trainer could make the role-play humorous through exaggeration, so much the better. For example, the trainer (role-playing the parent) would go out of the room and shout from a distance (e.g., kitchen) for the child (role-played by the parent) to put away the toys. This usually raised chuckles of recognition—there is no way for the parent to know whether the child registers the command or responds in any way. We believe that the trainer should take on the roles of ineffective parent or a misbehaving child, but not a competent parent; if the trainer demonstrates a high level of skill, parents may be reluctant to volunteer for fear of not measuring up to the trainer's example.

After the trainer had done the first role-plays, we then broke the parent group into pairs to practice particular skills. Later on, as groups became comfortable with each other, parents role-played a situation in front of the whole group—for example, role-playing the use of time-out with a "difficult child." In this case, one parent played the child and another parent the child's parent. The remainder of the group would act as coaches for the parent who was in the parent role. Sometimes it is helpful to "freeze frame" the role-play and then ask the group to brainstorm, "Now what should she do?" or, "What is the child trying to communicate or achieve by behaving like that?" Reluctant role players may be cast as a coach or partner to the parent who is doing the actual role-playing so that they can offer advice is needed but are not seen as central.

The content for the role-plays came from the parents themselves. For example, if a parent came to the group after a week of trying to ignore her son's whining and said, "I can't ignore him—it's much worse than anything you showed us on videotape," the trainer might respond, "Okay, you be your whining son, and Sally, why don't you demonstrate how you would try to ignore this." This role-play has the added advantage of helping the parent experience the strategy from the child's perspective—the withdrawal of attention, the refusal to engage in a struggle—in order to experience its effectiveness.

Home Assignments and Self-Management

A home assignment was given for every weekly group session. This usually involved asking parents to do some observing and recording of behaviors or thoughts at home and/or experimenting with a particular strategy. For example, one assignment asked parents to play one-on-one with their child each day for 15 minutes; another assignment was to record how often they praised between 5 and 6 P.M. for 2 days, and then to double their base rate for the remainder of the week. Another was for parents to keep track of their thoughts in response to a conflict situation with their child on two occasions. We regarded assignments as critical because they conveyed at least two important messages: namely, that participation in the group was not "magic moon dust" and that change was not the trainer's responsibility; parents had to collaborate with the trainer by working at home to make changes. The home assignments helped to translate theory (what is talked about in group session) into real life. They also provided a powerful stimulus for discussion at the subsequent session.

Parents will naturally resist these assignments, seeing them as one more stress in their lives, so it was essential to make a case for the usefulness of the assignments. Homework was presented to parents as an integral part of the learning process. When a parent failed to complete an assignment from the previous session, the reasons for this were explored. A collaborative approach involves questions such as "What made it hard for you to do the assignment?" "How have you overcome this problem in the past?" "What advice would you give to someone else who has this problem?" "Do you think it is just as hard for your child to learn to change as it is for you to change?" "What can you do to make it easier for you to complete the assignment this week?" "Do you think there is another assignment that might be more useful for you?" Often these questions were explored as a group discussion topic.

It is important to explore reasons why some parents might be having difficulty doing their home assignments; otherwise, parents may conclude that the trainer is not really committed to the assignments, or does not really want to understand their particular situation. The process of talking about the assignments and renegotiating assignments if parents feel they are too difficult or unrealistic (without making them feel a failure) is a key to motivating parents' engagement with the program.

In order to facilitate the self-management and home activity portion of the program we gave each parent a personal folder. Each week the trainer put the new assignment in the folder and reviewed the parents' assignment from the prior week. Trainers commented in writing on these assignments in the folder, sometimes giving a sticker or prize and discussing with the group a strategy that a parent has discovered. For shy group members, these folders became a private way to communicate with the trainer; the trainer was able to give personalized feedback by writing in the folders. Often a folder resulted in the leader discovering how engaged a nonverbal parent really was. Another benefit of the folders was that they were the one place where parents could tell the trainer private comments they might not want to share with the whole group. On the inside cover of the folder was a checklist where parents were asked to check off whether or not they did the weekly assignment. When the trainer reviewed a weekly folder she or he would call parents who had missed two consecutive weekly assignments. In our Head Start final program evaluation 83% of the parents reported the home assignments to be "useful" to "very useful" and fewer than 1% reported them to be "somewhat useless" to "very useless."

Readings and Tapes

Although we have noted that verbal training methods are less effective than performance-based methods, this does not mean that we eliminated all books and written materials. In fact, since people have varied learning styles, we believe that effective programs should utilize many different learning methods. In the PARTNERS program every parent received a copy of the author's *The Incredible Years: A Trouble-Shooting Guide for Parents of Children (ages 3–8 years)* (Webster-Stratton, 1992a) (or audiotapes for nonreaders) and were given a weekly reading assignment which dovetailed with the videotapes shown that week. For many parents this was the only parenting book they had ever read, and for the first time they saw the possibility of using books as a resource for parenting. There were times when parents came to sessions having read "ahead" and having tried out strategies not yet presented in class. Final evaluations indicated that 88.9% found the book to be a "very useful" learning method.

Trainer's Strategies

Many low-income parents have had primarily negative experiences with professionals (caseworkers, social service agency staff, teachers, therapists) in the past, and came to the PARTNERS program with some skepticism and even mistrust of the therapists and group leaders. Bearing this in mind, we theorized that there would be better parental engagement with the program if the trainers saw their role within the context of a "friendship relationship." A collaborative trainer was conceptualized as the kind of friend who listens, asks for clarification, is reflective and nonjudgmental, tries to understand what the parent is saying through empathy, helps problem solve and does not command, instruct, or tell parents how to do their job.

One of the ways the PARTNERS trainers showed their commitment to the family was through follow-up calls made during the week. Trainers "checked in" with a friendly call each week, asking how things were going and whether parents were having any difficulty with the home assignments. In the final evaluations of the training, parents commented that they were genuinely touched that a trainer "just called to see how I was doing." (These calls also aided the trainer by revealing how well parents were assimilating the material presented in group so that the trainer could attempt to clarify any misperceptions.) These calls allowed trainers and parents to get to know one another outside the group—particularly useful in the case of the quiet or reluctant parents—and promoted engagement with the program.

Self-Disclosure

As discussed earlier, the collaborative trainer renounces the role of an "expert" who has all the answers, an expert who stands apart from the families' problems. The trainer must be not only empathic, respectful and kind, but also genuine. These core conditions (as described by Carl Rogers, 1951) are the necessary underpinnings for the cognitive–behavioral methodology. One expression of genuineness is the trainer's willingness to be known—to share personal experiences, feelings and problems of his or her own. Trainers and therapists always have a rich array of stories, either from their own families or from work with other families, which they can draw upon at will.

Self-disclosure concerning one's personal issues and experience was, however, planned strategically. It cannot be overemphasized that the purpose of self-disclosure was not for clients to learn about the trainer's feelings and problems; rather, the purpose of self-disclosure was identical to the purpose of the training: to help parents learn to function more effectively in their role as parents. By sharing some personal experiences, the trainer could help families understand that parenting is, for everyone, a process of learning to cope and to profit from mistakes; it is not a process of achieving perfection. Thus the trainer's personal examples helped discredit the notion that there are perfect parents. They also served to normalize the parents' reactions and to give them permission to make mistakes. Moreover, this genuineness on the part of the trainers was designed to enhance the trainer's relationship with the group members, introducing openness and a degree of intimacy, and fueling the collaborative process.

Humor

Humor has value as a coping strategy and a training strategy. Trainers made deliberate use of humor to help parents relax and to defuse anger, anxiety, and cynicism. Parents need to be able to laugh at their mistakes; this is part of the process of self-acceptance. Humor helps them gain some perspective on their stressful situation, which otherwise can become debilitating. Some of the videotape scenes in our program were actually chosen more for their humor value than for their content value. Our trainers used humorous personal examples in the discussions, distributed humorous cartoons of parents and children (which are found in abundance in newspapers and magazines), and role-played situations in which they did everything wrong—that is, with lots of criticisms directed at the child, negative self-talk, and so on. Laughter helped build group spirit, strengthening parents' engagement.

Reframing

Therapeutic change depends on providing explanatory "stories," alternative explanations which help parents to reshape their perceptions of and their beliefs about the nature of their problems. Retraining by the trainer or therapist (cognitive restructuring) is a powerful interpretive tool for helping parents understand their experiences, thereby promoting change in their behaviors. It involves altering the parent's emotional and/or conceptual view of an experience by placing the experience in another "frame" which fits the facts of the situation well, thereby altering its meaning.

One common strategy in PARTNERS groups was for the trainer to help parents see the developmental needs represented by the child's behavior. Retraining a difficult child's behavior in terms of a psychological or emotional drive such as testing the security of limits, or reacting to the loss of the important parent, or moving toward independence, helps the parents see the behavior as appropriate or normal—in some cases even positive. Seen in this light, problematic behaviors are the expression of normal emotions and developmental stages. Viewing situations this way, parents can feel that they are participating in a process of growth for the child. This attitude enhances coping and decreases feelings of anger and helplessness. Understood in terms of children's needs to test the security of their environment or to test the love of their parents, parent–child conflicts become less overwhelming and parents are more able to remain committed to the hard work of being parents.

Positive Expectations

Parents are often skeptical about their ability to change, especially if they see in their behavior a family pattern, for patterns often seem fixed and irreversible. Thus another function of the trainer is to counter that skepticism with positive expectations for change. For example, one parent said, "My mother beat me, now I beat my children." In response, the trainer expressed her confidence in the parent's ability to break the family cycle. Each small step toward change—even the step of coming to a parent training program in the first place—can be pointed to as evidence that the problem is not fixed or irreversible.

PARTNERS trainers tried to convey optimism about the parents' ability to successfully carry out the strategies required to produce positive changes in the child's behaviors. According to Bandura (1977), efficacy expectations are thought to be the most important component. Thus, successful treatment depends on the ability of the trainer to strengthen parents' expectations of personal efficacy ("I am able to do it"). Citing examples of the success of other parents in similar situations proved to be a useful strategy.

Positive Reinforcement

Trainers tried to validate and reinforce parents whenever possible by noticing and commenting upon their use of effective strategies and their insights. One father reported the following incident:

> FATHER: I was just so frustrated with him! He wouldn't get dressed and was dawdling—I was going to be late for work. I got angrier and angrier. Finally, I went into his bedroom and shook him by the shoulders and yelled, "You want negative attention, you're going to get negative attention!" Then suddenly I thought, What am I doing? Where is this getting me? and walked out of the room.
>
> TRAINER: So, you were able to stop yourself in the middle of an angry tantrum. Good for you! That's remarkable. It sounds like your ability to stand back from the situation, to be objective and think about your goals, really helped you stop what you were doing. Is that true? What do you usually find helps you keep control of your anger? How would you replay the situation if it happens again?

In this example, the trainers reinforced the father's insight and drew attention to his coping skills during the conflict situation. The trainer also helped the father learn from the experience by rehearsing how he might respond in the future. These parents need to be reinforced through positive feedback for each change in their behavior, whether or not it results in improvement in their child's behavior. This affirming process helps parents gain confidence in their ability to sort out problems and to learn from their mistakes (Brown & Harris, 1978). The developmental literature suggests that mothers who have confidence in their child-rearing and who feel they have broad community support actually do better at parenting (Behrens, 1954; Herbert, 1987).

Because in most groups there are varying levels of educational background and communication skills, it is important for parents' engagement and for group cohesion that the trainer reinforce every parent for sharing his or her ideas regardless of the trainer's opinion of those ideas. Furthermore, PARTNERS trainers attempted to clarify for the group any unfocused or confusing statements made by parents so that they would not be ridiculed, ignored, or criticized because of something they had said. We called this "finding the kernel of truth" in what a parent has said: underscoring its value by showing how it contributes to the group's understanding of the topic under discussion. In our experience, if the trainer does not clarify and validate these statements, the parent who makes them is at risk for dropping out—and so might other parents who become disillusioned with the experience.

Other Strategies for Promoting Engagement

Identifying Goals of Group

At the initial parent group meeting, parents were asked to share some of their personal experiences with their children, as well as their goals for the training program. The goals for each parent were posted on the wall so that they could be referred to throughout the program. This initial discussion often produced immediate group rapport as parents realized they had similar difficulties and were working toward similar goals. Throughout the training, parents were given home assignments to write down the child behaviors they wanted to see increase or decrease. These targeted behaviors (e.g., go to bed at 8 P.M., not interrupt when on phone) became the focus of principle training. Several times during the program the trainer drew up a composite list of behaviors parents were working on so that group members could see the similarities among their issues. This promoted ongoing group cohesion, as well as attention to individual goals, thereby increasing parents' commitment to the program.

Ensuring Group Safety and Sufficient Structure

One of the most difficult aspects of the trainer's role is to prevent the group experience from becoming negative. If this should happen, dropout is a certainty. Therefore, during the first meeting we asked group members to generate rules that would help them feel safe, comfortable, and accepted in the group. These rules were kept posted on the wall to be added to or referred to if necessary during weekly sessions. Examples included (1) only one person may talk at a time, (2) everyone's ideas are respected, (3) anyone has a right to pass, (4) no "put downs" are allowed, and (5) confidentiality within the room.

For groups that were very verbal and tended to get sidetracked, it was helpful at the beginning of each session to select a parent to act as a co-trainer. The job of this parent co-trainer was to be a timekeeper, to make sure all vignettes were covered, to help identify participants who were sidetracking the discussion, and to keep the group focused on the main topics for the session. Our evaluations indicated that parents became frustrated and disengaged if the discussion wandered, and they appreciated having enough structure imposed to keep the discussion moving along. By rotating the job of co-trainer, the task of monitoring the group discussion became everyone's responsibility; everyone was committed to the group's functioning well.

The group process can also be disrupted by a participant who challenges the trainer's knowledge or advocates inappropriate child-rearing practices. It is important that the trainer not seem critical or frustrated with this person's comments, for this is the "coercion trap" many parents have experienced in the past. Instead, the trainer looked for the relevant points in what the person had said and reinforced them for the group. By conveying acceptance and warmth, even toward a parent who is an obviously difficult group member, trainers modeled acceptance and helped group members see that the goal was to understand and respect everyone.

Weekly Evaluations

Each week the parents were asked to evaluate the group session. This immediate feedback about how each parent was responding to the trainer's style, the group discussions, and the content presented in the session brought to light any engagement problems as the program was in progress—the parent who was dissatisfied with the group, the parent who was resisting a concept, the parent who did not see the relevance of a particular concept to his or her own situation, the parent who wanted more or less group discussion. Between sessions, trainers would call any parent who indicated a neutral to negative weekly evaluation on more than one occasion to discuss their concerns about the program. Sometimes the trainer would meet with parents individually to resolve these issues. If several participants were having difficulty understanding a particular concept, the trainer would bring it up in a subsequent session with the whole group. By responding to parents' evaluations with actions, trainers validated the collaborative nature of the program and fostered parental engagement. After the last session, the entire program was evaluated. This information was useful not only in planning future parent groups, but also in identifying parents who needed further help.

Managing Disengagement and Resistance

When a parent is resisting a basic concept or disengaging from the program, the trainer faces a dilemma. Should the trainer confront and challenge the parent regarding this, or just let it go in the interest of fostering collaboration and offering support? The trainer may be worried that confrontation will jeopardize the collaborative relationship. Yet this failure to address the issue really constitutes a kind of collusion with parents regarding their parenting practices. Therefore, how this resistance is handled by the trainer is crucial not only to the parents' level of engagement with the program, but also to the effectiveness of the training.

Resistance takes a variety of forms—failure to do homework, arriving late for group sessions, blaming the trainer, blaming the child or life circumstances, negatively evaluating the sessions, or challenging the material presented. Clients say such things as:

MOTHER: I feel I just can't absorb it all and I'm getting behind at home. I just can't do all this play stuff, there isn't anytime.

FATHER: Yeah, I go out of this group charged up, but when I get home I lose it. I don't start thinking about applying all this stuff until right before our group is to meet again.

To some extent, resistance is a necessary part of the change process for which trainers (and clients) need to be prepared. Patterson and Forgatch (1985) indicate that considerable resistance will peak midway through the intervention process. Resistance may be part of the parent's efforts to maintain self-efficacy and self-control in the face of changing family dynamics—in effect, the parent is "putting on the brakes." Or parents may resist out of discouragement—unrealistic expectations for change and lack of preparation for the long, hard work involved.

But in other cases, resistance is the client's legitimate and understandable response to aspects of the intervention or the trainership that are inappropriate, ill-conceived, or ineffective. Too often we refuse to entertain the possibility that client resistance or disengagement are evidence of flaws in our approach. Freudian tradition, of course, discourages us from doing so, viewing resistance as an element in the therapeutic relationship. Certainly this view of resistance has supported the prevalent skepticism about working with disadvantaged clients, the tendency to see them as unreachable due to their own circumstances rather than due to aspects of the training model, the training format, the trainer's role, and so on. Whatever the source of the resistance, the first task for the trainer is to put aside any notion that the resistance is a sign that the parent is noncompliant or unmotivated—a "difficult person." Perhaps the parent is resisting because his or her stressful life circumstances make it difficult to find the time to do the assignments. Perhaps the parent is disengaged because she or he perceives the trainer as patronizing or thinks the trainer is presenting "pat" answers and solutions without really understanding his or her situation. Or perhaps the trainer shows no sensitivity to the parents' culture, is using unfair language or foreign examples, or uses humor that makes the parent uncomfortable.

One aspect of PARTNERS that frequently inspired resistance was the use of time-out as an alternative to spanking.

FATHER: Well, all this time-out stuff is well and good, but in the final analysis I think spanking is what you really need to do. Especially when something bad happens, like a broken window.

TRAINER: So you really see spanking as the final "big gun"?

FATHER: I do. You know, I was spanked by my father and it didn't do me any psychological harm.

A collaborative trainer deals with resistance by starting from the premise that the parent's views are legitimate—in this case, respecting the parent's preference for spanking as legitimate. She then would explore this viewpoint with nonjudgmental questions such as, "Tell me how spanking works for you. How often do you use it?" "How do you feel afterwards?" "How does your child feel about it?" "How does it affect your relationship?" "Do you ever feel you lose control when you spank?" "What do you see as the advantages of spanking?" "Are there any disadvantages?" "How did it affect your relationship with your parent when you were spanked as a child?" Similar questions might then be asked about time-out. "Let's look at an alternative approach. What are the difficulties with time-out?" "What don't you like about it?" "What are its disadvantages?" "Are there any advantages?"

In our parent groups this kind of discussion between the trainer and a resistant parent tended to draw group members into the discussion, whereas a judgmental or authoritarian response would tend to result in silence. Direct confrontation is likely to increase the parent's defensiveness (Birchler, 1988). Furthermore, it devalues the parent in front of the other group members. In fact, in one of the few studies to do a microanalytic analysis of therapist–client interactions, Patterson and Forgatch (1985) found that resistance met by direct confrontation or teaching on the part of the therapist actually *increased* parents' noncompliance.

One technique we used for handling resistance to a behavioral strategy was to list the advantages and disadvantages, short-term and long-term consequences for the child and for the parent, on a blackboard. At the end of this discussion, the trainer summarized the ideas that were generated, clarified concepts, and added his or her own ideas if they had not already been raised. This group problem solving served to move people away from "absolutist" positions, opening them up to new ideas which they might not have considered previously, thus reducing resistance. This process of exploring the reasons behind (and not the psychological reasons *for*) the resistance, followed by the exercise of looking at the advantages and disadvantages of particular parenting strategies, is a kind of values clarification and problem-solving exercise which helped clarify feelings and experiences surrounding the issue. This strategy serves to join people rather than alienate them. It is more likely than direct confrontation to result in a gradual change in parents' perceptions and behaviors, especially if conducted in the context of a supportive relationship. On the other hand, a noncollaborative approach, in which the trainer directly confronted the parents' ideas, would create a conflict wherein trainer and parent each have to defend their own position in order to protect their integrity.

Another strategy for moving the parent from resistance to engagement is to invite the parent to consider a short experimental period.

> TRAINER: I understand your viewpoint regarding time-out and that you think children should be spanked for misbehaving. At the same time, Timmy seems to have been having more and more problems with being aggressive with his peers and at school and I know you are eager to help him with this problem. I'd like to suggest that we do an experiment. I'd like you to give it a try and act as if it will work. I'd like you to try doing time-out for a month and keep records, and then at the end of a month let's evaluate how it looks. You see, if it doesn't work, you can always go back to the way you have been doing things and won't have lost anything. What do you think about that?

In this example, the trainer does not attack the resistance by confronting it directly or repeating the reasons she or he thinks time-out is right (and why the parent is wrong to use spanking). Rather, the trainer engages in a process of gentle persuasion. Although she does not confront the resistance itself directly, she confronts the difference of opinion directly.

A collaborative response to resistance can reveal instances where the intervention needs to be adapted to the client. Once the trainer understands the reason for the resistance, then she or he can then modify the approach as necessary so that the treatment objectives are still foremost and the parent can cooperate with the intervention. For example, one parent said she could not put the child in a time-out room because she felt it would create bad feelings about the child's room and, more importantly, the child would feel abandoned. Further exploration by the trainer uncovered the fact that as a child this parent had been locked for hours in her bedroom by her own parents! As a result of this discussion, the trainer and parent devised a "calm-down" strategy using a chair in the corner of the living room rather than the bedroom. Over the course of future sessions, the trainer helped the parent understand that *short* time-outs, in which the parent reestablishes control, help children to feel more secure in their relationships with their parents, and that children whose behavior is not controlled by their parents actually may come to feel psychologically abandoned. By accepting the parent's objection, joining with her in coming up with an appropriate strategy, and then reframing the concept so that the parent perceived time-outs as a way of promoting security (rather than as abandonment), the trainer enabled the parent ultimately to accept the strategy for herself and her child.

Predicting resistance early in the training may also be helpful.

> TRAINER: Be prepared to feel awkward when you do this kind of play. Be prepared for yourself to resist wanting to do it because it does feel awkward. And be prepared for your child not to like it at first. Whenever someone learns a new behavior, there is a natural tendency for family members to resist this new behavior and to revert back to the status quo. In fact, some family members might actually try to pressure you to return to the old way of doing things.
>
> OR,
>
> You will probably feel awkward praising at first, especially if you haven't done much of this in the past. You may even feel your praise sounds phony. So don't wait for yourself to feel warmth toward your child in order to praise. Just get the words out, even if they are kind of flat. The feelings and genuineness will come later. The more you practice, the more natural it will become.
>
> OR,
>
> Lots of parents don't like time-out at first. Compared to spanking it's more time-consuming, it is harder to keep the self-control you need (especially if you want "revenge" with your child), and it feels awkward. But with practice it will become automatic and your child will learn exactly what to do. You will feel good because you are teaching your child a nonviolent approach to dealing with conflict.

When parents are prepared for resistance in advance, they are more able to remain engaged with the intervention, for they can reframe their reactions as part of the change process.

> FATHER: My wife made me come. The first night I couldn't wait for it to be over. I was real skeptical of 90% of the things they said in the class at first. I had never even heard of time-out. Before taking this class my idea of discipline was to spank and yell a lot—you know—hit first and ask later. I con-

centrated on the negative and that was the way I was brought up. Then about halfway through the classes I did a 360 degree turnabout—now I feel more in control, more confident, much happier as a parent now than I did before. I used to come home and think, God, what kind of trouble did they get into today? or What am I going to have to punish them for tonight? Now I appreciate them a lot more and can stand back and think, Well, jeez, they are pretty good kids. I like myself better now than I did before.

CONCLUSION

It has been stated that because low-income parents are "multiply entrapped" they will be unlikely to show up for parent groups, will most likely drop out of parent training programs, and/or will fail to show significant improvements in their parenting. In this chapter, we presented the notion that it is the characteristics of the intervention, not of the client, that determine the success of parent training with this population. We believe that successful parent training programs need to be community-based and to involve parents in planning, recruitment, co-leading groups, and setting priorities for program content. At the end of the school year we again asked the parents if they were interested in any other kinds of programs in the future. More than 70% said they wanted to continue the parent program throughout the kindergarten year. Forty percent wanted additional social skills training for their children during the summer months; 45% wanted training in anger management; 35%, training in enhancing partner relationships; and 35%, in controlling depression. Thus it would seem that, having had a successful experience with a parent program, these parents are ready for and interested in broadening the focus to other family issues that they see as needs for themselves.

Successful programs need not only to involve parents in determining priorities for the content but also need to be accessible and realistic given the practical constraints of parents living on welfare or the "working poor"—that means providing child care, transportation, food, and evening groups as well as daytime groups. The training program needs to be delivered in a collaborative way so that parents are given responsibility for developing solutions alongside the trained trainer. The training methods need to be responsive to a variety of learning styles and to utilize performance-based training methods such as videotape modeling, role-playing, and home assignments. Program content needs to be relevant and sensitive to individual parent needs and family circumstances. The group format not only is more cost-effective, but enhances support networks both within the family and within the community, ultimately leading to greater parent empowerment. We believe that these elements of an intervention lead to a higher level of parental engagement, and this involvement will result in parents gaining the knowledge, control, and competence they need to effectively cope with the stresses of parenting under conditions of poverty.

FATHER: Like I said, I was spanked as a child and I felt pretty worthless but still I yelled and hit my own kids a lot. There was no communication other than yelling. Now I see my children differently—as human beings you know not just kids. I see them as having their own personality traits and their own sense of who they are and what they want to do—rather than just kids who must do what I want them to do. I see them differently.

ACKNOWLEDGMENTS

The author would like to acknowledge the Head Start family service workers for their untiring commitment and caring for families, as well as the Puget Sound Head Start administrators and coordinators who provided continual support for both the research and intervention aspects of this program. Without this partnership between Head Start families, family service workers, administrators, and the research team, the successful implementation of this program would not have been possible. Special thanks to Lois Hancock for coordinating all aspects of this program, from data management to program implementation, and to Deborah Woolley for her editing and ideas regarding this paper. A portion of this paper was previously presented at the 1995 meeting of the Association for Advancement of Behavior Therapy, Washington, DC.

REFERENCES

Achenbach, T. M., & Edelbrock, C. S. (1991). *Manual for the Child Behavior Checklist and Revised Child Behavior Profile.* Burlington, VT: University Associates in Psychiatry.

Backeland, F., & Lundwall, L. (1975). Dropping out of treatment: A critical review. *Psychological Bulletin, 82,* 738–783.

Bandura, A. (1977). Self-efficacy: Towards a unifying theory of behavioral change. *Psychological Bulletin, 84,* 191–215.

Bandura, A. (1982). Self-efficacy mechanism in human agency. *American Psychologist, 37,* 122–147.

Bandura, A. (1989). Regulation of cognitive processes through perceiver self-efficacy. *Developmental Psychology, 25,* 729–735.

Barkely, R. A. (1987). *Defiant children: A clinician's manual for parent training.* London: Guilford Press.

Beck, A. T. (1979). *Cognitive therapy and emotional disorders.* New York: New American Library.

Behrens, M. L. (1954). Child rearing and the character structure of the mother. *Child Development, 25,* 225–238.

Belle, R. Q. (1990). Parent, child, and reciprocal influences. *American Psychologist, 34,* 821–826.

Bernal, M. (1984). Consumer issues in parent training. In R. Danzel & R. A. Polster (Eds.), *Parent training: Foundations of research and practice* (pp. 447–501). New York: Guilford Press.

Birchler, G. (1988). Handling resistance to change. In I. Falloon (Ed.), *Handbook of behavioral family therapy* (pp. 128–155). New York: Guilford Press.

Brown, G. W., & Harris, T. (1978). *Social origins of depression.* London: Tavistock.

Chilman, A. (1973). Programs for disadvantaged parents. In B. U. Caldwell & W. N. Riccuiti (Eds.), *Review of child development and research* (vol. 3). Chicago: University of Chicago Press.

Coie, J. D., Watt, N. F., West, S. G., Hawkins, D., Asarnow, J. R., Markman, H. J., Ramey, S. L., Shure, M. B., & Long, B. (1993). The science of prevention; A conceptual framework and some directions for a national research program. *American Psychologist, 48,* 1013–1022.

Dumas, J. E., & Wahler, R. G. (1983). Predictors of treatment outcome in parent training: Mother insularity and socioeconomic disadvantage. *Behavioral Assessment, 5,* 301–313.

Dweck, C. S. (1975). The role of expectations and attributions in the alleviation of learned helplessness. *Journal of Personality and Social Psychology, 31,* 674–685.

Eisler, R. M., Hersen, M., & Agras, W. S. (1973). Effects of videotape and instructional feedback on nonverbal marital interactions: An analogue study. *Behavior Therapy, 4,* 5510–5558.

Eyberg, S., & Johnson, S. M. (1974). Multiple assessment of behavior modification with families: Effects of contingency contracting and order of treated problems. *Journal of Consulting and Clinical Psychology, 42*(4), 594–606.

Farrington, D. P. (1992). Explaining the beginning, progress and ending of antisocial behavior from birth to adulthood. In J. McCord (Ed.), *Facts, frameworks, and forecasts: Advances in criminology theory* (Vol. 3, pp. 253–286). New Brunswick, NJ: Transactions.

Forehand, R., & McMahon, R. (1981). *Helping the noncompliant child: A clinician's guide to parent training.* New York: Guilford Press.

Glogower, F., & Sloop, E. W. (1976). Two strategies of group training of parents as effective behavior modifiers. *Behavior Therapy, 7*(4), 177–184.

Goldberg, I. D., Roghmann, K. J., McInerny, T. K., & Burke, J. D. (1984). Mental health problems among children seen in pediatric practice: Prevalence and management. *Pediatrics, 73,* 278–293.

Herbert, M. (1987). *Behavioral treatment of children with problems.* London, Academic Press.

Janis, I. L., & Mann, L. (1977). *Decision making: A psychological analysis of conflict, choice, and commitment.* New York: Free Press.

McMahon, R. J., & Forehand, R. (1984). Parent training for the noncompliant child: Treatment outcome, generalization, and adjunctive therapy procedures. In R. F. Dangel & R. A. Polster (Eds.), *Parent training: Foundations of research and practice* (pp. 298–328). New York: Guilford Press.

Medicine, I. O. (1994). *Reducing risks for mental disorders: Frontiers for preventive intervention research.* Washington, DC: National Academy Press.

Meichenbaum, D., & Turk, D. (1987). *Facilitating treatment adherence: A practitioner's guidebook.* New York: Plenum Press.

Patterson, G. R. (1982). *Coercive family process.* Eugene, OR: Castalia.

Patterson, G. R., Capaldi, D., & Bank, L. (1991). An early starter model for predicting delinquency. In D. J. Pepler & K. H. Rubin, (Eds.), *The development and treatment of childhood aggression* (pp. 139–168). Hillsdale, NJ: Erlbaum.

Patterson, G. R., & Forgatch, M. (1985). Therapist behavior as a determinant for client non-compliance: A paradox for the behavioral modifier. *Journal of Consulting and Clinical Psychology, 53,* 846–851.

Patterson, G. R., & Stouthanier-Loeher, M. (1984). The correlation of family management practices and delinquency. *Child Development, 55,* 1299–1307.

Radloff, L. (1977). The CES-D Scale: A self-report depression scale for research in the general population. *Journal of Psychological Measurement, 1,* 385–401.

Reid, J., Taplin, P., & Loeber, R. (1981). A social interactional approach to the treatment of abusive families. In R. B. Stuart (Ed.), *Violent behavior: Social learning approaches to prediction management and treatment* (pp. 83–101). New York: Brunner/Mazel.

Rogers, C. R. (1951). *Client-centered therapy.* Boston: Houghton Mifflin.

Rutter, M. (1980). *Changing youth in a changing society.* Cambridge, MA: Harvard University Press.

Saxe, L., Cross, T., & Silverman, N., Batchelor, W. F., & Dougherty, D. (1987). *Children's mental health: Problems and services.* Durham, NC: Duke University Press.

Schmaling, K. B., & Jacobson, N. S. (1987). *The clinical significance of treatment gains resulting from parent training interventions for children with conduct problems: An analysis of outcome data.* Paper presented at the meeting of the Association for the Advancement of Behavior Therapy, Boston.

Seligman, M. E. P. (1975). *Helplessness.* San Francisco: Freeman.

Spitzer, A., Webster-Stratton, C., & Hollinsworth, T. (1991). Coping with conduct-problem children: Parents gaining knowledge and control. *Journal of Child Clinical Psychology, 20,* 413–427.

Spoth, R., & Redmond, C. (1995). Parent motivation to enroll in parenting skills programs: A model of family context and health belief predictors. *Journal of Family Psychology, 9,* 294–310.

Twentyman, C. T., & McFall, R. M. (1975). Behavioral training of social skills in shy males. *Journal of Consulting and Clinical Psychology, 43,* 384–395.

Wahler, R. G. (1980). The insular mother: Her problems in parent–child treatment. *Journal of Applied Behavior Analysis, 13,* 207–219.

Webster-Stratton, C. (1984). Randomized trial of two parent-training programs for families with conduct-disordered children. *Journal of Consulting and Clinical Psychology, 52,* 666–678.

Webster-Stratton, C. (1985a). Predictors of treatment outcome in parent training for conduct disordered children. *Behavior Therapy, 16,* 223–243.

Webster-Stratton, C. (1985b). The effects of father involvement in parent training for conduct problem children, *Child Psychology and Psychiatry, 26,* 801–810.

Webster-Stratton, C. (1990). Stress: A potential disrupter of parent perceptions and family interactions. *Journal of Clinical Child Psychology, 19,* 302–312.

Webster-Stratton, C. (1992a). *The incredible years: A trouble-shooting guide for parents.* Toronto: Umbrella Press.

Webster-Stratton, C. (1992b). *The Parents and Children Videotape Series: Programs 1–10.* Seth Enterprises, 1411 8th Avenue West, Seattle, WA 98119, USA.

Webster-Stratton, C. (1995). *Preventing conduct problems in Head Start children: Short-term results of parent training intervention.* Unpublished manuscript.

Webster-Stratton, C., & Herbert, M. (1994). *Troubled families—Problem children. Working with parents: A collaborative process.* Chichester, England: Wiley.

Webster-Stratton, C., Hollinsworth, T., & Kolpacoff, M. (1989). The long-term effectiveness and clinical significance of three cost-effective training programs for families with conduct-problem children. *Journal of Consulting and Clinical Psychology, 57,* 550–553.

Webster-Stratton, C., Kolpacoff, M., & Hollinsworth, T. (1988). Self-administered videotape therapy for families with conduct problem children: Comparison with two cost-effective treatments and a control group. *Journal of Consulting and Clinical Psychology, 56,* 558–566.

Zigler, E., & Styfco, S. J. (1993). *Head Start and Beyond.* New Haven, CT and London: Yale University Press.

Part III

Treatment

This part offers a number of approaches to CAN across a number of areas: a training program for preschool children, multifaceted broad-scale service programs, injury prevention, youth violence prevention, teen parent programs, parent training for parents who have disabilities, and issues of treatment adherence.

A preschool socialization training program is described by Fantuzzo, Weiss, and Coolahan in Chapter 9. These authors address the importance of having the community participate in every level of service and research. The inner-city African-American community served by their work helped develop the assessment tools based on skills rather than on deviance, in contrast to most assessments. Further, they detail how to have community members recruit, be involved in treatment, and support each other. This chapter can be seen as a model for community involvement in CAN research and service whatever that community's ethnic or racial makeup.

Fantuzzo and his colleagues note that victims of CAN in poor communities are at high risk for psychopathology. Thus, teaching social skills as is done through the "Play Buddy" program may help prevent some of the psychological sequelae associated with poverty and CAN.

Large-scale, multifaceted services are the focus of chapters by Lutzker, Bigelow, Doctor, Gershater, and Greene and by Striefel, Robinson, and Truhn. Projects 12-Ways and SafeCare are described by Lutzker and associates. Project 12-Ways has been ongoing since 1979, offering ecobehavioral treatment to CAN families in rural southern Illinois. The term "ecobehavioral" means that families are seen as social ecologies in which CAN occurs as a function of multiple determinants within these ecologies. Thus, through direct treatment/training strategies (primarily through direct behavioral assessment), families receive several services, for example, parent training, stress reduction, problem solving, and home safety.

Project SafeCare is a systematic replication of Project 12-Ways, offering service to CAN and high-risk families in urban Los Angeles. Three salient services from Project 12-Ways (parent–child training, home safety, and child health care) are offered in a 15-week package. Project SafeCare has assessed video and found it useful for training these skills.

Striefel and his colleagues describe another multifaceted service known as a wraparound program, the Community Family Partnership Program (CFP). Like Projects 12-Ways and SafeCare, the CFP offers 10 services such as nutrition training, child care, prenatal care, and others and, like the program described by Fantuzzo et al., tries to empower the participating families through the families' active involvement in problem solving and helping each other in the CFP.

That "accident" is not a useful term in unintentional (or intentional) childhood injury is an important theme of Chapter 12, by Peterson and Gable. Injuries cause more deaths in children than all diseases combined. Thus, understanding risks and trying to prevent them is critically important for children's safety. Peterson and Gable explore these risks and note that many injuries are a result of CAN. They go on to suggest a number of strategies for reducing these risks for children.

Programs aimed at the prevention of youth violence make up Chapter 13, by Yung and Hammond, and Chapter 14, by Pittman, Wolfe, and Wekerle. In their chapter on preventing youth violence in African-American junior high school students, Yung and Hammond note that African Americans are overrepresented among the overall population as victims and perpetrators of violence. Thus, there is a compelling need for programs aimed at prevention. Described in this chapter is PACT, Positive Adolescent Choices Training Program, a hands-on, culturally sensitive program for seventh and eighth graders. PACT teaches social skills and anger management and provides education about violence. It is empirically driven, collecting important program evaluation data. In research comparing PACT adolescents with matched controls who were not involved in the program, the PACT adolescents displayed less verbal and physical aggression and other "misbehavior" in school.

Canadian adolescents are the subjects of the Youth Relationships Program (YRP) described by Pittman, Wolfe, and Wekerle. This program is aimed at adolescents who have experienced violence. Like the PACT, the YRP uses hands-on practice to teach nonviolent interpersonal skills.

Teenage mothers, whose numbers are increasing, are at particularly high risk for CAN. In Chapter 15, Budd, Stockman, and Miller report the results of surveys from service providers on how to engage teens in programs. In Chapter 16, Pinkston and Smith review several aspects of parent training, particularly for young, single parents.

Parents with developmental disabilities make up a higher proportion of CAN reports than their representation in the population, yet they receive very little attention in the CAN literature. Feldman describes his parent training program for parents with developmental disabilities in Chapter 17. His project makes use of developmentally appropriate materials for the parents that help the parents assist the children in gaining skills. In Chapter 18, Tymchuk addresses this issue in his description of the UCLA Parent/Child Health and Wellness Project. The project utilizes special assessment and training procedures adapted to the parents' reading levels and addresses their other skill deficits. As other authors here have suggested, Tymchuk favors direct behavioral assessment over more standard paper-and-pencil measures in assessing parents with developmental disabilities. The UCLA Project uses a specific parenting plan that incorporates parents' needs, as well as lesson plans and other very direct procedures.

Finally, Lundquist and Hansen note in Chapter 19 that the best treatment plans are only as good as the families' adherence to them. They detail the barriers to treatment adherence and suggest a number of strategies for improving it.

9

Community-Based Partnership-Directed Research

Actualizing Community Strengths to Treat Child Victims of Physical Abuse and Neglect

JOHN FANTUZZO, ANDREA DELGAUDIO WEISS, and KATHLEEN COYLE COOLAHAN

During the last two decades of the 20th century, the number of children reported abused or neglected has risen steadily. Nearly 3 million children were involved in maltreatment reports in 1993 (U.S. Department of Health and Human Services, 1995). Demographic data indicate that the likelihood of victimization is not equal for all children. The child victims of maltreatment are disproportionately young and from low-income households (Wolfner & Gelles, 1993). Fifty-one percent of the children reported abused or neglected in 1993 were 7 years old or younger, and almost one-third were between the ages of 3 and 7 (U.S. Department of Health and Human Services, 1995). Repeatedly, national incidence studies have indicated a strong relationship between low-income levels and a higher-than-average risk of child maltreatment (Pelton, 1994).

The maltreatment suffered by these young, vulnerable children places them at extremely high risk for developmental psychopathology (Cicchetti & Lynch, 1993). The research literature indicates that physical abuse and neglect disrupt mastery of the most important developmental task for preschool children—becoming competent in social relations with peers (Cicchetti & Carlson, 1989). Maltreated preschool children show significant difficulties in social functioning and peer

JOHN FANTUZZO, ANDREA DELGAUDIO WEISS, and KATHLEEN COYLE COOLAHAN • University of Pennsylvania, Philadelphia, Pennsylvania 19104.

Handbook of Child Abuse Research and Treatment, edited by Lutzker. Plenum Press, New York, 1998.

relationships relative to nonmaltreated children. Compared to control children, they display fewer socially competent behaviors in interactions with peers (Howes & Espinosa, 1984; Wolfe & Mosk, 1983), initiate fewer positive interactions with peers (Haskett & Kistner, 1991; Hoffman-Plotkin & Twentyman, 1984), and display more inappropriate responses to peers, such as aggression and withdrawal (Howes, 1987; Klimes-Dougan & Kistner, 1990).

Maltreated preschool children also display higher levels of problematic behaviors, which may increase the likelihood of being rejected or neglected by peers (Dodge, 1983) and perpetuate a cycle of social isolation. Victims of abuse and neglect show greater rates of externalizing problem behaviors, such as aggression, noncompliance, and impulsivity (Alessandri, 1991; Bousha & Twentyman, 1984; Hoffman-Plotkin & Twentyman, 1984). These children also experience increased levels of internalizing problems, such as social withdrawal, depression, anxiety, and avoidance (Egeland, 1991; Jaffe, Wolfe, Wilson, & Zak, 1986; Klimes-Dougan & Kistner, 1990). These findings indicate the negative impact of maltreatment on the social development of preschool victims.

In addition, maltreatment is associated with detrimental aspects of the child's larger ecology which may compound developmental risk. At the family level, there is a prevalence of stress indicators including young and single parenthood (Wolfner & Gelles, 1993), parental stress and social isolation (Garbarino, 1985), and domestic violence (McCloskey, Figueredo, & Koss, 1995). At the community level, there is an association between maltreatment and urban social disadvantage and disorganization, such as poverty (Pelton, 1994), unemployment (Wolfner & Gelles, 1993), juvenile delinquency, drug trafficking (Coulton, Korbin, Su, & Chow, 1995), and community violence (Osofsky, 1995).

Together, these findings make evident the complex, multidimensional nature of child abuse and neglect and the importance of designing and investigating treatment strategies for low-income preschool children living in socially and economically distressed communities (Garbarino & Kostelny, 1992). Developing comprehensive intervention strategies for multiple problems in a context of minimal resources raises serious questions about what methods can be used to treat large numbers of maltreated children. The development of these methods must include careful consideration of where treatment should take place and who should serve as the primary therapeutic agents.

Unfortunately, the response of the current mental health delivery system to these questions has been woefully limited in scope, resulting in services that are inadequate to meet the developmental and mental health needs of vulnerable children in these high-risk environments (U.S. Department of Health and Human Services, 1990). This inadequacy is due primarily to a dearth of tested mental health services available to children and families in impoverished urban settings (Children's Defense Fund, 1995; Kazdin, 1993). Little treatment outcome research is available to direct the design of treatment services for young victims of physical abuse and neglect (Cicchetti, Toth, & Bush, 1988; Kazdin, 1993; National Research Council, 1993). In a comprehensive review of the treatment literature, Wolfe and Wekerle (1993) found only five experimental studies of treatment interventions specifically developed for physically maltreated children, thus leaving professionals with a lack of empirically tested, effective strategies with which to address the developmental needs of child victims.

The inadequacy of the current treatment delivery system also stems from the unfortunate reality that the few services that do exist are often inappropriate and irrelevant to the life conditions of families in these settings (Crittenden, 1991; Fantuzzo, 1990). Traditional treatment approaches consist mainly of a narrow range of therapeutic strategies that are based primarily on the singular implementation of expert-directed intervention. This expert-directed approach is characterized by assessment strategies that focus primarily on deficiency and pathology and therapeutic practices that focus solely on providing services to individuals in clinic or office settings. Focusing on the individual without attending to the surrounding context implies that problems and their solutions lie solely within the individual (Rhodes & Englund, 1993). Energies are therefore directed at changing the individual without addressing precipitating conditions in the environment (Ryan, 1971). In all, these traditional treatment approaches suffer from a constriction of vision, a conceptual myopia, that severely limits the degree to which problems can be successfully identified, understood, and treated with this most vulnerable group of children and families.

A review of the community psychology literature reveals substantial support for these criticisms as well as recommendations for reforming the provision of treatment services with respect to complex social problems such as child maltreatment. First, treatment researchers are called to adopt a strengths or competence perspective (Duffy & Wong, 1996; Glenwick & Jason, 1993). This perspective asserts that mental health assessment and treatment practices should emphasize the identification and further cultivation of competence rather than focusing on deficiency and pathology (Weissberg, Caplan, & Harwood, 1991). Competence is defined as the ability to transact effectively with the environment, that is, coping with stressors and challenges in one's setting and maximizing opportunities. Intervention programs designed to enhance and capitalize upon these competencies are increasingly advocated as necessary alternatives to programs aimed merely at fixing problems (Zimmerman & Arunkumar, 1994).

Adopting a strengths perspective necessitates moving beyond a focus on individuals as the primary unit of analysis and considering the ecology in which individuals transact (Glenwick, Heller, Linney, & Pargament, 1990; Rappaport, 1990; Sarason, 1981; Trickett & Birman, 1989). An ecological perspective attends to person–environment transactions on multiple levels (Bronfenbrenner, 1977). The treatment of problems is conceptualized not as a process of altering the individual, but as a process of optimizing the fit between individuals and the multiple contexts in which they exist (Duffy & Wong, 1996).

Lastly, in place of unidimensional, expert-directed treatment methods that target individuals out of context (Tyler, Pargament, & Gatz, 1983), community-based researchers espouse the pursuit of comprehensive, divergent, multilevel strategies that are congruent with the complexity of social problems such as child abuse and neglect (Cowen, 1991; Kelly, 1990). To be ecologically valid and to mobilize community resources, such strategies should be used in natural settings and should be designed to engage natural helpers in the development of intervention strategies (Glenwick & Jason, 1993). This collaboration is characterized by a bidirectional flow of influence between researchers and natural helpers (both professionals and nonprofessionals), with both parties seen as having something to contribute and to learn (Tyler et al., 1983). In addition, treatment strategies must be much more comprehensive in scope than conventional individual-focused, expert-directed approaches. Interventions must be designed to address the most salient causes and consequences of child abuse and neglect that interact among various systems levels, including the individual, the family, the community, and the larger culture (Cicchetti & Toth, 1995; National Research Council, 1993).

The purpose of this chapter is to outline and illustrate a community-based approach for developing interventions for maltreated preschool children and their families. This strategy involves accessing and activating the capabilities of competent individuals who are natural participants in the multiple environmental systems that shape the development of young children. Designed to fit the circumstances of vulnerable participants and their high-risk natural surroundings, this approach calls for researchers to form a collaborative research team with resilient community members to plan, implement, and evaluate intervention methods at various system levels for maltreating families. In the following pages, we will (1) describe the process involved in developing community-based, partnership-directed intervention and (2) detail an application of this process designed to enhance the social functioning of low-income child victims and maltreating parents living in a large urban center.

DEVELOPING COMMUNITY-BASED
PARTNERSHIP-DIRECTED INTERVENTION STRATEGIES

The process of generating and implementing community-based, partnership-directed intervention methods consists of four major stages. In the following descriptions of these stages, the reader will note their recursive nature and the continuous, ongoing nature of the overall process that undergirds successful collaborations between researchers and community partners.

Stage 1: Forming Linkages with Community-Based Agencies
Serving Vulnerable Families with Young Children

The first stage involves strategically identifying appropriate agencies or institutions within the community that provide services to vulnerable families with young children and then forming working relationships with the administrators of these agencies. Well-established agencies that are located community-wide and are mandated to provide services to large numbers of families in the community are strategic sites for researchers to target. Specifically, the local Child Protective Services agency is an essential institution with which maltreatment researchers must form connections. Mandated by public law to identify and provide services to maltreated children, this agency has both the greatest responsibility to maltreating families and the greatest access to them. By working in concert with Child Protective Services staff, researchers can target intervention areas of a community that show evidence of the greatest incidence and most severe levels of child maltreatment. Other established community institutions that provide services to large numbers of families with young children include public schools and early intervention programs. Early intervention preschool programs typically offer a broad array of services to young children and families and can serve as attractive community-based sites for maltreatment prevention and treatment efforts.

For their part, researchers can bring to community-based treatment research enterprises a number of unique assets. First, they bring to the collaboration their expertise in research practices and methods. Most community agencies serving children and families lack the resources to conduct research and could profit greatly from empirically derived knowledge about the needs of their client base and the effectiveness of their services. Second, researchers can lend to the collaborative enterprise access to university or corporate technical, educational, and personnel resources. Third, researchers can spearhead efforts to procure external sources of finding to support maltreatment intervention development and research.

Stage 2: Partnering with Resistance

Unfortunately, wide cultural, socioeconomic, and political gaps often separate researchers, practitioners, and citizens. These gaps can be sources of mistrust and tension that may impede or block the conduct of research in community settings, as well as the use of research findings by members of the nonscientific community. This reality is most acute in the economically disadvantaged, politically disenfranchised pockets of society where the highest incidence of child maltreatment occurs. The greater the gaps are between researchers and other stakeholders, the higher the likelihood is that the efforts from "outside" investigators and "helpers" (researchers) will be mistrusted and rejected.

Against this backdrop of resistance, researchers must work to establish a foundation of trust upon which collaborative treatment research efforts can be built. Genuine partnership is possible only when a basis of trust has been established among all of the stakeholders in the partnership process—researchers, administrators, front-line staff (i.e., teachers and caseworkers), the recipients of services (i.e., parents), and concerned members of the community at large. Stakeholders' resistance should be viewed not as a bane or threat to the partnership process, but as a valuable and appropriate manifestation of their commitment to protecting the interests of their particular group. The partnership process should be grounded in an exchange of information and influence which allows each group of stakeholders to voice their needs, fears, and expectations with respect to the prospective collaboration. Rather than trying to avoid or squelch resistance, researchers should attempt to understand it from the perspective of the resisting party and respond to it by incorporating expressed concerns into the partnership agenda. The objective of this process is for the partnering groups to articulate and form a shared commitment to a constructive plan of action that addresses each group's concerns and therefore has a greater likelihood of being implemented successfully.

Stage 3: Creating a Multisystems Level Intervention Strategy

After addressing initial sources of resistance, researchers and community partners next engage in dialogue about the needs of vulnerable families and the community resources and strengths that can be marshaled to support these families. This dialogue is characterized by a two-way exchange of information designed to set the agenda for partnership activity. Together, researchers and community partners articulate common objectives for intervening with maltreating families on multiple levels and co-construct research methods to achieve these objectives. Because the risk factors for child physical abuse exist and interact at the individual, family, and community levels, researchers and community partners must create a comprehensive plan to intervene strategically at various system levels. Isolated treatment methods that target single systems are likely to be ineffective. Furthermore, effective interventions must be nested in therapeutic systems that support and sustain their existence.

Stage 4: Co-Implementation and Co-Evaluation

Following the co-construction of the research agenda and methods by researchers and community partners, the next stage in conducting community-based, partnership-directed treatment research is the co-implementation and co-evaluation of the partnership's research activities. Community partners are empowered to be researchers working in the interest of the community to investigate the implementation and efficacy of partnership-generated research methods. This empowerment derives from a recognition of their authority as "experts" on the conditions, culture, and politics of the community. Community partners can participate directly in research activities by assisting with data collection, acting as treatment agents, and helping the partnership team interpret the meaning of research findings. A consideration of the effectiveness of the strategies provides the team with an opportunity to come back together to refine treatment methods and reaffirm their partnership commitments.

In summary, the process described above consists of a series of continuous, cyclical stages that empower natural helpers to make substantial contributions to vulnerable members of their community. First, partners must honestly share fears and expectations of their prospective collaboration. This sharing should include disclosure of needs and feelings of mistrust. Out of this dialogue should come a recognition of the strengths that each partner brings to the collaboration and a commitment to cultivate these strengths. Second, there must be a genuine two-way flow of information to enable partners to learn the value of each other's unique perspectives and knowledge related to their joint venture. Partners must then translate their trust and knowledge base into useful assessment, intervention, and evaluation strategies. Finally, evaluation feedback informs a rethinking of the partnership's research objectives and strategies.

APPLICATION OF THE COMMUNITY-BASED
PARTNERSHIP-DIRECTED APPROACH

This section describes the application of the community-based, partnership-directed approach to intervention research for low-income, preschool victims of physical abuse and neglect and their families living in a large urban setting. This account describes the fruit of an intensive collaboration among the University of Pennsylvania, the Philadelphia Department of Human Services (DHS), the school district of the Philadelphia Prekindergarten Head Start Program, and Head Start parents. The following description includes an account of intervention development across a 4-year period and a brief summary of research findings at each stage of the process.

Forming Linkages with Community-Based Agencies to Establish a Context for Intervention

As stated, a critical community institution with which child abuse researchers must form a working partnership is the agency charged with identifying and providing services to child victims of abuse and neglect. We met with administrators of the Philadelphia Department of Human Service's (DHS) Office of Children, Youth, and Families and explained to them our interest in setting up and evaluating the effectiveness of three complementary types of maltreatment interventions. In these meetings, we presented a community-based, partnership-directed approach as our preferred modus operandi. We shared our belief that Head Start centers might be ideal sites for the interventions, since they are located throughout the poverty-stricken areas of the city and provide a wide range of comprehensive services for young children and families. Because we wanted to target the city communities that were most severely affected by child maltreatment, we worked with DHS administrators to identify regions in Philadelphia that contained the greatest number of indicated cases of physical abuse of preschool children. Not surprisingly, these were the regions with the highest concentration of vulnerable families (i.e., minority, single-female-headed households).

Next, we approached administrators of the largest Head Start grantee in the city, the school district of Philadelphia's Prekindergarten Head Start program. We expressed our desire to work collaboratively with them, the school district, and DHS to develop and test the effectiveness of community-based, partnership-directed intervention methods for maltreated Head Start children and their parents. As researchers, we brought to the partnership table a number of assets. First, we had done several preliminary studies showing the value of the Play Buddy Intervention (PBI) for enhancing the social functioning of maltreated preschool children (Fantuzzo & Holland, 1992). This line of research constituted the bulk of studies in the research literature on intervention methods for maltreated preschool children. Because the PBI had been tested only in clinic settings, we were eager to test its application to a natural setting such as Head Start. Fortunately, we were awarded grants from the National Center for Child Abuse and Neglect (NCCAN) and Head Start to conduct this investigation. We therefore were able to bring to the collaboration fiscal resources and a team of trained researchers to support the development and evaluation of the intervention, at no cost to our collaborators. The Head Start administrators decided to move forward with us, granting us a strategic community-based context in which to carry out the research. Based on the information from DHS, we chose 10 Head Start centers located in public school buildings in the highest-risk neighborhoods for child abuse, and began the critical entry process.

Partnering with Resistance

As outsiders to the highly stressed neighborhoods we had targeted, we were not initially welcomed by members of the community. Through the eyes of members of the low-income, African-American communities we were entering, we were white, middle-class scientists coming in to study them and document their deficiencies. Their considerable mistrust of our motives and methods made the process of physical and psychological entry a tremendous challenge at every level.

From the beginning, we encountered intense resistance from parents and community groups. The research team set up meetings with a committee of parents appointed by the Head Start Parent Policy Council to review our research objectives and methods. The first task for this community was to review the measures we would be asking parents to complete. The committee had very strong negative reactions to a number of the measures, and refused to permit several measures that are commonly used in maltreatment research—the Conflict Tactic Scales, Child Abuse Potential Inventory, Beck Depression Inventory, and Child Behavior Checklist—to be used. They found these measures to be overly negative, depicting the African-American family in a stereotypic way that emphasizes violence and deficiencies, but ignores strengths. Committee members informed us that in neighborhoods where residents have seen the Department of Human Services remove children from homes, people would not honestly answer questions posed by strangers about matters of family functioning. Instead, they would refuse to participate at all or would provide us with misinformation by giving what they perceived to be socially desirable responses. This airing of committee members' negative feelings about the measures led to a broader discussion of their many negative feelings and misunderstandings about the goals and objectives of the research project.

It soon became apparent that the prevailing sentiments in the community toward research, as it has typically been conducted in African-American communities, were extremely negative. Parents and community advocates described past experiences as research "subjects" whereby researchers pillaged the community for data but offered nothing in return except judgments of community members as deviant or degenerate. These outsiders, the parents explained, had no appreciation of the challenges they faced nor the resilience they demonstrated in the face of those challenges. Their opinions of research were so negative and the resistance they expressed was so intense that the survival of our research plan was in jeopardy.

Although the committee members' fierce protestations were somewhat daunting, we recognized that the intensity of the feelings they were expressing was an indication of the depth of their concern for the children and families in their community. We saw potential in this passion and chose to move toward the resistance rather than retreat from it. We validated the feelings of frustration and fear they were expressing, and conveyed to them that our primary commitment was not to a preconceived research agenda, but to working with them to co-construct and implement a shared agenda for intervening with vulnerable and isolated maltreating families. As an initial demonstration of this commitment, we offered to throw out any measures or procedures they found objectionable, and asked them to work with us to identify or develop more acceptable ones.

These early meetings served as the proving ground for an emerging researcher–citizen partnership. Through their resistance, members of the community adroitly tested our motives, methods, and values. Retreat on our part would have indicated that our allegiance was to enacting a preset agenda, not to the families living in the most high-risk, vulnerable communities. Standing our ground, we listened to the concerns of our community counterparts and responded by inviting them to work with us as research *partners*, not *subjects*. Empowering the community members to be partners transformed the threat they originally resisted into an opportunity for the community. The raw emotion underlying their resistance could now serve as a motive force fueling their active participation in the subsequent phases of the partnership process, that is, designing, implementing, and evaluating the effectiveness of various intervention strategies.

Creating a Multisystems Level Intervention Strategy

Creating a strategy to understand and treat child abuse requires researchers to attend to both the developmental status of child victims and adult perpetrators and the social ecology in which maltreatment occurs. Across ecological settings and developmental stages, child maltreatment is associated with a lack of social connectedness and support (Daro, 1988; Thompson, 1995). The ideal combination of intervention strategies should, therefore, function at multiple system levels to move individuals from social isolation to community. With this general goal in mind, the partnership team set out to identify community strengths and resources that could be cultivated, as well as potential obstacles. Assessment methods were developed to gather this essential information. Next, the data that were generated were used by the team to design three distinct, yet complementary, intervention strategies designed to reduce social isolation at the community, parent, and child levels.

At the community level, high levels of maltreatment have been found in socially disorganized neighborhood settings characterized by a breakdown of community and social cohesion (Barry, 1994; Coulton et al., 1995; Garbarino & Kostelny, 1994). We, therefore, sought an intervention strategy that would bring the most vulnerable families in these high-risk neighborhoods into Head Start, a nonstigmatizing, community-based setting in which children and parents could potentially be integrated into supportive social networks. We knew, however, that bringing these families into Head Start would not be sufficient; further effort would be necessary to pull them in from their likely positions on the social periphery and formally involve them in socially supportive networks. We created a second intervention strategy that would bring maltreating parents into consistent contact with resilient natural helpers and would provide moral support, information, and instrumental aid. Finally, we sought an effective strategy for intervening with the child victims of maltreatment. The research literature tells us that a major consequence of maltreatment at preschool age is an impaired ability to master the developmentally salient task of forming positive relationships with peers (George & Main, 1979; Hoffman-Plotkin & Twentyman, 1984). Developmentally appropriate interventions for children at this age should therefore target the strengthening of peer social skills and integrate children into supportive peer networks (Thompson, 1995).

These three intervention strategies are outlined in the following discussion. The first, the Reach Out Intervention, involved using natural helpers (Head Start parents) to recruit as many maltreating families as possible into the Head Start setting. This effort would allow us to offer community-based intervention services to greater numbers of the most needy families. The other two interventions, Community Outreach through Parent Empowerment (COPE) and Play Buddy, were designed to employ natural helpers to enhance the social connectedness of

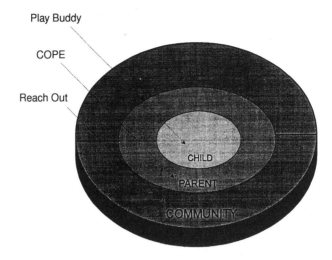

Figure 1. Multisystems level intervention.

maltreating parents and their children, respectively. These interventions represent co-constructed strategies for linking vulnerable parents and children to supportive social networks in Head Start.

Implementation and Evaluation of the Multisystems Level Intervention

Subsequent to drafting a comprehensive research plan, the partnership team activated this plan by carrying out the following sequence of research activities. These activities were aimed at enrolling vulnerable isolated children and families in Head Start, assessing the needs and strengths of the Head Start community, and developing viable parent and child intervention strategies to enhance the social functioning of both parents and children.

Reach Out

Initially, we discovered that there was a very small number of maltreated children in Head Start, even though the targeted centers were located in neighborhoods with the highest density of preschool physical abuse and neglect. We learned from our community partners that there were many more children in these neighborhoods who were eligible for Head Start than there were available openings. Therefore, the families most capable of completing all the steps in the Head Start enrollment process were the ones who were first to be enrolled. Typically, these families were the ones with the best social networks and the most adequate family support systems. Parents in Head Start alerted their friends when there were openings and helped them with entry procedures and politics (i.e., attending all the required appointments, filling out all the forms, getting medical examinations, and navigating the interviews with the social service staff). As a result, socially isolated maltreating families facing many stressors were at a distinct disadvantage in competing for the limited number of slots.

Therefore, our first intervention activity (at the community level) was to create a pipeline to Head Start centers for socially isolated maltreating parents and to enroll child victims and families in Head Start. We created a community liaison research position for a former Head Start parent with extensive experience in Head Start parent leadership and parent advocacy groups in the community. This team member helped us arrange focus groups to develop the Reach Out intervention, a strategy for bringing isolated, maltreating families into Head Start. There were two major aspects to the Reach Out intervention: (1) developing methods to contact isolated maltreating parents with children eligible for Head Start and to offer them Head Start enrollment, and (2) helping vulnerable parents complete the multistep enrollment process. To accomplish the first objective, our team had a number of meetings with parents' rights groups in the community and DHS leadership to develop sensitive contact procedures that offered enrollment opportunities to parents while protecting their confidentiality. Names and phone numbers of highly vulnerable families who were eligible for enrollment and interested in receiving information were given to our team. Small groups of very capable parents from targeted Head Start centers and doctoral level psychology graduate students were hired for a short-term job to participate in a "Head Start recruitment drive." The partnership team developed a simple phone contact strategy and trained the participating Head Start parents and the students to carry it out. To test the hypothesis that the Head Start parents would be more effective in establishing contact than the graduate students, phone contact numbers were randomly assigned to either Head Start parents or graduate student staff ($N = 200$ for each). In order to protect the confidentiality of these families, and to ensure that staff were blind to abuse status, staff were informed that the contact telephone numbers were obtained from Head Start for recruitment purposes. Forty-two percent of the targeted parents were successfully contacted (191 of 400); of these parents, 48.2% said they were interested in Head Start for their children (92 of 191). Ultimately, 43% of the interested parents enrolled their children in Head Start (40 of 92)—10% of the total population of abused preschoolers (40 of 400). Not surprisingly, parents were significantly more successful at contacting other parents ($n = 127$ for parents and $n = 64$ for graduate students, chi square = 5.5, $p < .05$).

To help vulnerable families complete the enrollment process, we worked with groups of Head Start parents and Head Start social service staff to study the process and identify potential obstacles and possible solutions. Three major obstacles included getting medical and dental screenings in a timely manner, completing all the paperwork, and attending an interview with Head Start social service staff. Our team approached the dental and medical schools at the University of Pennsylvania and identified pro bono services they provided that met Head Start's screening requirements. Additionally, during the second year of the Reach Out intervention, parent team members who were trained to make telephone contacts helped parents complete forms and accompanied parents to their Head Start interview. With these additional resources and experience, parent team members were able to contact 73% of identified families (397 of 540), of whom 60% were interested in enrolling their child in Head start (243 of 397); of this number, 42% were enrolled in Head Start (101 of 243). This was 19% of the identified cases, an increase of 153% from the efforts in the first year. The proportion of abused children in the Head Start centers we targeted increased from a baseline of 5% (4 of 80 children) to 20% in a two-year period (16 of 80 children).

Assessment

As discussed above, the parent leadership in Head Start, in conjunction with other community parent advocacy groups, summarily rejected many of the deficiency- or pathology-oriented measures that are typically used in clinic, hospital, or university-based child maltreatment research. Therefore, we worked with our Head Start and community partners to identify acceptable parent, family, and preschool social competency measures and, where needed, developed and tested measures for use with this population. This productive research effort yielded many useful assessment measures (Fantuzzo & Atkins, 1995). The first set of measures that was developed related to our initial partnership commitment to connect isolated child victims and maltreating parents to existing child and parent social communities in Head Start.

To accomplish this task, we needed assessment methods that would identify social needs and strengths in Head Start children and families. For the children, we focused on interactive peer play for two basic reasons: (1) becoming competent in social relations with peers is one of the most important developmental tasks for preschool children, and (2) during the preschool years, peer social interactive skills are developed primarily in the context of peer play. Initially, children identified by observation and teacher report who displayed the "highest" and "lowest" levels of interactive play across a representative sample of 800 Head Start children were videotaped during classroom free-play sessions. In conjunction with parents and teachers, we studied the videotapes of more than 25 of the highest-rated and 25 of the lowest-rated children. We used this process to develop an observational coding system for peer play interactions (Peer Social Interactions Observational Coding System; Fantuzzo & Atkins, 1995) and a teacher rating scale (Penn Interactive Peer Play Scale; Fantuzzo, Sutton-Smith, Coolahan, Manz, Canning, & Debnam, 1995). We also tested the Social Skills Rating Scale (SSRS; Gresham & Elliott, 1990), a teacher rating measure of preschool social competency, for use with this population. We found that the SSRS yielded three useful overall social skills scales (Interpersonal Skills, Self-Control, and Verbal Assertion) and two global problem behavior scales (Internalizing and Externalizing problem behaviors).

For the parents, we created life events scales that indicated "Blessings" (i.e., events that were uplifting, hopeful, and supportive to the parent and family) and "Burdens" such as stressful events that were discouraging and taxed parental resources (Fantuzzo & Atkins, 1995). To ensure that events reflected the realities of this population of parents, items for these scales were derived from surveys conducted with representative groups of Head Start parents. We also developed a context-specific method of assessing the degree to which a parent was an active participant in the social network of parents in their Head Start center (Parent Head Start Social Network; Fantuzzo & Atkins, 1995). This measure involved parents rating each parent at their center (approximately 80 parents) on the degree to which they talked to the parent, participated in Head Start activities with the parent, and participated in social activities outside of Head Start with the parent.

Thus far, the partnership team had successfully expanded the number of maltreated children and families attending Head Start and had identified and tested a number of social competence assessment strategies for use with this population. We next set out to use these measures to learn about the unique needs of child victims and maltreating parents and the strengths evident in these high-risk environments. This information would be used by the team to help design the parent and child interventions.

Large-scale assessment studies comparing child and parent peer social functioning in maltreating and nonmaltreating families were conducted with teachers, parents, and research assistants blind to maltreatment status. The child study involved 54 children with a history of maltreatment and 54 demographically matched nonmaltreated children. Comparisons between the two groups revealed that, compared to the nonmaltreated children, the maltreated children exhibited significantly less self-control in social interactions and significantly more internalizing adjustment problems and disconnection in peer play. An additional comparison was made between the levels of interactive peer play displayed by maltreated and nonmaltreated children who were referred by teachers (blind to maltreatment status) as candidates for intervention because they exhibited poor interactive peer play skills. This comparison revealed that the maltreated children showed significantly lower levels of interactive peer play and significantly more isolated play behaviors than the nonmaltreated children who were referred for intervention. The assessment also identified a group of resilient children who displayed high levels of interactive play despite being exposed to the same high-risk environment as their classmates. As rated by teachers, these children were leaders who directed other children without being bossy, contributed creative play ideas, encouraged others to join in play, and helped settle peer conflicts.

The parent assessment study involved 116 African-American Head Start patents. Seventy-six participants were identified by Head Start staff as isolated and vulnerable, as evidenced by the nature of their contact with Head Start. The remaining 40 participants were parents with a history of maltreatment involving their Head Start child (these parents registered their child in Head Start as a result of our Reach Out intervention). Parent assessments revealed that the maltreating parents were identified by their peers (who were blind to maltreatment status) as being among the most socially isolated parents in Head Start. For example, on average more than 85% of the parents at the center reported that they had never spoken to the maltreating parents. The maltreating parents also reported significantly lower levels of social support and higher levels of stress than nonmaltreating parents. The assessment also identified parents with incredible social resources and skill, evidenced by extensive peer networks in Head Start.

Parent Intervention

Being a parent of young children is a very challenging part of adult development (Duvall, 1977; Olson & Lavee, 1989). Adults with children in the infancy and early childhood years have been found to report higher levels of familial and marital conflict and lower levels of well-being than have adults with older children or with no children (Belsky & Rovine, 1990). In addition, research has shown that low levels of social support are associated with problematic parenting. Socially isolated parents have been found to exhibit dysfunctional parenting behaviors such as restrictiveness and punitiveness. In contrast, parents with high levels of social support have been found to display nurturant, responsive parenting behaviors (Jennings, Stagg, & Connors, 1991; Webster-Stratton, 1990), which are associated with positive social outcomes for children (McLoyd, 1990; Travillion & Snyder, 1993). Social support may ease the stresses of parenting young children by providing a forum for information exchange and emotional support (Cohen & Wills, 1985).

Parents commonly receive social support from naturally existing social networks, primarily extended kin (Gunnarsson & Cochran, 1990). For many families, however, non-kin, neighborhood-based relationships may be more prominent sources of social interaction, particularly if family relations are strained. For families at risk of child maltreatment, the U.S. Advisory Board on Child Abuse and Neglect has recommended strengthening these neighborhood supports (1991, 1993). Due to the often transient and unreliable nature of neighborhood contacts (Belle, 1982), social connections should be provided through settings with consistent daily contact with other parents (Thompson, 1995). Schools and early intervention programs such as Head Start represent ideal contexts for building social networks for isolated families.

For these reasons, the parent intervention was designed for implementation in a natural community setting: Head Start. It was intended to offset parents' social isolation, to build natural community-based supportive networks, and to provide culturally relevant information regarding parent management strategies. There were three main steps in the development of the parent intervention: (1) co-construction of the intervention with parents, (2) piloting the intervention strategies and content, and (3) large-scale implementation and evaluation of the intervention.

Co-construction of the intervention was accomplished through collaborative relationships in which parents were active participants in designing and formatting the intervention. It was our hypothesis that community-based and culturally relevant activities would be more respected, more acceptable, and more useful in improving parental psychological and societal adjustment than more traditional parent training interventions. An especially important component of co-construction was to identify content that was relevant to parents and a format that encouraged active participation. Our parent intervention was given the acronym COPE (Community Outreach through Parent Empowerment).

The first step was to develop and test the COPE intervention. Prior to planning the intervention, considerable effort was made to identify additional parents referred from the Philadelphia Department of Human Services for physical abuse and to enroll these children in Head Start. Subsequently, parents' needs were explored through focus group discussions. The first planning groups were held at two Head Start centers also participating in the child intervention. Assisted by parents who had contributed to our Head Start recruitment (Reach Out), we held brief parent support groups which were available to all parents with children at those centers. At the initial meeting, the rationale for the intervention was described as "connecting parents with other Head Start parents" and identifying effective strategies that parents can use to manage their daily stressors. At the recommendation of parent leaders, we began the meetings with short skits depicting difficult parenting situations. The specific content of the skits (e.g., dropping a child off at preschool, grocery shopping with a young child) was suggested by parents in each group. These dramatizations appeared to be effective in engaging parents and encouraging active discussion.

These brief parenting groups provided us with important information for the second stage of the intervention, running a year-long pilot implementation of parent groups for eight Head Start classes. Based on focus group discussions with project staff and Head Start parents, several key elements were identified for conducting the groups: (1) the use of parents as co-facilitators, (2) the use of culturally expressive presentation styles (e.g., role-plays), (3) an emphasis on team-building and empowerment activities, (4) the purposeful inclusion of topics related to specific neighborhood issues (e.g., violence and trauma), and (5) the building of peer support relationships through Head Start. These five elements formed the basis of the intervention format.

Next, we integrated what we learned about parents' needs from the focus groups into an intervention curriculum that would fit the above format. We believed that it was important to address self-development issues before parent roles or community relationships could be explored. The curriculum involved three major interdependent topics that were sequenced according to a hierarchy of needs and skills: Parent as Change Agent for Self, Parent as Change Agent in the Child's Presence, and Parent as Change Agent in School/Community Contexts. Discussions on the first topic involved building trust and addressing mistrust between parents and facilitators and identifying personal strengths and weaknesses, stressors and coping mechanisms, and goals and barriers to reaching those goals. Partnership at this stage was defined as helping the individual (in collaboration with others) to identify personal life issues that contribute to stress and to identify personal assets that can be mobilized to combat the hassles of daily life. Topics of discussion included relationships with family and friends, race, poverty, gender issues, social isolation, stress, physical health, and emotional well-being. Particular emphasis was placed on how to develop friendships and community with other isolated parents. *Parent–parent* collaborations were especially encouraged.

The second topic area, Parent as Change Agent in the Child's Presence, focused more directly on the role of parenting, relationship with the child, parental competence, and intimacy. Here, empowerment was identified as understanding how one's responses to stress when children are present contribute to the exacerbation of that stress, how parent–child relationships contribute to educational failure or low motivation in young children, and how children's behavior can be managed effectively. Supportive *parent–child* interactions were encouraged.

The third topic area, Parent as Change Agent in School/Community Contexts, informed parents on how to transact effectively with school systems and other community agencies, with a specific focus on increasing parents' involvement in their child's education. Empowerment was defined as the active engagement of the parent in the contexts of school and community. Topics included the politics of advocacy for children's education, understanding the world of the teacher, and learning negotiation and conflict resolution skills. *Parent–teacher* collaborations were encouraged and developed in this module.

After the initial stages of planning and piloting, the COPE parent intervention was implemented on a large scale. First, support groups were set up by two intervention teams consisting of a Head Start parent leader and a graduate student. These teams identified eight Head Start classrooms that contained pilot participants and then randomly assigned them to intervention and control conditions. Next, these teams spent volunteer time in classrooms to become familiar with the staff and parents. Once the teams were accepted by the staff and parents, they set up a room in the Head Start center, with refreshments, two mornings a week and invited targeted parents to drop in. These meetings provided an informal link for isolated parents who may have been initially unwilling or unable to attend more intensive parent training sessions, and supplied a context for participation in the COPE sessions.

Evaluation of the COPE intervention showed that the first module, "Parent as Change Agent for Self," was very well received. More than 100 Head Start parents participated in the intervention: 76 isolated and vulnerable families and 40 families with a history of maltreatment (32 of which were enrolled in Head Start through our Reach Out efforts). It was especially encouraging that the DHS-referred parents showed high participation; for the most vulnerable parents, we achieved attendance rates approaching 67%. This figure exceeds those for other published parent interventions for maltreating parents by as much as 50%.

We learned a great deal from implementing the COPE intervention. To assess its effectiveness in increasing parents' levels of positive social contact with other Head Start parents and reducing daily stress levels, maltreating and nonmaltreating parents in both intervention and control groups were assessed posttreatment. The results of our assessments with respect to parental supports and stressors indicated significantly lower levels of perceived stressors and higher levels of perceived parental supports in the treatment group. Differences were also found with respect to parent ratings of isolation and social support. Parents in the treatment group were rated significantly higher by other Head Start parents as being a parent who talks with other parents in Head Start, engages with others in Head Start activities, and has social contact with other Head Start parents outside of Head Start than were parents in the control group. In short, the COPE intervention was found to be effective as a strategy for offsetting parents' social isolation and providing culturally relevant information regarding parent management strategies.

Play Buddy Intervention

In the preschool years, acquiring social competencies to participate fully in play activity with peers and to be accepted by them is a primary developmental task. Child maltreatment can disrupt the acquisition of these competencies (Aber & Cicchetti, 1984; Main & George, 1985). Our own assessment data indicate that, compared to their nonmaltreated counterparts, maltreated children exhibit significantly more adjustment problems, general social competence difficulties, and problems in peer play interactions. These data comport with similar findings in the research literature and highlight the importance of targeting play as a natural and developmentally salient context for intervention with maltreated preschool-aged children.

Our strategy for intervening involved extending the development of a peer-mediated intervention called the Play Buddy Intervention (PBI). Guided by a developmental–ecological model, this intervention is designed to capitalize on the natural potency of peers as treatment agents and to utilize play as a context for enhancing the social competence of preschool child victims. At the heart of this strategy is the Play Buddy, a resilient peer who displays exceptionally high levels of positive play interactions even though he or she comes from the same high-risk environment as the child victim (Fantuzzo & Holland, 1992).

PBI was developed and tested in a university-based lab school for maltreated preschool children. Studies were conducted to determine the effectiveness of this treatment strategy for socially withdrawn maltreated preschool children. The first study was a small-scale investigation involving four withdrawn, maltreated children and two peers who displayed high levels of prosocial behavior (Fantuzzo, Stovall, Schachtel, Goins, & Hall, 1987). Dyadic play sessions were conducted, which involved providing a maltreated child with opportunities to play with a socially competent child ("Play Buddy") in a supportive and safe context. The social behavior of the withdrawn children was recorded during these play sessions and during free-play time in the children's classrooms. The PBI resulted in increases in positive social behavior in both treatment (playroom) and generalization (classroom) settings. Next, a larger-scale replication study was conducted to assess the relative effects of resilient peers versus familiar adults as treatment agents (Fantuzzo et al., 1988). In this study, 36 withdrawn, maltreated preschoolers were randomly assigned to one of three experimental groups: peer-treatment (PBI), adult-treatment, or control conditions. The PBI condition involved training high-functioning, maltreated peers to involve socially withdrawn participants in their play activity. The adult-treatment condition substituted a familiar adult for the competent child. Findings indicated that children in the PBI condition showed significant increases in positive social behaviors in treatment and generalization settings, whereas children in the adult-treatment group displayed a significant decrease in social behavior in both contexts after treatment. Furthermore, the children in the PBI condition showed decreases in problem behavior from pre- to posttreatment assessment on indices of psychological adjustment, whereas participants in the adult-treatment and control conditions actually evidenced significant increases in these behaviors over time.

These initial studies demonstrated the therapeutic potential of the PBI, but fell short of establishing its ecological validity. Three factors qualified its generalizability: (1) because PBI was studied in a university lab, its applicability to a real-world, community-based agency such as Head Start was unknown; (2) parents, teachers, and other members of the community were not involved in the design and implementation of the intervention; and (3) PBI was not implemented in the natural classroom setting, but was conducted as a "pull-out" intervention where children were removed from their classroom and supervised by university research assistants. A primary objective of the partnership team was to adapt the PBI for use in Head Start classrooms and to conduct multisite randomized field tests to determine its effectiveness. Efforts to enhance ecological validity included modifying the PBI for use in Head Start centers, conducting the intervention in the natural classroom, and training natural helpers (Head Start staff and parents) to conduct the intervention.

To adapt PBI for use in Head Start classrooms and maximize its effectiveness, the research team worked closely with Head Start staff and parent leaders. First, assessment instruments were developed, as described previously, to improve our ability to identify children who were particularly effective in promoting play interaction with ineffective players. Second, a substantial amount of time was spent working with Head Start teachers to conceptualize how the PBI could take place concurrently with natural free-play activities in the classroom. Third, a specific role was created for a parent volunteer, the Play Supporter, who was responsible for the daily implementation of the dyadic play sessions in the classroom. These parents were trained to support the Play Buddy's attempts to draw the Play Partner into play by praising his efforts at the end of the play session.

The adapted form of the PBI session included the following steps. First, the play supporter entered the classroom and set up the Play Corner (an area of the classroom designated for the dyadic play sessions). Next, the play supporter talked individually with the play buddy in preparation for the 20-minute play session with the play partner. During this conversation, the play supporter concretely identified the play activities that the play buddy had previously engaged in with the play partner that resulted in positive play interactions. During the play sessions, the play supporter observed the play interactions from outside the play corner. At the session's end, the play supporter made supportive comments to the play partner and the play buddy about their interactive play. The intervention involved, on the average, 20 play sessions spread over an 8-week period (three sessions/week).

Two studies were conducted to test the effectiveness of this adapted version of the PBI for increasing the level of interactive play engaged in by socially withdrawn maltreated and nonmaltreated Head Start children. The initial study involved 46 socially withdrawn African-American Head Start children, 24 of whom had a documented history of physical abuse, ranging from minor to moderate physical injuries (Fantuzzo et al., 1996). These children were identified as socially isolated by teacher ratings and direct observation of free-play sessions. Each of the 46 children was randomly assigned to either the PBI or Attention Control condition. Designed to control for the extra attention of being paired with a peer and spending time with this peer in a special play corner under the supervision of a parent volunteer, the control condition involved pairing a target child with a classmate of average interactive play ability (rather than an exceptionally competent play buddy). Children in the control condition met in the same play corners with the same set of toys for the same number of dyadic play sessions. Their play conditions were identical to the children in the PBI condition except that they were not paired with a play buddy and the play supporter only supervised their play and did not prompt or encourage interactive peer play between dyad members. During a 2-week period before and after the series of intervention sessions, videotapes were made of the participants during regular play sessions. Raters, blind to group assignments and abuse status, used the Peer Social Interactions Observational Coding procedure to rate the play sessions. Two months posttreatment, the social functioning of the children was rated by teachers using the Social Skills Scales and the Problem Behavior Scales of the Social Skills Rating System.

Results from this first treatment outcome evaluation supported the effectiveness of the PBI. Controlling for pretreatment levels of play, both maltreated and nonmaltreated socially withdrawn Head Start children showed a significant increase in positive interactive peer play behavior and a decrease in solitary play behavior as a result of the PBI. In addition, treatment gains in observed social interactions were validated by teacher ratings of classroom social functioning on the

SSRS two months following treatment. Maltreated and nonmaltreated children who received the PBI were found to exhibit significantly higher Self-Control and Interpersonal Skills and lower Internalizing and Externalizing problem behaviors than children in the control condition. Furthermore, a 91% treatment integrity evaluation (i.e., treatment carried out as planned), a 100% rate of cooperation from participating Head Start staff, and an 89% rate of successful PBI play session attempts are testimony to the value of our partnership base and efforts to increase the ecological validity of the intervention.

The second treatment outcome study involved 82 socially ineffective Head Start children, 37 of whom had a documented history of abuse or neglect. The findings of the first study were replicated. A post-only comparison of the peer interaction behavior children randomly assigned to either the treatment or attention control condition revealed that treatment children showed significantly higher levels of observed peer play interaction and significantly lower levels of solitary play than children in the control group. In addition, teacher ratings of social skills and interactive play were significantly greater for children in the treatment group. Treatment children also showed significantly lower incidence of behavior problems. These findings strongly support the effectiveness of the PBI as a strategy for increasing the level of interactive play of socially withdrawn maltreated and nonmaltreated Head Start children.

Coming Back Together

After this 4-year research effort was completed, the research team worked with the leadership in Head Start and the Department of Human Services to explore how these productive efforts could lead to improved services. Two major initiatives stemmed from these efforts: First, Head Start created a position on their advisory board for a representative from Child Protective Services. This created a formal channel of communication between the two community agencies and increased the possibility of future collaborations. Currently, they are considering ways to share information and reach out to more vulnerable families in these high-risk neighborhoods to prevent maltreatment and to enhance children's and families' well-being. Second, the University of Pennsylvania researchers in conjunction with the Head Start administration wrote a grant proposal to seek funds to further develop the partnership-directed model and institute it across the entire 3,000-family Head Start program. The team successfully competed for a 5-year Head Start Teaching Center demonstration grant to incorporate the research model into the program-wide training model to improve child and family services. Partnering strategies and specific intervention and assessment methods resulting from the above research have already been incorporated successfully into this large-scale training effort (Fantuzzo et al., 1996).

CONCLUSIONS

After over three decades of investigating child abuse and neglect, researchers and practitioners are faced with enormous challenges. These challenges are a direct function of both the major accomplishments of research enterprises and the realities of translating research findings into achievable treatment and prevention strategies. On the one hand, researchers and practitioners have sensitized the public to this problem, resulting in mandatory reporting laws and government systems to identify and investigate maltreatment. This progress has provided an avenue for identifying research participants and has made possible hundreds of empirical studies examining causes and consequences of various forms of maltreatment. These research efforts have expanded our understanding of the multidimensional nature of this problem, and have produced intricate and more refined models for explaining how traumatic events affect various pathways of child development and how parental and environmental characteristics mitigate or potentiate ill effects (Cicchetti & Toth, 1995). Furthermore, researchers have scrutinized their own work and, having identified substantial flaws, have prescribed more rigorous and precise scientific methods.

On the other hand, it is widely recognized that a relatively small amount of this research has found its way into the neighborhoods of our most vulnerable families. Despite the development of intricate, multifaceted models, little treatment outcome research is available that demonstrates the translation of these models into comprehensive interventions and tests their effectiveness with young, low-income, minority children victimized by child physical abuse and neglect (Kazdin, 1993; Wolfe & Wekerle, 1993). This unfortunate situation is aggravated by the systematic dismantling of federally funded research specifically targeting child abuse and neglect. Since 1981, funding for research and demonstration projects through the National Center on Child Abuse and Neglect (NCCAN) has decreased 44% (Thompson & Wilcox, 1995), and currently there is no funding for field-initiated research through NCCAN.

Researchers addressing this complex, life-threatening national problem are thus faced with the predicament of having to expand the scope, sophistication, and precision of treatment and prevention research while working with fewer resources. The purpose of this chapter was to present and demonstrate a community-based, partnership-directed research approach to child physical abuse and neglect that is designed to maximize the strength of natural resources that exist within high-risk environments. The overall message that we hope the chapter imparts is that attending to the "Where," "Who," and "How" of treatment *(where* treatment takes place, *who* participates in the design and implementation of treatment, and *how* treatment research is conducted) is critical to translating heuristic models of child maltreatment into effective research and to developing a sustainable research process that will generate a more precise and authentic knowledge base. Highlighted in the remaining paragraphs are the "Where," "Who," and "How" factors that we believe hold great promise for large-scale treatment and prevention research.

Where

Head Start is an ideal natural national laboratory for conducting child abuse and neglect treatment and prevention research (National Research Council, 1993). Without question, it is the largest and most far-reaching program serving low-income families with young children. In 1993, Head Start served approximately 721,000 children and their families in more than 35,000 classrooms, in all 50 states, the District of Columbia, U.S. territories, and in nearly 150 Tribal Nations (U.S. Department of Health and Human Services, 1993). Across the nation, Head Start is charged with serving even greater numbers of children and families with a set of comprehensive services that are more responsive to their needs. Furthermore, Head Start has expanded its mission to include a 0–3-year-old program (Early Start) and to fund transition projects that create programmatic links between Head Start and public elementary schools (U.S. Department of Health and Human Services, 1993).

In addition to its size and expansiveness, a number of other factors make Head Start a strategic location for maltreatment intervention research. First, the program's overall philosophy emphasizes the significance of the parent–child relationship in children's development and encourages direct parental involvement in program activities and decision making. Second, Head Start's relative success has won it continued (and at times expanded) fiscal support. Unlike NCCAN, Head Start has weathered periods of governmental belt-tightening and enjoys a favorable prognosis for future funding. Finally, the architects of Head Start's future recognize that, in order to respond to the varied needs of increasing numbers of families, the program must forge partnerships with key community institutions to provide effective, coordinated services. Research that spurs the formation of such partnerships and evaluates the effectiveness of resulting services for children and families is an urgent priority for Head Start. We have demonstrated that researchers can form linkages between Head Start and Child Protective Services and create research opportunities that benefit child victims and maltreating parents.

Who

Treatment outcome research efforts should identify resilient individuals who are indigenous to early childhood classrooms and community settings and capitalize on their talents. Resilient children and parents are those who display high levels of adaptive social functioning in challenging, high-risk environments. These individuals can serve as excellent models for child victims and maltreating parents. Social learning theory underscores the important role that competent peers play in learning new behaviors (Bandura, 1977). Research in social learning shows that being exposed to familiar, successful models in the natural setting and having opportunities for practice, feedback, and social reinforcement maximize learners' performance of new skills (Kanfer & Goldstein, 1991). We have demonstrated that, within a supportive community-based agency (Head Start), researchers can successfully identify resilient peers and develop a therapeutic context that promotes peer learning opportunities for vulnerable peers.

How

Research should be conducted in genuine partnership with community-based agencies and natural helpers from the community. We have learned from the research efforts detailed above that genuine partnership is realized as researchers face the mistrust of practitioners and participants, co-construct assessment and intervention strategies with these community partners, and co-implement and co-evaluate these strategies. In other words, partnering is happening when researchers are understanding their community partners' *passions* (pro and con) about research and "outside helpers," eliciting *ideas* from community partners about problems and possible solutions, and engaging in conjoint research *actions*. Overall, this entire process is designed to shift from an exclusively expert-directed approach to intervention research to a partnership-directed learning process. Accordingly, the emphasis changes from *what* we do to *whom* to *how* we do what *with whom*.

ACKNOWLEDGMENTS

This research project was supported in part by grants received from the U.S. Department of Health and Human Services' Head Start Bureau and the National Center for Child Abuse and Neglect.

A special thanks goes to our collaborators, Dr. Raymond Meyers of the Department of Human Services, Ms. Rosemary Mazzatenta and her Head Start staff, and a team of resilient Head Start parents. Our work with this outstanding group helped us to define genuine partnership-directed research.

REFERENCES

Aber, J. L., & Cicchetti, D. (1984). The social–emotional development of maltreated children: An empirical and theoretical analysis. In H. Fitzgerald, B. Lester, & M. Yogman (Eds.), *Theory and research in behavioral pediatrics* (pp. 147–205). New York: Plenum Press.

Alessandri, S. M. (1991). Play and social behavior in maltreated preschoolers. *Development and Psychopathology, 3*, 191–205.

Bandura, A. (1977). *Social learning theory.* Englewood Cliffs, NJ: Prentice Hall.

Barry, F. D. (1994). A neighborhood-based approach: What is it? In G. B. Melton & F. D. Barry (Eds.), *Protecting children from child abuse and neglect: Foundations for a new national strategy* (pp. 14–39). New York: Guilford Press.

Belle, D. (1982). Social ties and social support. In D. Belle (Ed.), *Lives in stress* (pp. 133–144). Beverly Hills, CA: Sage.

Belsky, J., & Rovine, M. (1990). Patterns of marital change across the transition to parenthood. *Journal of Marriage and the Family, 52*, 5–19.

Bousha, D. M., & Twentyman, C. T. (1984). Mother–child interactional style in abuse, neglect, and control groups: Naturalistic observations in the home. *Journal of Abnormal Psychology, 93*, 106–114.

Bronfenbrenner, U. (1977). Toward an experimental ecology of human development. *American Psychologist, 32*, 513–531.

Children's Defense Fund (1995). *The state of America's children*, Washington, DC: Author.

Cicchetti, D., & Carlson, V. (Eds.). (1989). *Child maltreatment: Theory and research on the causes and consequences of child abuse and neglect.* New York: Cambridge University Press.

Cicchetti, D., & Lynch, M. (1993). Toward an ecological/transactional model of community violence and child maltreatment: Consequences for children's development. *Special Issue: Children and violence. Psychiatry: Interpersonal and Biological Processes, 56*, 96–118.

Cicchetti, D., & Toth, S. (1995). A developmental psychopathology perspective on child abuse and neglect. *Journal of the Academy of Child and Adolescent Psychiatry, 34*, 541–565.

Cicchetti, D., Toth, S., & Bush, M. (1988). Developmental psychopathology and incompetence in childhood: Suggestions for intervention. In B. Lahey & A. Kazdin (Eds.), *Advances in clinical child psychology.* New York: Plenum Press.

Cohen, S., & Wills, T. A. (1985). Stress, social support, and the buffering hypothesis. *Psychological Bulletin, 98*, 310–357.

Coulton, C. J., Korbin, J. E., Su, M., & Chow, J. (1995). Community level factors and child maltreatment rates. *Child Development, 66*, 1262–1276.

Cowen, E. (1991). In pursuit of wellness. *American Psychologist, 46*, 404–408.

Crittenden, P. (1991). Treatment of child abuse and neglect. *Human systems: The Journal of Systemic Consultation & Management, 2,* 161–179.

Daro, D. (1988). *Confronting child abuse.* New York: Free Press.

Dodge, K. A. (1983). Behavioral antecedents of peer social status. *Child Development, 54,* 1386–1399.

Duffy, K.G., & Wong, F. Y. (1996). *Community Psychology.* Boston: Allyn and Bacon.

Duvall, E. (1977). *Marriage and family development.* New York: Lippincott.

Egeland, B. (1991). A longitudinal study of high-risk children: Educational outcomes. *Special Issue: New directions in risk and early intervention research. International Journal of Disability, Development, and Education, 38,* 271–287.

Fantuzzo, J. W. (1990). Behavioral treatment of the victims of child abuse and neglect. *Behavior Modification, 14,* 316–339.

Fantuzzo, J. W., & Atkins, M. S. (1995). *Resilient peer training: A community-based treatment to improve the social effectiveness of maltreating parents and preschool victims of physical abuse.* (NCCAN Publication No. 90-CA-147103). Washington, DC: National Center on Child Abuse and Neglect.

Fantuzzo, J., Childs, S., Stevenson, H., Coolahan, K., Ginsburg, M., Gay, K., Debnam, D., & Watson, C. (1996). The Head Start teaching center: An evaluation of an experiential, collaborative training model for Head Start teachers and parent volunteers. *Early Childhood Research Quarterly, 11,* 79–100.

Fantuzzo, J. W., & Holland, A. (1992). Resilient peer training: Systematic investigation of a treatment to improve the social effectiveness of child victims of maltreatment. In A. W. Burgess (Ed.), *Child trauma I: Issues and research.* New York: Garland.

Fantuzzo, J. W., Jurecic, L., Stovall, A., Hightower, A. D., Goins, C., & Schachtel, D. (1988). Effects of adult and peer social initiations on the social behavior of withdrawn, maltreated preschool children. *Journal of Consulting and Clinical Psychology, 56,* 34–39.

Fantuzzo, J. W., Stovall, A., Schachtel, D., Goins, C., & Hall, R. (1987). The effects of peer social initiation on the social behavior of withdrawn maltreated preschool children. *Journal of Behavior Therapy and Experimental Psychiatry, 18,* 357–363.

Fantuzzo, J. W., Sutton-Smith, B., Atkins, M., Meyers, R., Stevenson, H., Coolahan, K., Weiss, A., & Manz, P. (1996). Community-based resilient peer treatment of withdrawn maltreated preschool children. *Journal of Consulting and Clinical Psychology, 64,* 1377–1386.

Garbarino, J. (1985). An ecological approach to child maltreatment. In L. H. Pelton (Ed.), *The social context of child abuse and neglect* (pp. 228–267). New York: Human Sciences Press.

Garbarino, J., & Kostelny, K. (1992). Child maltreatment as a community problem. *Child Abuse & Neglect, 16,* 455–464.

Garbarino, J., & Kostelny, K. (1994). Neighborhood-based programs. In G. B. Melton & F. D. Barry (Eds.), *Protecting children from child abuse and neglect: Foundations for a new national strategy.* New York: Guilford Press.

George, C., & Main, M. (1979). Social interactions of young abused children: Approach, avoidance, and aggression. *Child Development, 50,* 306–318.

Glenwick, D. S., Heller, K., Linney, J. A., & Pargament, K. I. (1990). Criteria of Excellence I. Models for adventuresome research in community psychology: Commonalities, dilemmas, and future directions. In P. Tolan, C. Keys, F. Chertok, and L. Jason, (Eds.), *Researching community psychology: Issues of theory and methods* (pp. 76–90). Washington, DC: American Psychological Association.

Glenwick, D.S., & Jason, L.A. (1993). Behavioral approaches to prevention in the community: A historical and theoretical overview. In D. S. Glenwick and L. S. Jason (Eds.), *Promoting health and mental health in children, youth, and families* (pp. 3–16). New York: Springer.

Gresham, F. M., & Elliott, S. N. (1990). *The Social Skills Rating System.* Circle Pines, MN: American Guidance Services.

Gunnarsson, L., & Cochran, M. (1990). The support networks of single parents: Sweden and the United States. In M. Cochran, M. Larner, D. Kiley, L. Gunnarsson, & C. R. Henderson (Eds.), *Extending families: The social networks of parents and their children* (pp. 105–116). Cambridge, England: Cambridge University Press.

Haskett, M. E., & Kistner, J. A. (1991). Social interactions and peer perceptions of young physically abused children. *Child Development, 62,* 979–990.

Hoffman-Plotkin, D., & Twentyman, C. T. (1984). A multimodal assessment of behavioral and cognitive deficits in abused and neglected preschoolers. *Child Development, 55,* 794–802.

Howes, C. (1987). Social competence with peers in young children: Developmental sequences. *Developmental Review, 7,* 252–272.

Howes, C., & Espinosa, M. A. (1985). The consequences of child abuse for the formation of relationships with peers. *Child Abuse & Neglect, 9,* 397–404.

Jaffe, P., Wolfe, D., Wilson, S., & Zak, L. (1986). Similarities in behavioral and social maladjustment among child victims and witnesses to family violence. *American Journal of Orthopsychiatry, 56,* 142–146.

Jennings, K. D., Stagg, V., & Connors, R. E. (1991). Social networks and mothers' interactions with their preschool children. *Child Development, 62,* 966–978.

Kanfer, F., & Goldstein, A. (1991). *Helping people change,* New York: Pergamon.

Kazdin, A. E. (1993). Psychotherapy for children and adolescents: Current progress and future research directions. *American Psychologist, 48,* 644–657.

Kelly, J. G. (1990). Changing contexts and the field of community psychology. *American Journal of Community Psychology, 18,* 769–792.

Klimes-Dougan, B., & Kistner, J. (1990). Physically abused preschoolers' responses to peers' distress. *Developmental Psychology, 26,* 599–602.

Main, M., & George, C. (1985). Responses of abused and disadvantaged toddlers to distress in agemates: A study in the day care setting. *Developmental Psychology, 21,* 407–412.

McCloskey, L., Figueredo, A. J., & Koss, M. P. (1995). The effects of systemic family violence on children's mental health. *Child Development, 66,* 1239–1261.

McLoyd, V. C. (1990). Minority children: Introduction to the special issue. *Child Development, 61,* 263–266.

National Research Council (1993). *Understanding child abuse and neglect.* Washington, DC: National Academy Press.

Olson, D. H., & Lavee, Y. (1989). Family systems and family stress: A family life cycle perspective. In K. Kreppner and R. M. Lerner (Eds.), *Family systems and life span development* (pp. 165–195). Hillsdale, NJ: Erlbaum.

Osofsky, J. D. (1995). The effects of exposure to violence on young children. *American Psychologist, 50,* 782–788.

Pelton, L. H. (1994). The role of material factors in child abuse and neglect. In G. B. Melton & F. D. Barry (Eds.), *Protecting children from child abuse and neglect: Foundations for a new national strategy.* New York: Guilford Press.

Rappaport, J. (1990). Research methods and the empowerment social agenda. In P. Tolan, C. Keys, F. Chertok, and L. Jason, (Eds.), *Researching community psychology: Issues of theory and methods* (pp. 51–63). Washington, DC: American Psychological Association.

Rhodes, J., & Englund, S. (1993). School-based interventions for promoting social competence. In D. S. Glenwick and L. S. Jason (Eds.), *Promoting health and mental health in children, youth, and families* (pp. 17–32). New York: Springer.

Ryan, W. (1971). *Blaming the victim.* New York: Vintage Press.

Sarason, S. B. (1981). *Psychology misdirected.* New York: Free Press.

Thompson, R. A. (1995). *Preventing child maltreatment through social support: A critical analysis.* Thousand Oaks, CA: Sage.

Thompson, R. A., & Wilcox, B. L. (1995). Child maltreatment research: Federal support and policy issues. *American Psychologist, 50,* 789–793.

Travillion, K., & Snyder, J. (1993). The role of maternal discipline and involvement in peer rejection and neglect. *Journal of Applied Developmental Psychology, 14,* 37–57.

Trickett, E. J., & Birman, D. (1989). Taking ecology seriously: A community development approach to individually-based preventive interventions in schools. In L. A. Bond and B. E. Compas (Eds.), *Primary prevention and promotion in the schools* (pp. 361–390). New York: Sage.

Tyler, F. B., Pargament, K. I., & Gatz, M. (1983). The resource collaborator role: A model for interactions involving psychologists. *American Psychologist, 38,* 388–398.

U.S. Advisory Board on Child Abuse and Neglect (1991). *Creating caring communities: Blueprint for an effective federal policy on child abuse and neglect.* Washington, DC: U.S. Government Printing Office.

U.S. Advisory Board on Child Abuse and Neglect (1993). *Neighbors helping neighbors: A new national strategy for the protection of children.* Washington, DC: U.S. Government Printing Office.

U.S. Department of Health and Human Services (1990). *National plan for research on child and adolescent mental disorders.* Washington, DC: Author.

U.S. Department of Health and Human Services, Administration on Children, Youth, and Families (1993). *Creating a 21st century Head Start: Final report of the advisory committee on Head Start quality and expansion.* Washington, DC: Author.

U.S. Department of Health and Human Services (1995). *Child Maltreatment. 1993: Reports from the states to the National Center on Child Abuse and Neglect.* Washington, DC: Author.

Webster-Stratton, C. (1990). Stress: A potential disruptor of parent perceptions and family interactions. *Journal of Clinical Child Psychology, 19,* 302–312.

Weissberg, R. P., Caplan, M., & Harwood, R. L. (1991). Promoting competent young people in competence-enhancing environments: A systems-based perspective on primary prevention. *Journal of Consulting and Clinical Psychology, 59,* 830–841.

Wolfe, D. A., & Mosk, M. D. (1983). Behavioral comparisons of children from abusive and distressed families. *Journal of Consulting and Clinical Psychology, 51,* 702–708.

Wolfe, D. A., & Wekerle, C. (1993). Treatment strategies for child physical abuse and neglect: A critical progress report. *Clinical Psychology Review, 13,* 473–500.

Wolfner, G. D., & Gelles, R. J. (1993). A profile of violence toward children: A national study. *Child Abuse & Neglect, 17,* 197–212.

Zimmerman, M. A., & Arunkumar, R. (1994). *Resiliency research: Implications for schools and policy* (pp. 1–19). Social Policy Report, Society for Research in Child Development, Vol. 8. Ann Arbor: University of Michigan Press.

10

An Ecobehavioral Model for the Prevention and Treatment of Child Abuse and Neglect
History and Applications

JOHN R. LUTZKER, KATHRYN M. BIGELOW,
RONALD M. DOCTOR, RONIT M. GERSHATER,
and BRANDON F. GREENE

HISTORY

The term *ecobehavioral* was coined in the 1970s when a dialogue was published in the *Journal of Applied Behavior Analysis* between ecological psychologists and applied behavior analysts. The ecological psychologists suggested that while behavioral psychology had much to offer in the way of empirically based treatments, especially with children and their families, the field at that point had ignored social ecological factors between treatment and outcome (Willems, 1974). That is, although behavioral psychology had prided itself on direct observation methodologies of assessment and treatment, as opposed to reliance on indirect measures, observations tended to be narrow in focus, restricted in environments, and temporally proximate. Thus, in examining parent–child interactions, the behavior analyst of the time might have observed mother–child interactions in a clinic setting and drawn conclusions about the parent–child relationship based upon the behavioral antecedents and consequences to each molecular interaction in that setting. A more ecological approach would be to observe the mother and child in a more natural and treatment-specific

JOHN R. LUTZKER • Department of Psychology, University of Judaism, Los Angeles, California 90077-1599.   KATHRYN M. BIGELOW and RONIT M. GERSHATER • University of Kansas, Lawrence, Kansas 66045.   RONALD M. DOCTOR • California State University, Northridge, California 91330.   BRANDON F. GREENE • Behavior Analysis and Therapy Program, Southern Illinois University, Carbondale, Illinois 62901.

Handbook of Child Abuse Research and Treatment, edited by Lutzker. Plenum Press, New York, 1998.

setting such as the home. Further, it was suggested that if treatment in some form was applied to parent–child interactions, data should be collected on how that treatment may have affected other aspects of the parent–child relationship.

Thus, the "eco" in ecobehavioral stems from a notion that the family social ecology must be considered in any examination of parent–child relationships and in developing effective behavioral intervention treatment strategies.

The "behavioral" piece of ecobehavioral comes from the methodology of applied behavior analysis. That is, to be behavioral is to operationalize behavior such that it can be observed reliably and that observation and treatment can be described in a manner sufficient for replication. Treatment strategies therefore are direct, relevant, and based on data collection methods that will generate appropriate and effective results. In a retort to the concerns expressed by the ecological psychologists during this early dialogue, it was suggested that comprehensive social ecological assessment in the absence of directive treatment strategies would be irresponsible (Baer, 1974). Thus, ecobehavioral approaches were born from this tentative (at the time) marriage of ideas between ecological and behavioral psychology.

Applying an ecobehavioral approach to the prevention and treatment of child abuse and neglect seemed a practical and logical tack when Project 12-Ways (described later) was created. When the contract to create Project 12-Ways was written in 1979, the treatment literature contained only a few case studies using either simple behavioral parent training or behavioral stress reduction techniques for parents involved in child abuse and neglect. Although each approach seemed to have merit, the newly developing ecological theories of child abuse and neglect (Belsky, 1980) suggested that a broader-based conceptualization and treatment approach might be more effective. That is, in looking at the child maltreatment phenomenon, a number of questions arose. First, although parent training seemed a reasonable strategy, researchers questioned whether poor parenting strategies alone were responsible for child abuse and neglect. This question is especially relevant given that many parents may lack good behavior management skills, but they do not harm or neglect their children.

Another question was whether child maltreatment was exacerbated by stress that the parent could not manage. Again, although this seemed logical, there were countless parents able to cope with serious stressors without harming their children. Finally, the emerging sociological theories about child abuse and neglect suggested that variables such as poverty, joblessness, social isolation, and skill deficits of the children (child factors) were risk factors. Thus, it also seemed to follow that a truly comprehensive ecobehavioral approach should provide multifaceted comprehensive assessment and treatment. It was from this perspective that Project 12-Ways was created.

PROJECT 12-WAYS

Project 12-Ways has continually provided services in rural southern Illinois since 1979 (Lutzker, Frame, & Rice, 1982). Referrals to Project 12-Ways come from the Illinois Department of Children and Family Services and recently from private agencies with whom the Department has contracted to manage services. Typically, the parents have been reported for child abuse and neglect or are considered at risk of perpetrating such harm. Services are delivered in situ, mostly in the families' homes, but also in other community and educational settings. The unusual name for the project came from the 12 services that were described in the original proposal: parent–child training, stress reduction for parents, basic skill training for the children, money management training, social support, home safety training, multiple setting behavior management (in situ services), health and nutrition, problem solving, marital counseling, alcohol abuse referral, and single mother services.

Originally, it was thought that staff would be specialists in one or two services and that families would receive services from an appropriate combination of these specialists. It was immediately apparent, however, that this was completely impractical because families expressed discomfort at having several specialists serve as interventionists. Therefore, each staff member was trained in each service component and became a generalist. Almost all of the staff members have been graduate students in the Behavior Analysis and Therapy Program in the Rehabilitation Institute of Southern Illinois University at Carbondale. Accordingly, they are steeped in academic coursework and practical, supervised training in behavioral psychology, with an emphasis on behavioral assessment, single-case research design, behavioral principles, and treatment strategies as they pertain to children and families.

The primary reasons for in situ services are (1) the belief that in situ delivery of services increases the likelihood of generalization of newly learned skills across behaviors, settings, and time, and (2) the fact that families involved in child abuse and neglect, or young, single mothers, are not likely to find their way to a university clinic for services. Thus, the Project 12-Ways services described here typically are not delivered in a clinic or office setting.

Data from single-case research designs have documented the effectiveness of the ecobehavioral approach to child maltreatment by showing skill development in parent training (Dachman, Halasz, Bickett, & Lutzker, 1984), stress reduction (Campbell, O'Brien, Bickett, & Lutzker, 1983), marital counseling (Campbell et al., 1983), home safety assessment and hazard reduction (Tertinger, Greene, & Lutzker, 1984; Barone, Greene, & Lutzker, 1986), infant stimulation and health care skills (S. Z. Lutzker, J. R. Lutzker, Braunling-McMorrow, & Eddleman, 1987; Delgado & Lutzker, 1988), affect training (Lutzker, Megson, Webb, & Dachman, 1985), home cleanliness, and nutrition (Sarber, Halasz, Messmer, Bickett, & Lutzker, 1983). Program evaluation data have consistently shown that when compared to a matched comparison group in the same region, families who receive services from Project 12-Ways are significantly less likely to be reported again for child abuse and neglect up to 4 years after services (Lutzker & Rice, 1984). Also, in one evaluation, it was determined that Project 12-Ways families were more severe than comparison families prior to treatment. This was independently confirmed by workers through anecdotal reports.

It seems clear that the ecobehavioral model, with its multifaceted assessment and treatment techniques, is effective in treating and preventing child maltreatment. Less clear is whether this model could be replicated with other populations. There have been at least two attempts to replicate; however, in each case, the services provided in the replications were provided by graduate assistants. Thus, although child abuse and neglect was successfully treated and prevented in these replications, researchers question whether other ways to present the model and to deliver services more efficiently would also be effective. With those issues in mind, two replications have evolved: Project Ecosystems, aimed at families who have children with developmental disabilities, and Project SafeCare, aimed at providing more efficient services, using persons other than graduate assistants.

PROJECT ECOSYSTEMS

Project Ecosystems was created to systematically replicate Project 12-Ways by asking whether the ecobehavioral model could be applied to families who have children with developmental disabilities, in an urban setting, and using graduate assistants who were not so steeped in behavior analysis and therapy as is the staff from Project 12-Ways. That is, the staff for Project Ecosystems are recruited from several universities around southern California (Lutzker & Campbell, 1994). Children with developmental disabilities are at high risk for child abuse and neglect and for placement into more restrictive living arrangements. The children served by Project Ecosystems are at particular risk because of their severe behavioral excesses or deficits.

The in situ services provided by Project Ecosystems are parent–child training, stress reduction for parents and children, basic skill training for the children, problem-solving training for the parents, and behavioral pediatrics. The parent–child training takes the form of planned activities training (PAT), which focuses on preventing challenging child behavior by teaching parents to plan and structure activities for their children, to state the rules and expectations of activities (which include not only "fun" activities, but everyday activities such as getting ready to go to school and to prepare for mealtimes), and to use incidental teaching, feedback, and consequences (Huynen, Lutzker, Bigelow, Touchette, & Campbell, 1996).

Stress reduction in the form of behavioral relaxation training (BRT) (Poppen, 1988) teaches parents or children to assume 10 postures known to produce relaxation. Practice in this technique allows the individual to relax quickly in stress-related situations in the natural environment. For parents, this is useful when they are about to embark on PAT or when attempting to be patient during an incident of challenging behavior by the child. BRT has also been successfully used with children who have developmental disabilities. For example, Kiesel, Lutzker and Campbell (1989) used it to reduce seizures and their antecedents (hyperventilation) in a child with severe mental retardation.

Basic skill training involves teaching the children directly or teaching the parents to teach skills such as functional communication, simple hygiene, or feeding skills. Problem-solving strategies are systematically taught by using a model described by Borck and Fawcett (1982). These skills have been used by parents to help them receive better services for their children and to arrange respite care for themselves (Lutzker & Campbell, 1994). Behavioral pediatrics is the provision of services as adjuncts to medical issues. For example, Lutzker and Campbell (1994) described a child with Down's syndrome who displayed phobic behavior related to medical stimuli. She was successfully treated through symbolic modeling in the form of specially tailored and personalized stories containing increasingly descriptive medical situations. Lutzker and Campbell (1994) also described the case of a child who feared going to the dentist. This child was successfully treated with simple modeling and reinforcement procedures.

Clearly, the ecobehavioral model has been successfully replicated and extended with families who have children with developmental disabilities. Case studies, single-case experiments (Bigelow, Huynen, & Lutzker, 1993), and program evaluation data have attested to the success of this model. The California State Council on Developmental Disabilities conducted an evaluation that determined that families who received services from Project Ecosystems required fewer collateral services from other agencies and thus the project was less costly than other services.

PROJECT SAFECARE

Project SafeCare was proposed and designed to validate three new intervention components with identified abusive, neglectful, and at-risk parents that were patterned after three critical areas and strategies of intervention from Project 12-Ways. Project SafeCare examined the issues of (1) efficiency of treatment, (2) medium of parent training, (3) types of trainers, (4) possible individual difference variables associated with maltreatment, and (5) potential cultural differences on all of these factors.

More specifically, Project 12-Ways found that not all 12 intervention strategies and areas of intervention were equally critical in preventing child abuse. In Project SafeCare we extracted three salient means of intervention in parental behavioral deficiencies associated with abuse. These three areas of emphasis were (1) infant and child health care, (2) home safety, and (3) stimulation/bonding or parent–child interaction. New intervention programs patterned after similar components in Project 12-Ways were developed and tested on the Project SafeCare parent population. The ultimate goals are reduction of recidivism (in the case of abusive and neglectful parents) and prevention (for at-risk parents). Current program evaluation is ongoing for this information. Although randomized, because of the realities of providing service, all three components were presented to each parent and were therefore nested within subjects' population. Consequently, it was not possible to separate components and study their particular effects on abuse. We can, however, look at the effectiveness of training within components and can study the combined effect of all three components on abuse.

A second major question raised by Project SafeCare was whether intervention could be streamlined to 15 sessions for all components together without losing the level of effectiveness found by Project 12-Ways. In other words, can parents be trained to criterion on each component in five sessions for each component (15 for all three components) without loss of effectiveness on critical targets, particularly subsequent abuse?

A third consideration in Project SafeCare had to do with the provider of service or training. Almost all behavioral intervention studies with abusive or at-risk parents utilized graduate students as sources of training. But how effective might other types of trainers be with child abuse and neglect families? This represents an issue of dissemination. Project SafeCare examined and compared graduate student interventionists with child care protective service workers, nurses, and video programs for effectiveness of training to performance criteria and affect on subsequent abusive behavior.

Finally, it was possible within the research design to examine several important issues and questions from the child abuse literature that could be derived from the richness of contact, follow-up and sample sizes available in Project Safe-Care populations. For example, each parent was given an extensive array of self-report measures to correlate with abuse, neglect and at-risk group membership and with training success and abuse reports. In addition, because Project SafeCare had an extensive Latina population referred for services, it was possible to compare Spanish-only speakers with English speakers on all variables, but particularly the self-report scores, training effectiveness, and mode of training on abuse.

As an additional note regarding design and research issues, we should emphasize that our populations were divided into "abusive" and "neglectful" parents with nonoverlapping criteria. It was therefore possible to independently study abuse and neglect populations on all independent and dependent variables. In many respects, such comparisons between neglect and abuse allows us to develop differential measures for assessment of these categories and to test intervention results on these subpopulations. There is considerable evidence that parents involved in abuse and those involved in neglect are quite separate populations, but are often lumped together as "abusive" parents in research studies (Lutzker, 1990). Analysis of differences could prove to be a valuable first step in fully separating these populations for empirical study. The at-risk group served as a comparison population to determine the predictive validity of any differential selection criteria and the effects of treatment on prevention of abuse and neglect.

Indirect and Direct Measures

Infant and Child Health Care

Project SafeCare's infant and child health care component was designed to teach parents to prevent illness, identify symptoms, and provide appropriate treatment (Delgado & Lutzker, 1988). Parents' knowledge of basic health care information was assessed using a 10-item true/false quiz. Because parents' knowledge of health care information may not necessarily reflect their actual behavior when treating children's symptoms, parent behavior was also assessed during a role-play situation. A validated task analysis of the steps required when identifying and treating symptoms was used to evaluate parent behavior.

Prior to training, parents were given a written scenario (Spanish versions were also available) that described a child with symptoms of a particular illness. This was read aloud to parents with limited reading ability. The parent was then asked to tell the counselor what she believed the problem was, and show the counselor what she would do to treat the symptoms. The task analysis involved steps such as identifying symptoms correctly, consulting medical reference materials, reading instructions on medications, checking symptoms again, and ending treatment when appropriate.

Following assessment, parents were provided with a validated health manual and symptom guide which provided information on how to use the manual, planning and prevention, caring for children at home, calling the physician, and urgent care. The symptom guide presented information specific to each illness, such as whether the illness required urgent care, what the parent should do to treat the illness, and what the physician might do if consulted. Parents were also provided with basic health supplies, such as a mercury thermometer, a medicine dropper, and antibiotic ointment.

Health training involved instructions, modeling, parent practice, and feedback, with positive practice of those steps completed incorrectly. Following a discussion of the steps of the task analysis and their rationales, the counselor modeled each step of the task analysis while treating an illness depicted on a role-play scenario card, and then asked the parent to practice the same steps. Feedback was then provided, and parents were asked to practice the steps completed incorrectly again until demonstrated correctly. During each session, parents practiced using their health materials while role-playing the treatment of a variety of symptoms requiring either treatment at home, calling the physician, or urgent care. Following training in the use of the task analysis during the first four sessions, the counselor and parent discussed information presented in the health manual. Specific activities such as record keeping, taking a temperature, and administering medication were taught. When possible and appropriate, the child was involved in these activities and the health care scenarios. Dolls were used when it was inappropriate to involve the child, such as when administering medication.

During the fifth training session, parents were provided with several opportunities to meet the 100% training criterion in health role-play scenarios involving self-treatment, calling the physician, and seeking emergency treatment. Following training, a social validation questionnaire was administered to determine parents' opinions about the training program and their skills following training.

Home Safety

The home safety component was designed to teach parents to identify and eliminate accessible hazards within their home. The number of accessible hazards in the living room, kitchen, bathroom, and child's bedroom was measured using the Home Accident Prevention Inventory–Revised (HAPI-R), a revalidated version of the Home Accident Prevention Inventory (Tertinger et al., 1984, 1988). The HAPI-R is a safety checklist that includes the following hazards: fire and electrical hazards, suffocation by mechanical means, suffocation by ingested objects, guns, poisonings by solids and liquids, falling hazards, and drowning hazards. After obtaining consent from the parent, the observers looked through the home for hazards falling into these categories, in order to obtain the number of accessible hazards. An accessible hazard was one within the reach of the tallest child while standing on the floor, or on a surface to which the child could climb.

For families demonstrating a need for cleanliness training, home cleanliness was assessed using the Checklist for Living Environments to Assess Neglect (CLEAN; Watson-Perczel, Lutzker, Greene, & McGimpsey, 1988). Each room was divided into item areas, and a score assigned to each area rating the cleanliness, number of items of clothing or linen not belonging, and the number of other objects belonging. The scores for each area were summed and divided by the number of item areas, yielding a percentage clean score for each room. Most families have not demonstrated a need for this component. All counselors, however, were trained to assess home cleanliness and conduct clean training.

Home safety training involved instructions, counselor modeling, parent practice, and feedback. Parents were also provided with drawer and cupboard latches and outlet covers, and were taught to install these safety devices throughout their home. Training began in the room with the greatest number of hazards, and subsequent sessions focused on each of the remaining rooms in turn. During each session, feedback on remaining hazards in previously trained rooms was provided to the parent, with instructions to make any remaining hazards inaccessible.

Some families participated in video home safety training. Four videos addressing home safety in the living room, kitchen, bathroom, and bedroom presented examples of hazards common to those rooms, and provided descriptions and demonstrations of parents identifying hazards and making them inaccessible. During each training session, the Project SafeCare counselor asked the parents to watch one video, accompanied by a written supplement describing the hazards common to each room and ways to make the hazards inaccessible. Parents participating in video training also received home safety supplies. Following training, parents were asked to complete a social validation questionnaire which assessed parents' opinions of the training program and their skills in making their homes safe following training.

Bonding

The bonding component is comprised of two distinct training protocols: parent–child interactions training (children 8–10 months to age 5), and parent–infant interactions training (birth to 8–10 months). Both were designed to increase positive interactions between parent and children.

Parent–child interactions training primarily consisted of Planned Activities Training (PAT; Sanders & Dadds, 1982; Lutzker, Huynen, & Bigelow, 1998). PAT involves planning activities in advance, explaining rules and activities, engaging children in activities, and providing feedback in order to increase positive interactions and prevent challenging child behavior. Parent–child interaction skills were assessed using a 10-second observe, 5-second record partial-interval time-sampling procedure. The behaviors assessed were found by 11 child development specialists (teachers, child care directors, clinicians, and researchers) to be important to assess when measuring the parent–child relationship, and included parent leveling (positioning oneself at the physical level of the child), touch, attending, verbalizations, and instructions. The child behaviors consisted of verbalizations, affect, aggression, and following instructions. Composite scores of appropriate and inappropriate parent and child behavior were obtained from these observations. A checklist was used to assess parent use of Planned Activities Training. These behaviors included preparing for activities in advance, explaining activities, explaining rules, using incidental teaching, and providing feedback and consequences.

Training was conducted over five sessions, and consisted of discussion of the steps involved in PAT and their rationale, modeling, parent practice, and feedback. During the discussion of PAT, the counselor and the parent filled in the PAT checklist with information specific to the activity at hand. For example, when discussing playtime, parents were asked to describe their specific concerns about their child's behavior, or to give examples of play activities their children particularly enjoy. This information was added to their PAT checklist, so that the materials were tailored to their own needs. Training took place during play activities as well as activities such as getting dressed, bath time, and mealtime.

Parents were also provided with a set of play activity cards which depicted a variety of stimulating play activities in which parents and children could engage. These activity cards were incorporated into PAT; counselors modeled and parents practiced PAT during activities depicted on the activity cards. Assignments provided to parents at each session involved asking parents to use PAT, positive interaction skills, and activity cards to provide more engaging activities for their children.

Parent–infant interactions training was designed for parents of children from birth to 8–10 months, and involved teaching parents to plan and engage in stimulating play activities and use appropriate interaction skills with their infants. Parent and infant behaviors were also found by 11 child development specialists to be important to assess when evaluating parent–infant interactions. A partial-interval time-sampling procedure was used to assess parent and child behaviors during play and other daily living activities. The parent behaviors included smiling, looking, verbalizations, touch, play, and imitation. The infant behaviors included smiling, looking, verbalizations, touch, play, imitation, and crying. Composite scores for appropriate and inappropriate parent and child behavior were obtained from these observations.

Each parent–infant interaction training session focused on a specific set of skills. These included physical interactions, verbal interactions, guided play, and PAT. These skills and their rationales were discussed, and then the counselor modeled the target behaviors in play or other activities with the child. The parent was then asked to practice these skills with the child. Feedback was provided by the counselor, and then additional practice in the skills needing improvement was conducted.

Parents participating in this component also received a set of activity cards depicting a variety of play and daily living activities. These cards provided parents with suggestions and served as prompts to engage in planned activities with their children, and they were incorporated into training; target behaviors were modeled and practiced during activities depicted on the cards. Assignments involved asking parents to use the newly practiced interaction skills and activity cards during their daily interactions with their child.

Video Training

Home safety, parent–child interactions, and parent–infant interactions training videos were designed and filmed by Project SafeCare. These videos were also translated into Spanish. Initially, videos were to be presented as the primary mode of training for parents designated to participate in video training. Some parents' performances improved to criterion; some improvements were less dramatic. In cases in which video training did not result in criterion level performance, research assistants provided additional training and feedback.

Indirect Measures

Although direct observation of the parent and child behavior involved in health, safety, and parent–child interactions is the optimal method for evaluating changes in parent behavior following treatment, indirect measures may provide a secondary measure of the effects of treatment.

Project SafeCare uses seven questionnaires to assess a host of parent and child characteristics. These questionnaires are administered to all participating mothers and fathers, and are completed prior to training, following the completion of training, and at six-month follow-up intervals. Their primary purpose is to provide standardized descriptive information about Project SafeCare families, and to evaluate change in parent-reported information following the completion of Project SafeCare services.

All parents complete the Child Abuse Potential Inventory (CAP; Milner 1986, 1994), the Parenting Stress Index (PSI; Abidin, 1990), and the Beck Depression Inventory (BDI; Beck & Steer, 1993). The CAP Inventory has been used as a screening device to assess risk for physical child abuse. A Spanish translation of the CAP Inventory is available for research purposes, but no data are currently available demonstrating the ability of the Spanish version to screen for physical child abuse in this population. Because a majority of the families served on Project SafeCare speak Spanish, the CAP Inventory has not been used by Project SafeCare to classify parents.

The PSI (Abidin, 1990) assesses stressors associated with parent characteristics and child characteristics, and other stressors within the parenting role. It has been used to assess stress levels among parents who are at risk for or reported for child abuse, among other populations. While research has not independently demonstrated the validity of PSI-Short Form, it is likely that it is as valid as the full-length version because it is a direct derivation of the longer form. The BDI (Beck & Steer, 1993) assesses the presence of depressive symptoms in the parent, and is also used to evaluate change in parents' reports of depression following treatment.

In addition to these measures, four devices are used with parents with older children. The Parent Behavior Checklist (Fox, 1994) is used to assess parental discipline, nurturing, and expectations in parents of children age birth to 4 years of age. The Eyberg Child Behavior Inventory (Eyberg & Colvin, 1994) provides a measure of parent-reported child behavior problems. This measure assesses disruptive behaviors in children ages 2 to 16 on an Intensity Scale, which indicates the frequency of the problem, and a Problem Scale, which identifies the specific behaviors that are current problems for the parent. The Conners' Ratings Scale (Conners, 1989) is used to characterize patterns of problem behavior in children 3 to 17 years of age. It includes scales for conduct disorder, anxious–shy behavior, restless–disorganized behavior, learning problems, psychosomatic symptoms, obsessive–compulsive behavior, antisocial behavior, and hyperactive-immature behavior. It also includes a 10-item hyperactivity index which measures the extent to which the child displays behaviors indicative of Attention-Deficit/Hyperactivity Disorder (ADHD). The Parental Anger Inventory (PAI; DeRoma & Hansen, 1994) was designed to assess anger experienced by abusing parents in response to challenging child behavior. Parents are asked to rate child-related situations as problematic or nonproblematic and then indicate the magnitude of anger elicited in each situation using a 5-point scale.

These self-report measures are conducted with all parents when appropriate, and are used primarily to assess parent and child behavior and to provide a pre/post measurement of the intervention's effectiveness. The data collected from these measures are secondary to direct observation data, however, in that self-report data may be influenced by a variety of factors. Direct observation data provide the most accurate measure of parent and child behavior.

Outcome

Changes of Plans

Before active training began on Project SafeCare, several modifications were made to the original design. One primary research question asked, "What is the best means of delivering these services?" Training was to be provided by research assistants, caseworkers, nurses, and in a video format to equal numbers of families across the first three years of the project. During the first year of Project SafeCare, the funding that was to have been provided for public-health nurses was lost by the agency that was to provide the nurses to Project SafeCare. Consequently, nurses, who would have been paid by the agency, were not available to provide training to Project SafeCare families. In order to examine the question as to whether a nurse could effectively provide Project SafeCare services, a recent nursing-school graduate was hired, and successfully provided training in the health component to two families. Additional funds were not available, however, to hire more nurses, or nurses with several years of experience. Because of this departure from the original design, the 36 families originally designated to be involved in the nurse training condition were reassigned to either the caseworker, research assistant, or video training condition.

Similarly, deviations from the original plan were made in the caseworker training condition. As part of the agreement between Project SafeCare and DCFS, three caseworkers were provided with reduced caseloads in return for conducting training with 36 Project SafeCare families. Two of these caseworkers were supposed to conduct training, and one was to be an alternate. During the months following their training in how to conduct parent training in the three components, it became clear that even with reduced caseloads, it was not possible to have caseworkers provide weekly training sessions in a consistent manner to families. Although their caseloads had been reduced, the number of children for whom the caseworkers were responsible was still more than optimal according to DCFS standards. With the court appearances, home visits, and on-call time required of caseworkers, their availability for training sessions with PS families was significantly limited. In fact, there were many instances in which the caseworkers cancelled their scheduled appointments with PS families because of these responsibilities. This was a substantial obstacle; nonetheless, several families were able to complete training in the health component conducted by a caseworker.

Only months later, however, both caseworkers took leaves. Families initially assigned to this condition were reassigned to other modes of training. While one of the original caseworkers returned to conduct additional training, another offered his resignation. With only one caseworker available to conduct training, families were no longer assigned to the caseworker condition. In an effort to resolve this ongoing problem, DCFS supervisors provided Project SafeCare with a full-time caseworker to conduct training. This caseworker no longer had a caseload, but was employed by the department. Although she met the training criteria for each component, when conducting training with parents, she did not demonstrate training skills in the appropriate manner. These deficits in her training skills resulted in parents not meeting training criteria.

Following a change in the supervision of the department, this specially assigned caseworker was transferred, and one unit of caseworker trainees was designated to work with Project SafeCare. Although it had been stipulated that the caseworkers' caseloads would be reduced, their caseloads remained equivalent to that of other caseworkers. Again, their primary responsibilities impeded their ability to consistently meet with Project SafeCare families. Thus, the caseworker training condition was also omitted from the original design, and these families were reassigned to either a "partially trained by a caseworker" condition, or to the research assistant or video condition.

Although the effectiveness of training conducted by caseworkers was not clearly demonstrated, it was apparent that their responsibilities prevented them from having the consistent contact and involvement with Project SafeCare families necessary to effectively complete training. Reduced caseloads were supposed to be provided, but any reduction they did receive failed to provide them with the flexibility needed to attend weekly sessions with families. The caseworkers' availability was further limited by their responsibility to be available for emergency situations.

In some cases, the training provided by a caseworker did not meet the necessary standards. This appeared, however, to be a specific problem with only one caseworker. The original design required that 36 families receive nurse training, and 36 required caseworker training. These two goals were not met.

The original program design called for evaluating the effectiveness of four different modes of training with a specified number of families over four years. The aim was to reach more families, in the most direct and efficient manner. Presumably, many families already receiving services provided by social workers or nurses would benefit from additional training provided by these types of professionals. Based upon these findings, however, it was determined that the competing responsibilities of the caseworkers prevented a thorough evaluation of this mode of presentation.

Attrition also became an obstacle that, while expected, was much greater than anticipated. Parents in the at-risk group were voluntary, making the attrition in this group higher than that in the abuse group. While attrition among at-risk families who agreed to participate in the program was high, a large number of parents declined to participate in the project before signing the initial informed-consent form. This can be attributed to the nature of families involved in, or at risk for, child abuse and neglect, but it may also be related to characteristics of the program. It appeared that the considerable assessment conducted with families prior to, as well as during training, may have resulted in some families dropping out of the program. Future research should continue to evaluate the factors that are necessary to engage families in services.

Parents' attendance at scheduled sessions was addressed by implementing an appointment calendar system involving reminders and gold stars for attendance. A slight improvement in some parents' attendance was observed upon the implementation of the calendars, but this increase was not statistically significant. From attendance and attrition patterns seen in Project SafeCare, it is apparent that making participation more engaging and rewarding to families and reducing the burden placed on them may reduce attrition.

Other departures from the originally planned protocol involved discarding caseworker social validation of the effects of training. From an original sample of social validation forms mailed to caseworkers following the completion of training with families they had referred, none were returned completed. Only a few caseworkers returned the forms, and all of these included notes from the caseworker indicating that the family was no longer in their caseload or that the case had been closed.

Throughout the project, several of the original objectives necessarily had to be revised in order to adjust to the natural circumstances of the agencies and families who participated. Some of these circumstances required more extensive adjustments than others; obstacles such as these must be met with flexibility and the ability to adapt to changing circumstances in the community.

Group Data

Despite the adjustments and revisions made to the originally proposed project, group outcome data have clearly answered most of the proposed research questions. The first question was, "Can the three services most often provided by Project 12-Ways be made more efficient and be more effectively provided in 15 sessions?" When provided in five sessions by research assistants, these services have been effectively delivered. In the bonding component, parents' use of PAT has improved from 43% to 86% (Figure 1). Observations of the validated parent and child interaction skills indicated that the number of intervals in which appropriate parent behavior was observed increased from 64% to 70% following training. The instructions provided by the parents to the children were also assessed. The percentage of instructions that were stated appropriately increased from 89% to 95%. Further, among a smaller group of parents who participated in follow-up observations, appropriate parent interaction skills increased from the baseline of 64% to 74% and appropriate instructions increased to 99%. Thus, parents who have participated in research assistant training have demonstrated substantial improvements in their parent interaction skills and their use of Planned Activities Training. Further, parent interaction skills and instructions improved from posttraining to follow-up observations. Corresponding improvements in child behavior have also been observed (Figure 2). In the research assistant training group, appropriate child behavior increased from 71% of intervals to 79%, posttraining. Instruction following increased from 65% of instructions to 82% at posttraining. As with parents, child behavior also improved from posttraining to follow-up. Data collected during activities in which training was not conducted indicate that the improvements in parent (Figure 3) and child behavior (Figure 4) generalized to novel activities.

Similar improvements were observed among four parents who participated in video PAT (Figure 5). Their use of PAT increased from 61% to 94%, and the

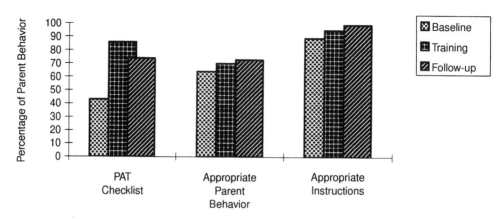

Figure 1. Percentage of parent use of PAT, parent appropriate interaction skills, and appropriate instructions during activities in which training was conducted.

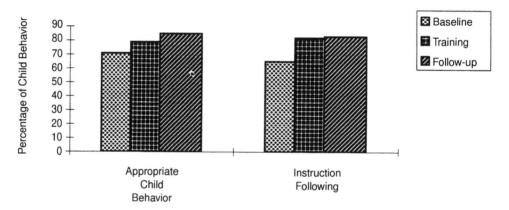

Figure 2. Percentage of child appropriate behavior and instruction following during activities in which training was conducted.

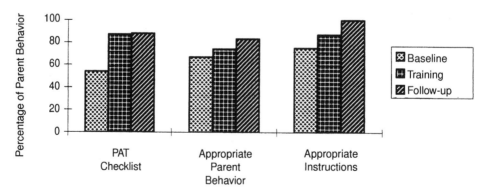

Figure 3. Percentage of parent use of PAT, parent appropriate interaction skills, and appropriate instructions during generalization activities.

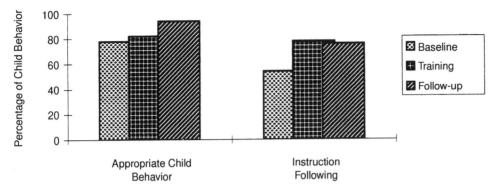

Figure 4. Percentage of child appropriate behavior and instruction following during generalization activities.

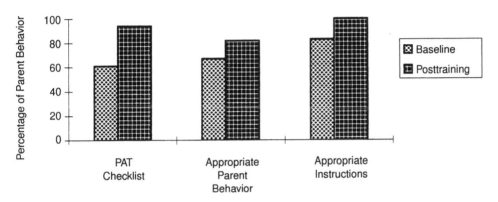

Figure 5. Percentage of parent use of PAT, parent appropriate interaction skills, and appropriate instructions during activities in which video training was conducted.

percentage of intervals in which appropriate interaction skills were demonstrated increased from 67% to 82%. The percentage of instructions that were stated appropriately increased from 83% to 100%. Appropriate child behavior increased from 73% of intervals to 86%, posttraining. Instruction following increased from 55% to 100% (Figure 6). Thus, PAT provided in a video format is effective in increasing parent use of PAT and improving parent and child interaction skills. An additional improvement was seen in the quality of instruction provided to children, and their instruction following. In addition to demonstrating the effective use of PAT with parents at risk for or reported for child abuse and neglect, these results lend support to the use of video parent training with this population.

Parents' health care skills also significantly improved. Of parents who received health training provided by either research assistants, caseworkers, a nurse, or combinations of a caseworker and research assistant, or in a video format with research assistant, 86% met the 100% training criterion in role-play scenarios requiring self-treatment, calling the physician, and emergency treatment (Figure 7).

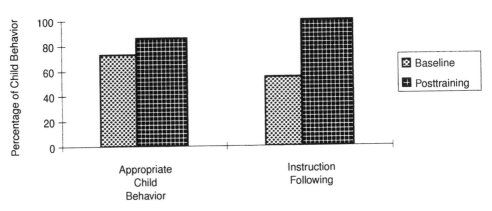

Figure 6. Percentage of child appropriate behavior and instruction following during activities in which video training was conducted.

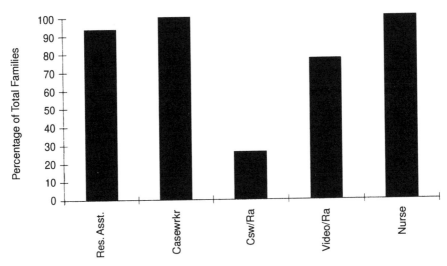

Figure 7. Percentage of parents who met the 100% training criterion on self-treat, call the physician, and emergency treatment role-play scenarios across each mode of training.

Of the parents who did not meet the training criterion, there was an improvement of at least 80% in parent performance (Figure 8).

In addition to improvements in the bonding and child health care components, reductions in the number of hazards were observed among families participating in this component. Across all groups, the average reduction in hazards from baseline to posttraining was 68%.

The second research question was, "What is the relative effectiveness of these services when provided by research assistants, a nurse, DCFS caseworkers, and in a video format?" In its systematic replication of Project 12-Ways, Project Safe-Care sought to evaluate the effectiveness of these training protocols when delivered by DCFS caseworkers and a nurse, as well as in a video format. It has been demonstrated by Project 12-Ways that research assistants can effectively provide

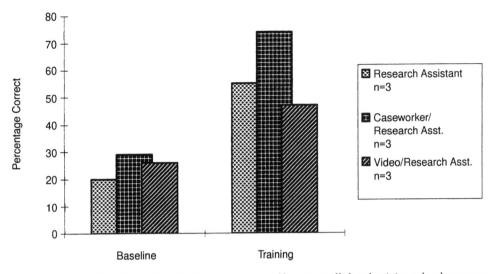

Figure 8. Average baseline and posttraining scores on self-treat or call the physician role-play scenarios across each mode of training for parents who did not meet the 100% training criterion.

these training components to families reported for child abuse and neglect. This result has been replicated by Project SafeCare in a very different, urban community. The remaining question was whether caseworkers and nurses can provide these services, and whether video is an effective medium. One nurse provided health training to two parents as effectively as research assistants. Both parents met the 100% training criterion, and these improvements were maintained at follow-up observations.

Caseworkers, as described above, provided training only in a somewhat incomplete manner to a handful of families, and in half of these cases, training started by a caseworker was concluded by a research assistant. Four parents completed health training with caseworkers, and all four met the training criterion. There were also four families who began health training with a caseworker and finished training with a research assistant. Only one of these families met the training criterion. Of the parents who did not meet the criterion, however, there was still a 155% improvement in parent performance on health role-play scenarios. Thus, although only 5 of the 8 parents who had any contact with caseworkers in the health component met the training criterion, there were significant improvements in parent performance following training.

Neither caseworkers nor the nurse provided training in the bonding or home safety components. Research assistants and video training were the two modes of training provided in these components, and some families received a combination of these modes of training. Video parent–child interactions training, as discussed previously, was effective in increasing parents' use of PAT and positive parent and child interaction skills. Video home safety training was also effective in improving the safety conditions of homes (Table 1). Following video training, parents reduced accessible hazards from baseline to posttraining by 65%. Parents who participated in training by research assistants reduced hazards by 71%. Thus, the difference in outcome between parents who received

Table 1. Percentage Reduction in Hazards from Baseline to Posttraining
across Modes of Training and Referral Group

	n	Video	Research asst. (R.A.)	Video/R.A.	Total
Abuse	13	72.1%	83.9%	46.3%	74.5%
Neglect	14	39.4%	69.7%	n/a	66.3%
At-risk	5	76.0%	49.2%	79.6%	54.5%
Total reduction		64.7%	71.4%	57.4%	68.3%

research assistant training and those who received video training alone was not substantial. Some parents who received video training, however, did not reduce hazards to an acceptable level with video training alone, so additional training and feedback were provided by a research assistant. These parents reduced accessible hazards by 57%. This average reduction, which was lower than the reduction observed in other groups, may be attributed to individual characteristics of these families who, even with additional research assistant training, did not reduce accessible hazards as much as families who received only research assistant training. These results suggest that video training, although effective with some families, may not be suitable for other families. Further examination of the factors which make video training more appropriate for some families and less appropriate for others is needed.

Single-Subject Evaluation

Although group data answer many questions about the overall effectiveness of these training procedures, single-subject data are more effective when an individual's behavior change over time is of interest. Figure 9, an example of clinical data, depicts the percentage of correct steps on health role-play scenarios for one parent who received video and research assistant training in the health component. With the presentation of the health manual and symptom guide (written materials), and then the introduction of the health video, the parent's performance did not improve. With the introduction of research assistant training, which included modeling, practice, and feedback, the parent immediately met the 100% training criterion. Thus, while the training video included much of the same information as presented by the research assistant, the modeling and feedback provided by the research assistant and the practice required of the parent resulted in immediate improvements in parent performance which were maintained throughout the remainder of research assistant training. At follow-up, however, the number of steps correctly performed in a self-treat/call the physician role-play scenario decreased to 69%. Parent performance on an emergency treatment scenario, however, remained at 100%.

Figure 10, an example of single-case experimental data with one family, depicts parent use of PAT, appropriate interaction skills, and appropriate instructions. PAT was provided by a research assistant to a Spanish-speaking mother referred for neglect after one of her children drowned. With training, her use of

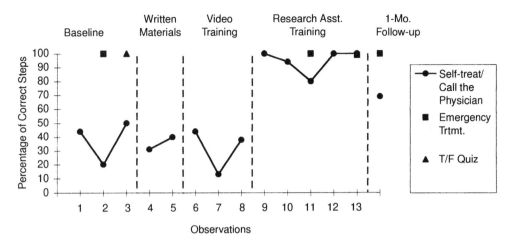

Figure 9. Percentage of correct steps on role-play scenarios for one parent who participated in video health training supplemented by research assistant training. Supplemental training was introduced when the parent's performance remained at baseline levels following video training.

PAT increased in training and generalization activities. Increases in parent appropriate interaction skills were observed during bath and meal. In all activities, parent inappropriate behavior was negligble. Figure 11 depicts child behavior, which maintained or increased improvement slightly following training with the mother.

Figure 12, another example of single-case experimental data with one family, shows the number of hazards across four rooms in the home of a Spanish-speaking mother referred because her child had fallen from an open second-story window. Prior to training, the number of hazards was low in the bedroom and living room, but the number of hazards in the bathroom and kitchen posed a risk to the children in the home. Home safety training was initially introduced in the bathroom, resulting in an immediate decrease in the number of hazards to nearly zero. During the next session, training was conducted in the kitchen. Again, the number of hazards decreased to nearly zero. In the living room, the number of hazards decreased during baseline, but in the bedroom, baseline hazards were variable. Following training in these rooms, however, the parent reduced the number of hazards to zero. Thus, the safety conditions of a home which contained a significant number of hazards prior to training was improved dramatically after three training sessions.

Single-case experimental designs can also be used to demonstrate the external validity or generality of a training package by evaluating its use with more than one individual. Figure 13 shows the effectiveness of health training with two parents. Training was provided by research assistants, resulting in improvements in parents' use of the correct steps in identifying symptoms and providing appropriate treatment. Both parents met the 100% training criterion on role-play scenarios requiring self-treatment, consulting the physician, or seeking emergency treatment.

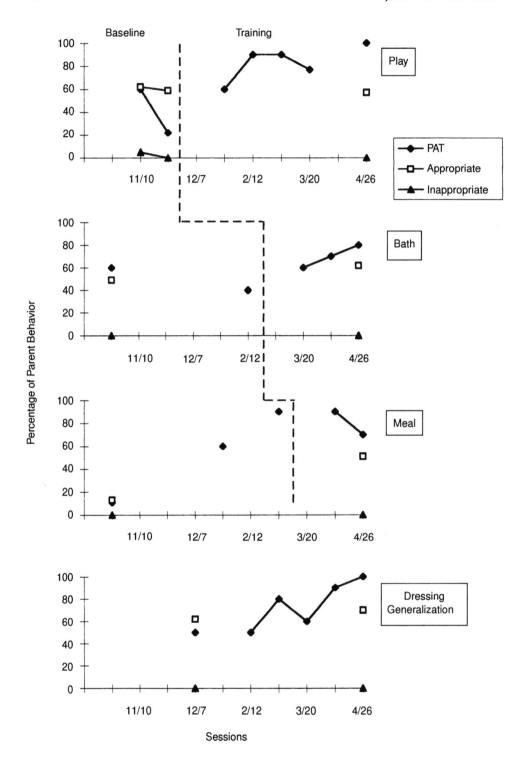

Figure 10. Percentage of appropriate and inappropriate interaction skills and correct use of PAT for one parent who participated in PAT provided by a research assistant.

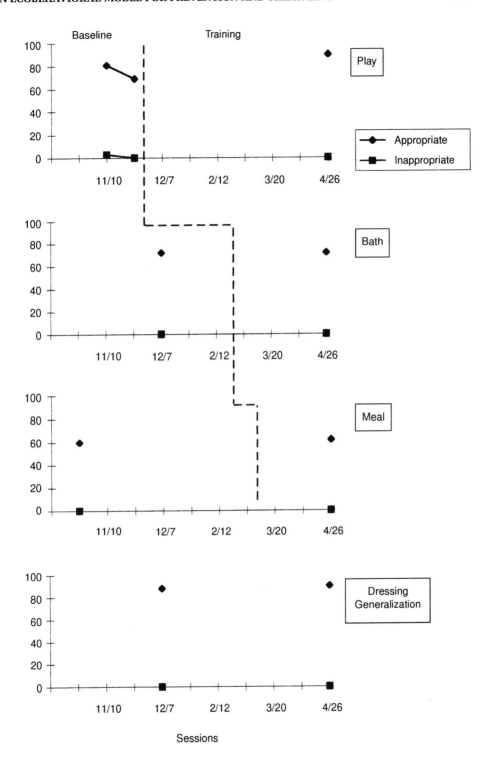

Figure 11. Percentage of appropriate and inappropriate child interaction skills for the child of a parent who participated in PAT provided by a research assistant.

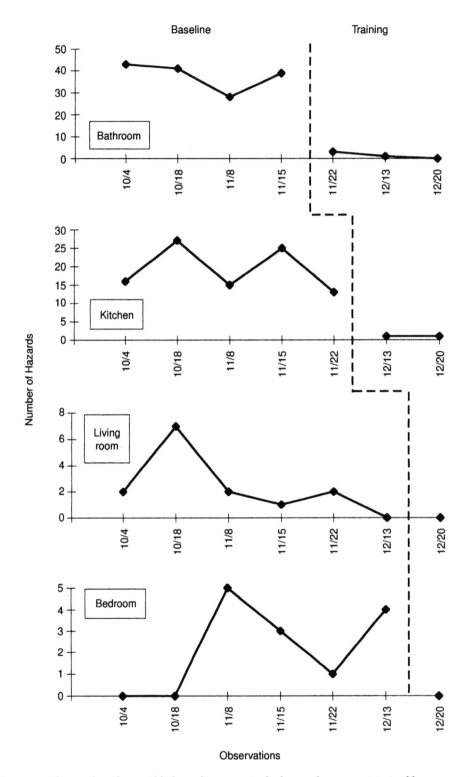

Figure 12. The number of accessible hazards present in the home of one parent trained by a research assistant.

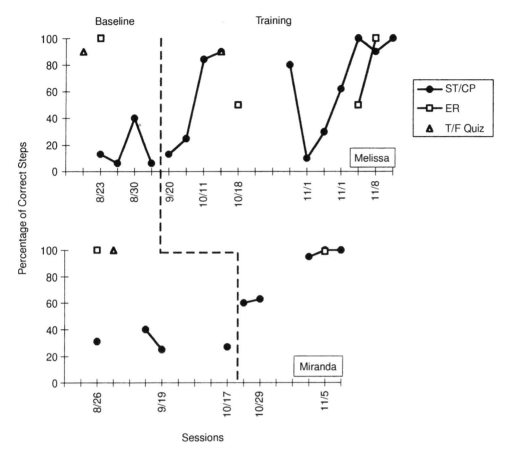

Figure 13. Percentage of correct steps on role-play scenarios for two parents who participated in health training provided by research assistants.

PROGRAM EVALUATION

Program evaluation is the process by which a treatment, research, or service program is examined to determine the clinical efficacy of the treatment procedures, the cost-effectiveness of the program, and the social validation by its consumers. Program evaluation is considered an extremely important component of any treatment program, as it allows researchers to examine significant questions about the program and to modify the interventions accordingly. Some researchers consider it unethical not to conduct program evaluations, as an absence of evaluations could lead to the continuation of ineffective interventions with a lack of cost-effectiveness (Lutzker & Campbell, 1994).

There are various forms that program evaluations can take. The first level is examination of clinical data. Clinical data can provide useful information regarding any observable change in behavior, and whether this change meets the goals of the program. In addition, these data can be used when reporting to agencies, and in supervision (Lutzker & Campbell, 1994). There are clinical data from individual families on Project SafeCare that illustrate the effectiveness of combined video and graduate assistant training in the identification and correct treatment of common childhood illnesses (cf., Figure 9). In these cases, the families increased from a baseline level of 38% correct responses to 100% correct identification of illness and appropriate treatment.

The second level of evaluation is case studies. These reports usually reflect a dramatic change in behavior of one individual as a result of an often novel treatment, where other means of treatment have not been successful (Lutzker & Campbell, 1994). On Project SafeCare, Planned Activities Training has been used to improve the positive interactions between a parent and her child (cf., Figures 10 and 11). As part of the training procedure, this parent improved her interactional skills and learned how to prepare for an activity in such a way as to maximize child involvement and minimize maladaptive behavior.

The third level of program evaluation is single-case experiments. For example, multiple baseline designs were developed to allow researchers to examine the effect of a treatment across settings, subjects, or behaviors without having to withdraw the treatment to establish control. Multiple baseline designs were used across families in Project SafeCare to demonstrate the efficacy graduate training in childhood health management (cf., Figure 13). Parents once again reached the criterion of 100% correct responses across all types of scenarios that called either for home treatment, for calling and visiting a physician, or for seeking emergency treatment.

The most extensive level of evaluation is program evaluation in which larger questions are examined that pertain to the overall clinical efficacy of the program, the cost-effectiveness, and consumer satisfaction with the services provided (Lutzker & Campbell, 1994). This type of program evaluation is ongoing and is currently being conducted by Project SafeCare.

The treatment approach of Project SafeCare is based on an ecobehavioral approach that views child abuse and neglect as a multifaceted problem in need of multiple social/ecological modifications (Lutzker, Wesch, & Rice, 1984). Therefore, Project SafeCare utilizes a multitude of direct and indirect outcome measures that will allow a complete evaluation of the variables present in abusing and neglectful families, as well as the clinical efficacy of the interventions.

Previous program evaluations have been conducted on Project 12-Ways and Project Ecosystems (Lutzker & Rice, 1984; Lutzker & Rice, 1987). Like Project Safe-Care, both of these projects use an ecobehavioral approach to treat families who have been reported for child abuse and/or neglect, or who have children with developmental disabilities. The results of these evaluations have clearly demonstrated the clinical efficacy of these treatment programs. For example, families that received services from Project 12-Ways were less likely to have recidivism (reincidences of abuse and neglect) than were comparison families (Lutzker, & Rice, 1984, 1987; Wesch & Lutzker, 1991). Families seen by Project Ecosystems are unlikely to have their children placed in a more restrictive setting (Lutzker & Campbell, 1994).

Project SafeCare focuses primarily on the health, safety and well-being of young children. Parents are taught to recognize and report illnesses (and to discriminate between illnesses that can be treated at home and those that need a physician's attention); to make their homes hazard proof for their children; and to increase parent–infant bonding through stimulation and scheduled activities. One of the major undertakings of Project SafeCare was to replicate these three training areas from services delivered in Project 12-Ways and consolidate them into smaller, more efficient treatment packages that would ideally be delivered in 5 sessions. In addition, an examination and evaluation of the efficacy of three possible treatment modes (graduate assistant training, video training, and caseworker training) was conducted. Another major goal of Project SafeCare was to find preventive means to intervene with families that have been identified as being at high risk for abuse and/or neglect of their children.

There are many areas of interest in a service program such as Project SafeCare. One of the most important and significant indicators of success of a treatment program such as Project SafeCare are low recidivism rates. Recidivism is defined as abuse and/or neglect following the termination of services by a treatment program. Such an evaluation is conducted by collecting abuse and neglect reports from the Department of Child and Family Services on each family that is referred to the project. The frequency of abuse reports posttreatment is compared to pretreatment frequencies of abuse. Data are also collected regarding the number of emergency room visits that the child made pre- and posttraining. In addition, these data are compared with that of families that did not receive services from Project SafeCare. If safety and health training are successful, the incidence of injuries, illnesses, and household accidents should decrease posttreatment. In addition, abuse reports should decrease posttraining if Project SafeCare has been successful at improving the bond and increasing the positive interactions between parents and children.

As part of the program evaluation of Project SafeCare, a comprehensive statistical evaluation of all indirect and direct measures will be conducted. All analyses will be conducted across the three groups: those reported for child abuse, those reported for neglect, and those determined to be at-risk for child maltreatment. Of particular interest, as well, is whether there is a significant difference in scores between English-speaking and Spanish-speaking families.

The direct measures are the data collected during health, safety, and bonding training. Multivariate analyses will be used to evaluate these (grouped) data collected from direct observation of parent performance in all three training areas. These data are examined to determine the change in scores and competency of the parents in these areas after training has been completed. Of those families who do not meet criterion or complete training, an analysis will be conducted to assess the change in scores with incomplete training. In addition, an analysis of the reason for attrition will be conducted. The indirect measures such as the Child Abuse Potential Inventory, the Beck Depression Inventory (BDI), and the Parenting Stress Index (PSI) will be analyzed to determine whether scores increase or decrease posttraining.

Project SafeCare utilizes a demographic form that compiles information about the families served, on more than 200 variables. These include factors such as race, household income, number of children, admission versus denial of child abuse and neglect, and extensive information about the parents' childhood. Some of the factors are of considerable importance. For example, Zuravin and DiBlasio (1996) identified 11 characteristics associated with neglect and 4 associated with abuse that enabled them to correctly place the parent in either group approximately 80% of the time. Characteristics such as having been sexually abused as a child, having run away from home, having committed a crime, being placed in foster care, having had abortions and premature babies, having more than 2 children before age 18, suffering from depression, and low levels of education were associated with neglect. On the other hand, abusive mothers were more likely to have had a mother with emotional problems, more likely to have been antisocial as a child, more likely to be receiving AFDC support, and less likely to be positively attached to their own mothers. The results of earlier studies are consistent with these findings (Parke & Collmer, 1975; Wolock & Horowitz, 1977).

When conducting the evaluation of Project SafeCare, certain demographic characteristics are of specific interest. For example, all analyses will be conducted across the three groups (abuse, neglect, and at-risk) and across languages (English-speaking families versus Spanish-speaking families). In addition, such characteristics as the type of abuse suffered by the mother as a child (if any), the age of the mother at the birth of her first child, admission/denial of any abusive/neglectful behavior, number of children in the family, level of education, and socioeconomic status are of interest and will be compared to the outcome of both the direct and indirect measures.

Finally, the overall effectiveness, as well as the social acceptability, of the programs will be evaluated by examining social validity data. A questionnaire with questions regarding the professionalism and empathy of the staff, as well as the training procedures, is given to each family upon completion of the program. This is a very important area when dealing with parents who have been reported for abuse and neglect, because they may be in denial or embarrassed about their situation and thus may be resistant to treatment. Therefore, it is crucial that our staff behave in a manner that the families find approachable and nonthreatening, and that the services are delivered effectively and in a meaningful way. The social validation questionnaire asks the parents to rate the staff as well as the services. In addition to this questionnaire, parents are asked to rate the staff and the training at the end of each session in the home. These questionnaires allow the investigator to determine whether the program has social significance for the individuals being served.

By the end of its first four years, the staff of Project SafeCare will have served more than 120 families living in Los Angeles County. It is crucial that all aspects of the program be examined and evaluated to determine the efficacy of the program, the cost-benefit ratio, and the consumer satisfaction with the services. The incidence of child abuse and neglect has risen dramatically and a remedy for this vast problem is greatly needed. Program evaluations can aid in this process by providing researchers with valuable information regarding the characteristics of such parents. This information could ultimately lead to more effective programs that could identify potentially abusive or neglectful parents in their teens, and provide training that could reduce the likelihood of abuse occurring. Thus, such evaluations are an important aspect of any large research project.

SUMMARY

The ecobehavioral model has been successfully used to provide services for child maltreating families in rural southern Illinois. Questions concerning replication have been addressed by Project Ecosystems, which has extended the model to developmental disabilities with adults and children and in an urban community. Project Ecosystems serves a broader socioeconomic range than Project 12-Ways, thus suggesting replicability across SES. Project SafeCare serves the urban San Fernando Valley of Los Angeles and has a majority of Latinas/Latinos among its families who also are characterized by low SES. Project SafeCare has demonstrated that videos can be effective adjuncts to providing these services and that a nurse and caseworkers can also be taught to deliver ecobehavioral services.

The ecobehavioral model embodies an attempt to address the social/ecological concerns that place children at risk. Replication provides confidence in efficacy and allows for exploration of systematic changes of the model.

ACKNOWLEDGMENTS

The writing of this chapter was funded, in part, by a grant from The California Wellness Foundation. We are grateful for the assistance of Randi Sherman.

REFERENCES

Abidin, R. R. (1990). *Parenting Stress Index* (2nd ed.). Charlottesville, VA: Pediatric Psychology Press.

Baer, D. M. (1974). A note on the absence of a Santa Claus in any known ecosystem: A rejoinder to Willems. *Journal of Applied Behavior Analysis, 7*, 167–168.

Barone, V. J., Greene, B. F., & Lutzker, J. R. (1986). Home safety with families being treated for child abuse and neglect. *Behavior Modification, 10*, 93–114.

Beck, A. T., & Steer, R. A. (1993). *Beck Depression Inventory: Manual*, San Antonio, TX: Psychological Corporation.

Belsky, J. (1980). Child maltreatment: An ecological integration. *American Psychologist, 35*, 320–335.

Bigelow, K. M., Huynen, K. B., & Lutzker, J. R. (1993). Using a changing criterion design to teach fire escape skills to a child with developmental disabilities. *Journal of Developmental and Physical Disabilities, 5*, 121–128.

Borck, L. E., & Fawcett, S. B. (1982). *Learning counseling and problem-solving skills.* New York: Haworth.

Campbell, R. V., O'Brien, S., Bickett, A., & Lutzker, J. R. (1983). In-home parent-training, treatment of migraine headaches, and marital counseling as an ecobehavioral approach to prevent child abuse. *Journal of Behavior Therapy and Experimental Psychiatry, 14*, 147–154. Indexed in the *Inventory of Marriage and Family Literature.*, Vol. X, Family Resource Center, 1984.

Conners, C. K. (1989). *Manual for Conners' Rating Scales.* New York: Multi-Health Systems.

Dachman, R. S., Halasz, M. M., Bickett, A. D., & Lutzker, J. R. (1984). A home-based ecobehavioral parent-training and generalization package with a neglectful mother. *Education and Treatment of Children 7*, 183–202.

Delgado, L. E. & Lutzker, J. R. (1988). Training young parents to identify and report their children's illnesses. *Journal of Applied Behavior Analysis, 21*, 311–319.

DeRoma, V. M., & Hansen, D. J. (1994, November). Development of the parental anger inventory. Poster presented at the Association for the Advancement of Behavior Therapy Convention, San Diego.

Eyberg, S., & Colvin, A. (1994, August). Restandardization of the Eyberg Child Behavior Inventory. Poster presented at the annual meeting of the American Psychological Association, Los Angeles.

Fox, R. A. (1994). *Parent Behavior Checklist.* Brandon, VT: Clinical Psychology Publishing.

Huynen, K. B., Lutzker, J. R., Bigelow, K. M., Touchette, P. E., & Campbell, R. V. (1996). Planned activities training for mothers of children with developmental disabilities: Community generalization and follow up. *Behavior Modification, 20*, 406–427.

Kiesel, K. B., Lutzker, J. R., & Campbell, R. V. (1989). Behavioral relaxation training to reduce hyperventilation and seizures in a profoundly retarded epileptic child. *Journal of the Multihandicapped Person, 2*, 179–90.

Lutzker, J. R. (1990). Behavioral treatment of child neglect. *Behavior Modification, 14*, 301–315.

Lutzker, J. R., & Campbell, R. V. (1994). *Ecobehavioral family interventions in developmental disabilities.* Pacific Grove, CA: Brooks/Cole.

Lutzker, J. R., Frame, R. E., & Rice, J. M. (1982). Project 12-Ways: An ecobehavioral approach to the treatment and prevention of child abuse and neglect. *Education and Treatment of Children, 5,* 141–155.

Lutzker, J. R., Huynen, K. B., & Bigelow, K. M. (1998). Parent training. In V. B. Van Hasselt & M. Hersen (Eds.), *Handbook of psychological treatment protocols for children and adolescents* (pp. 467–500). Hillside, NJ: Erlbaum.

Lutzker, J. R., Megson, D. A., Webb, M. E., & Dachman, R. S. (1985). Validating and training adult–child interaction skills to professionals and to parents indicated for child abuse and neglect. *Journal of Child and Adolescent Psychotherapy, 2,* 91–104.

Lutzker, J. R., & Rice, J. M. (1984). Project 12-Ways: Measuring outcome of a large-scale in-home service for the treatment and prevention of child abuse and neglect. *Child Abuse & Neglect, 8,* 519–524.

Lutzker, J. R., & Rice, J. M. (1987). Using recidivism data to evaluate Project 12–Ways: An ecobehavioral approach to the treatment and prevention of child abuse and neglect. *Journal of Family Violence, 2,* 283–290.

Lutzker, J. R., Wesch, D., & Rice, J. M. (1984). A review of Project 12-Ways: An ecobehavioral approach to the treatment and prevention of child abuse and neglect. *Advances in Behaviour Research and Therapy, 6,* 63–73. Indexed in the *Inventory of Marriage and Family Literature.* Vol. XI, Family Resource Center, 1985.

Lutzker, S. Z., Lutzker, J. R., Braunling-McMorrow, D., & Eddleman, J. (1987). Prompting to increase mother–baby stimulation with single mothers. *Journal of Child and Adolescent Psychotherapy, 4,* 3–12.

Milner, J. S. (1986). *The Child Abuse Potential Inventory: Manual* (2nd ed.). Webster, NC: Psytec.

Milner, J. S. (1994). Assessing physical child abuse risk: The Child Abuse Potential Inventory. *Clinical Psychology Review, 14,* 547–583.

Parke, R., & Collmer, M. (1975). Child abuse: An interdisciplinary analysis. In M. Hetherington (Ed.), *Review of Child Development Research* (Vol. 5, pp. 509–590). Chicago: University of Chicago Press.

Poppen, R. (1988). *Behavioral relaxation training.* New York: Pergamon.

Sanders, M. R., & Dadds, M. A. (1982). The effects of planned activities training and child management procedures in parent training: An analysis of setting generality. *Behavior Therapy, 13,* 452–461.

Sarber, R. E., Halasz, M. M., Messmer, M. C., Bickett, A. D., & Lutzker, J. R. (1983). Teaching menu planning and grocery shopping skills to a mentally retarded mother. *Mental Retardation, 21,* 101–106.

Tertinger, D. A., Greene, B. F., & Lutzker, J. R. (1984). Home safety: Development and validation of one component of an ecobehavioral treatment program for abused and neglected children. *Journal of Applied Behavior Analysis, 17,* 159–174.

Watson-Perczel, M., Lutzker, J. R., Greene, B. F., & McGimpsey, B. J. (1988). Assessment and modification of home cleanliness among families adjudicated for child neglect. *Behavior Modification, 12,* 57–81.

Wesch, D., & Lutzker, J. R. (1991). A comprehensive evaluation of Project 12-Ways: An ecobehavioral program for treating and preventing child abuse and neglect. *Journal of Family Violence, 6,* 17–35.

Willems, E. P. (1974). Behavioral technology and behavioral ecology. *Journal of Applied Behavior Analysis, 7,* 151–166.

Wolock, I., & Horowitz, B. (1977). *Factors relating to levels of child care among families receiving public assistance in New Jersey.* Final report to the National Center on Child Abuse and Neglect (DHEW Grant 9-C-418). Washington, DC: National Clearinghouse on Child Abuse and Neglect Information.

Zuravin, S. J., & DiBlasio, F. A. (1996). The correlates of child physical abuse and neglect by adolescent mothers. *Journal of Family Violence, 2,* 149–166.

11

Dealing with Child Abuse and Neglect within a Comprehensive Family-Support Program

SEBASTIAN STRIEFEL,
MICHAELLE ANN ROBINSON,
and PAT TRUHN

Since 1989, the Community–Family Partnership (CFP) program in northern Utah has provided comprehensive services to families living in poverty. Such families are at increased risk for child abuse and neglect due to the many stresses associated with poverty (Gaudin, 1993; Tower, 1992). Within the two counties served by the program, the incidence rate of substantiated child abuse and neglect cases in 1994 was 0.3% ($n = 355$), slightly less than in the state of Utah (0.5%; $n = 10,430$) (Utah Children, 1996) and the United States (0.4%; $n = 1,036,000$) (National Committee to Prevent Child Abuse, Utah Chapter, 1995; Peterson & Urquiza, 1993).

This chapter describes the CFP program and how it provides comprehensive family support services to low-income families. Its central focus is on how CFP staff, in partnership with low-income families and staff from other agencies, provide comprehensive family support services which prevent and remediate child abuse and neglect. Lessons learned, evolution of policies and procedures, and outcomes achieved are discussed.

To understand the impact of comprehensive services on families living in poverty and, specifically, how these services can affect child abuse and neglect, one must understand the context within which the services are provided (Love,

SEBASTIAN STRIEFEL • Center for Persons with Disabilities and Psychology Department, Utah State University, Logan, Utah 84322-6800. MICHAELLE ANN ROBINSON and PAT TRUHN • Center for Persons with Disabilities, Utah State University, Logan, Utah 84322-6800.

Handbook of Child Abuse Research and Treatment, edited by Lutzker. Plenum Press, New York, 1998.

1983). The Community–Family Partnership program in northern Utah is one of the original Comprehensive Child Development Programs (CCDPs) funded by the Administration for Children and Families between 1989 and 1994. The CFP program thus includes both a federal and a local context.

FEDERAL CONTEXT

Authorized by Congress in 1988, the Comprehensive Child Development Program (CCDP) is designed to address the pervasive needs of low-income children and families and to combat the fragmentation of existing programs that serve them. Its objective is to promote educational achievement and economic and social self sufficiency through the provision of intensive, comprehensive, and continuous support to both children and families from a child's birth until entry into school. (Smith & Lopez, 1994, p. 1).

Federal Goals

The goals of the CCDPs are fourfold:

1. To help poverty-level families maximize the development of each child in the home under school-age to prevent educational failure. This includes prevention and elimination of child abuse and neglect by intervening as early as possible to prevent and alleviate the negative impact on child development.
2. To help each family move toward social and economic self-sufficiency, thus preventing welfare dependency. This includes training parents in skills that will help prevent abuse and neglect, such as child management and mental health treatment.
3. To work as partners with other community agencies in achieving the two previously stated goals. This includes helping families access services from community agencies for problems that contribute to the occurrence of abuse and neglect, for example, substance abuse treatment.
4. To identify policy issues useful for welfare reform. This includes support for unified efforts to address problems such as child abuse and neglect through integrating services, such as interagency efforts to alleviate poverty and its negative effects and thus decreasing the stress often associated with poverty that leads to abuse and neglect.

Federal Mandates

The mandates of CCDPs are to (1) help families use existing services whenever possible (e.g., Aid to Families with Dependent Children), (2) work with other agencies to identify gaps in services and find ways to fill these gaps (e.g., working to create needed mental health services for children because few such services exist), (3) provide some direct services (e.g., in-home parent training in child development and basic nutrition), and (4) serve as the payer of last resort for some services (e.g., paying for needed family health care services when no one else will pay).

Program Evaluation

The CCDPs are probably the most comprehensive child and family service demonstration projects ever funded by the Federal Government. Therefore, they have extensive evaluation components, including a federal third-party impact evaluation, a federal third-party process evaluation, a federal qualitative ethnographic evaluation, and a local formative and summative evaluation. (For more information on the programs' evaluation see Smith & Lopez, 1994.)

Core Services

The intent of the legislation establishing the CCDPs was that enrolled families would receive services for five years. The law required certain services to be available to families directly, or indirectly by brokerage of the services with other community agencies and programs (Smith & Lopez, 1994). The mandated core services included

1. Early childhood education and development services for all children under school age
2. Early intervention for children with or at risk for developmental delays or disabilities
3. Nutritional services for children and families
4. Child care that meets state licensing standards
5. Child health services (medical and dental)
6. Prenatal care for pregnant women
7. Mental health services for children and adults
8. Substance abuse education and treatment
9. Parental education in child development, health, nutrition, and parenting
10. Vocational training and other education related to obtaining employment or employment that pays more, has a benefit package, or both (Smith & Lopez, 1994, pp. 4–5).

Compliance Standards

The federal funding agency established a number of family and service compliance standards during the seven years of the CFP's existence. For example, each child under the age of 5 was to participate in 3, 30-minute, in-home, developmental learning activities per month with their parent, or a minimum of 12 half-day sessions per month in a center-based early childhood education program. Licensed child care was to be paid for all children of parents who were employed or enrolled in a training/education program regardless of family income. Federal policy regarding compliance standards evolved and changed from time to time. Achievement of compliance was monitored for 5 years via a quarterly computer download of CFP data.

LOCAL CONTEXT

Local Program Description

The CFP program at Utah State University in Logan, Utah, began in October, 1989. At any given time, it serves 60 families from Cache and Box Elder counties in northern Utah. The counties served cover roughly 7,000 square miles and have a population of about 108,000. Several mountain ranges, a desert, the Great Salt Lake, and the rural nature of the area require many program families and CFP staff to travel some distance to access or deliver services. Eighty-three percent of the population is Caucasian. The other 17% of the population is made up relatively equally of Hispanics, Asians, and Native Americans (Utah Department of Health, 1987).

Eligibility

To be eligible for CFP services a family's income needs to be below the Federal Poverty Guideline (below $18,220 for a family of five in 1996). In addition, the family must include either a pregnant woman or an infant less than one year of age. This child is known to the CFP as the "focus child." To date, the program has served 127 families.

Recruiting Families

Initially, CFP staff recruited families by sharing information about the program with advisory board members and other community agency personnel. In addition, flyers about the program were posted in laundromats, grocery stores, and other locations likely to be frequented by low-income families. Staff members also visited low-income neighborhoods and knocked on doors to inform families about the program and its services. Later, recruitment included the dissemination of brochures, referral of new families by families already served by the program, and referrals from community agencies.

During initial interviews, family members often said that they enrolled in the program because they needed help in specific areas such as getting a job, child care, or helping their children. Some families wanted many services, some only a few, and others did not know what they wanted besides help in getting their lives and those of their families to improve. Some demographic information on the 127 families served to date is shown in Table 1.

Comprehensive Services

For CFP staff, comprehensive services means making services available to families directly or indirectly (i.e., through brokering any service needed) to maximize child development or to help families move toward social or economic self-sufficiency. CFP services, therefore, include more than the federally mandated core services; they may include, for example, legal assistance, car repairs, rent payments, and assistance with immigration issues.

Table 1: Demographic Information for All Families Ever Enrolled in CFP
(Number of Families Served = 127)

Variable	Number	Percent	Mean
Marital status of mother			
Married	75	59.1	
Single	21	16.5	
Widowed	1	.8	
Divorced	14	11.0	
Separated	11	8.7	
Single, living with partner	5	3.9	
Total	127	100.0	
Ethnicity of family			
American Indian or Alaskan Native	12	9.4	
Asian or Pacific Islander	4	3.1	
Black, not of Hispanic origin	1	.8	
Hispanic	12	9.4	
White, not of Hispanic origin	98	77.3	
Total	127	100.0	
Primary language of family			
American Indian	4	3.1	
Asian	2	1.6	
English	111	87.4	
Spanish	10	7.9	
Other	0	.0	
Total	127	100.0	
Years of education			
Father	95		10.6
Mother	127		10.6
Parent ages (in years)			
Father	95		31.1
Mother	127		29.7
Number of adults (age 18 and over)	244		
Number of children	393	100.0	
0–1 year	28	7.1	
1–2 years	21	5.4	
2–3 years	26	6.6	
3–4 years	22	5.6	
4–5 years	33	8.4	
5–6 years	55	14.0	
6–18 years	208	52.9	
Average family size			5.05

Staffing Patterns

The primary contact person for each family is a home visitor called a family consultant, who works with a maximum of 10 families. Family consultants, in partnership with families, have the primary responsibility for many services including (1) needs assessment, (2) development and implementation of family and individualized service plans, (3) home-based parent training in child development, child management, self-concept building, stress management, nutrition, budgeting, and so on, (4) such case management functions as helping families access services from other agencies or CFP staff, and (5) assessing progress on goals set. Family consultants work closely with several CFP specialists who provide consultation or direct assistance in obtaining such services as licensed child care, employment and training, and mental and physical health care. Additional specialists facilitate involvement of fathers, provide group parent education opportunities, and staff a preschool classroom in each county for 3-year-olds.

Staff Training

All service staff in the CFP program, with the exception of one home visitor and some preschool teaching assistants, have at least a bachelor's degree. During initial staff recruitment, care was taken to hire people with different training backgrounds, because no one discipline possessed all of the knowledge and skills required to provide the needed services. Staff members had degrees in such disciplines as social work, child development, psychology, education, nursing, and health education. The diversity of disciplines allowed for cross-training of skills using existing staff, and for a broader prospective when problem solving. All initial staff received more than a month of training in several content areas, including child and family development, health and safety, nutrition, budgeting, and community resources. Initial training also included a broad range of such skills as establishing rapport and partnerships, conducting standardized needs assessments, defining goals in measurable terms, conducting training with parents, accessing community agencies and programs, and risk management (including dealing with suspected child abuse and neglect). Staff members hired later receive similar training; much of this training is accomplished through reading, listening to audiotapes, watching videotapes, and being paired with staff members already doing a similar job. Supervisors periodically accompany staff members on home visits to observe them providing services. Such home visits serve to assess staff skills and to determine the need for other specific training. Staff training is ongoing and is based on staff and administratively identified training needs. Individual and group supervisory sessions are held weekly. Twice per year 5 staff, family, or advisory board members attend three-day CCDP training sessions in Washington, D.C. These meetings provide opportunities to learn how other CCDP projects deal with similar family and program issues.

Partnership and Empowerment

Partnership

The program's name, Community–Family Partnership, was selected jointly by staff and an advisory board of parents and representatives from community agencies, businesses, and the university. To these groups the name reflected the philosophy that if families were to make meaningful progress they needed to be equal partners in the service process. Implicit in the concept of partnership is a relationship between persons having a joint interest and a common purpose. Partners collaborate and cooperate with each other in an effort to achieve a common purpose that has mutual benefits.

In a practical sense this means that each partner

1. Brings something to the relationship (strengths)
2. Gets something from the relationship (needs met)
3. Agrees to work toward a common purpose (goal)
4. Understands that by working together, more can be accomplished than by working alone (complementary and additive strengths)
5. Understands that compromise will sometimes be necessary (give and take)
6. Understands that power and authority are shared (knowledge and expertise rather than titles are the key)
7. Understands that establishing and maintaining these relationships takes ongoing time and effort to assure that the partnership works (that a win-win situation occurs)
8. Understands that a cost-benefit balance must be maintained (no one partner should carry an excess burden)
9. Understands that partnerships are on a continuum, ranging from those that work extremely well to those that don't seem to work at all (each partner must do their share)

The concept of partnership means that family members are involved in decisions having an impact on them. For example, interagency staffings held to solve a particular family's problems occur with the family "sitting at the table" either as the lead partner or as an equal member of the group. When decisions are made about a family without their participation, the partnership has broken down.

Empowerment

Empowerment exists when one helps oneself or others produce or prevent change, as in, for example, controlling some aspect of one's life by making choices (Striefel, 1991). Empowerment is the direct opposite of paternalism, a practice of making decisions for or about another under the guise of knowing best what is right for him or her. Empowering others includes exploring the pros and cons of each possible alternative to a problem or behavior and then respecting the person's right to make the final decision. It also includes being supportive of the person even when disagreeing with the decision made.

Empowerment is a difficult process to implement with individuals who have abused or neglected their child, because they have demonstrated that they do not make the kinds of decisions expected by society. Yet abuse and neglect often occur because the perpetrator does not recognize other options as viable alternatives for achieving their personal goals. Abuse and neglect laws are designed to control inappropriate behavior and to protect children. They also serve to disempower individuals who use their power in ways unacceptable to society.

Services Integration

Working with families in which children are at risk for abuse and neglect has afforded yet another opportunity for community agencies and programs to collaborate in building a more integrated system of services for families. Konrad (1996) defined services integration as a "process by which two or more entities establish linkages for the purpose of improving outcomes for needy children, individuals, and families" (p. 1). Ideally, comprehensive and integrated services assure enhanced accessibility and continuity of services, facilitate prevention as well as intervention, increase accountability for quality of services, and reduce the duplication, waste, inefficiency, and cost of services (Wingspread, 1993).

From its inception, the CFP has actively pursued services integration through a variety of activities. The advisory board which was formed during the grant-writing phase to give input into the planning of the CFP model evolved into a group of very active subcommittees which continue to pursue innovative solutions to fill gaps in community resources and services for families.

Annually updated, written interagency agreements define shared costs and services between the CFP and a broad group of community agencies including mental health providers, state social service agencies, sexual abuse treatment programs, child and family support centers, health clinics, child care providers, and housing agencies. The more factors (e.g., costs, services) shared, the stronger the partnership and the better services are integrated.

Educational forums sponsored by the CFP bring local and state experts together to address gaps in service such as lack of affordable housing and health care, or to problem-solve such difficult systems issues as the gap between welfare and family economic self-sufficiency. At the individual family level, the brokering process helps families access community services; follow-up and ongoing interagency collaboration resolves problems of turf or personality conflicts, and maximizes the benefits of comprehensive, integrated services to families.

CFP Service Model

The CFP service model provides the framework for implementing partnerships with families and empowering family members. The model includes four major dynamic processes: (1) comprehensive assessment of family and family member needs, (2) formulation of a family service plan and an individualized development plan for each child under the age of 5, (3) implementation of the plans, and (4) evaluation of the progress made by the family and family members toward achievement of their plans.

The service model also defines the approach taken by staff in working with families. Staff members are trained to be sensitive to family issues, to interact with families in ways that establish functional relationships with them, and to coordinate their activities with those of other staff members so that families feel empowered rather than overwhelmed and fragmented by multiple services. Staff members are also trained to combine respect for a family's pace and encouragement of the family members to push themselves toward their chosen family goals.

Needs Assessment

Upon enrollment in the CFP, and every four months afterward, the family and their assigned family consultant work together in completing a needs assessment which asks a series of family-friendly questions in each of 11 domains of family life, including

1. Employment, job retention, career exploration, education, and training
2. Housing
3. Financial management
4. Physical health, dental and mental health
5. Family functioning
6. Parenting skills
7. Social self-sufficiency
8. Homemaking skills
9. Transportation
10. Public assistance and overall well-being
11. Transitioning out of the CFP

It is not unusual for some family-defined needs to require a more in-depth assessment. Staff specialists in health, mental health, and economic self-sufficiency are available to join the family and family consultant partnership in that process. For example, both parents of one family enrolled in CFP identified a high level of marital stress as significantly contributing to their ability to care for their children's basic needs. In addition, the mother identified feeling depressed and the father was concerned about the frequency of losing his temper. With the parents' permission, the family consultant asked a CFP mental health specialist to administer the SCL-90-R (Derogatis, 1994), a mental health screening instrument, which resulted in the identification of moderately severe mental health problems. These mental health problems were then addressed with appropriate services.

Methods used for assessing developmental needs of the children vary depending on the age of the child. The Hawaii Early Learning Program (HELP) activity sheets developed by Parks (1991) are used in the home to assist parents in assessing and identifying the developmental needs of their infants and toddlers. The HELP assesses skills in cognitive, expressive language, gross motor, fine motor, social–emotional, and self-help domains of development. When children turn 3 years of age and enter the CFP center-based early childhood program, the Revised Brigance Inventory of Development (Brigance, 1991) is used to assess developmental needs of children 3–5 years of age in the following areas: gross-motor skills and behaviors, fine-motor skills and behaviors, self-help skills, speech and language skills, general knowledge and comprehension, social and emotional development, reading readiness, manuscript writing, and basic math skills. More intensive, specific, assessment of identified developmental delays is conducted when indicated by results of the HELP or Brigance.

Individualized Service Plan

Once the needs assessment has been completed, the family consultant assists the family in developing a Family-Based Support Plan (FBSP) by prioritizing needs, choosing those to be worked on during the next four months, converting them into goals, and planning activities aimed at achieving each goal. During this process, the family consultant encourages each family to identify its own strengths and resources that can be used to achieve each goal. Other resources, for example, services from CFP specialists or community agencies, responsibilities of each partner, and time lines for completion of activities, are identified. This information is documented in written form.

Information obtained about each child from the HELP and Brigance assessments is reviewed with parents and converted into a written Individualized Child Development Plan (ICDP) with developmental goals for the next four months. When children are less than 3 years of age, the parents work with the family consultant to specify goals. When children are older than 3 years, the parents work with the child's preschool teacher.

Children who have developmental disabilities, or delays sufficient to warrant enrollment in specialized programs, are referred to special needs, early intervention programs within the community. The family consultant and staff specialists help the family to enroll their child in the program which best fits the child's needs. In these situations, the educational plan used by the other agency for the child's program serves as the ICDP for the CFP.

Implementation

Once the FBSP or ICDP has been written, the family consultant and other CFP staff work closely with the family and staff from many different community agencies to implement the family's service plans. Goals, activities, time lines, and responsibilities are changed upon agreement of all members of the partnership.

Evaluation of Progress

Family and family member effort, and progress toward goal achievement, is recorded as it occurs. At the end of each 4-month FBSP or ICDP period, a formal assessment of progress is conducted by the parent(s), the family consultant, and other appropriate staff. Shortly following this evaluation, the needs assessments and service plan development begin again.

CFP Computerized Information System

Documentation of all components of the individualized service plans occurs through a computerized system of interactive data bases. The system generates a series of working forms and documents that are both partnership-friendly and efficient. For example, from information obtained from a family's completed needs assessment the computerized system prints the family's complete FBSP including the parents' identified goals and activities. Separate listings of family goals and activities can be printed for specialists working with a family. From the HELP and Brigance data, a specific ICDP is produced for each child, along with data monitoring sheets for recording a child's daily behavior and progress. The CFP computerized system used the federally required and other locally defined data to produce reports used by both direct service and administrative staff to monitor the quality and management of program services for families and to identify and remedy problems early. For example, monthly reports are generated summarizing services provided, progress made, and family status on several dimensions such as health, mental health, child development, and economic self-sufficiency.

EXAMPLES OF THE IMPACT OF COMPREHENSIVE SERVICES
ON FAMILY ABUSE AND NEGLECT

What follows are examples of how CFP staff and their community and family partners implemented the comprehensive family support services of the CFP services model to deal with issues of child abuse and neglect.

Family Example 1

Background

Family 1 participated in CFP for a period of 5 years. The mother had Mild Mental Retardation and the father was diagnosed with Attention-Deficit Disorder and learning disabilities. The father had worked unsuccessfully at a series of part-time jobs; the mother had never worked outside the home. At the time of enrollment in CFP, this couple had an infant daughter. A second child was born two years later.

Family Issues

Relevant family issues included (1) the failure of the first child to gain weight during infancy, (2) the identification of developmental delays in both children, (3) the mother's lack of homemaking skills in food preparation and storage, cleaning and maintaining the home, and money management, (4) the parents' lack of knowledge and skills to care for and nurture infants and toddlers, (5) the lack of parenting and behavior management skills, (6) the lack of adequate finances to support the family, (7) the mother's low self-esteem, (8) the father's poor social skills, (9) the lack of family transportation, (10) the lack of social network and extended family support, (11) a history of poor job retention skills, and (12) the developmental pace of the children exceeding the parents' acquisition of new parenting skills.

Services Provided to Family

The family received weekly visits from their family consultant. Together, needs were identified, goals developed, and activities planned to address the identified issues. The parents received training in child management, appropriate activities to encourage child development, parenting skills, and child health and nutrition. The father, with CFP assistance, applied for and received Social Security Disability benefits. Money management and budgeting skills were taught by CFP staff through activities such as jointly identifying all expenses and all income, setting up a budget, and paying critical bills like rent and utilities before buying extras. The staff also assisted the family weekly with shopping and homemaking skills, including nutrition and meal preparation, by helping the mother develop nutritious meal menus, providing her with simple recipes from children's cookbooks, and showing her how to prepare meals until she could do so by herself. The parents attended group social and educational programs planned at further developing skills that would assist them in forming a social network. In addition, the children received weekly services for developmental delays from an early intervention program.

The community health nurse was involved with the family initially, providing information and training about infant nutrition and monitoring the growth of the first child. CFP health, men's issues, and economic self-sufficiency staff members worked with the family. Job skills counseling to maintain employment, job search assistance, and emotional supports were provided to the father as he looked for part-time employment. The family was assisted with the process of purchasing, licensing, insuring, and maintaining a vehicle. The family also received support from the weekly contacts with a variety of staff members.

Abuse/Neglect Incident

As the children grew, their need for parenting grew faster than the parents' ability to acquire the skills needed to be competent parents. During the fifth year of participation in CFP, the parents appeared overwhelmed by the increasingly complex demands of parenting. Skills that they had had used to provide for their infants' and toddler's safety were no longer appropriate for active, verbal, independent preschoolers. The children were not well monitored within the home or neighborhood; this raised concerns about their safety. Even with intensive assistance, the parents were unable to set limits, reward positive behavior, and deal with verbally resistant behavior. Soon the children were in control and their parents became ineffective in accomplishing even such simple tasks as bathing, getting and keeping the children dressed in appropriate clothing, or getting the children to eat nutritious foods instead of a diet of candy and fast food. As the frustration of the parents increased with their decreased control, indicators of inappropriate physical management appeared. At the same time, the conditions in the home deteriorated. The home became unsafe and unsanitary as the children created more "messes." Feeling helpless, the parents did little, even with support, to correct the problems. The combination of inadequate parenting skills and lack of sufficient daily living skills necessary to maintain a healthy and safe environment for the children resulted in a neglect report being made by CFP staff and the subsequent removal of the children from the home.

Interagency Collaboration and Impact

Although CFP staff had worked intensively with the family and collaboratively with other agencies providing services to the family prior to the neglect report, collaborative efforts were intensified following the removal of the children from the home. CFP staff facilitated a series of interagency staffings involving the family's social worker from the Division of Family Service (DFS) and staff from other agencies involved with the family. Working within the framework of the family's DFS treatment plan, staff members from the agencies working with the family, and representatives from the community, specifically from the Mormon church, defined their roles and the services that each would provide, thus maximizing service delivery without duplication of efforts.

The highlight of the collaborative effort was the creativity of the individuals involved in moving beyond their typical roles to provide innovative services utilizing approaches geared to help the family achieve the goals identified as necessary for their children to be returned to the home. One added service was mental health treatment for both parents provided by CFP mental health staff. The mother was hospitalized with severe depression and suicidal ideation following the placement of the children in foster care. Follow-up treatment was provided by a CFP therapist who was a specialist in providing mental health treatment to individuals with mental retardation.

The father's work with his CFP therapist addressed issues of temper control, inappropriate physical management of the children, and guilt about the impact of his behavior upon his family. DFS initiated family preservation services to work on homemaking skills with the parents in their home, using staff from an agency trained to work with individuals who have mental retardation.

Additionally, each agency coordinated visits to the home so that the parents received regular reinforcement for the homemaking skills they were learning throughout the week. The father was assisted in informing his parents, who had been unaware of any parenting problems, of the removal of the children from the home. Other services already in place for the children and family continued.

Parental rights were terminated one year after the placement of the children into foster care. Although intensive, comprehensive, collaborative services provided over 5 years did not facilitate the reunification of this family, it did assist in finding an alternative resolution that assured the safety of the children and the continued involvement of the parents in the lives of their children. The grandparents became actively involved and were awarded custody of the children. The biological parents moved out of state to be near the children's grandparents. The grandparents have supported, encouraged, and carefully monitored the ongoing involvement of the biological parents with the children. The children are safe, healthy, and have a relationship with both their grandparents and biological parents in a way that minimizes the likelihood of future abuse or neglect.

Family Example 2

Background

This mother was single and pregnant when she enrolled in CFP 4 years prior to this description. Her son was born soon after enrollment. The mother married the child's father 2 years later. A second child was born the same year.

Family Issues

The family issues included (1) the mother's lack of a high school education, (2) initial concerns about parenting skills and the child's safety when with his father, (3) threats directed by the father toward the mother, (4) an inadequate income, fears of applying for public assistance, and poor budgeting skills, (5) interfering and controlling behaviors by parents of both the mother and father, (6) the father's history of being abused as a child and depression as an adult, (7) parental disagreement regarding appropriate parenting and discipline practices, and (8) adjustment problems of the oldest child to having his father reside in the home following the parents' marriage.

Services Provided to Family

The family consultant visited this family weekly and provided training in child development and behavior management using such commercially available resources as the HELP Activity Sheets (Parks, 1991) and the SOS manual (Clark, 1985). Some examples of the specific behavior management skills taught included identification of reinforcers and how to deliver them contingently, the use of appropriate, non-abusive discipline techniques, and how to give appropriate verbal instructions. The family consultant worked collaboratively with the social services case worker to address the safety concerns of the mother so that she could obtain financial support. Problem-solving skills were taught and implemented by the mother to address budget issues, housing needs, and relationship issues with the child's father and the mother's extended family. The skills taught included identifying the problem and the options for dealing with the problem, identifying the pros and cons for each option, selecting what seems to be the most desirable option and carrying it out, and evaluating the outcomes.

The father actively participated in the CFP program following his marriage. He addressed with the family consultant relationship issues with his wife and extended family and was involved with learning the same behavior management and child development skills that had been taught to his wife. CFP assisted him in obtaining and paying for mental health treatment in the community.

Abuse/Neglect Incident

The oldest child in this family attended the CFP preschool. One morning the preschool teacher observed bruise marks on the child's neck. When the child was asked about the marks, he stated that his father had choked him.

Interagency Collaboration and Impact

A CFP initiated abuse report was made to DFS. As a result of the long collaborative working relationship, the DFS investigator contacted the family consultant to obtain information regarding family functioning. The family consultant had input into the interventions that were recommended for the family. Although the stepfather was angry and expressed his feelings of betrayal by CFP staff when initially contacted by DFS regarding the abuse report, the family consultant provided support to him, reminded him why the report had to be made, and helped him see the positive outcomes that could occur as a result of the report. The father agreed voluntarily to participate with DFS recommendations, thus avoiding a court appearance to face an abuse complaint. He began participation again in therapy, addressing both his personal issues and parenting issues, and the family remained intact.

Family Example 3

Background

This family consisted of a pregnant mother with an 8-month-old infant at the time of enrollment in CFP. The mother had an ongoing relationship with the father of the children and they periodically lived together. After 3 years, the father became an active CFP participant.

Family Issues

The family issues included (1) the mother's unemployment, the mother's poor job retention skills, and inadequate finances; (2) the mother's substance abuse; (3) the lack of appropriate parenting and child development skills; (4) an oldest child with significant developmental delays; (5) the involvement of the mother with the legal system because of check forgery; (6) the mother's initial lack of commitment to active participation in CFP; and (7) the mother's dependency upon her parents, combined with serious mental health issues in the extended family.

Services Provided to Family

This family received weekly visits from their family consultant. Initial services consisted of assisting the mother in obtaining public assistance and housing. Child development and behavior management were taught by the family consultant. The family consultant verbally confronted the mother about inconsistencies in her behavior and the verbal reports of others (for example, the reasons for repeatedly losing jobs). Eventually the mother admitted having a substance abuse problem. The family consultant was supportive of the mother when she entered treatment by being available to her when needed and by helping her plan for the future. She also supported the mother when she confronted the father about his unwillingness to provide financial support to the family.

Abuse/Neglect Incident

The children in this family were at high risk for abuse and neglect. Both parents lacked parenting skills and had unrealistic expectations of their children. Substance abuse was occurring. Multiple stressors such as poverty, joblessness, homelessness, relationship problems, and a child with developmental delays were present. The emotional needs of both parents were not being met. Thus, the parents found it difficult to demonstrate empathy and be nurturing toward the children.

Interagency Collaboration and Impact

Ongoing collaborative relationships facilitated the family consultant's work with public assistance programs to reach services that would meet the basic needs of the family. Working relationships with an early intervention program and the public school system facilitated access to specialized developmental services for the child with disabilities. Relationships with social services facilitated the mother's referral to an inpatient and outpatient substance abuse treatment program. Foster care for the children while the mother was in jail was avoided as a result of collaboration with DFS staff.

After 6 years of participation in CFP, these parents demonstrate competency in parenting, nurturing, and managing the behavior of their children. The father volunteers in the CFP preschool and shows very positive and appropriate interactions with the children and teachers. Parents now nurture and demonstrate affection toward their children. The mother continues with substance abuse counseling and has been substance free for one and one-half years. Both parents are employed. The parents have become active advocates within the public school system for their daughter with disabilities. Although the parents have yet to fully address their dependency issues with their parents, or their money management issues, the children are no longer at risk for abuse or neglect.

LESSONS LEARNED

When a comprehensive family support program works exclusively with families experiencing the many stresses of poverty, the likelihood is high that staff members will be actively involved in helping parents change patterns of behavior toward their children. The intensity and frequency of staff contact with families increases the possibility that staff members will be aware of risk for, or existence of, child abuse and neglect. Clearly, staff members must deal with abuse issues as an integral part of their ongoing work with many families. As a result, CFP staff has learned a number of useful lessons about family, staff, agency, and administrative issues. Some of these lessons are identified in the following discussion.

Lessons Learned about Families

Limits of Confidentiality

One lesson learned is that it is important to review limits of confidentiality with families (American Psychological Association, 1992) at the beginning of the partnership and periodically afterwards. Doing so builds a framework of information against which the staff–family partnership can process reports of child abuse and neglect. A document defining the limits of confidentiality, including legal responsibility of staff members to report suspected child abuse and neglect, should periodically be read, comprehended, and signed by parents.

Informing Families that a Report Is Being Made

Another lesson centered around the question of when, who, and how to inform a family that an abuse/neglect report is being made by a CFP staff member. Opinions voiced on this issue were grounded in two differing perspectives and required staff discussion followed by the setting of administrative policy. Proponents of prior notification base their arguments on the principle that a professional who has a strong working relationship with a family should demonstrate trust in the family's ability to work through the difficulties of knowing that a report is being made, rather than breach trust by creating secrets (Brosig & Kalichman, 1992). In some situations a family member may be empowered by the professional to make the report; this may begin the therapeutic process of change and healing. Thus, the professional can be most helpful by assisting the family to anticipate, understand, and make positive changes as a result of coping with the investigative process and outcomes. Proponents of not informing the family of an impending report cite strong concerns that forewarning family members will interfere with the investigation, result in destroyed evidence, and put the child at further risk (Besharov, 1990). CFP policy is to inform the family and try to work through the issues unless there is a clear indication of risk of harm to a family member, staff member, or the investigative process.

Reducing the Risk of Abuse Requires Intensive Resources

Families enrolled in comprehensive family support programs who are at risk for child abuse and neglect need intensive staff resources, major commitments of time, and continual support from staff. During 6 years of providing comprehensive services to families, the CFP staff has learned that many, but not all, parents experienced developmental and emotional impoverishment and/or abuse as children. Results of mental health screening tests administered by CFP staff indicate that more than 40% of the parents served grapple with mental health problems that significantly interfere with their providing good parenting and a safe environment for their children. Along with high needs for core services such as mental health counseling, these families likely need assistance in coping with a child abuse report, rebuilding trusting relationships with CFP and other agency staff, and making any required changes in parenting and family life identified during the abuse investigation, often doing this difficult work with limited personal and family resources. When serious disabilities are present in the family, and when the cost of needed intensive services is prohibitive or those kinds of services are not available in the community, the challenges are even greater. For example, it became clear to CFP staff that, because of their cognitive disabilities, one set of parents needed the intensive support and parent training that a structured family living program could provide. None was available.

Small Steps

Sometimes, when parents are very needy, have multiple difficulties, are reluctant to engage in partnerships with staff, and are limited in utilizing the available services for themselves, family progress appears to be very slow. Patient but firm and consistent efforts to connect with a family at their pace often leads to gains. Families often must be carefully taught to take small steps and to recognize their successes. Sometimes recognizing the impact of services on their children builds successes for parents, prevents abuse and neglect, and empowers parents to move ahead in addressing their issues.

Lessons Learned about Staff Needs

Staff Safety

The safety of family support staff must be explicitly addressed when the risk is high for child abuse and neglect. Factors to be assessed are (1) potential danger to staff, including family history of violence, threats, and other responses to stress, (2) degree of physical isolation of the family's home, (3) accessibility of assistance from others, and (4) staff members' knowledge and understanding of how to effectively use risk management procedures. The resulting conclusion of potential harm requires action to assure staff safety. Possible options include provision of services in an alternate and safe environment, pairing of staff for visits with the family, and, in cases of high risk, a temporary end to services until resolution of the crisis.

External Training and Consultation

Family support staff members need periodic consultation and training from community practitioners experienced with child abuse. Training provided by qualified child abuse and neglect professionals assists staff members in understanding the roles and perspectives of staff members of other agencies. It helps build a more sophisticated knowledge base to guide observations and interpretations of family dynamics and experience. It also contributes toward more refined decision making about the need for prevention, reporting, intervention, and helping the family through human service, legal, and other community systems.

Internal Training and Supervision

Family support staff members also need training from their own supervisors. Ongoing training from trusted and respected supervisory staff is essential to assisting with strategies for working with families' reactions, methods of rebuilding trust, ensuring one's own safety, and coping with such professional and personal dilemmas as setting boundaries, issues that so often arise in complex and multineed family situations (Walker, Harris, & Koocher, 1989).

Group Support

Family support staff derive benefits from group supervision and a professional support group. Group supervision meetings provide the opportunity for problem solving, peer support, and coming to grips with dilemmas. For example, the concept of empowering parents is a critical part of the CFP philosophy and one the direct service staff works very hard to implement. They are, however, acutely cognizant that abusing and neglectful parents have demonstrated decision making that is harmful to children and thus clearly at odds with society's expectations. Child abuse and neglect laws which define professionals' roles are designed to control inappropriate behavior and protect children. These laws also serve to disempower individuals. Another kind of dilemma experienced by staff occurs when the action deemed by another agency to be in the best interest of the child is in direct conflict with the philosophy of a comprehensive family support program that works to maximize the strength of the entire family unit. Group discussions help staff members to clarify the realities of such dilemmas and to generate ideas about intervention strategies aimed at meeting family and program goals.

A support group led by a qualified group leader outside the program staff provides a confidential environment in which direct family service staff can process professional issues and dilemmas including those associated with child abuse and neglect. For example, staff members bring their personal experiences, values, and beliefs about child abuse and neglect to their employment setting. The support group provides an arena in which commonly experienced conflicts between personal perspective and the complex realities of working with families can be articulated, clarified, and resolved.

Lessons Learned about Interagency Collaboration

Guidelines for Mutual Collaboration

Families at risk for child abuse and neglect are best served when guidelines for mutual consultation and collaboration with staff from other agencies are developed and used. One positive outcome of inviting staff members of the children's protective agencies to provide training about abuse and neglect was the development of an agreement for mutual consultation and collaboration. The agreement acknowledges the unique roles and expertise of each agency and the services provided by its staff. CFP staff may request consultation at any time, either by telephone or in a joint staffing, about the advisability of filing a report, the steps of and a probable time frame for an investigation, and the final disposition. Outcomes of the collaboration have included a better consensus about indications for filing reports, better information about specific investigations (which allows better planning for supporting families), better implementation of more cohesive family service plans, and more productive joint staffings with families resulting in better resolutions for the family unit.

Written Interagency Agreements

Written interagency agreements provide for consistency of processes across all involved staff. Formal agreements define roles and responsibilities of each agency, guide the collaborative working relationship when a family receives services from both, and provides policy to guide decisions in the case of conflict (see a sample of interagency agreement in the Appendix).

Lessons Learned about Administrative Support

Written Risk Management Policies and Procedures

Clearly defined risk management policies and procedures, including those related to child abuse and neglect, must be available to provide clear and accurate guidance for program staff. Consultation with appropriate legal experts helps to ensure consistency with state child abuse and neglect laws. One caveat, however, is that specific guidance provided by legal experts may depend on the agency with which they are affiliated. For example, the opinion of an attorney from the department of human services may vary substantially from that of the attorney representing a professional mental health organization. Another caveat is that although interagency collaboration during the reporting and investigation process has been stressed as productive for families and staff, administrative policies, procedure, and practices must clearly support an individual staff member's legal right and perceived professional responsibility to independently file a report of suspected child abuse and/or neglect. Kalichman (1993) has reported the development of a Report Decision Making Model which the reader is encouraged to review if interested in this topic. It is also an administrative responsibility to ensure that staff is trained, supervised, and supported in carrying out program risk management policies and procedures, including those of ensuring personal safety.

Active Administrative Support

Active administrative support is essential for the empowerment of staff to function effectively in meeting the complex challenges of working with families in which child abuse and neglect is at issue. Support includes ensuring adequate budget, procedures, and legitimization for the intensity of effort and comprehensive services required by families; support also, includes ensuring staff training, outside leadership for staff support groups to deal with professional and emotional issues, ongoing supervision, needed consultation with outside experts, and ongoing joint collaboration with other agency staff.

APPENDIX

Interagency Cooperative Agreement
Community–Family Partnership
Center for Persons with Disabilities
Utah State University, Logan, UT 84322-6800

This is an agreement made on _____, between the Community–Family Partnership (CFP) and Department of Human Services, Division of Family Services (DFS), hereafter referred to as the Cooperating Agency.

General Information
A. The term of this agreement shall be one year. The agreement may be terminated by either party at any time in advance of expiration upon 30 days written notice.
B. The agreement is automatically renewable upon subsequent renewals of CFP federal funding.
C. This agreement specifically applies to the cooperative working relationship between CFP staff and DFS staff in those instances when children of CFP families are placed in foster care under the care and supervision of DFS staff.

Scope of Services:
Community–Family Partnership
CFP provides services aimed at enhancing child, parent, and family development and ameliorating the impact of poverty. Among the CFP services available to children are home-based child development, CFP preschool for 3 year old children, and periodic assessment and referral for appropriate medical and developmental services. Additionally, training in parenting and skills necessary to support parenting is available.

1. Upon notification of placement of a CFP child(ren) into foster care, CFP staff shall obtain written consent from the biological parents to exchange information with DFS and provide a copy of the release to DFS.

2. With parental consent, CFP will provide information such as developmental status, health history, and child functioning in the home and school environments to DFS to assist in the transition of the child(ren) to the foster home, to assist in completion of DFS records, and to assist in the care and supervision of the children while in DFS custody.

3. Upon placement into foster care, CFP staff shall mail information to the foster parents describing the CFP program and services available to children in foster care.

4. Within two weeks of foster placement, a meeting with the foster parent(s), DFS case worker, CFP family consultant, and guardian ad litem is scheduled by CFP staff. During the meeting, CFP services that have been provided for the child(ren) in the past are reviewed and CFP services available to the child(ren) while in foster care are presented. The participants are encouraged to make recommendations regarding continued participation in CFP and level of service recommended. It is expected that the level and frequency of participation of CFP child(ren) in ongoing CFP services will be individualized to meet both the needs of the child(ren) and the needs of the foster family.

5. If the foster parent(s) agree with continued participation of the foster child(ren) in CFP, the following CFP documents are signed by the participants: "Foster Family Service Agreement" and "Permission to Serve a Minor Child In Foster Care".

6. CFP staff will work cooperatively with DFS to facilitate implementation of the DFS Treatment Plan for the biological parents. Any areas of the treatment plan for which CFP shall have primary responsibility shall be negotiated during an interagency staffing.

7. Although routine interactions and communication regarding the child's participation in CFP occurs between the foster parent(s) and family consultant, the DFS case worker must give consent for evaluations conducted by CFP. Copies of results of any assessments or evaluations conducted while CFP children are in foster care will be provided to DFS as well as to the biological parents. Any other permission forms or consents needed for the child(ren) for CFP participation will be forwarded to the caseworker for signature. The DFS case worker will be invited to participate in any staffings or conferences, such as parent–teacher conferences, regarding the child(ren). Any concerns or observations about the child or the child's adjustment or development while in foster care, will be directed to the DFS case worker.

8. CFP staff will meet with DFS staff, upon request, to coordinate service plans and service delivery.

Division of Family Services

The Division of Family Services is charged by the State of Utah and the judicial system with responsibility for care and treatment of the children placed in foster care. In this role, DFS assumes most of the role of parent for the children in their care. In this role, DFS makes decisions about the placement, care, and treatment of the children in their custody.

1. (Optional) Upon placement of a CFP child(ren) into foster care, and *with permission* of the foster parent(s) DFS staff will notify CFP of the placement and provide CFP staff with the name and address of the foster parent.

2. DFS staff will inform the foster parents that a interagency meeting will be scheduled within two weeks following placement to discuss ongoing participation of the child(ren) in CFP. DFS staff will encourage foster parent(s) participation in this meeting.

3. Prior to the interagency meeting to discuss the ongoing participation of the child(ren) in CFP, DFS staff shall discuss with the biological parents their wishes for ongoing participation of their child in CFP. The parents wishes about participation in CFP shall be presented during the interagency staffing when continued participation in CFP is discussed. DFS staff shall be supportive of continued participation of the child(ren) in CFP, *especially* in those cases where the focus is to return the child to their biological parents.

4. DFS staff will meet with CFP staff upon request to coordinate service plans and service delivery. The listed services shall be provided in a timely, efficient, and expeditious manner, to the extent possible. A cooperative and coordinated approach within the boundaries of this services agreement will increase the effectiveness of services to children jointly served by DFS and CFP.

5. Regardless of the foster parents decision to participate in CFP, DFS will facilitate completion of a yearly developmental assessment by CFP staff. This assessment is generally scheduled in the month following the child's birthday. DFS will also facilitate the yearly assessment of the child by the CFP third party evaluator. This evaluation is usually scheduled in the month of the child's birthday.

Other

A. The CFP reporting requirements include providing information to the CFP project regarding frequency of utilization and description of services utilized by CFP children in foster care. This information will be provided, upon request, in a manner consistent with rules and regulations governing confidentiality and privacy.

B. Individuals representing the cooperating agencies shall demonstrate the skills and/or qualifications necessary to meet the scope of services outlined in Section A. All cooperating personnel shall be licensed or credentialed to perform the duties expected by their appropriate regulatory or licensing board.

C. Compensation: Not applicable.

D. CFP and the cooperating agency will designate an individual to be the primary contact person for management of this contract.

Contact Person for CFP: _____

Contact Person for Cooperating Agency: _____

_____   _____
        Director   Director
   Cooperating Agency   Community–Family Partnership

_____   _____
          Date   Date

ACKNOWLEDGMENT AND NOTE

The program discussed in this chapter was funded by grant number 90-cc0039 from the Administration for Children and Families in the Department of Health and Human Services. The views expressed are those of the authors and should not be construed as official or as the views of the funding agency.

REFERENCES

American Psychological Association. (1992). *The ethical principles of psychologists and code of conduct.* Washington, DC: Author.

Besharov, D. J. (1990). *Recognizing child abuse: A guide for the concerned.* New York: Free Press.

Brigance, A. H. (1991). *Revised Brigance diagnostic inventory of early development.* North Billerica, MA: Curriculum Associates.

Brosig, C. L., & Kalichman, S. C. (1992). Child abuse reporting decisions: Effects of statutory working of reporting requirements. *Professional Psychology: Research and Practice, 23,* 486–492.

Clark, L. (1985). *SOS! Help for Parents.* Bowling Green, KY: Parents Press.

Derogatis, L. R. (1994). *SCL-90-R symptom checklist-90-R: Administration, scoring, and procedure manual.* Minneapolis, MN: National Computer Systems.

Gaudin, J. M. (1993). *Child neglect: A guide for intervention.* Washington DC: National Center on Child Abuse, U.S. Department of Health and Human Services.

Kalichman, S. C. (1993). *Mandated reporting of suspected child abuse.* Washington, DC: American Psychological Association.

Konrad, E. (1996). A historical perspective and framework for evaluation of integrated service systems. In J. M. Marquart & E. Konrad (Eds.), *New directions for program evaluation: Evaluation of integrated service systems* (pp. 1–15). San Francisco: Jossey-Bass.

Love, A. J. (1983). The organizational context and the development of internal evaluation. In A. J. Love (Ed.), *Developing effective internal evaluation: New directions for program evaluation,* no. 20 (pp. 1–23). San Francisco: Jossey-Bass.

National Committee to Prevent Child Abuse, Utah Chapter. (1995). Telephone conversation. Salt Lake City, UT: Author.

Parks, S. (1991). *HELP . . . at home: Activity sheets for parents.* Palo Alto, CA: Vort.

Peterson, M. S., & Urquiza, A. J. (1993). *The role of mental health professionals in the prevention and treatment of child abuse and neglect.* McLean, VA: The Circle.

Smith, A. N., & Lopez, M. (1994). *A comprehensive child development program: A national family support program.* Interim report to Congress. Washington, DC: U.S. Department of Health and Human Services.

Striefel, S. (1991, March). Empowerment and Success. *CFP News, 2,* 1–2.

Tower, C. C. (1992). *The role of educators in the prevention and treatment of child abuse and neglect.* Washington, DC: National Center on Child Abuse, U.S. Department of Health and Human Services.

Utah Children. (1996). *Child well-being in Utah, 1996.* Salt Lake City, UT: Author.

Utah Department of Health. (1987). *Utah vital statistics: Annual report* (Technical Report #119). Salt Lake City, UT: Author.

Walker, C. E., Alpert, J., Harris, E., & Koocher, G. (1989). State licensing boards consider requiring child abuse knowledge base for purpose of licensure and relicensure. In *Report to the APA board of directors from the ad hoc Committee on Child Abuse Policy.* Washington, DC: American Psychological Association.

Wingspread Conference. (1993). *Going to scale with a comprehensive services strategy* (Summary Notes). New York: National Center for Services Integration, Columbia University.

12

Holistic Injury Prevention

LIZETTE PETERSON and SARA GABLE

Some readers will immediately recognize the relevance of a chapter on childhood injury prevention to the field of child abuse and neglect, whereas others will be surprised at its inclusion in such a book. One of the goals of this chapter, therefore, is to make all interested readers aware of the important connections between these two fields, and to convince researchers that each area has much to contribute to the other. The leading killer of children in this nation is trauma. Children experience physical trauma in a variety of ways, most of which are related to how our nation, states, communities, and families protect children and to what we believe about protecting children. This chapter argues that because of common etiological factors, difficulty in actively distinguishing among types of trauma, and similarity in effective interventions, efforts to unite these research endeavors can strengthen both areas and serve to more adequately protect children in the future from injury, the foremost threat to their health and welfare.

TWO TRADITIONAL AREAS OF RESEARCH

Unintentional Injury

Traumatic injury necessitates emergency treatment for 16 million children each year, of whom 600,000 require extended hospital care and at least 30,000 will experience permanent disability. Injuries kill more children than cancer, AIDS, heart disease, chronic illnesses, and acute illnesses combined (Dershewitz & Williamson, 1977). Childhood injury research has received far less scientific attention and funding than the other major threats to children's health, although with increased efforts and heightened public awareness, this trend may be shifting (Scheidt & Workshop Participants, 1988).

LIZETTE PETERSON • Department of Psychology, University of Missouri at Columbia, Columbia, Missouri 65211.   SARA GABLE • Human Development and Family Studies Extension, University of Missouri at Columbia, Columbia, Missouri 65211.

Handbook of Child Abuse Research and Treatment, edited by Lutzker. Plenum Press, New York, 1998.

There are a variety of reasons for the shortage of research on children's injuries. First, injury has been recognized as a significant source of threat to children and adults only since the 1940s (De Haven, 1942), and sound conceptual models of injury were not presented until the 1970s (Haddon, 1970, 1972). Before that time, injuries were regarded as a product of fate rather than the subject of scientific inquiry. Most laypersons and some scientists continue to think of "accidental injury" as if some number of bad things will fortuitously happen to children and there is little anyone can do to prevent their occurrence. Even among those who recognize scientific laws operating in the etiology of inadvertent injury, there has been a tendency to limit research to only part of the spectrum of causes for injury.

One area of early success was environmental modification to reduce child injury. Cribs that strangled infants because the bars allowed their heads to pass through and become trapped were banned from production (Consumer Product Safety Commission, 1979), as were refrigerators whose doors locked children inside their airless chambers (Robertson, 1983). Mandatory use of flame retardants in clothing, particularly in children's pajamas, resulted in decreases in the number of nonhousefire burns in children (Smith & Falk, 1987). Similarly, poisonings were reduced by limiting the dosage in any one bottle and by child-resistant packaging (Walton, 1982). Thus, public health approaches dominated the area of unintentional injury for decades and demonstrated an impressive number of successful interventions. Despite such effective endeavors, however, injuries to children in our country have not decreased concurrently with other causes of childhood mortality and morbidity (Baker, O'Neill, Ginsburg, & Li, 1992), and injuries remain considerably higher in the United States than in many other industrialized countries (Fingerhut & Kleinman, 1989).

One possible reason for continued high rates of injury and for the continued lower than desirable rate of research in this area has been resistance to focusing on the more behavioral aspects of injury. Injuries occur when the child and the environment collide in a violent or dangerous fashion. Altering the environment to entirely avoid injuries (as in putting a barrier on the stairs to avoid child falls) or to limit the extent of damage (as in using shock-absorbing materials under children's play equipment) are both sensible strategies. However, the other part of the childhood injury phenomenon includes the child's behavior, which is influenced both by inherent child characteristics and by the responsiveness of the child's caregiver. There has been strong resistance to focusing injury prevention interventions on children, as if to do so is to blame the victim (Pless, 1978). In addition, public health approaches that target the caregiver have typically involved broad educational interventions that result in increased knowledge, but fail to yield increased injury prevention efforts (e.g., Colver, Hutchinson, & Judson, 1982). As will be discussed later in this chapter when interventions are considered, there has been a recent shift in research strategies within the area to include more ecologically valid behavioral interventions. These interventions focus both on children and on their caregivers, in the context of their daily environment, and thus allow for a more holistic "ecobehavioral" approach (Lutzker & Rice, 1984) toward injury reduction, an approach which considers both environmental and behavioral bases of injury.

It may be ironic that the injury reduction area has avoided an individualized approach to the caregiver, whereas the area of abuse and neglect has historically adopted an individual psychopathology approach to intervention to the exclusion of other viewpoints (e.g., Helfer, 1977). Similar to the area of injury research just sur-

veyed, however, one of the important movements in research on child abuse and neglect has involved contextualizing problematic parent–child interactions and recognizing that interventions will be more effective if they are broadened to include
environmental determinants (Garbarino, 1988). In this fashion, although the clinical
and research traditions of these two research areas overlap minimally, the areas are
moving together toward a common goal in terms of the growing recognition in both
areas of the importance of a more holistic approach, as is seen in the next section.

Child Abuse and Neglect

Similar to the epidemiological reports of unintentional injury, research on
child abuse and neglect documents that large numbers of children are involved.
Each year, more than a million cases of child abuse and neglect are substantiated
and at least 150,000 children are seriously injured by caregiver abuse and neglect
(National Center on Child Abuse and Neglect, 1993). Of these, 18,000 children are
permanently disabled (Baladerian, 1991). The 2,000 infants and children who
make up estimates of fatal abuse and neglect (MacKeller & Yanagishita, 1995) most
likely represent only a small portion of caregiver-related fatalities. Childhood injuries from abuse have occurred throughout recorded history, but were not recognized as a problem requiring intervention and investigation until the 1940s
(Caffey, 1946). Moreover, it was not until the 1960s that "the battered child syndrome" was officially labeled a focus for research (Kempe, Silverman, Steele,
Droegemueller, & Silver, 1962). Again, parallel to the injury field, early research
focused either on describing the syndrome (e.g., Schmitt & Kempe, 1974) or suggesting untested interventions. In stark contrast to the environmental approach
taken by public health to injury reduction, however, early interventions to curb
child abuse and neglect focused on a psychiatric model which viewed abuse as a
result of parental immaturity and psychopathology (Cohen, Raphling, & Green,
1966). These early interventions did not show evidence that such treatment was
effective in reducing neglect or abuse, and currently individual psychotherapy is
regarded as offering limited success to maltreating families (Daro, 1988).

Research with abusive parents, however, has revealed that certain life situations experienced by parents tend to pose risks for abuse. Limited emotional and
material resources were frequently seen in maltreating families (Gelles, 1973).
From knowledge of such setting conditions, a more ecological approach evolved
which suggested the need to consider parenting behaviors in the context of the
skills and abilities of the parent, as well as the stresses and supports of the community in which the parent resided (e.g., Garbarino, 1977, 1982). This shift, in
turn, resulted in the current ecobehavioral approach to the problem of child abuse
and neglect, which nicely parallels the advances in the injury prevention area.

TWO DISTINCT AREAS?

The label "unintentional injury" is preferred by scientists as a replacement for
"accidental injury" because accidents are largely viewed as unfortunate products of
fate, unpredictable and unpreventable. There is another connotation of the concept
of "accident," however. "Accident" suggests that the injury was not inflicted and
was not anyone's fault. The concepts of deliberate injury and of blameworthiness

are implicit in the boundaries currently maintained by both the unintentional injury area and the area of abuse and neglect.

One significant yet frequently unasked question is the extent to which intended and unintended injuries can be accurately classified by legal and medical authorities. The research community has assumed that each of these areas has its own conceptual integrity and that each area can be readily discriminable from the other area. However, these assumptions are not based on evidence that unintentional injuries can be reliably differentiated from injuries resulting from caregiver abuse and neglect. In fact, some evidence that exists suggests that a sizable proportion of injuries currently classified as unintentional injuries are actually the product of child maltreatment. Ewigman, Kivlahan, and Land (1993) and others (e.g., National Research Council, 1993) recently examined medical examiner reports, fire investigation reports, and Division of Family Service ratings and found compelling evidence that child maltreatment fatalities are often miscategorized as unintentional injury. In Ewigman and colleagues' study, for example, a third of the cases classified in the state records as unintentional injury were designated by "blind" raters as definite maltreatment and another third were classified as possible maltreatment. Only 11% were clearly cases of unintentional injury in which the caregiver played no significant role. Such data provided the impetus for forming child death review teams nationwide, to investigate the etiology of child deaths. Current data suggest that such investigations may destroy our illusion of the fine boundaries between injury that is not deliberately inflicted and that is not neglectful (truly unintentional childhood injury) and child abuse and neglect. It seems time to consider whether it is most accurate to view the inflicted/intentional versus noninflicted/nonintentional distinction as a dichotomy or whether these categories are better conceptually represented by a continuum. Similarly, the extent to which caregivers should be considered blameworthy or blameless, because of their inaction or failure to protect the child, may be more effectively considered as a matter of degree rather than an absolute. The next two sections discuss the "inflicted" and "failure to protect" dimensions of childhood injury.

Inflicted Injury as a Continuum

A parent impatiently motions for the child to come across the street and is then horrified as the child dashes in front of an oncoming car (a not uncommon etiology for child pedestrian injury; Christoffel, 1986). The injury is clearly unintended, yet it is caused by the action of the parent. Another parent playfully tickles the child, who jerks backward quickly, crashing his chair through a window—parental action resulting even more directly in injury. A 2-year-old pulls the hair of his 8-month-old sibling and the parent swats his bottom, unintentionally knocking him into the edge of the table, splitting open his scalp. Does this cross the line into inflicted injury, because the parent struck the child? Recall that more than 90% of parents accept and practice this form of discipline (Wauchope & Straus, 1990). Does the unfortunate presence of the table and the child's poor balance automatically shift this from an unintentional into an inflicted injury?

What of the parent who, frustrated with the infant's crying, shakes or throws the baby onto a soft mattress, causing permanent brain damage or death, without any knowledge that such actions could cause harm? What of the parent who tries to stop a toddler from biting by inserting red pepper into the mouth, only to have the child aspirate the pepper and die? Or the parent who, frustrated with toileting accidents, draws a hot bath and scalds her child, without knowing that a young child's skin will burn in water that an adult's hand will easily tolerate? All of these adult actions result in child injury that is unintended, yet all are caused by parental action and most are inflicted, in the sense that the parent aggressively handled the child. Graziano (1994) persuasively pointed out that there are extremely varying criteria among parents concerning what qualifies as acceptable punishment. Even if our society can agree on the inflicted versus not inflicted distinction, the extent to which the discipline is likely to be viewed as unacceptable will vary greatly both among parents and among child oriented professionals. It thus seems unlikely that there is strong consensus either within the community or within the arenas of clinical practice and research concerning what constitutes uninflicted versus inflicted injury. Rather, factors such as knowledge, intended outcome, and predictability of actual outcome, all influence the point on the continuum of action at which a given injury might be placed.

Neglect as a Continuum

If abusive or inflicted injuries are evaluated on some continuum representing intentional parent action, it also makes sense to evaluate injuries resulting from neglect on a continuum, a continuum of inaction. Parents assume a number of fundamental responsibilities when raising a child. Beyond guaranteeing economic success and fostering social skills, morality, and intellectual achievement, insuring the child's physical survival is the paramount assignment for parents (LeVine, 1974). Protecting the child from hazards in the environment requires both environmental changes and active supervision by parents. Although only a small number of studies have examined naturalistic injury prevention styles in parents, it appears that once children are mobile, parents intervene more often to keep the child from playing with potentially dangerous objects (or to keep objects safe from the child) than for any other purpose (Gralinski & Kopp, 1993). Some studies suggest that parents of toddlers perform such interventions more than 5 times per hour in a typical day (Power & Chapieski, 1986).

Such active supervision is extraordinarily labor intensive. Many factors influence how much supervision is necessary to insure child safety in a given situation. In addition to characteristics of the individual child, the danger in the immediate situation (a busy street, a hot pot of coffee) as it interacts with the developmental level of the child (a 6-month-old versus a 6-year-old in the bathtub) form some of the relevant parameters.

To intervene preventively, the parent must be physically present and relatively vigilant. Regarding supervision as a dichotomy (acceptable versus neglectful) rather than a continuum, implies a high degree of agreement on what level of supervision is required in given situations with children of various ages. Research and legal standards that describe child maltreatment often suggest that care that fails to meet "community standards" constitutes maltreatment (Christoffel et al., 1992). However, such community standards are not available in any existing literature, and research examining the judgments of community mothers, division of family service workers, and physicians suggests that there is a striking lack of consensus across groups of raters, situations varying by environmental risk, and a range of child ages (Peterson, Ewigman, & Kivlahan, 1993). In many cases, Peterson and colleagues (1993) found that the standard deviation for minutes that respondents judged children at various ages could safely be left alone was larger than the means. Said simply, there appears to be little agreement among laypersons or experts as to what constitutes adequate supervision. Given these data, and considering the problem logically, we think that the continuum of caregiver inaction is a compelling way to conceptualize one of the major process variables for children's injury.

In addition to our documented inability as a science to differentiate abuse and neglect from unintentional injury, there are other epidemiological and etiological characteristics which unite these two research areas. A review of the determinants and consequences of unintentional injury and of child abuse and neglect will thus be considered in the next section.

EPIDEMIOLOGY AND PATTERNS OF INJURY

Risk Factors

Peterson and Brown (1994) posited a working model to understand factors that are linked to injury risk for children. This model separated environmental factors, caregiver-based variables, and child-based variables for risk. At the broadest level, low-income status is the environmental factor most strongly associated with both unintentional injury (Nersesian, Petit, Shaper, Lemieux, & Naor, 1985) and abuse and neglect (Pelton, 1977). Even within a low-income background, children from families reporting high family chaos and confusion are more likely to experience injuries listed as unintentional (Matheny, 1993) or related to abuse and neglect (Straus, Gelles, & Steinmetz, 1980) than are children whose families experience less chaos and more predictability and organization.

Frequent residential relocation is associated with both unintentional injuries (Beautrais, Fergusson, & Shannon, 1982) and with abusive and neglectful parenting (Altemeier, O'Connor, Vietze, Sandler, & Sherrod, 1984). Similarly, crowding, both within households and in neighborhoods, has been linked to unintentional injury (Rivara & Barber, 1985) and to maltreatment (Gray, Cutler, Dean, & Kempe, 1977). Chaos, moving, and overcrowding are all salient sources of environmental stress, likely to be related both to the presence of an unusual number of hazards and to disruptions in caregiving and increases in children's risk-taking behaviors. Additional stressors in the form of negative life events are often related to injuries such as unintentional poisoning (Beautrais et al., 1982) and burns, fractures, and even motor vehicle crashes (Beautrais, Fergusson, & Shannon, 1981). Similarly, loss of a key relationship, illness, or increased child-care responsibilities have been shown to result in increased abusive discipline (Green, Gaines, & Sandgrund, 1974). One potential mechanism for these effects is an absence of social support, which logically is related to both unintentional injury (Pearn & Nixon, 1977) and child abuse and neglect (Giovannoni & Billingsley, 1970).

These environmental factors may have more extensive impact on some mothers than on others. In addition, some specific maternal factors have been linked to abuse (note that the literature has focused on maternal over paternal factors; more research is needed in this area). Younger mothers have children at higher risk for injury, both unintentional (McCormick, Shapiro, & Starfield, 1981) and maltreatment related (Lynch, 1975). Single mothers' children are injured unintentionally more often (Rivara & Barber, 1985) as well as because of abuse and neglect (American Association for Protecting Children, 1988). Finally, mothers who abuse substances (unintentional injury, Bijur, Kurzon, Overpeck, & Scheidt, 1992; maltreatment, Berkeley Planning Associates, 1983) or who are depressed (unintentional injury, Brown & Davidson, 1978; maltreatment, Garbarino, Kostelny, & Dubrow, 1991) have children at high risk for injury.

Children themselves often show characteristics that appear to be related to higher potential for injury. In general, externalizing behavior problems seem potentially risky. Having irregular eating and sleeping habits is associated with both unintentional (Matheny, 1987) and abusive (Herrenkohl & Herrenkohl, 1979) injuries. Being distractible is similarly linked to a variety of unintentional injuries (Zuckerman & Duby, 1985), as well as to abuse (Egeland, Sroufe, & Erickson, 1983). Children with higher activity levels experience more frequent serious unintentional injuries (Hartsough & Lambert, 1985) and experience more abusive discipline (Daro, 1988). Disruptive behavior also appears to increase contact with both hazards that produce injuries (Cataldo et al., 1992) and with abusive discipline (Lorber, Felton, & Reid, 1984). Although research in both areas has found a strong negative reaction to any study that appears to blame the child-victims for their own injuries, recognizing the variables that place children at greater risk is important in planning interventions to protect these children.

In summary, the great majority of etiological factors of child maltreatment, whether they are characteristics of the environment, the parent, or the child, are also found to predict unintentional injury. The child maltreatment literature is drawn from a very different tradition than is the literature on unintentional injury. Thus, the commonality in precursors to both kinds of injury is particularly compelling. It also may be useful to consider how both areas of injury may be influenced by the consequences of the event.

Consequences

Although the bulk of the epidemiological literature on children's injury has focused on describing the antecedents to children's injuries, it seems sensible to consider briefly the consequences of children's injury as well. One of the most potent myths in both areas is that identification of a case of injury somehow removes or reduces the risk for the child. The aphorism in the unintentional injury literature is "once burned, twice shy." In point of fact, there is no literature to suggest that this is the case. Moreover, although serious injury is a relatively low base rate event, certain at-risk children have repeated injuries (e.g., Hartsough & Lambert, 1985); such data should be compelling evidence that one injury will *not* prevent another. At-risk children clearly remain at risk following an injury. Cataldo and associates (1992), for example, definitively established that previously injured children had *higher*, not lower, rates of hazard contact in a simulated injury situation. Similarly, Daro (1988) noted that families employing abusive discipline tend to continue to escalate that strategy, even after reports of abuse to authorities. In a review of 89 demonstration projects, Cohn and Daro (1987) reported that more than a third of the families continued to abuse or neglect their children during the treatment and more than half were believed to maltreat their children following treatment. In essence, injury predicts future injury, not later safety.

Similarly, parents appear not to realize that the experience of an injury connotes an at-risk situation. Although little empirical work has been done, one naturalistic observation study suggested that parents tended not to use children's injury experiences as an occasion for teaching to avoid further injuries in children. Specifically, 80% of the time, parents followed a minor injury of their 8-year-old child with no consequence whatsoever; 14% of the time, they gave a lecture (note that children reported hearing lectures only about 3% of the time, suggesting that these communications were not even registered by the children as interventions); and parents changed rules or delivered consequences less than 3% of the time (Peterson, Bartelstone, Kern, & Gillies, 1995). Parents apparently believed the physical consequences of the injury would result in the child not repeating the injury risk behavior. Similarly, abusive parents often proceed as if they believe their harsh discipline will halt the objectionable behavior and the need for further abuse, although it seems to have just the opposite effect on a child (Reid, Taplin, & Lorber, 1981). In other words, these parental suppositions regarding the effects of injury and of parents' behavior on children's learning appear to be dangerously false.

Bimodal Patterns of Injury

Some injuries are predictable because they involve steadily escalating risky behavior. For example, consider children who are reported by witnesses to repeatedly enter busy streets, and thus being struck by a car seems predictable (K. K. Christoffel personal communication, July 15, 1992), or children whose caregiver begins with spanking and then inflicts soft-tissue injuries, and then fractures, and ultimately even more serious injuries (O'Neill, Meacham, Griffin, & Sawyers, 1973). In contrast, other injuries occur in situations that the parent and child have never encountered before. The classic unintentional child drowning occurs when the caregiver goes to answer the telephone for "just a minute," and the child slips in the bathtub or gets out the back door where the pool or hot tub is located. Similarly, inflicted injury sometimes happens when a normally nonaggressive caregiver responds violently. A caregiver throws, strikes, or shakes a small child, not recognizing his or her own strength or the child's physical vulnerability. Although both situations result in an injury that is completely predictable after the fact, prospectively guarding against such injuries is especially challenging.

This and the previous section have documented underlying conceptual similarities for unintentional and for maltreatment injuries. These arguments suggest that our current conceptualization of injury serves as a barrier to more effective research and to interventions that could prevent injuries that are inflicted versus unintentional, or neglectful versus not. Our inability as a science to differentiate these forms of injury, their logical continuity, their similar environmental, parental, and child-based risk factors, and the same bimodal patterns of occurrence argue for a more unified approach. In addition to the political, conceptual, and methodological barriers that may be present to block such unification, there are other significant and recurrent societal barriers to injury prevention that deserve consideration.

SOCIETAL IMPEDIMENTS

This chapter began with concern about the rates of injury in the United States in recent years in comparison with other industrialized countries (Fingerhut & Kleinman, 1989). Countries reporting greater success in reducing all kinds of children's injury have been able to unite nationwide, community level, and individual family approaches to injury prevention (see Bergman & Rivara, 1991, for example, for a description of Sweden's successful response to the threat of childhood injury). In contrast, concerns in our nation about individual rights, as well as a lack of clarity in our mandate to protect children, leave our children more vulnerable to injury.

Safety Legislation

Berger (1981) described the "serious misconception" held by many Americans that the federal government is proactive in removing potentially hazardous products from the marketplace. Although there has been a small amount of successful legislation (discussed earlier in this chapter) to prevent child strangulation, asphyxiation, burns, and poisonings, such legislation has tended to be the exception, rather than the rule (Peterson & Roberts, 1992). For example, Rivara (1982) describes the illogical reasoning underlying the continuing marketplace support for children's minibikes, "toys" that travel up to 50 miles per hour. One reason cited for failing to approve legislation halting the manufacture of such vehicles was that there is no proof that faster speeds result in more severe injuries!

Berger (1981) cited similar hesitancy in legislation to block the manufacture of toys that pose serious threats of blindness due to the small projectiles that they fire. Current legislation requires that such toys display only a small warning label on the flaps of the boxes noting that eye damage could result. Fireworks-related injuries in some states have decreased when local ordinances were passed banning them and have risen again as the ordinances were repealed (Smith & Falk, 1987).

Consider the large plastic bags that continue to surround our drycleaning and to asphyxiate children. Many low-income families use them to cover babies' crib mattresses (Baker & Fisher, 1980). Rather than outlawing this asphyxiation hazard, our legislators have offered a printed warning on each cover, announcing that this container can produce a fatal injury for a baby or a toddler. Implicit in this announcement is the awareness that our society recognizes this danger but views convenience for drycleaners and consumers as more significant. Finally, some researchers estimate that as many as 42% of medically attended injuries to children under one year of age may be due to "baby walkers" (O'Shea, 1986), which continue to be manufactured despite their lack of developmental advantage and their danger to children. These are only a few examples in which our government has chosen free enterprise over the health and safety of children.

The U.S. culture has not reached a comfortable balance between protection of children and citizens' individual rights (Garbarino, 1988). Moreover, as will be seen in the next section, our concern for parents' rights to discipline their children, even in potentially harmful ways, continues to overshadow our sense of responsibility for the physical and emotional safety of our children.

Right to Discipline

In our culture, both legal and some religious traditions support the rights of parents, and to some extent teachers and principals, to physically punish children (Graziano & Kunce, 1992). It is ironic that even child abuse legislation has explicitly supported the rights of parents to inflict corporal punishment, by stating that "nothing in the statute should be construed as interfering with the rights of the parents to use physical punishment" (Straus, 1991, p. 140).

Our society finds itself in a steady escalation of violence, which we tend to regard with a blend of horror and jaded desensitization. Although our country advocates for humane treatment of animals, national samples of parents suggest that more than 90% have physically punished their children (Straus et al., 1980; Wauchope & Straus, 1990). Retrospective studies report similarly that more than 90% of college-age participants report having experienced physical discipline when growing up (Bryon & Freed, 1982; Graziano & Namaste, 1990). These parental actions are supported by underlying parental beliefs; a 1988 National Opinion Survey reported that of the parents in the United States surveyed, more than 80% either agreed or strongly agreed that "It is sometimes necessary to discipline a child with a good, hard spanking" (Flynn, 1994). Four out of five young adults believe in the right of parents to spank (Graziano & Namaste, 1990). Further, even those charged with safeguarding children's health believe in spanking; McCormick (1992) reported that 67% of physicians advocated spanking when children refused to go to bed, ran into the street, or struck a playmate.

Even within the child abuse and neglect research community, there are mixed feelings concerning the acceptability of physical punishment with children. Yet there is clear evidence of the link between physical discipline and child abuse (Burns, 1993). Natural histories of spanking practices reveal a patterned shift from spanking to soft-tissue injuries, then to broken bones, and later to other more serious kinds of abuse. These data suggest that abuse is a logical progression from physical discipline to injury (O'Neill et al., 1973). Graziano and Namaste (1990) noted that corporal punishment under certain conditions of pressure, stress, and negative reinforcement of child–parent behavior patterns can escalate to abusive discipline. In essence, any parent who uses physical discipline may, under the right setting conditions, escalate to abuse. A sizable number of reported and unreported cases of physical abuse begin with corporal punishment, according to Hay and Jones (1994).

Because physical discipline appears undeniably linked to physical abuse, parents' rights to use physical discipline could be questioned. In addition, subabusive physical discipline is positively correlated with an extensive number of child behavior problems, including aggression, depression, and eventual substance use and problems with the law (Straus & Gimpel, 1992; Weller, Romney, & Orr, 1987). Even if the child is not actively abused, parental use of physical punishment is clearly not in the child's best interest.

We must also question a society in which unnecessary physical force is outlawed in all human actions between adults, but not between adults and children (Graziano & Namaste, 1990). The United Nations Conventions on the Rights of the Child articulates the rights of children not to live in fear of physically inflicted pain and violence. More than 200 other countries have adopted this policy; the United

States has not. This societal inaction marks another major barrier to the prevention of injuries and the promotion of physical and emotional health in children.

Understanding the conceptual, policy-oriented, legal, and societal barriers to effective injury prevention research may be a first step toward more effective interventions. It seems sensible, as a next step, to examine what these molar impediments to progress may tell us about what types of interventions are needed. Said differently, at the parental level, how do the societal beliefs and attitudes the parents hold, and the parents' own skills and resources, lead to situations that create the risk of child injury? The next section explores examples of setting events that may contribute to the risk of injury and the final section will consider what this means in terms of suggestions for effective prevention.

MODEL OF BEHAVIORAL RISK FACTORS

The epidemiological risk factors described earlier provide insight concerning the families likely to be at greatest risk for both unintentional injury and injury due to neglect and abuse. Yet such data do not identify junctures for effective intervention. It is difficult or impossible to rectify low-income status or to alter mothers' youth or single marital status. Moreover, risk factors such as substance abuse or depression are extremely challenging to treat in isolation and offer little information about the routine, day-to-day parenting difficulties experienced by these mothers (Lief, 1985; Luther & Walsh, 1995).

An important new direction in descriptive research on abuse and neglect risk factors has been a shift toward the examination of the specific behavioral patterns of parent–child interactions that afford the opportunity for active intervention. Figure 1 shows a hierarchical parenting model which can assist in organizing parenting needs suggested by the literature. First, there is a clear need for parenting skills to avoid injury and maltreatment. Underlying the use of skills, however, the parents' awareness (or the lack thereof) of the child's developmental status and abilities influences the degree to which parents can interpret and effectively guide the child's behavior. Similarly, parental beliefs about childrearing and children will likely influence how much energy they invest in activities such as child supervision and how much control they feel the need to exert over their child's misbehavior. Negative emotions such as depression or anger that parents may experience during routine caregiving can create the risk that harsh discipline will escalate to abuse. Similarly, a depressed parent may lack energy to effectively interact with and protect the child. In addition, the view of one's own efficacy influences the effectiveness of child protection. Then, at the most basic level, the parent's willingness to assume the role of the parent (to be responsible for the child's needs and safety) and the role of mother or father (to nurture, love, and enjoy the child) underlies the degree of success at all of the levels of parenting. Finally, at the most basic level, the quality of personal resources and belief in one's own worth and abilities provide the foundation on which successful parenting interventions can be built.

Much of the past literature and many chapters in the current handbook focus on teaching the parenting skills that are needed. Peterson and Brown (1994) described a comprehensive curriculum of such skills. This chapter will focus on the

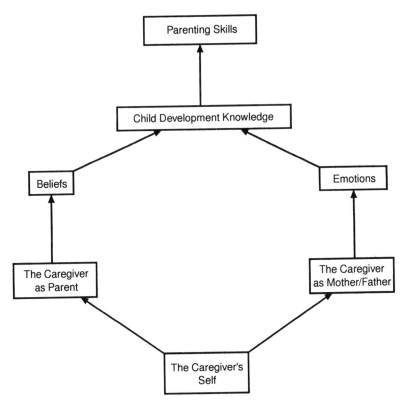

Figure 1. Multilevel conceptual model of parenting.

immediately underlying areas instead—the need to increase developmental awareness, to alter problematic parental beliefs, and to decrease negative emotions. The role of parent and mother/father, and ultimately the personal resources of the self will also be considered briefly as a comprehensive part of a preventive intervention for child maltreatment and injury.

DEVELOPMENTAL UNDERSTANDING RELEVANT TO SUPERVISION

Underestimating Infants' Abilities

Most parents are aware that infants can be seriously injured by falling down stairs or out of windows, poisoned by cleaning substances, solvents, or pesticides, or drowned in bathtubs, cleaning buckets, or ponds. Despite most parents' awareness, such injuries routinely take the lives of children under two years of age in this country. Falls often result when parents do not believe the child has the motor control to crawl to the stairs or climb to the window, poisonings occur when parents do not understand how quickly the child can reach cleaning solutions under the sink or do not believe the child has the fine motor control to open the containers, and drownings occur when parents do not understand that the top-heavy toddler can easily fall into any standing body of water and drown. In general, parents need a more veridical picture of how early and in what ways children can change location and contact hazards, and they need to recognize items within the household that do not pose a hazard to an adult but do to a small child (e.g., water which merely feels very warm to an adult can result in scalding burns to an infant).

Overestimating Preschoolers' Abilities

Ironically, the same parents who are unaware of their baby's ability to move into contact with injury hazards are often the very ones who expect their preschooler to remember complicated household rules, to be able to hold the rule in mind despite salient distractions, and to have "internalized" the rule so that it effectively controls the preschooler's behavior in the absence of an adult caregiver. Parents also often assume that because a child of 3 or 4 has fairly mature receptive and expressive language skills, the child's memory for language-based rules is equally mature. Further, parents expect children to be able to screen out salient, often visual stimuli (e.g., a ball one is chasing across the grass, rolling onto the sidewalk, over the curb, into the road) in favor of the memory of a verbally based rule for behavior (e.g., never run into the street). Such control begins to be consolidated in elementary-school-age children, but is unlikely in preschoolers (Kendall & Wilcox, 1979). Finally, knowing the rule and reciting it and having the rule exert internalized control over one's behavior are two very different things for the preschool-age child. Verbally based teaching only gradually comes to exert behavioral control in the absence of a caregiver (Zettle & Hayes, 1982). Most parents overestimate the ages at which such control is achieved.

Overestimating Elementary School Children's Knowledge of Safety Rules

When parents of elementary-school-age children are asked how they prevent injury in their children, one of their most common responses is that they insure safety by teaching the children rules (Peterson, Farmer, & Kashani, 1990). However, little research has been done to examine the extent to which family safety rules actually may be preventive. The results that do exist are equivocal. In one study, 8-year-old children (the majority of whom spent some time alone at home) and their parents were asked to name their family's safety rules in a set of open-ended questions about kitchen rules, encountering strangers, and dealing with emergencies. Respondents were then asked yes or no questions about the existence of specific rules (Peterson, Mori, & Scissors, 1986). The parent–child dyads showed very little correspondence in their open-ended rules and scarcely better than chance agreement on many of the dichotomous (yes or no for the rule) choices. Yet most of the parents believed the child was well prepared to stay at home alone and that the child knew the family rules. If this single Midwest study is any indication of how well children understand and live by family rules, such rules would not seem to have the strong preventive power parents believe them to have.

In contrast, we recently examined rules in a different way, by counting the number of rules a family said they endorsed from a checklist and then assessing the relationship between naturally occurring minor injuries experienced by the 8-year-old child participants during a 1-year observation period (Peterson & Saldana, 1996). Families reporting a greater number of safety rules had children with fewer injuries.

Whether these results suggest that safety rules themselves may be preventive in some molar fashion or whether there are other explanations (e.g., families with high injury awareness and concern have more rules) remains a question for future research.

Intervention Suggestions

For many years, physicians have utilized anticipatory guidance, a systematic effort to prepare parents for the next step in their toddler's growth (Roberts & Wright, 1982) to point out the emerging possibilities for child injury. However, many at-risk parents never receive such assistance. Thus, increasing parents' awareness of the developing infants' capabilities and the resulting requirements for parenting seems an important first step for intervention. In addition, parents need to be aware that a child's verbal recitation of a rule does not mean that the rule will be remembered accurately at a later date, and that mere words may not be able to exert potent control over a highly motivated response such as chasing a soccer ball into the street or a beach ball into a pool. Having children physically act out various safety scenarios around the house may provide parents with a more accurate appraisal of their child's actual safety knowledge and skill rather than the ability to merely reiterate rules. Observing the child's behavior under conditions requiring mature judgment and impulse control may further inform parents about children's actual competence in potentially risky situations. In general, parents need to increase their supervision and injury prevention instructions for children of all ages. Data exist on how to assist parents to implement these precautions (e.g., see the parental instruction outlines in Peterson, Mori, Selby, & Rosen, 1988), but more research is needed to reveal how best to involve parents in such teaching.

DEVELOPMENTAL UNDERSTANDING
RELEVANT TO DISCIPLINE PRACTICES

There are many commonalties between the mistaken beliefs about children's abilities that increase the risk for unintentional injuries and the erroneous parental beliefs that lead to abusive discipline. Clearly, parents who anticipate that children can remember rules, apply them in the presence of distracting stimuli, and use them to override impulses are going to feel the need to use more physical discipline than are parents who understand that the child is unable to exert such control. In addition, parental expectations that children can manage their own clothing and food needs, and can provide reciprocal emotional support to the parent, sets up a chain of parental frustration, child acting out, harsh parental discipline, and child injury that extends well beyond the issues raised in previous sections. These issues are discussed in detail below; after the difficulties are contemplated, potential interventions are briefly considered.

Overestimating Children's Impulse Control

Parents who attribute the child's rule breaking to intentional misbehavior are more likely to punish harshly than parents who view the child's behavior as representative of his or her developmental level. In addition to unreasonable beliefs concerning children's self-control, the literature also suggests that abusive and neglectful parents have inappropriate expectations for preschool children's ability to reguide their emotions, to amuse themselves if the mother is not well, and to deal effectively with physical self-care, for example, getting up on time and getting dressed (Azar, Robinson, Hekimian, & Twentyman, 1984). Note that these unrealistic expectations do not involve parents' inaccurate knowledge of developmental milestones, as we argued was the case in the section on infants' unintentional injuries. These inaccurate parental beliefs have to do with overestimating the child's ability to integrate cognitive and affective processes, with the subsequent attribution of causality to the child (e.g., she misbehaved on purpose), the assumption of the need for strong discipline (e.g., she needs to learn better and I must hurt her to teach her), and subsequent aggression toward the child (Azar & Rohrbeck, 1986).

Overestimating the Child's Ability to Take Perspective

A second area of unrealistic parental expectations for preschool children concerns the parents' belief that the child can understand and effectively meet the parents' emotional needs. At the simplest level, this implies that the parent believes the child is capable of understanding and responding to one of the parents' physical needs (e.g., the parent is tired, so the child should play quietly for prolonged periods while the parent sleeps). At another level, it suggests that the parent anticipates that the child can empathize with the parent's emotional neediness and effectively comfort the parent. Such expectations include the child giving up his or her own developmental tasks (e.g., school for an older child) in order to provide care for the parent. Thus, the child is put at risk both by the parent's inability to understand the perspective of the child (Newberger & Cook, 1983) and by the parent's belief that the child can engage in perspective taking concerning the parent's instrumental and emotional needs.

Specific Developmental Triggers

The two areas just described, childhood impulse control and children's ability to perspective take, are the most general categories for which at-risk parents lack awareness of developmental status and needs. There are also some very specific developmental behaviors that may serve as triggers for abuse. Toileting errors (wetting or soiling clothing or furnishings) are often found to be the specific trigger for abuse (Daro, 1988). Similarly, having the child tell the parent "no" elicits high levels of frustration in abusive populations (Bauer & Twentyman, 1985). Failing to share when asked, cursing, and lying are also specific child behaviors reported by parents at risk for abuse as particularly anger provoking (Peterson et al., 1993).

Intervention Suggestions

Problems of children's low impulse control, lack of perspective taking, and specific developmental triggers that provoke parental anger should all be the subject of parental education concerning developmental abilities. However, parents' failures to correctly interpret these child behaviors are more likely to elicit abusive and neglectful responding from parents. Rather than simply teaching parents about holding more accurate developmental beliefs, it may be necessary to reprogram several problematic beliefs held by at-risk parents before they can accept more accurate developmental descriptions. Peterson, Gable, Doyle, and Ewigman (in press) offered a table of developmentally problematic behaviors that children engage in, the corresponding parental belief that puts the child at risk, the angry or neglectful cognition that the belief yields, and then a more developmentally appropriate cognition. For example, a parent makes a request and the child responds "no." The parental belief that follows may be "A parent should be able to control the child and should not tolerate disobedience"; the angry cognition is "How dare he defy me, I'll teach him to do what I say"; the developmentally appropriate cognition is "Children at this age often say 'no' as a way of defining themselves as a person, separate from their mother. It is annoying, but it is a normal developmental behavior." Then parents are taught to use distraction, offering choices, basic compliance training to deal with the child's behavior, and anger management to deal with their own responses. It seems important to address the underlying emotions (anger) and cognitions ("How dare he") before trying to teach at-risk parents about the developmental appropriateness of the behavior. However, all of this conjecture requires empirical confirmation in the future.

EXPECTATIONS FOR PARENTING

Parents' beliefs about their children's cognitive and behavioral abilities must underlie their own expectations for what constitutes appropriate parenting. Thus, it may be necessary not only to alter parents' awareness of their children's developmental status and abilities, but also to follow through with information about how this understanding can be translated to safe and effective parenting behaviors. Two logical targets for such preventive interventions include developing more appropriate expectations concerning the need for supervision and the development and implementation of safety rules.

Failure to Supervise Adequately

In order to protect an infant from environmental hazards, there seems to be universal agreement that either the child must be removed from the hazard or the hazard must be removed from the child's environment (Gralinski & Kopp, 1993). Knowing when a child can motorically put herself or himself at risk by contacting a hazard (climb, crawl, manipulate a latch) and then removing the hazard before that time is essential, given that continuously vigilant parental supervision is extremely difficult to maintain. "Child proofing" homes is much more popular now than in the past, and yet most safety checks, especially in low-income homes, continue to show many environmental hazards which could easily be altered or removed. Further, there are some situations that involve hazards that cannot be completely removed and thus necessitate effortful parental supervision (e.g., busy streets, bathing in the bathtub).

Increasing parental vigilance may be easier in some ways for caregivers with infants than for parents of older children. As was argued earlier, the parental belief that young children can control their own impulses may result in seriously negligent supervision patterns around high-traffic areas, bodies of water, and sources of heat (e.g., coffeepots and space heaters). Although the absence of any kind of norms for active supervision of children at various ages would seem to make assisting parents with such decisions even more difficult, we would argue that supervision standards should not be established by community norms. Rather, research on children's abilities and risk for injury should dictate caregiver supervision practices. For example, it is normative for parents to allow children to cross streets independently when they enter elementary school, even though data suggest that children of this age are not capable of accurately making the discriminations necessary for such crossing. Although crossing guards are often present at the streets nearest the school, young children often must cross several streets by themselves on their way from home to school and back again. It is not surprising to find that the hours before and after school are among the times of highest risk for pedestrian injury to young children (Christoffel et al., 1991). More research is needed concerning the developmental period at which children are cognitively capable of the judgments necessary for safe crossing. In addition, we need research on how to make crossing the street as straightforward a task as possible. As one example, children currently are cautioned against midblock crossing, but midblock crossing may actually be easier to safely execute, as it involves cars in only two directions. Children are often hit in crosswalks by a car turning right or left onto the children's crossing street. In such cases, simply carrying out a simplistic, memorized rule (e.g., look left, look right, look left, cross) to assess oncoming traffic will not be protective.

Overreliance on Rules

As was noted earlier, parents report relying on family safety rules to be a primary method for protecting children (Peterson et al., 1990). Unfortunately, there has been very little research conducted on the effectiveness of family rules in preventing childhood injury. Thus, parents need to be aware that expecting the child to adhere to safety rules should never suffice in preventing preschoolers' injuries. Even older children tend not to recall or even recognize family safety rules when the rules are presented (Peterson et al., 1986), and preschool children's memory for such abstract statements (often beginning with "don't") is less than their elementary school counterparts. Further, even when the rule is recalled, it is unlikely to override the preschooler's impulses. Thus, parents must either learn to effectively utilize environmental methods (e.g., such barriers as fences, child gates, cabinet locks) or must rely on vigilant supervision to protect very young children. Understanding *why* high-effort care is essential may help to provide the motivation for parents' continued vigilance.

Having access to respite caregiving for single parents also seems important in maintaining adequate levels of supervision, as does the caregivers' emotional acceptance of the parental role and all the responsibilities entailed. Finally, the transfer of control from vigilant caregiving to the child's own impulse control needs to be a gradual process dictated not by environmental exigencies, but by the child's developmental abilities and motivation. At some point, safety rules must stand as proxies for parental presence, as children are afforded more freedom, as well as more responsibility. This topic is considered in more detail in the next subsection.

Intervention Suggestions

More than any of the other areas, it is difficult to offer empirically validated suggestions to deal with supervision and rule issues. As has been noted, there is no consensus concerning how much supervision is required to keep children safe at different ages and very little is known about how rules function to protect children. The most important suggestion that this chapter can offer is to increase the research directed toward both areas. In the meantime, it appears that most parents underestimate the amount of supervision necessary and overestimate the effectiveness of rule instruction. Such knowledge may assist parents in balancing the maintenance of parental control over risky behavior against the child's own needs and abilities.

CONSEQUENCES FOR RULE BREAKING AND UNINTENTIONAL INJURY

Parents tend to follow most child injuries (80%) with no consequences, and to use weak consequences such as lectures the rest of the time (following 14% of injuries; Peterson et al., 1995). However, one of the best predictors of the use of some form of consequence following an injury was the presence of a family rule pertaining to the injury. Parents of 8-year-old children in Peterson and colleagues' naturalistic observation study enacted consequences following two-thirds of the injuries in which children broke family rules. It is up to the reader to decide if the glass is two-thirds full or one-third empty here—most often when the child broke a rule, the parents did respond with a lecture, discipline, or other intervention. However, fully one-third of the injuries that occurred because the child had broken a safety rule (i.e., injuries which could not have occurred if the child had not broken a safety rule) were not followed by any kind of consequence. Clearly, the most effective teaching experiences for altering risky behavior are parents' following rule violations with clear and consistent consequences.

As noted earlier, this recommendation can be a two-edged sword. Lack of consequences leaves the child's risky behavior unchanged and the child a likely candidate for an injury. On the other hand, harsh punitive consequences can lead to coercive cycles of discipline and ultimately to inflicted injury. What is required is that the child make a firm connection between risky behavior and an immediate negative outcome. Time-out for a young child provides a time for reflection and moves the child toward the self-control parents ultimately wish the child to develop. For an older child, loss of privilege is a logical consequence of risky behavior—if you cannot ride the bike safely, you lose the privilege of riding for a few days. If you play with a sharp or hot appliance, you are too young to use it and can reapply for safe use after a week of being banned. Where loss of the risky activity is unlikely to be perceived as punishing, withdrawal of other privileges that imply maturity (use of stereo, choice of television programs, trips to a friend's house) seem logical consequences. Thus, the key elements for the effective use of negative behavioral consequences include informing children of parental expectations regarding children's safe and risky behavior, explaining the inherent dangers of children's risky activity, teaching children to select alternative safe behaviors, and, perhaps most importantly, following up children's safety violations with predictable and consistent consequences.

The research that exists suggests that this is not how most parents socialize injury in middle childhood, although few researchers have studied how parents effect safety rule implementation and adherence. The American Academy of Pediatric Medicine recently began a campaign advocating that parents use firm disciplinary measures to insure that their children wear bicycle helmets consistently. To what extent do parents follow such recommendations? In a new exploratory study (Peterson, Saldana, & Schaeffer, 1997), mothers of second- and eighth-grade children were asked to imagine that their family had a rule requiring helmet use whenever the child rode a bike. Then, the mothers role-played several scenarios in which the child appeared to be leaving the home on his or her bicycle without the helmet.

Initially, parents tended to use open-ended reminders (e.g., "Aren't you forgetting something?") or simple commands (e.g., "Get your helmet") more often than they imposed consequences (e.g., "You may not ride the bike if you do not wear the helmet"). Parents were more likely to shift from reminders and commands to consequences during the role-play if the child persisted in refusing to wear the helmet. Mothers of the children at highest developmental risk (i.e., eighth-grade boys) tended to use consequences more than mothers of younger children. Nonetheless, even with the high social desirability demands of this role-play, a disturbing number of parents said they would let the child ride without a helmet even if such action broke a family rule.

It would appear that parents need first to understand that children wield potent contingencies for parents. Then, parents need to be aware that if children learn that when they use hostile refusal or threaten a tantrum, parents tend to withdraw the safety rule, children will be more likely to challenge parents than to obey many safety rules. It is also important for parents to understand that specific safety rules (e.g., "Look both ways when crossing the street") will not be sufficient to keep the child safe. Instead, providing children with a more complex and flexible understanding of potential injury situations (e.g., not all cars slowing for a stop sign actually stop; drivers may make a sudden right turn with no signal) in combination with specific safety rules may be more effective in preventing injuries.

RULES AND PROTECTION FROM UNINTENTIONAL INJURY

To what extent can injuries be prevented by following safety rules? Currently, there are no good answers to this question. Peterson and Schick (1993) examined records describing more than 1,000 child injuries and abstracted safety rules that would have prevented the injuries. One requirement was that rules not impose constant, general child vigilance (e.g., "Look where you are going at all times") and that they be reasonable in terms of daily life (e.g., wearing a helmet at all times might prevent some forms of head injury but would not be viewed by most people as a reasonable rule). The Peterson and Schick (1993) study found that approximately one-third of the minor injuries that occurred would have been prevented by the safety rules that were empirically derived from the injuries.

Another perspective on the problem can be found by taking common family safety rules and seeing how many injuries would be prevented by those commonly used rules. Peterson and Saldana (1996) asked naive coders to apply 75 family safety rules gathered from the unintentional injury literature to the same set of 1,000 child injuries, and again found that about one-third of the injuries would have been prevented by adherence to these rules. Sometimes the child was injured because the family did not impose the rule. Sometimes the child was injured because the family did accept the rule but the child had not adhered to it.

Consistent rule application has been suggested here as an important aspect of injury prevention. However, Peterson and Saldana (1996) found that parents who reported their child's risky behavior as unacceptable, even if there was no explicit family rule against that behavior, had children with marginally fewer injuries ($r = -.25$, $p < .096$). Although this finding described only a modest relationship and did not reach conventional levels of statistical significance, it offers an intriguing suggestion. Parents with high general safety expectations may instill more general safety consciousness in their children, even in the absence of teaching specific isolated rules. Future research may profitably consider how to further investigate this finding, as the results could have important implications for understanding the significance of safety rules and other aspects of parenting behavior for preventing childhood injuries.

EXCESSIVE CONSEQUENCES FOR RULE BREAKING

Throughout this chapter, we have advocated viewing parenting beliefs and behaviors as a continuum rather than as a dichotomy. The past two sections have focused on one end of the continuum and have argued that inadequate consequences both for specific safety rules and general safety behavior put the child at risk for unintentional injury. Paradoxically, not only too few and too weak consequences but consequences that are too many and too harsh on the other end of the continuum also put the child at risk. Abusive parents typically feel the need to exert greater and more frequent control over their children than do nonabusive parents (Herrenkohl, Herrenkohl, & Egolf, 1983). This excessive need to dictate the child's behavior is often coupled with coercive attempts to regain control, which are met with increased resistance from the child, cueing even more aggressive discipline from the parent (Reid et al., 1981). Such strong parental needs for control have been linked directly to child abuse (Monroe & Schellenbach, 1989).

Ironically, one of the child misbehaviors that is most likely to cue parental anger and harsh discipline is unsafe behavior, such as running away from a parent toward a busy street (Peterson et al., 1993). Some experts have even suggested that abusive discipline may be cued by desires to keep the child safe (Crittenden, 1995), although this viewpoint is not shared by most individuals in the field of child maltreatment research. In any case, if physical discipline is a precursor to child abuse, then the need for tight control over the child's behavior and the use of physical discipline as a method of obtaining this tight control may be predictive of child injury. If a parent prematurely believes that a young child's behavior should be controlled by knowledge of family rules (both safety rules and rules dealing with social and moral obligations), then the parent is also more likely to use negative consequences to correct lapses in control, rather than to increase supervision and teaching to alter the child's behavior. In addition, negative attributions of responsibility to the child are likely to provoke more angry or depressed emotions in the parent, which are themselves the source of more intemperate discipline, as will be seen in the following section.

EMOTIONS

Anger

The emotion mentioned most often as an immediate precursor to child maltreatment is anger (Berkeley Planning Associates, 1983). Abusive parents experience more anger and frustration in response to child misbehavior than do other parents (Bauer & Twentyman, 1985). In fact, instead of experiencing feelings of empathy and concern in response to an infant's crying, abusive parents more often experience anger (Milner, Halsey, & Fultz, 1995). Anger both amplifies the parent's physical response to the child and limits the parent's tendency to monitor her or his response. Thus, anger recognition and management techniques are frequently mentioned as vital components of any treatment program for abusive and at-risk parents (Wolfe, 1994).

Depression and Helplessness

Parental depression may result in the withdrawal of appropriate levels of supervision and rule application, culminating in child injury (Garbarino et al., 1991). Depression can also be related to increases in harsh discipline techniques (Lahey, Conger, Atkeson, & Treiber, 1984) and, subsequently, to child abuse. The feelings of helplessness that accompany depression may trigger the need to obtain control over some aspect of the parent's life and thus lead to an increase in attempts to alter the child's behavior. Negative parental affect results in less parental patience and increased frustration with child misbehavior (Dix, 1991). Thus, it may sometimes be necessary to deal effectively with the parents' emotional difficulties in addition to their parenting limitations to prevent both unintentional injury and maltreatment.

"PARENTING" VERSUS "MOTHERING" OR "FATHERING"

Several times during this chapter, we have made reference to the responsibilities that must be accepted by anyone who attempts to raise a child. Within our model (see Figure 1), we have artificially separated such instrumental activities as providing food and shelter and maintaining physical safety (which we arbitrarily label "parenting") from the socioemotional activities such as enjoying, loving, and psychologically nurturing the child (which we label "mothering" or "fathering"). This separation seems necessary because some of the individuals we serve seem prepared to "parent" or assume physical responsibility for the child, but not to "mother" or "father" the child in terms of establishing a strong emotional bond with the child. Other individuals (particularly very young mothers or mothers with psychiatric or substance abuse problems) seem emotionally bonded to their child but not able or willing to incur responsibility for the child's physical care. Clearly, a child needs both a parent and a mother/father for healthy development. Our hierarchy suggests that acceptance of both of these roles is more likely if negative emotions are controlled and beliefs about childrearing are consonant with effective practice, if the individual is aware of the child's developmental proclivities and abilities, and if effective parenting skills are present. Our society needs to focus more on the discrete responsibilities for keeping children safe that are part of effective parenting, and the use of a strong mother–child or father–child bond as a motivator for such performance. Finally, acceptance of these roles is more likely to be successful if the caregiver's own basic needs are met and an intact sense of self-worth, self-esteem, and self-efficacy are present.

SELF-EFFICACY AND CAREGIVING

Very little has been written on the potential positive motivation that may result from enhanced self-efficacy and the internal rewards derived from effective parenting. However, continuous supervision, effective child guidance using distraction and redirection, and punishing the child by using time-out or reinforcement of other behaviors rather than physical force all require extra effort and energy. It seems likely that parents who feel they are effective and who derive satisfaction and happiness from engaging in demanding parenting challenges are more likely to persist in such behaviors than parents who perceive fewer positive outcomes resulting from encounters with their children. For example, Peterson et al. (1990) found that beliefs in one's own ability to influence child safety predicted the number of interventions parents made to avoid child injury. Similarly, maltreating parents typically have a poor sense of their efficacy as parents (Daro, 1988). Thus, another important area for focus in preventing child injury and maltreatment may be consolidating each parent's sense of efficacy and increasing the degree to which parents are able to derive enjoyment and rewards from successful parenting.

AWARENESS, EXPECTATIONS, EMOTIONS, AND ROLES

Throughout this chapter, the links between parents' cognitions and their emotions have been stressed. For example, a lack of awareness of a preschooler's limitations in memory and impulse control is likely to be related to parental expectations that the preschooler can regulate his or her own negative emotions according to a set of parental rules. Parental anger and depression are the likely result when the child fails to live up to such expectations. The coercive cycles these setting events create predicts the occurrence of future abuse (Reid et al., 1981).

Similarly, failing to be aware of an infant's expanding motor abilities seems related to parental expectations that the child does not yet need to be vigilantly supervised. Hopelessness or depression may also negatively influence a parent's inclination and ability to engage in effortful supervision, and ineffective parenting is likely to potentiate negative affect and block positive, motivating affect. The cycle of the parent's inability to predict the child's behavior, with subsequent poor outcomes, creates a similar downward spiral of perceived parental inadequacy and resulting hopelessness. Effective intervention should meet all of the levels suggested earlier in the hierarchical model, and should treat the parent at each level, not only teaching parenting skills, but also increasing developmental knowledge, altering inappropriate parenting beliefs, decreasing negative emotions, facilitating acceptance of parenting plus mothering/fathering roles, and enhancing view of the self.

IMPLICATIONS FOR PREVENTION

The more the parent is aware of the child's developmental needs and abilities, the easier effective parenting will be. However, teaching parents about all the nuances of cognitive, affective, and motor development would be challenging indeed. Further, it is clear that maltreating parents do not hold different beliefs about developmental milestones than other parents (Azar et al., 1984). Thus, it seems sensible to focus on those parental expectations for their children that are likely to trigger neglectful supervision or abuse. As noted earlier, Peterson, Gable, and colleagues (in press) provided an example of intervention for such expectations by outlining a set of cognitions parents may have, and describing how the child behavior (e.g., saying "no") may evoke an angry cognition ("How dare he say 'no' to me. I need to teach him who is boss"). Then, a therapist can suggest a more appropriate, developmentally based cognition ("This is a sign of autonomy. He is taking more responsibility for his choices"). To facilitate substituting developmental awareness statements for angry child-based attributions, parents need to be aware that the child has not chosen deliberately to have faulty memory, poor impulse control, or a short attention span—that all of these characteristics are normative characteristics of a given developmental level.

Clear specification of the behaviors that constitute appropriate parenting need to be a part of any maltreatment program. Rather than articulating community norms, interventions need to link the child's developmental capabilities and needs to the behaviors that are required from the parents to keep the child safe. Parents should feel that they can effectively meet the child's needs. It may also prove helpful to encourage parental self-reinforcement and rewards from significant others for engaging in high-effort parenting, in order to assist in maintenance of such behavior.

Most interventions for child maltreatment have focused on anger management skills. Such intervention seems very sensible, particularly if linked to common developmental triggers and parenting skill challenges (e.g., appropriate use of such parenting techniques as ignoring or time-out is likely to initially involve high levels of frustration for parents). Anticipating this and teaching methods of coping with the negative affect seems an important part of any parenting program. Parental awareness of how their own emotional problems are likely to negatively influence their parenting may assist in limiting the negative effects of emotional problems or maternal addiction. Direct treatment of parental substance abuse or emotional problems may also be indicated (Smith, Dent, Coles, & Falek, 1992).

CONCLUSION

Much of this handbook outlines state-of-the-art treatment for maltreating families. Interventions at the national, state, community, and individual family levels are articulated. We concur with recommendations that suggest ecological changes, both for the physical environment (e.g., safe places to play) and the psychosocial environment (e.g., networking among low-income, isolated women). We support parenting interventions (e.g., Wolfe, 1994) that teach parents disciplinary skills and anger management, as well as those which emphasize strengthening the parental bond to the child. We also urge teaching developmental awareness, altering problematic parental beliefs and expectations, and treating parental disorders such as depression and substance abuse.

This chapter emphasizes the relationship between childrearing and the two literatures on injury that still exist as disconnected entities. We have documented the difficulty in appropriately labeling most forms of injury, the common etiology, patterns, and consequences of unintentional injury and of injury related to abuse and neglect. Finally, we have shown how parents' developmental awareness leads to specific expectations on the part of the parent, and have articulated how these expectations may decrease appropriate supervision and increase harsh discipline. We have presented information on parental negative affect and its role, as well as the role of self-efficacy and the parenting plus the mother/fathering roles. Our ultimate message is that theoretical and empirical gains will be made from placing childhood injuries on the continuum of parent beliefs, behaviors, and intentions rather than considering injuries as a dichotomy. We suggest that effective interventions will enhance parents' knowledge and understanding of child development, encourage parental use of more effective and positive methods of child discipline, reduce parents' negative affect, and facilitate effective anger management. Such interventions will have the maximum likelihood of keeping children safe from all forms of traumatic injury.

REFERENCES

Altemeier, W. A., O'Connor, S., Vietze, P., Sandler, H., & Sherrod, K. (1984). Prediction of child abuse: A prospective study of feasibility. *Child Abuse & Neglect, 8*, 393–400.

American Association for Protecting Children. (1988). *Highlights of official child neglect and abuse reporting, 1986*, Denver, CO: American Humane Association.

Azar, S. T., Robinson, D. R., Hekimian, E., & Twentyman, C. T. (1984). Unrealistic expectations and problem-solving ability in maltreating and comparison mothers. *Journal of Consulting and Clinical Psychology, 52*, 687–691.

Azar, S. T., & Rohrbeck, C. A. (1986). Child abuse and unrealistic expectations: Further validation of the parent opinion questionnaire. *Journal of Consulting and Clinical Psychology, 54*(6), 867–868.

Baker, S. P., & Fisher, R. S. (1980). Childhood asphyxiation by choking or suffocation. *Journal of the American Medical Association, 244*, 1343–1346.

Baker, S. P., O'Neill, B., Ginsburg, M. J., & Li, G. (1992). *The injury fact book* (2nd ed.). New York: Oxford University Press.

Baladerian, N. J. (1991). *Abuse causes disabilities: Disability and the family.* Culver City, CA: SPEC-TRUM Institute.

Bauer, W. D., & Twentyman, C. T. (1985). Abusing, neglectful, and comparison mothers' responses to child-related and non-child-related stressors. *Journal of Consulting and Clinical Psychology, 53,* 335–343.

Beautrais, A. L., Fergusson, D. M., & Shannon, D. T. (1981). Accidental poisoning in the first three years of life. *Australian Paediatric Journal, 17,* 104–109.

Beautrais, A. L. Fergusson, D. M., & Shannon, D. T. (1982). Childhood accidents in a New Zealand birth cohort. *Australian Paediatric Journal, 18,* 238–242.

Berger, L. (1981). Childhood injuries: Recognition and prevention. *Problems in Pediatrics, 12,* 1–59.

Bergman, A. B., & Rivara, F. P. (1991). Sweden's experience in reducing childhood injuries. *Pediatrics, 88,* 69–74.

Berkeley Planning Associates. (1983). *The exploration of client characteristics, services, and outcomes. Evaluation of the clinical demonstration projects on child abuse and neglect.* Contract No. 105-78-1108. Washington, DC: National Center on Child Abuse and Neglect.

Bijur, P. E., Kurzon, M., Overpeck, M. D., & Scheidt, P. C. (1992). Parental alcohol use, problem drinking, and children's injuries. *Journal of the American Medical Association, 267,* 3166–3171.

Brown, G. W., & Davidson, S. (1978). Social class, psychiatric disorder of mother, and accidents to children. *Lancet, 1,* 378.

Bryon, J. W., & Freed, F. W. (1982). Corporal punishment: Normative data and sociological and psychological correlates in a community college population. *Journal of Youth and Adolescence, 11*(2), 77–87.

Burns, N. M. (1993). *Literature review of issues related to the use of corrective force against children.* Ottawa: Department of Justice, *Working Document WD 1993-6e.*

Caffey, J. (1946). Multiple fractures in the long bones of infants suffering from chronic subdural hematoma. *American Journal of Roentgenology, 56,* 163–173.

Cataldo, M. F., Finney, J. W., Richman, G. S., Riley, A. W., Hook, R., Brophy, C. J., & Nau, P. A. (1992). Behavior of injured and uninjured children and their parents in a simulated hazardous setting. *Journal of Pediatric Psychology, 17,* 73–80.

Christoffel, K. K. (1986). Childhood pedestrian injury: A pilot study concerning etiology. *Accident Analysis and Prevention, 18,* 25–35.

Christoffel, K. K., Schofer, J. L., Lavigne, J. V., Tanz, R. R., Wills, K., White, B., Barthel, M., McGuire, P., Donovan, M., Buergo, F., Shawver, N., & Jenq, J. (1991). "Kids n' cars," an ongoing study of pedestrian injuries: Descriptive and early findings. *Children's Environments Quarterly, 8,* 41–50.

Christoffel, K. K., Scheidt, P. C., Agran, P. F., Klaus, J. F., McLoughlin, E., & Paulson, J. A. (1992). *Standard definitions for childhood injury research.* Washington, DC: U.S. Department of Health and Human Services.

Cohen, M., Raphling, D., & Green, P. (1966). Psychological aspects of the maltreatment syndrome of childhood. *Journal of Pediatrics, 69,* 279–284.

Cohn, A. H., & Daro, D. (1987). Is treatment too late: What ten years of evaluative research tells us. *Child Abuse & Neglect, 11,* 433–442.

Colver, A. F., Hutchinson, P. J., & Judson, E. C. (1982). Promoting children's home safety. *British Medical Journal, 285,* 1177–1180.

Consumer Product Safety Commission. (1979). *Impact of crib safety activities on injuries and deaths associated with cribs.* Washington, DC: Author.

Crittenden, P. (1995). Violence within the family. Paper presented at the conference *Violence Against Children in the Family and the Community,* Los Angeles, January 26–28.

Daro, D. (1988). *Confronting child abuse research for the effective program design.* New York: Free Press.

De Haven, H. (1942). Mechanical analysis of survival in falls from heights of fifty to one hundred and fifty feet. *War Medicine, 2,* 539–546.

Dershewitz, R. A., & Williamson, J. W. (1977). Prevention of childhood household injuries: A controlled clinical trial. *American Journal of Public Health, 67,* 1148–1153.

Dix, T. (1991). The affective organization of parenting: Adaptive and maladaptive processes. *Psychological Bulletin, 110,* 3–25.

Egeland, B., Sroufe, A., & Erickson, M. (1983). The developmental consequence of different patterns of maltreatment. *Child Abuse & Neglect, 7,* 459–469.

Ewigman, B., Kivlahan, C., & Land, C. (1993). The Missouri child fatality study: Underreporting of maltreatment fatalities among children under five years of age, 1983–1986. *Pediatrics, 91,* 330–337.

Fingerhut, L., & Kleinman, J. (1989). Trends and current status in childhood mortality, United States, 1900–1985. *Vital Health Statistics, 26,* 1–44.

Flynn, C. P. (1994). Regional differences in attitudes toward corporal punishment. *Journal of Marriage and Family, 56,* 314–324.

Garbarino, J. (1977). The human ecology of child maltreatment: A conceptual model for research. *Journal of Marriage and Family,* 721–735.

Garbarino, J. (1982). *Children and families in the social environment.* New York: Aldine.

Garbarino, J. (1988). Preventing childhood injury: Developmental and mental health issues. *American Journal of Orthopsychiatry, 58,* 25–36.

Gabrarino, J., Kostelny, K., & Dubrow, N. (1991). *No place to be a child: Growing up in a war zone.* Lexington, MA: Lexington Books.

Gelles, R. J. (1973). Child abuse as psychopathology: A sociological critique and reformulation. *American Journal of Orthopsychiatry, 43,* 611–621.

Giovannoni, J. M., & Billingsley, A. (1970). Child neglect among the poor: A study of parental adequacy in families of three ethnic groups. *Child Welfare, 49,* 196–204.

Gralinski, J. H., & Kopp, C. B. (1993). Everyday rules for behavior: Mothers' requests to young children. *Developmental Psychology, 29,* 573–584.

Gray, J. D., Cutler, C. A., Dean, J. G., & Kempe, C. H. (1977). Prediction and prevention of child abuse and neglect. *Child Abuse & Neglect, 1,* 45–58.

Graziano, A. M. (1994). Why we should study subabusive violence against children. *Journal of Interpersonal Violence, 9,* 412–419.

Graziano, A. M., & Kunce, L. J. (1992). Effects of corporal punishment on children. *Violence Update, 1,* 8–10.

Graziano, A. M., & Namaste, K. A. (1990). Parental use of physical force in child discipline: A survey of 679 college students. *Journal of Interpersonal Violence, 5*(4), 449–463.

Green, A. H., Gaines, R. W., & Sandgrund, A. (1974). Child abuse: Pathological syndrome of family interaction. *American Journal of Psychiatry, 131,* 882–886.

Haddon, W., Jr. (1970). On the escape of tigers: An ecologic note. *American Journal of Public Health, 60,* 2229–2234.

Haddon, W., Jr. (1972). A logical framework for categorizing highway safety phenomena and activity. *Journal of Trauma, 12,* 193–207.

Hartsough, C. A., & Lambert, N. M. (1985). Medical factors in hyperactive and normal children: Prenatal, developmental, and health history findings. *American Journal of Orthopsychiatry, 55,* 190–201.

Hay, T., & Jones, L. (1994). Societal interventions to prevent child abuse and neglect. *Child Welfare, 73,* 379–403.

Helfer, R. E. (1977). On the prevention of child abuse and neglect. *Child Abuse & Neglect, 1,* 502–504.

Herrenkohl, E., & Herrenkohl, R. C. (1979). A comparison of abused children and their nonabused siblings. *Journal of the American Academy of Child Psychology, 18,* 260–269.

Herrenkohl, R. C., Herrenkohl, E. C., & Egolf, B. P. (1983). Circumstances surrounding the occurrence of child maltreatment. *Journal of Consulting and Clinical Psychology, 51,* 424–431.

Kempe, C., Silverman, F., Steele, B., Droegemueller, W., & Silver, H. (1962). The battered child syndrome. *Journal of the American Medical Association, 181,* 17–24.

Kendall, P. C., & Wilcox, L. E. (1979). Self-control in children: Development of a rating scale. *Journal of Consulting and Clinical Psychology, 47,* 1020–1029.

Lahey, B. B., Conger, R. D., Atkeson, B. M., & Treiber, F. A. (1984). Parenting behavior and emotional status of physically abusive mothers. *Journal of Consulting and Clinical Psychology, 52,* 1062–1071.

LeVine, R A. (1974). Parental goals: A cross cultural view. *Teachers College Record, 76,* 226–239.

Lief, N. R., (1985). The drug user as parent. *The International Journal of the Addictions, 20,* 63–97.

Lorber, R., Felton, D. K., & Reid, J. (1984). A social learning approach to the reduction of coercive processes in child abusive families: A molecular analysis. *Advances in Behavior Research and Therapy, 6,* 29–45.

Luther, S. S., & Walsh, K. G. (1995). Treatment needs of the drug-addicted mothers: Integrated parenting psychotherapy interventions. *Journal of Substance Abuse Treatment, 12,* 341–348.

Lutzker, J. R., & Rice, J. M. (1984). Project 12-Ways: Treating child abuse and neglect from an ecobehavioral perspective. In R. F. Dangel & R. A. Polster (Eds.), *Parent training: Foundations of research and practice* (pp. 260–293). New York: Guilford Press.

Lynch, M. A. (1975). Ill-health and child abuse. *Lancet, 2,* 317–319.

MacKeller, F. L., & Yanagishita, M. (1995). *Homicide in the United States: Who is at risk?* (Vol. 21). Washington, DC: Population Reference Bureau.

Matheny, A. P., Jr. (1987). Psychological characteristics of childhood accidents. *Journal of Social Issues, 41*(2), 45–60.

Matheny, A. P., Jr. (1993, May). *Gender differences for unintentional injuries of opposite-sex twins: Implications and injury control.* Paper presented at the Second World Conference on Injury Control, Atlanta, GA.

McCormick, K. F. (1992). Attitudes of primary care physicians toward corporal punishment. *Journal of American Medical Association, 267*(23), 3161–3165.

McCormick, M. C., Shapiro, S., & Starfield, B. H. (1981). Injury and its correlates among 1-year-old children. *American Journal of Diseases of Children, 135,* 159–163.

Milner, J. S., Halsey, L. B., & Fultz, J. (1995). Empathic responsiveness and affective reactivity to infant stimuli in high- and low-risk for physical child abuse mothers. *Child Abuse & Neglect, 19,* 767–780.

Monroe, L. D., & Schellenbach, C. J. (1989). Relationship of Child Abuse Potential Inventory scores to parental responses: A construct validity study. *Child and Family Behavior Therapy, 11,* 39–58.

National Center on Child Abuse and Neglect. (1993). *Study findings: National study of the incidence and severity of child abuse and neglect.* Washington, DC: U.S. Government Printing Office.

National Research Council. (1993). *Understanding child abuse and neglect.* Washington, DC: National Academy of Sciences.

Nersesian, W. S., Petit, M. R., Shaper, R., Lemieux, D., & Naor, E. (1985). Childhood death and poverty: A study of all childhood deaths in Maine, 1976 to 1980. *Pediatrics, 75,* 41–50.

Newberger, C. M., & Cook,, S. J. (1983). Parental awareness and child abuse and neglect: A cognitive developmental analysis of urban and rural samples. *Journal of Orthopsychiatry, 53,* 512–524.

O'Neill, J. A., Meacham, W. F., Griffin, P. P., & Sawyers, J. L. (1973). Patterns of injury in the battered child syndrome. *Journal of Trauma, 13,* 332–339.

O'Shea, J. S. (1986). Childhood accident prevention strategies. *Forensic Science International, 30,* 99–111.

Pearn, J., & Nixon, J. (1977). Prevention of childhood drowning accidents. *Medical Journal of Australia,1,* 616–618.

Pelton, L. (1977) *Child Abuse and neglect and protective intervention in Mercer County, New Jersey: A parent interview and case record study.* Trenton, NJ: Bureau of Research, New Jersey Division of Youth and Family Services.

Peterson, L., Bartelstone, J., Kern, T., & Gillies, R. (1995). Parents, socialization of children's injury prevention: Description and some initial parameters. *Child Development, 66,* 224–235.

Peterson, L., & Brown, D. (1994). Integrating child injury and abuse–neglect research: Common histories, etiologies, and solutions. *Psychological Bulletin, 116,* 293–315.

Peterson, L., Ewigman, B., & Kivlahan, C. (1993). Judgments regarding appropriate child supervision to prevent injury: The role of environmental risk and child age. *Child Development, 64,* 934–950.

Peterson, L., Farmer, J., & Kashani, J. H. (1990). Parental injury prevention endeavors: A function of health beliefs? *Health Psychology, 9,* 177–191.

Peterson, L., Gable, S., Doyle, C., & Ewigman, B. (in press). Beyond parenting skills: Battling barriers and building bonds to prevent child abuse and neglect. *Cognitive and Behavioral Practice.*

Peterson, L., Mori, L., & Scissors, C. (1986). "Mom or Dad says I shouldn't": Supervised and unsupervised children's knowledge of their parents' rules for home safety. *Journal of Pediatric Psychology, 11,* 177–188.

Peterson, L., Mori, L., Selby, V., & Rosen, B. N. (1988). Community interventions in children's injury prevention: Differing costs and differing benefits. *Journal of Community Psychology, 16,* 188–204.

Peterson, L., & Roberts, M. C. (1992) Complacency, misdirection, and effective prevention of children's injuries. *American Psychologist, 47,* 1040–1044.

Peterson, L., & Saldana, L. (1996). Accelerating children's risk for injury: Mothers' decisions regarding common safety rules. *Journal of Behavioral Medicine, 19,* 317–331.

Peterson, L., Saldana, L., & Schaeffer, C. (1997). Maternal intervention strategies in enforcing children's bicycle helmet use. *Journal of Health Psychology, 2,* 225–230.

Peterson, L., & Schick, B. (1993). Empirically derived injury prevention rules. *Journal of Applied Behavioral Analysis, 26,* 451–460.

Pless, I. B. (1978). Accident prevention and health education: Back to the drawing board? *Pediatrics, 62,* 431–435.

Power, T. G., & Chapieski, M. L. (1986). Childrearing and impulse control in toddlers: A naturalistic investigation. *Developmental Psychology, 22,* 271–275.

Reid, J. R., Taplin, P., & Lorber, R. (1981). A social interactional approach to the treatment of abusive families. In R. B. Stuart (Ed.), *Violent behavior: Social learning approaches to prediction management. and treatment* (pp. 83–101). New York: Brunner/Mazel.

Rivara, F. P. (1982). Minibikes: A case study in underregulation. In S. B. Bergman (Ed.), *Preventing childhood injuries* (Report of the 12th Ross Round Table on Critical Approaches to Common Pediatric Problems, pp. 61–63). Columbus, OH: Ross Laboratories.

Rivara, F. P., & Barber, M. (1985). Demographic analysis of childhood pedestrian injuries. *Pediatrics, 76,* 375–381.

Roberts, M. C., & Wright, L. (1982). Role of the pediatric psychologist as a consultant to pediatricians. In J. Tuma (Ed.), *Handbook for the practice of pediatric psychology* (pp. 251–289). New York: Wiley-Interscience.

Robertson, L. S. (1983) *Injuries: Causes, control strategies, and public policy.* Lexington, MA: Lexington Books.

Scheidt, P. C., & Workshop Participants. (1988). Behavioral research toward prevention of childhood injury. *American Journal of Diseases of Children, 142,* 612–617.

Schmitt, B., & Kempe, C. (1974). The battered child syndrome. In R. Gelles & J. Kagen (Eds.), *Current pediatric therapy* (7th ed., pp. 102–104). Philadelphia: Saunders.

Smith, G. S., & Falk, H. (1987). Unintentional injuries. In R. W. Ambler & B. Dold (Eds.), *Closing the gap* (pp. 143–163). New York: Oxford University Press.

Smith, I. E., Dent, D. Z., Coles, C. D., & Falek, A. (1992). A comparison study of treated and untreated pregnant and postpartum cocaine-abusing women. *Journal of Substance Abuse Treatment, 9,* 343–348.

Straus, M. A. (1991). Discipline and deviance: Physical punishment of children and violence and other crime in adulthood. *Social Problems, 38,* 133–154.

Straus, M., Gelles, R., & Steinmetz, S. (1980). *Behind closed doors: Violence in the American family.* Garden City, NY: Anchor Press/ Doubleday.

Straus, M. A., & Gimpel, H. S. (1992). *Corporal punishment by parents and economic achievement: A theoretical model and some preliminary empirical data.* Paper presented at the meeting of the American Sociological Association, Durham, NH: Family Research Laboratory, University of New Hampshire.

Walton, W. W. (1982). An evaluation of the Poison Prevention Packaging Act. *Pediatrics, 69,* 363–370.

Wauchope, B., & Straus, M. A. (1990). Physical punishment and physical abuse of American children: Incidence rates by age, gender, and occupational class. In M. A. Straus & R. J. Gelles (Eds.), *Physical violence in American families: Risk factors and adaptations to violence in 8,145 families.* New Brunswick, NJ: Transaction Books.

Weller, S. C, Romney, A. K., & Orr, D. P. (1987). The myth of a subculture of corporal punishment. *Human Organization, 46*(1), 39–47.

Wolfe, D. A. (1994). The role of intervention and treatment services in the prevention of child abuse and neglect. In G. B. Melton & F. D. Barry (Eds.), *Protecting children from abuse and neglect: Foundations for a new national strategy* (pp. 182–223). New York: Guilford Press.

Zettle, R. D., & Hayes, S. C. (1982). Rule-governed behavior: A potential theoretical framework for cognitive–behavioral therapy. In P. C. Kendall (Ed.), *Advances in cognitive–behavioral research* (Vol. 1, pp. 73–118). New York: Academic Press.

Zuckerman, B. S., & Duby, J. C. (1985). Developmental approach to injury prevention. *Pediatric Clinics of North America, 32,* 17–29.

13

Breaking the Cycle
A Culturally Sensitive Violence Prevention Program for African-American Children and Adolescents

BETTY R. YUNG and W. RODNEY HAMMOND

INTRODUCTION

Although our knowledge of violence prevalence is far from complete, there is virtually no question that male and female African Americans of all ages are consistently overrepresented as the victims and perpetrators of interpersonal violence. This fact appears to hold true across the continuum of severity, from relatively inconsequential fights among school children to the violent deaths reflected annually in national mortality data. Evidence further suggests that within African-American families and communities there is a greater reported incidence of violent acts affecting all types of relationships (spouse/partner, parent/child, and youth and their peers) than is found among all other groups.

The immediate human, social, and economic costs of violence present a compelling case for prevention. The case is made still stronger by consideration of the potential for cyclical perpetuation of violence by those who experience or habitually witness it. Within some African-American communities, the exposure to deadly neighborhood violence is so routine that even very young children demonstrate acute awareness of gunfire danger and the need for self-protection. In interviews with young children living in a public high-rise in Chicago, Dubrow and Garbarino (1989) reported that all of their child subjects had witnessed a shooting before the age of 5. They also observed that during the interviews these children dropped to the floor in fear at the slightest loud noise. African-American children and adolescents living in such dangerous situations frequently respond to the risks within their

BETTY R. YUNG • School of Professional Psychology, Wright State University, Dayton, Ohio 45407. **W. RODNEY HAMMOND** • National Center for Injury Prevention and Control, Centers for Disease Control, Atlanta, Georgia 30341-3724.

Handbook of Child Abuse Research and Treatment, edited by Lutzker. Plenum Press, New York, 1998.

environment by arming themselves in self-defense (Harris, 1993; Yung & Hammond, 1995). Ironically, the decision to carry a gun often places them at much higher risk for becoming victims of violence or for killing or injuring others in a dispute.

Although the need for prevention efforts cannot be challenged, the pathway to prevention is less clear. Not only is the etiology of violence poorly understood, literature on interpersonal violence risk and prevention/intervention strategies tends to be compartmentalized into separate bodies of work which study child abuse, domestic violence, and youth assaultive violence as discrete phenomena (Finklehor & Dzuiba-Leatherman, 1994; Hampton, 1987; Jenkins, 1995). This fragmentation tends to obscure the common threads linking diverse manifestations of family and community violence as well as presenting the interventionist with a confusing array of logical time points and targets for prevention efforts.

Acknowledging that there is no single perfect prevention focus, this chapter will present a culturally sensitive prevention model which intervenes at a critical juncture with African-American adolescents as they are entering the period of greatest vulnerability for violence in their developing relationships with friends, neighborhood acquaintances, classmates, adult authority figures, and romantic partners. The chapter emphasizes expressive violence occurring in the context of conflict arising in interpersonal relationships because this manifestation of violence is the most common source of threat for African-American families. We exclude discussion of instrumental violence that occurs as a by-product of another crime such as robbery, nor do we cover violence related to psychopathology or sexual assault. Following a brief review of what is known about the nature and extent of expressive violence in African-American families and communities, we will describe the conceptual foundation and components of a youth violence prevention program we have been operating since 1989. Special attention will be placed on ethnic/cultural adaptations to program techniques and materials. The chapter will end with a discussion of evaluation methods, summary results, and limitations of the approach.

VIOLENCE PREVALENCE AMONG AFRICAN AMERICANS

Homicide Victimization and Perpetration

There are more reliable data on homicides than on all other degrees of violence (Rosenberg & Mercy, 1991). For at least the past three decades, health statistics have documented higher homicide rates for male and female African Americans of all ages than for other ethnic minorities or Caucasians (Centers for Disease Control [CDC], 1990; U.S. Department of Justice [USDOJ], 1994). For African Americans between the ages of 15 and 34, homicide is the leading cause of death (CDC, 1990). In 1992, murder rates of African-American men ages 15 to 24 were nearly 9 times higher than those of their same-age Caucasian male peers. In recent years the sharp rise in homicides among 15- to 19-year-old African-American males has been particularly troubling—from a rate of 48.64 per 100,000 in 1980 to a 1992 rate of 128.82 (CDC, 1996).

Similar increases have been reported in the commission of homicides by young African-American men as reflected in criminal justice statistics. Between 1985 and 1992, arrests for homicides among 14- to 17-year-old African-American males rose 300% (Council on Crime in America, 1996). Of the 25,180 homicide offenders arrested in 1992, 90% were male, 50% were ages 15 to 24, and 55% were African-American (USDOJ, 1994). Arrest rates for lethal violence carried out by African-American women, although much lower than those of same race males, typically exceed those of Caucasian men and women (Goetting, 1988; Kruttschnitt, 1993).

Child Physical Abuse

Studies of the extent of physical abuse of African-American children and adolescents have shown mixed results. National and regional estimates during the 1970s and 1980s suggested that families reported for physical child abuse and neglect were disproportionately drawn from poor, less educated, and African-American families (Hampton & Newberger, 1985; also see reviews in Hampton, 1987, and in Hampton & Yung, 1995). Other studies, including the first National Study of the Incidence and Severity of Child Abuse and Neglect ([NIS], 1981 cited in Hampton, 1987) and a more recent national self-report survey of children and adolescents (Finklehor & Dzuiba-Leatherman, 1994) estimated physical child abuse rates for African-American families that were slightly elevated above those of Caucasian families, but not at levels of statistical significance. However, other recent research has reported family victimization levels for African-American children that were six times higher than national prevalence estimates (Richters & Martinez, 1993). Also secondary analyses of NIS data found significant cultural differences in child disciplinary practices among African-American and Caucasian families. African-American parents were more likely to use belts, cords, straps, and switches to punish their children and to employ more severe levels of punishment (Hampton, 1987; Hampton & Yung, 1995; Lassiter, 1987). The extreme forms of these well-intentioned, but potentially dangerous, acts can result in serious injury or death, and indeed young African-American children are disproportionately represented in cases of fatal caretaker abuse, inflicted most often by parents attempting to control behavior such as crying or disobedience (Crittenden & Craig, 1990).

Spouse/Partner Abuse

Several studies suggest higher levels of spouse and romantic partner abuse among African Americans. The Second National Family Violence Survey found that African-American women were 1.23 times more likely than Caucasian women to experience minor domestic violence and more than twice as likely to be the victims of severe violence (Hampton & Yung, 1995). An Atlanta study estimated that fatal and nonfatal victimization rates from family and intimate assaults were three times higher for African Americans than for Caucasians (Saltzman et al., 1990). Although in nonfatal episodes of domestic violence, women are more frequently the victims, studies of fatal violence patterns among spouses have found that African-American males are at greater risk for spouse homicide than are African-American women or Caucasians of either sex (Dawson & Langan, 1994; Mercy & Saltzman, 1989).

Community Violence and Youth as Victims, Perpetrators, or Witnesses

The upsurge in youth violence has generated a proliferating body of research which attempts to gauge the extent of violence experienced, witnessed, or committed by young people in the community. The amount of physical fighting in which youngsters engage and their patterns of weapon-carrying are now measured annually in self-reports gathered through the Youth Risk Behavior Surveillance System (YRBSS) developed by the Centers for Disease Control. The YRBSS, which includes questions related to violent behavior, is widely used in school systems throughout the country. Other studies have examined the extent of violence exposure among young people living in high-crime urban settings, and many such studies include analyses of the correlations of this exposure to the perpetration of violence. Almost without exception, these studies have found substantially higher levels of victimization, physical fighting, routine gun carrying, self-reported and officially documented assaults on others, and witnessing of violent acts among African-American youth than have been found among Caucasian or other ethnic minority children and adolescents (for a more complete review, see Yung & Hammond, 1997).

Carrying of guns by African-American male adolescents is an area of particular concern. African-American boys and young men exceed their male and female peers in the carrying of guns, off and on school property, at rates ranging from 12.6% to 20.9% (Kann et al., 1995; Valois, McKeown, Garrison, & Vincent, 1995; U.S. Department of Health and Human Services [USDHHS], 1995). Studies that have focused primarily or exclusively on African-American youth living in inner-city neighborhoods have shown much higher rates, with two studies reporting that about 40% of the African-American survey population had carried guns at some time in their lives (DuRant, Prendergast, & Cadenhead, 1994; Webster, Gainer, & Champion, 1993) and one finding that about 16% carried guns virtually every day (Webster et al., 1993).

The high levels of concern about violence among African-American boys and young men tend to overshadow the severity of the problem among African-American girls and young women. Although rates for all types of violence risks and experiences are consistently higher for male youth, African-American female children and adolescents witness and experience within-family and community violence at rates that exceed those of Caucasian or other ethnic minority females. Several studies have also reported physical fighting among African-American female adolescents at rates that were 1.5 to 2 times higher than those of other females (DuRant et al., 1994; Kann et al., 1995; Valois et al., 1995) and were relatively close to those of males (DuRant et al., 1994).

Newer research is also beginning to examine the phenomena of child exposure to chronic violence in troubled communities. Most such studies have focused on a predominantly African-American child or adolescent sample in large urban communities such as Chicago (Bell & Jenkins, 1993, Shakoor & Chalmers, 1991), Baltimore (Lorion & Saltzman, 1993), Detroit (Schubiner, Scott, & Tzelepis, 1993), New Orleans (Osofsky, Wewers, Hann, & Fick, 1993), and Washington, D.C. (Richters & Martinez, 1993). The level of violence seen by children and adolescents in these studies is shockingly high, perhaps none more so than the results reported by Richters and Martinez (1993), who found that 47% of the first- and second-graders interviewed had seen someone shot. One study compared the violence exposure of inner-city African-American youth to groups of Caucasian suburban and rural youth, finding that 42% of the minority metropolitan sample reported having seen someone shot, in contrast to 4% of the comparison group (Gladstein, Slater-Rusonis, & Heald, 1992).

Links between Family and Community Violence

The victims and perpetrators of most family and community violence show striking similarities. The demographic profile of the aggressor, that is, the person most likely to abuse an intimate partner, to carry a gun, to assault or kill an acquaintance, or to commit serious or fatal physical abuse against his children or stepchildren, is a young African-American male of low socioeconomic status living in an inner city (DuRant, Getts, Cadenhead, & Woods, 1995; Mercy & Saltzman, 1989; Saltzman et al., 1990; Stark & Flitcraft, 1991). An individual with this profile is also the most likely person to witness lethal violence in the community, to be the victim of child physical abuse, and to die by by spousal homicide or other violent means (Hammond & Yung, 1993; Hampton, 1987; Rosenberg & Mercy, 1991). All adult victims and perpetrators are more likely than nonvictims and nonperpetrators to be unemployed, welfare-dependent, school dropouts, and residents of public or substandard housing (Crittenden & Craig, 1990; Hampton, 1987; Stark & Flitcraft, 1991). All child and adolescent victims and perpetrators of violence are also more likely to have come from low-income families and to be performing poorly in school, suggesting future risk for poor employment and other related negative socioeconomic outcomes (Cotten et al., 1994; Kulig, Valentine, & Steriti, 1994; Schubiner et al., 1993).

Many adult and adolescent perpetrators of violence have co-varying problem behaviors, including alcohol abuse, use or sale of illegal drugs, and involvement in other criminal activities. Both batterers and their victims are likely to be abusers of alcohol (Stark & Flitcraft, 1991) and high blood alcohol levels have been found in both homicide victims and their killers in a majority of domestic and non-domestic fatalities (Hammond & Yung, 1993). Use and sale of drugs has been found to be a strong predictor of victimization of youth and their carrying of guns for aggressive purposes. Gun carriers are also prone to associate with deviant peers, especially other gun carriers, to fight with peers and strangers more often, and to have arrest records (Sheley, McGee, & Wright, 1992; Webster et al., 1993).

Much expressive violence is likely to show persistence over time, with a strong probability of escalation unless an intervention occurs. A history of battering is a frequent antecedent to violent death, resulting either in the killing of the victim or a revenge slaying of the offender (Mercy & Saltzman, 1989; Stark & Flitcraft, 1991). A majority of child abuse fatalities were preceded by earlier complaints and investigations of maltreatment (Crittenden & Craig, 1990). Many incidents of youth homicide began as arguments, increased in intensity over time, and ultimately turned into a lethal confrontation (Jenkins, 1995).

Research on expressive violence among African Americans shows strong correlations among the various manifestations of violence. Previous victimization and witnessing of violence are predictors of youth fighting, gun carrying, and the killing of others as well as other negative outcomes (Bell & Jenkins, 1993; DuRant et al., 1994; Schubiner et al., 1993). Many child abusers were themselves abused as children and/or came from families where there was violence between their parents. Similarly, many batterers and their victims experienced and/or witnessed violence in their homes as they grew up (Stark & Flitcraft, 1991).

None of these risk factors or personal characteristics represents a direct causal relationship to violent behavior or victimization. The majority of African Americans who live in disadvantaged circumstances do not engage in violent behavior (Hammond & Yung, 1993); nor do the majority of abused children or child witnesses to domestic violence grow up to be violent or to be the victims of abuse although they are more likely to have such involvement than those who were not victims or witnesses of within-family violence (Oliver, 1993; Spatz-Widom, 1989). Perhaps highest on the continuum of risk for future violence perpetration, children who have both witnessed violence between their parents and have been victims of family violence show more antisocial and aggressive behavior than do nonwitnesses, nonvictims, or those who have been witness only or victim only (Hughes, 1988).

The demographic similarities between violence victims and aggressors suggests that some risks for family and community violence clearly fall into the category of environmental factors, chiefly the conditions frequently associated with poverty (e.g., limited resources, residence in communities with high crime rates, and adverse future prospects). Attar, Guerra, and Tolan (1994) determined that neighborhood disadvantage and community-level stress were significantly related to the development of aggressive behavior in young African-American children. Elliott (1994a, b) has argued that the conditions of poverty contribute to the perpetuation of violent behavior once initiated. In his longitudinal study of chronic violent offending among males, he found few ethnic/racial differences in early propensity for violence (Elliott, Huizinga, & Morse, 1986). However, African Americans were more likely than Caucasian youth to continue violence into young adulthood; in his view this is attributable to the difficulties they experience in moving into conventional work and family roles. Racial/ethnic differences in treatment by law enforcement and the criminal justice system further contribute to the difficulties of breaking out of a pattern of violent and other criminal behavior. African-American adolescents and young adults are more likely than all other groups to be arrested for violent crimes and to receive harsher sentences (Jones & Krisberg, 1994; Office of Juvenile Justice and Delinquency Prevention [OJJDP], 1993).

The mutual interactions between risk factors and the cumulative effects of multiple risks are additional influences on the development and maintenance of violent behavior, particularly as related to the formation of dysfunctional behavioral scripts that can cyclically breed more violence. Physically abused children, child witnesses of domestic and community violence, and children exposed to early harsh discipline are more likely to develop cognitive beliefs and behavior patterns that support the perpetration of violence, for example, an inability to conceptualize solutions to conflict other than violence and a propensity to attribute hostile intent to others (Dodge, Bates, & Pettit, 1991; Weiss, Dodge, Bates, & Pettit, 1992). Such beliefs are characteristic of youth with histories of aggressive behavior and carrying guns (Dodge, Price, Bachorowski, & Newman, 1990; Slaby & Guerra, 1988; Webster et al., 1993). An accumulation of risk factors contributes to the greater probability of engaging in a variety of aberrant behaviors, and various studies have found more overall exposure to risk factors for African-American children and adolescents than for other youth samples (Catalano et al., 1993; Vega, Zimmerman, Warheit, Apospori, & Gil, 1993).

The complexity of the dynamics and risk factors related to violence suggests that many avenues to violence prevention should be pursued, including changes in law and policy related to gun regulation and treatment of violent offenders in the criminal justice system; better service programs and protection for the victims of family and community violence; screening for victimization; improvements in the policing of violent neighborhoods; community development programs; and the use of environmental strategies to make schools and communities safer. Among the types of interventions vitally needed are programs to help youth develop positive skills that will enable them to develop and maintain violence-free relationships. This is the focus of the Positive Adolescent Choices Training (PACT) program.

DESCRIPTION OF THE PACT PROGRAM

Overview and History

In collaboration with the local public school system, PACT began as a demonstration project to determine whether social skills training would be an effective violence prevention or reduction strategy for high-risk African-American adolescents. After a brief pilot with older adolescents, the program selected as its target population adolescents in 7th or 8th grades (typically ranging in age from 12 to 16) who were identified by teachers as having mild to moderate histories of aggression, to have been victims or witnesses of violence, and/or to have social skills deficits. The PACT program has been partnered with the same middle school since 1989 and is now incorporated into the school's regular schedule as part of the health education curriculum. It serves between 50 to 60 adolescents annually. Youth receive their violence prevention training in small groups of 6 to 8 students who meet twice a week for one class period and the training is completed during a school semester.

The content of the program has undergone some evolution since its beginning. Initially, we relied on the use of the ASSET program (Hazel, Schumaker, Sherman, & Sheldon-Wildgen, 1981), which trained youth on seven social skills introduced to them by videotapes of peer models demonstrating the target skills. Although we liked the video format, the skills training procedures, and some of the evaluation procedures of this program, the videos themselves were problematic in that they did not show African-American role models and were less relevant to African-American youth in terms of language, dress, scenario content, mannerisms, and cultural "feel." We addressed this by developing our own youth videotape training aids, a three-set video program called *Dealing with Anger: Givin' It, Takin' It, Workin' It Out* (Hammond & Yung, 1991). For this series, we selected three target social skills, decreased and simplified the component steps in the skill, and used near-age African-American role models to demonstrate the correct use of the skills as well as modeling participation in the group training process. We also began to blend in exercises and activities from other model curricula, including the Violence Prevention Program of Prothrow-Stith (1987) and anger management components adapted from Feindler and Ecton (1986) and Goldstein and Glick (1987). We further added companion therapeutic games to reinforce student learning, to appeal to different learning styles, and to add fun and variety to the curriculum.

Today the principal components of the PACT approach are

1. Training on three social skills
   - Giving negative feedback (Givin' It)
   - Receiving negative feedback (Takin' It)
   - Negotiation (Workin' It Out)

The prosocial skills training component helps participants learn to express anger, frustration, or disappointment constructively, to listen and react appropriately to the criticism or anger of others, and to go through a problem-solving and compromise process to work out persistent disagreements.

2. Anger management training

Here participants learn to recognize anger triggers, to understand their anger responses, to think through consequences of their behavioral responses to anger, and to call upon techniques to control their anger.

3. Education/information about violence

In this component we stress dispelling myths about violence risk and raising awareness of the dynamics of violence, including experiences which occur within the participants' own environment. Emphasis is also placed on helping youngsters gauge potentially harmful situations and plan strategies to reduce their risk.

Rationale and Conceptual Foundation for the PACT Approach

PACT trains adolescents in safer, more appropriate, socially effective ways of interacting with others. Essentially it offers instruction and practice directed to helping participants add new behaviors, or to substitute for the behaviors that are likely to lead to physical conflict, ones which generate less antagonism. The model also works toward helping adolescents learn to recognize and control the powerful emotional reactions which can interfere with the performance of these positive behaviors.

The PACT approach is based on concepts and techniques drawn from social learning and anger control theory and research. It is also compatible with social interactionist constructs as applied to the situational precipitators and dynamics of violence.

Originating in the work of Bandura (1969, 1977), social learning theory maintains that social behaviors is learned by observing what other people do and what consequences their actions bring. Such learning is further shaped by positive and negative reinforcement that results from behaving in particular ways. Social behavior related to violence may be learned and maintained through a variety of influences which may include the following:

Modeling

Significant individuals in the child's life—parents, family members, other adults in the neighborhood, and peers—may have modeled behaviors of aggression or victimization that the child imitates in his or her own relationships. As noted earlier, research suggests a strong correlation between experiencing or witnessing violence and later demonstration of that behavior in the victim and/or witness (Busch, Zagar, Hughes, Arbit, & Bussell, 1990; DuRant et al., 1995; Patterson, 1982; Sheley et al., 1992; Spatz-Widom, 1989, 1990). The behavior modeling perspective strongly emphasizes the role of family members in training the child to initiate and retain coercive behaviors (Forehand, King, Peed, & Yoder, 1975; Patterson, 1982). The impact of the negative family modeling may be exacerbated by a lack of training for prosocial skills (Patterson, DeBaryshe, & Ramey, 1989). Many believe that the exposure of children and youth to other live models of aggressive behavior in the community and to violent role models in the media contributes substantially to the maintenance of aggression (DuRant et al., 1995; Slaby & Roedell, 1982).

Reinforcement Patterns

Parents and other adults may have failed to provide positive reinforcement for the performance of appropriate social behaviors and/or may have inadvertently reinforced negative behaviors by providing attention for aggressive behavior (Patterson, 1982). When youngsters continue to follow the coercive "scripts" they have learned at home or in the community in their interactions with other children, they may continue to be reinforced for such behavior. High-status peers, particularly those with similar aggressive tendencies, may reward coercive behavior such as being "tough" or bullying to take another child's possession. Victims may reward the behavior by showing fear or passively submitting to demands. Thus, an act of violence is reinforced as a source of power, status, control, or obtaining some material object that is desired (Epanchin, 1987; Patterson, Reid, & Dishion, 1992).

Cognitive Patterns and Responses

Particular patterns of faulty cognitive processes have been found to be more common both to aggressive and victimized children than to their peers (Coie, Dodge, Terry, & Wright, 1991; Dodge et al., 1990; Dodge et al., 1991; Slaby & Guerra, 1988). For example, such children are less able to problem-solve, to self-regulate their behavior, and to see things from another's perspective. They are also more likely to:

- Pay less attention to social cues
- Misread situations
- Make more negative evaluations of others
- Believe that others' intentions are hostile
- Believe that victims don't suffer
- Believe that victims deserve what they get
- Generate fewer alternatives to problem situations
- Report that they would respond with aggression to a problem situation
- Attribute hostile intentions to others, even in a neutral situation

Emotional Factors

Poorly controlled negative moods or states such as anxiety, anger, or depression can impair the performance of positive social behavior and contribute to responses of aggression. Anger in particular can be a strong trigger for aggression. If its intensity is not mediated by physical, cognitive, or behavioral control techniques, anger may prevent reasonable decision making as to how to handle a provocation nonaggressively (Feindler and Ecton, 1986; Novaco, 1976; Nelson, Hart, & Finch, 1993). Aggressive responses to anger can also be reinforced and maintained by social and psychological payoffs such as feelings of power and control a person may have when he or she becomes violent (Rokach, 1987).

Precipitators and Situational Dynamics of Confrontation

Social interactionist theory proposes that aggressive behavior is goal-directed and that an individual engages in acts of violence in order to control others' behavior, to achieve retribution, or to preserve self-image. An individual who lacks skill in using persuasion or verbal strategies may resort to coercion to get something he or she wants, for example, a behavior change in others. Similarly, a person may turn to violence in an attempt to "restore justice" in retribution for a perceived wrong or injury or to save face when his or her image has been challenged by a signal of disrespect (Felson & Tedeschi, 1993). This perspective may be especially informative in helping to advance understanding of violence among African-American youth, particularly male adolescents who are quick to fight over what many adults would consider trivial matters—putdowns, name-calling, insults about appearance, bumps, staring "too long," or other minor affronts. The ethnographer Anderson (1994) provides a particularly eloquent explanation of the issue of respect among young African-American men:

> There is a generalized sense that very little respect is to be had, and therefore everyone competes to get what affirmation he can of the little that is available. The craving for respect that results gives people thin skins. Shows of deference by others can be highly soothing, contributing to a sense of security, comfort, self-confidence, and self-respect. Transgressions by others which go unanswered diminish these feelings and are believed to encourage further transgressions. . . . Among young people, whose sense of self-esteem is particularly vulnerable, there is an especially heightened concern with being disrespected. Many inner-city young men in particular crave respect to such a degree that they will risk their lives to attain and maintain it. (p. 93)

Methods Used in the PACT Program

The PACT model is built around social skills and anger management training methods which assume that participants can learn new and more effective interpersonal skills and cognitive–behavioral scripts through systematic instruction introduced by models and reinforced through guided practice (Goldstein & Glick, 1987). Anger management interventions focus in particular on the development of self-control skills and substitute behaviors such as evaluating anger responses, behaviors, and consequences or using self-instructions or relaxation methods to calm down in order to help participants "unlearn" aggressive responses to anger that have been accepted through modeling and conditioning (Feindler & Ecton, 1986; Rokach, 1987). Training methods used in the PACT program also address the situational dynamics and immediate precipitators of violent acts. Learning a new skill involves not only performing the steps making up the skill, but understanding the rationale for using the skill and its individual component steps. These rationales can be especially persuasive if cast as a means of empowering youth with tools to help them get what they want from others. In addition, the group training sessions teach participants how to better interpret the verbal and nonverbal cues of others. Acquiring the ability to accurately observe and process social information reduces the tendency to presume hostile intent by others where it may not exist. Finally, teaching youth face-saving ways to address the complaints and verbal hostility of others and to back down through compromise decreases the possibility that a physical confrontation will break out over a trivial insult or slight.

A brief explanation of specific training methods used in the PACT program follows. A more detailed description of the model is available in the PACT Program Guide (Yung & Hammond, 1995).

Social Skills Training

The PACT program follows well-established methods traditionally used in social skills training programs; that is, it provides adolescent participants with observation of models who exhibit the behavior skillfully; opportunity for practice on the specific target skill through role-plays; feedback from others on the demonstration of the skill; and positive reinforcement as a favorable consequence for a skillful performance. Attention is given to following the principles of good modeling (Goldstein, Apter, & Harootunian, 1984; Kazdin, 1984). Our videotape vignettes show both near-perfect models and coping models in which youngsters show less than perfect performance. They also feature ethnically similar performers and emphasize the component skill steps visually and verbally. Group facilitators routinely conduct live modeling of the skills and the group participants conduct several role-plays of each skill as well as observing and giving feedback to each other during the role-play sequence. In addition, we videotape each session and frequently replay the videos so that participants may observe themselves performing the target skill. These modeling opportunities provide abundant opportunities for "overlearning," which is believed to contribute to the potential for retaining the skills and generalizing their use to nontraining situations (Goldstein et al., 1984).

For each target skill, the same sequence is followed:

- An initial videotape display of the skill
- Live role modeling by the group facilitators
- Group discussion of the rationale for each skill step
- Role-plays by each group member with coaching by facilitators as needed
- Self-evaluation of the role-play by the actors
- Feedback by group members and the group facilitator on the role-play performance

After completing classroom role-plays, participants are assigned "homework" in which they are encouraged to try the skill in a real-life situation and come back to the next session with a report on what happened. We attempt to make real-world use of the skills go more smoothly by a series of preparatory, processing, and reinforcing activities which emphasize anticipating and planning for possible reactions by others, teaching reinforcing self-talk for trials that may not have been entirely successful, and providing strong rewards for effort.

Anger Management

Several sessions are formally devoted to anger management, beginning with an introduction to what anger is, how it feels, and how to recognize it. We teach adolescents to be aware of such physiological signs of anger as muscle tension and breathing changes. One exercise that we have found to be helpful in developing this awareness is to have group members conduct a nonverbal role-play in which they demonstrate a feeling of anger without using words. We next introduce participants to the ABC exercise developed by Feindler and Ecton (1986) and also used in the Aggression Replacement Training program of Goldstein and Glick (1987). Through this exercise adolescents learn to analyze specific incidents as to the *anger trigger* (i.e., what provoked the feeling of anger), the *behavior* that followed the feeling of anger, and the *consequences* that resulted from the behavior. Special care is taken to help adolescents understand the distinction between anger and aggression. They are also taught simple cool-down techniques to help them calm down. Although we spend only a limited amount of time laying this foundation (2 to 3 sessions), related content is integrated throughout the entire program. For example, natural events occurring during training, for example, disputes between group members in which tempers flare, provide excellent opportunities to reinforce understanding of the anger/aggression distinction, the signals of anger, the use of cool-down techniques, and analysis of the feelings and behaviors which surrounded the incident.

Violence Risk Education

We believe there is value to dispelling common myths that adolescents may hold about violence (e.g., beliefs that carrying a gun will make you safer). In a survey of attitudes and knowledge about gun-related violence, Price, Desmond, and Smith (1991) found that there were distinct gender and ethnic differences in the beliefs of adolescents about the sources of violence risk. For example, African-American male adolescents were more likely than others to believe that African-American men who die violently are most often killed in a confrontation with police.

In the violence risk education provided in PACT, we teach our group members to understand the difference between expressive and other types of violence and the situational elements that may contribute to high risk (e.g., alcohol, guns, and bystander influences.) We use a web chart exercise adapted from Prothrow-Stith (1987) as one of the techniques for generating discussion about the common circumstances and characteristics of violence. We also teach participants to evaluate risk in particular situations through a checklist called "Scoping the Scene." This checklist prompts adolescents to consider power differentials between themselves and the person with whom they are in conflict, the impact of peer pressure during a confrontation, the likelihood of the other person carrying a weapon, and other factors which would help to determine the safest course of action. The exercise familiarizes them with "red flag" situations in which it would be better to walk away, seek adult help, or ignore a provocation.

Similar to anger management content, information about violence risk is integrated throughout the program. It is especially important to deal openly with violent events happening in the group setting, in the school, or in the broader community which may be of concern to the participants. Adolescents need the opportunity for cognitive processing of incidents such as a violent assault or murder of a classmate or neighbor. Newspaper articles or video news clips from local media can be used as discussion prompts. Using real events occurring in the group members' own lives as teaching tools helps to keep the training relevant.

We do not believe that violence risk education by itself would be sufficient as a prevention strategy. As substance abuse prevention programs have demonstrated, awareness of risk does not give youngsters either the tools or the motivation to avoid health risk behavior. However, we believe that this awareness-raising is valuable as part of a prevention package which includes skill-building and incentives for behavior change.

Therapeutic Games

We intersperse therapeutic and educational games at various points in the program and consider them helpful as motivators and reinforcers. Some games we use emphasize team-building and learning to cooperate in groups. Others reinforce special social skill training needs less directly addressed in the curriculum (e.g., learning to notice and interpret nonverbal signals or to give positive feedback). We also use games as a check of learning. For example, instead of a paper-and-pencil test of students' knowledge of the target social skills, we have them play "PACT Jeopardy." As in the television show, in this game students have to answer questions about the skill or its components or identify from video clips what skill was or should be used in a particular situation. They are awarded points and prizes for correct responses.

Reinforcement Systems

We recommend a structured reinforcement system to motivate youngsters to maintain good attendance and make progress in skill development. At minimum the system should include liberal use of praise and ideally it should incorporate social or material reinforcers such as field trips, parties, certificates of accomplishment, or food treats. Because we are typically operating at a secondary level of prevention with a student population already exhibiting some behavior problems, we use a formal incentive system in the PACT program. Participants are awarded token dollars for accomplishments such as getting to class on time, following instructions, volunteering for an activity, completing homework, and performing well in role-plays. They may exchange these dollars in the "PACT Store" for inexpensive items such as candy or sports cards, or save for more valuable items such as radios, basketballs, or watches. An end-of-the-year field trip is contingent upon good attendance and positive teachers reports.

Other Practices

We use other methods in the PACT program which we believe contribute to success in student motivaton, progress, and retention and to smooth integration into the environment at our host school. We pay particular attention to casting the program in a positive light to student participants. In our outreach materials, we focus on skill and leadership development and health and safety promotion rather than on the prevention of negative behavior. At school the program is referred to as the PACT Club. We allow students to develop the rules for expected behavior in the group sessions, to select their own team names and colors and to choose incentives for which they would like to work. We consider opening day an especially important session, as it shapes the program image in the participants' minds. If students do not gain an immediate positive perception, they are likely not to return after the first session. On the first day of class we turn the video camera toward the door so that students can see themselves on the monitor as they walk by or come into the room. We explain program purposes, logistics, and the incentive system, but spend a good portion of the session playing getting-to-know-you games. We later sponsor whole-school assemblies at which our group members do live skill demonstrations in order to demystify for their classmates what goes on in the PACT Club.

Our program is staffed by doctoral-level clinical psychology students who serve as the group co-facilitators. As a program "imported" to the school from outside, we have a critdical need to have excellent communication and cooperation from the school administration, teachers, and other school personnel. We provide an orientation for teachers to familiarize them with PACT program content, structure, referral processes, and expected outcomes. It is particularly important that teachers and other referral sources understand that a relatively brief social skills and anger management training program will not produce magical behavioral transformation in a youngster who is a chronic fighter or class disrupter. The more realistic expectation may simply be that after participation in this program he or she will fight less often and will be more open to discussing problems calmly. We maintain ongoing communication with teachers about student progress through progress notes and teachers' meetings. We also let the school know if there are going to be visitors to observe the program, or other unusual activities. We send thank-you notes and small gifts to demonstrate our appreciation for the school's cooperation. We welcome school administrator or teacher visits to our class and encourage them to participate in activities such as role-plays if they desire. Evidence of the success of these special efforts became apparent when the program and budget committee of our partner school voted to contribute to the funding of the PACT program. Although their support is modest, to us its major importance was the affirmation of the program as a tradition of the school.

Cultural Sensitivity in the PACT Program

Neither the theoretical models on which our prevention approach is based nor the intervention techniques in themselves are unique to work with African-American youth. We share the viewpoint expressed by Coatsworth, Szapocznik, Kurtines, and Santisban (1997), which recommends beginning with sound conceptual models and empirically tested methods and rendering them more acceptable, relevant, and accessible to ethnic minority youth through the use of culturally compatible content. Program content must take into account how ethnic-specific influences may affect the development and maintenance of the problem behavior. For example, an interventionist working with African-American youth in the area of violence must understand the issue of resepect and disrespect as a frequently present element influencing what happens in an angry confrontation.

We believe that success in work with African-American adolescent groups is inevitably linked to the participants' perceptions that what is being taught is applicable, and to their comfort with the daily activities and atmosphere of the program. Paying special attention to ethnic/cultural issues can produce more positive perceptions and better fit between the program and the participants. In the following sections we summarize how we have operationalized cultural sensitivity in the PACT program.

Environmental Features

We attend closely to creating a positive program image and a pleasant physical and social environment. We make special efforts to avoid a connotation of stigma associated with participating in the program. This reflects our understanding that African-American adolescents frequently feel they are singled out for prevention programs because of their potential or actual problem behavior. We stress positive peer culture and group behavior management techniques to avoid making participation aversive. Our walls are filled with positive slogans, artwork reflecting ethnic/cultural heritage, pictures of participants and other symbols of group identity, and records of group and individual accomplishments.

Ethnically Similar Role Models

Positive African-American role models are very visible in our program. They are shown in the video vignettes, on wall posters, and in the staffing of the program. Historically at least one of the group facilitators has been African-American and in most years we have had two. We recognize that shared ethnic background is not in itself a guarantee of cultural sensitivity but we believe that it promotes good rapport and a positive modeling effect. For programs that are not able to provide an ethnically similar group facilitator, we recommend that they make use of African-American parents or volunteers in some capacity.

Language

In all aspects of the program, we stress the use of concrete, familiar expressions that young African-American adolescents will understand. It is important for group facilitators to become familiar with the slang used by African-American adolescents, and where appropriate, to use these expressions in processing role-plays or in explaining concepts to the participants. An exception is vulgar or profane language. We understand that profanity is unfortunately a common feature of the language heard and used by urban African-American adolescents but we do not permit it in our groups.

Reality Base

The vignettes used in the videos which introduce the target skills were developed with consumer input around common sources of adolescent conflict ("he said/she said" rumors, disputes between family members, accusations of theft, etc.). All other scenarios role-played by the participants are based on conflict situations in their own lives. This aspect of the training method in itself gives a base of reality and relevance to program content. In addition, we make use of contemporary school or community issues as teaching tools for violence risk education.

Facilitator Preparation

There are several levels of preparation needed for maximum effectiveness as a facilitator for adolescent groups that are exclusively or predominantly African-American. Foremost is the need for prospective staff to examine their beliefs and assumptions about the participants—their goals, behavior patterns, characteristics, abilities to learn—and to look for any negative stereotypes or prejudices that would block effectiveness or convey low expectations. Staff of violence prevention programs also have particular need for honest self-examination of their views on violence among minority and/or disadvantaged youth, especially any erroneous beliefs around its ethnic/cultural origins and its acceptance or inevitability within the ethnic or cultural group. It is also critical for group facilitators to understand the culture and subcultures of the adolescents in their group; that is, common stressors, neighborhood attributes such as gang activity, whether interracial conflict is a major problem within the school or community, and other facets of the youngsters' immediate environment. Group leaders also need to become familiar with broader cultural influences, such as images of African-American youth in music and popular media. In addition, they need to be aware of and prepare for their role in the spotlight as positive models for the youth in their groups. They must keep in mind that they will convey messages with both their verbal and nonverbal behavior and that their use of the skills must be evident in all interactions with the adolescents.

Evaluation of the PACT Program

We use diverse measures of process, outcome, and impact of the PACT approach on the behavior of our young participants. In this section of the chapter, we will describe the evaluation methods used and highlight some of the findings as well as calling attention to the limitations of the evaluation design. Related data on program outcomes are available in other studies (Guerra, Tolan, & Hammond, 1994; Hammond & Yung, 1991; U.S. General Accounting Office, 1995). Instruments used in the program evaluation are published in the PACT Program Guide (Yung & Hammond, 1995).

Each year the referral list generates more students we can serve in the program. We do not carry out random assignment but instead select participants on the basis of availability to participate, as a function of fit with their academic schedules or involvement in other programs. Youngsters who are referred but who are unable to participate become the comparison group. Participation in the program is voluntary, but annually we have only a very small percentage (less than 1%) of youth who refuse to participate. All the outcome methods listed in the section that follows are tracked both on participant and control groups.

Observer Ratings

We use blind ratings by neutral observers of videotapes of individual adolescents demonstrating use of each of the three target skills in a role-play scenario acted out with an adult facilitator at pre- and postintervention levels. Ratings are done on a behavioral checklist specifying the presence or absence of each component skill step; skill step scores are averaged for a total performance score on a particular skill. This measure assesses these questions: Did the participating youth acquire the target skills? How did their skill change compare to that of the untrained youth?

Ratings by Teachers, Parents, or Other Significant Adults

We collect pre/post ratings by teachers, parents, or other significant adults on a more global measure of prosocial and anger management skills, measuring the three skills taught in addition to other, more "generic" prosocial skills. The instrument we use involves a Likert-scale rating and is modeled closely after the evaluation tools developed by Hazel, et al. (1981). This measure captures information as to whether the acquisition of the target skills has generalized to performance outside of training. It also enables us to determine whether the participating youth have acquired and demonstrated additional social skills and how adult perceptions of them compare to those toward untrained youth.

Self-Ratings

Using an adaptation of the global social skill instrument given to adults, we collect pre/post youth self-ratings to determine whether the intervention makes them feel more confident in their general levels of social skill performance and their ability to perform the three target social skills. In addition, we compare their perceptions with those of untrained youth.

School Behavioral Records

Each year we examine school disciplinary records, emphasizing actual *behavior* of students rather than *dispositions* such as suspensions or expulsions. Although we initially looked at the latter, experience has taught us that there are many variables affecting whether or not a student is suspended; for example, prior history of misbehavior, parental cooperation, alternative resources available, and other factors less directly indicative of the seriousness of the offense. Our process involves recording reports, kept in the principal's office, which document behavior problems exhibited by students in class, on school grounds, or on the school bus. Each incident notes the student's name, date of the incident, nature of the incident, and disposition. We categorize disciplinary incidents into three types:

1. *Physical aggression*—hitting, pushing, shoving, kicking, biting, spitting, or using a weapon. We also include throwing objects such as books which hit or could hit another person. Physical aggression has to be directed toward a person (e.g., if an adolescent slams a fist into the wall but his or her act is not threatening to someone else, we would code such an act as an "other misbehavior").
2. *Verbal intimidation or aggression*—threatening physical violence, profanity, or behavior described by teacher as "unruly" or "disruptive" or "mouthing off" but without any description of physical aggression as defined above.
3. *Other misbehavior*—skipping school, cutting class, refusal to do work, leaving school or class without permission, being in halls without hall pass, smoking in the bathroom, or miscellaneous negative behavior.

We track school disciplinary records for the entire school year during the period of participation. This tracking helps us to assess whether the behavior of participating youth at school changed during or after receiving training and how it compared to the behavior of untrained youth with similar characteristics.

Juvenile Court Records

We also examine charges recorded by the local juvenile court system, again emphasizing the underlying behavior as opposed to the disposition, which can be affected by previous court records, availability of good legal counsel, verbal or nonverbal behavior in the court hearing, and other variables. We categorize arrest charges into three categories:

1. *Violence-related offenses*—e.g., assault, homicide or attempted homicide, weapons-related, domestic violence, rape, menacing.
2. *Other criminal acts*—e.g., burglary, theft, drug offenses, vandalism, trespassing, probation violations.
3. *Status offenses*—acts for which youth may be charged because of their status as minors; includes truancy, running away from home, and incorrigibility

We track the entire pre/post juvenile court records of all participants and control youth, and we are able to continue this teaching up to age 18. This gives us valuable information as to whether the effects of training on violent or other criminal behavior are maintained over time and how the postintervention community behavior of trained youth compares to that of untrained youth.

Summary Results

Early studies demonstrated that African-American youth who completed training demonstrated improvement in the target skills as measured by pre- to post-observation of behavior by teachers and by youth trainers and that teachers perceived greater gains in targeted skills for PACT-trained youth than for untrained youth (Hammond & Yung, 1991). More recent analyses of school behavior records has shown that youngsters who received violence prevention training demonstrated a significant reduction in physical aggression at school; that their behavior improved during the course of training and was maintained beyond their participation in the program; and that youngsters who were referred on similar criteria but who did not receive training typically showed no reduction or increased levels of such incidents over the same time (Yung & Hammond, 1993). As one specific example, second-semester participants in the PACT program in 1993 ($n = 20$) had 15 pretraining incidents of physical aggression at school in comparison to 9 such incidents for comparison youth ($n = 19$). During and after their participation in PACT, incidents among the experimental group youth decreased to 7 whereas for comparison group youth, the number of aggressive incidents increased to 14 during the same time. There were slight differences in pre/post levels of verbal aggression in favor of trained youth, but these differences were not significant, nor were there any significant differences in other types of misbehavior such as cutting class.

Results of juvenile court record checks indicate that, over the course of time, untrained comparison youth have had higher general levels of involvement with juvenile court, more violence-related charges, and a higher per-person rate of offending than PACT-trained youth during the period of time that corresponds to postintervention for trained youth. In addition, untrained youth have also shown a trend of greater involvement in more serious types of criminal activity which carry greater risk of death or injury either to themselves or to others (e.g., breaking and entering, burglary, and criminal trespass). The proportion of untrained compared with trained youth engaging in violent and other criminal offenses has been about 2 to 1. We have also examined year-to-year changes in arrest records to determine maintenance effects of the PACT intervention. We have found that there is some worsening of behavior (i.e., increase in charges) for both trained and untrained youth over time but that the arrests of untrained youth are still double that of PACT-trained youth, even two years beyond the time of the intervention. For example, the numbers of violence-related charges for PACT youth increased from 3 in 1992 to 8 in 1993. However, for the comparison youth, such charges increased from 12 in 1992 to 21 in 1993 (Yung & Hammond, 1993).

Limitations of the Evaluation Design

There are limitations to our evaluation design: no random assignment, long-term follow-up on only one measure (juvenile court records), no attention placebo group, no structured way to capture data on victimization, selection of participants and controls from a single site, and no testing of the efficacy of a particular component vs. a different component (e.g., effects of using an incentive system vs. no use of material rewards). Ideally, a long-term follow-up would also include interviews or surveys that would capture information on self-reported aggression as well. As our former PACT participants enter adulthood, it would be very useful in the future to examine impact on relationships with domestic partners and children.

CONCLUSIONS

Just as there are limitations to our evaluation design, there are limitations as to what a time-limited prosocial skills training approach alone can do to diminish all of the risk factors that may contribute to violence in interpersonal relationships. Although not a direct cause, the chronic stressors of poverty certainly make it more likely that individuals will have fewer general resources to help them cope with frustration and conflict. A lack of such supports may make them more prone to lash out physically when angry. We note that many of our participants are experiencing academic as well as behavioral problems; this increases the probability that they will join the ranks of school dropouts and the unemployed. It is also clear that good short-term outcomes for some of our graduates are lost if they become enmeshed in drug use or sales. Our intervention approach addresses neither of these very real risks. However, we have experienced successes in reducing violent and other criminal behavior among high-risk youth and are encouraged that these nonviolent behaviors have been maintained over time. Our experiences lend merit to the idea that the cycle of violence can be broken.

REFERENCES

Anderson, E. (1994). The code of the streets. *Atlantic Monthly, 273*(5), 81–94.

Attar, B., Guerra, N., & Tolan, P. (1994). Neighborhood disadvantage, stressful life events, and adjustment in urban elementary-school children. *Journal of Clinical Child Psychology, 23*, 391–400.

Bandura, A. (1969). *Principles of behavior modification*. New York: Holt, Rinehart, and Winston.

Bandura A. (1977). *Social learning theory*. Englewood Cliffs, NJ: Prentice Hall.

Bell, C., & Jenkins, E. (1993). Community violence and children on Chicago's Southside. *Psychiatry, 56*, 46–54.

Busch, K., Zagar, R., Hughes, J., Arbit, J., & Bussell, R. (1990). Adolescents who kill. *Journal of Clinical Psychology, 46*, 472–485.

Catalano, R., Hawkins, D., Krenz, C., Gillmore, M., Morrison, D., Wells, E., & Abbott, R. (1993). Using research to guide culturally appropriate drug abuse prevention. *Journal of Consulting and Clinical Psychology, 61*, 804–811.

Centers for Disease Control. (1990). Homicide among young black males—United States, 1978–1987. *Morbidity and Mortality Weekly Report, 39*, 869–873.

Centers for Disease Control. (1996). *Injury mortality: National summary of injury mortality data, 1986–1994*. Atlanta, GA: Author.

Coatsworth, J., Szapocznik, J., Kurtines, W., & Santisban, D. (1997). Culturally competent psychosocial interventions with antisocial problem behavior in Hispanic youth. In D. Stoff, J. Breiling, & J. Maser (Eds.), *Handbook of antisocial behavior* (pp. 395–403). New York: Wiley.

Coie, J., Dodge, K., Terry, R., & Wright, V. (1991). The role of aggression in peer relations: An analysis of aggression episodes in boys' play groups. *Child Development, 62*, 812–826.

Cohen, N., Resnick, J., Browne, D., Martin, S., McCarraher, D., & Woods, J. (1994). Aggression and fighting behavior among African-American adolescents: Individual and family factors. *American Journal of Public Health, 84*, 618–622.

Council on Crime in America. (1996). *The state of violent crime in America*. Washington, DC: New Citizenship Project.

Crittenden, P., & Craig, S. (1990). Developmental trends in the nature of child homicide. *Journal of Interpersonal Violence, 5*, 202–217.

Dawson, J., & Langan, P. (1994). *Bureau of Justice Statistics special report: Murder in families*. Washington, DC: U.S. Department of Justice.

Dodge, K., Bates, J., & Pettit, G. (1991). Mechanisms in the cycle of violence. *Science, 250*, 1678–1683.

Dodge, K., Price, J., Bachorowski, J., & Newman, J. (1990). Hostile attributional biases in severely aggressive adolescents. *Journal of Abnormal Psychology, 99*, 385–392.

Dubrow. M., & Garbarino, J. (1989). Living in the war zone: Mothers and young children in public housing development. *Child Welfare, 68*, 3–20.

DuRant, R., Getts, A., Cadenhead, C., & Woods, E. (1995). The association between weapon-carrying and the use of violence among adolescents living in or around public housing. *Journal of Adolescence, 18*, 579–592.

DuRant, R., Pendergrast, R., & Cadenhead, C. (1994). Exposure to violence and victimization and fighting behavior by urban Black adolescents. *Journal of Adolescent Health, 15*, 311–318.

Elliott, D. (1994a). Serious violent offenders: Onset, developmental course, and termination—the American Society of Criminology 1993 presidential address. *Criminology, 32*, 1–21.

Elliott, D. (1994b). Longitudinal research in criminology: Promise and practice. In E. Weitekamp & H. Kerner (Eds.), *Cross-national longitudinal research on human development and criminal behavior* (pp. 189–201). The Netherlands: Kluwer Academic.

Elliott, D., Huizinga, D., & Morse, B. (1986). Self-reported violent offending: A descriptive analysis of juvenile violent offenders and their offending careers. *Journal of Interpersonal Violence, 1*, 472–514.

Epanchin, B. (1987). Aggressive behavior in children and adolescents. In B. Epanchin & J. Paul (Eds.), *Emotional problems of childhood and adolescents* (pp. 109–140). Columbus, OH: Merrill.

Feindler, E., and Ecton, R. (1986). *Adolescent anger control*. New York: Pergamon.

Felson, R., & Tedeschi, J. (1993). A social interactionist approach to violence: Cross-cultural applications. *Violence and Victims, 8*, 295–308.

Finklehor, D., & Dzuiba-Leatherman, J. (1994). Children as victims of violence: A national survey. *Pediatrics, 94*, 413–420.

Forehand, R., King, H., Peed, S., & Yoder, P. (1975). Mother–child interactions: Comparison of a noncompliant clinic group and a non-clinic group. *Behavior Research and Therapy, 13*, 79–85.

Gladstein, J., Slater-Rusonis, E., & Heald, F. (1992). A comparison of inner-city and upper-middle-class youths' exposure to violence. *Journal of Adolescent Health, 13*, 275–280.

Goetting, A. (1988). Patterns of homicide among women. *Journal of Interpersonal Violence, 3*, 3–20.

Goldstein, A., Apter, S., & Harootunian, B. (1984). *School violence*. Englewood Cliffs, NJ: Prentice-Hall.

Goldstein, A., & Glick, B. (1987). *Aggression replacement training: A comprehensive intervention for aggressive youth*. Champaign, IL: Research Press.

Guerra, N., Tolan, P., & Hammond, R. (1994). Prevention and treatment of adolescent violence. In L. Eron, J. Gentry, & P. Schlegel (Eds.), *Reason to hope: A psychosocial perspective on violence and youth* (pp. 383–403). Washington, DC: American Psychological Association.

Hammond, R., & Yung, B. (1991). Preventing violence in at-risk African-American youth. *Journal of Health Care for the Poor and Underserved, 2*, 359–373.

Hammond, R., & Yung, B. (1993). Psychology's role in the public health response to assaultive violence among young African-American men. *American Psychologist, 48*, 142–154.

Hampton, R. (1987). Family violence and homicide in the black community: Are they linked? In R. Hampton (Ed.), *Violence in the black family* (pp. 135–156). Lexington, MA: D.C. Heath & Company.

Hampton, R., & Newberger, E. (1985). Child abuse incidence and reporting by hospitals: Significance of severity, class, and race. *American Journal of Public Health, 75,* 56–60.

Hampton, R. L., & Yung, B. (1995). Violence in communities of color: Where we were, where we are, where we need to be. In T. Gullotta, R. Hampton, & P. Jenkins (Eds.), *When anger governs: Preventing violence in America* (pp. 53–86). Newbury Park, CA: Sage.

Harris, L. (1993). *A survey of experiences, perceptions, and apprehensions about guns among young people in America.* Boston: Harvard School of Public Health. Survey 930018 prepared by LH Research, Inc. for the Harvard School of Public Health under a grant from the Joyce Foundation.

Hazel, S., Schumaker, J., Sherman, J., & Sheldon-Wildgen, J. (1981). *ASSET: A social skills program for adolescents.* Champaign, IL: Research Press.

Hughes, H. (1988). Psychological and behavioral correlates of family violence in child witnesses and victims. *American Journal of Orthopsychiatry, 58,* 77–90.

Jenkins, P. (1995). Threads that link community and family violence: Issues for prevention. In T. Gullotta, R. Hampton, & P. Jenkins (Eds.), *When anger governs: Preventing violence in America* (pp. 33–45). Newbury Park, CA: Sage.

Jones, M., & Krisberg, B. (1994). *Images and reality: Juvenile crime, youth violence and public policy.* San Francisco: National Council on Crime and Delinquency.

Kann, L., Warren, C., Harris, W., Collins, J., Douglas, K., Collins, M., Williams, B., Ross, J., & Kolbe, L. (1995). Youth Risk Behavior Surveillance—United States, 1993. *Journal of School Health, 65,* 163–170.

Kazdin, A. (1986). *Behavior modification in applied settings.* Homewood, IL: Dorsey.

Kruttschnitt, C. (1993). Violence by and against women: A comparative and cross-national perspective. *Violence and Victims, 8,* 253–270.

Kulig, J., Valentine, J., & Steriti, L. (1994). A correctional analysis of weapon-carrying among urban high school students: Findings from a cross-sectional survey. *Journal of Adolescent Health, 15,* 90. Abstract of a Presentation at the Annual Meeting of the Society for Adolescent Medicine, March 16–20.

Lassiter, R. (1987). Child rearing in black families: Child-abusing discipline. In R. Hampton (Ed.), *Violence in the black family* (pp. 3–20). Lexington, MA: D.C. Heath & Company.

Lorian, R., & Saltzman, W. (1993). Children's exposure to community violence: Following a path from concern to research to action. *Psychiatry, 56,* 55–65.

Mercy, J., & Saltzman, L. (1989). Fatal violence among spouses in the United States, 1976–85. *American Journal of Public Health, 79,* 595–599.

Nelson, W., Hart, K., & Finch, A. (1993). Anger in children:A cognitive behavioral view of the assessment–therapy connection. *Journal of Rational–Emotive and Cognitive–Behavior Therapy, 11,* 135–150.

Novaco, R. (1976). The functions and regulations of the arousal of anger. *American Journal of Psychiatry, 133,* 1124–1128.

Office of Juvenile Justice and Delinquency Prevention. (1993). *Juveniles and violence: Juvenile offending and victimization.* Fact Sheet #3, July, 1993. Washington, DC: U.S. Department of Justice.

Oliver, J. (1993). Intergenerational transmission of child abuse: Rates, research, and clinical implications. *American Journal of Psychiatry, 150,* 1315–1324.

Osofsky, J., Wewers, S., Hann, D., & Fick, A. (1993). Chronic community violence: What is happening to our children? *Psychiatry, 56,* 36–45.

Patterson, G. (1982). *A social learning approach.* Vol. 3. *Coercive family process.* Eugene, OR: Castalia.

Patterson, G., DeBaryshe, B., & Ramsey, E. (1989). A developmental perspective on antisocial behavior. *American Psychologist, 44,* 329–335.

Patterson, G., Reid, J., & Dishion T. (1992). *Antisocial boys.* Eugene, OR: Castalia.

Price, J., Desmond, S., & Smith, D. (1991). A preliminary investigation of inner city adolescents' perceptions of guns. *Journal of School Health, 61,* 255–259.

Prothrow-Stith, D. (1987). *Violence prevention curriculum for adolescents.* Teenage Health Teaching Modules. Newton, MA: Education Development Center.

Richters, J., & Martinez, P. (1993). The NIMH Community Violence Project. I: Children as victims and witnesses to violence. *Psychiatry, 56,* 7–21.

Rokach, A. (1987). Anger and aggression control training: Replacing attack with interaction. *Psychotherapy, 24,* 353–362.

Rosenberg, M., & Mercy, J. (1991). Assaultive violence. In M. Rosenberg & J. Mercy (Eds.), *Violence in America: A public health approach* (pp. 14–50). New York: Oxford University Press.

Saltzman, L., Mercy, J., Rosenberg, M., Elsea, W., Napper, G., Sikes, K., & Waxweiler, R. (1990). Magnitude and patterns of family and intimate assault in Atlanta, Georgia, 1984. *Violence and Victims, 5,* 3–17.

Schubiner, H., Scott, R., & Tzelepis, A. (1993). Exposure to violence among inner-city youth. *Journal of Adolescent Health, 14,* 214–219.

Shakoor, B., & Chalmers, D. (1991). Co-victimization of African American children who witness violence: Effects on cognitive, emotional, and behavioral development. *Journal of the National Medical Association, 83,* 233–237.

Sheley, J., McGee, Z., & Wright, J. (1992). Gun-related violence in and around inner-city schools. *American Journal of Diseases of Childhood, 146,* 677–682.

Slaby, R., & Guerra, N. (1988). Cognitive mediators of aggression in adolescent offenders. I: Assessment. *Developmental Psychology, 24,* 580–588.

Slaby, R., & Roedell, W. (1982). The development and regulation of aggression in young children. In J. Worrell (Ed.), *Psychological development in the early years* (pp. 97–149). New York: Academic Press.

Spatz-Widom, C. (1989). Does violence beget violence? A critical examination of the literature. *Psychological Bulletin, 106,* 3–28.

Spatz-Widom, C. (1990). The cycle of violence. *Science, 244,* 160–166.

Stark, E., & Flitcraft, A. (1991). Spouse abuse. In M. Rosenberg & J. Mercy (Eds.), *Violence in America: A public health approach* (pp. 123–157). New York: Oxford University Press.

United States Department of Health and Human Services. (1995). *Health-risk behaviors among our nation's youth, 1992* (DHHS 95-1520). Hyattsville, MD: Author

U.S. Department of Justice (1994). *Violent crime.* NCJ-147486. Washington, DC: Bureau of Justice Statistics.

United States General Accounting Office. (1995). *School safety: Promising initiatives for addressing school violence* (GAO/HEHS-95-106). Washington, DC: Author.

Valois, R., McKeown, R., Garrison, C., and Vincent, M. (1995). Correlates of aggressive and violent behaviors among public high school students. *Journal of Adolescent Health, 16,* 26–34.

Vega, W., Zimmerman, R., Warheit, G., Apospori, E., & Gil, A. (1993). Risk factors for early adolescent drug use in four ethnic and racial groups. *American Journal of Public Health, 83,* 185–189.

Webster, D., Gainer, P., & Champion, H. (1993). Weapon carrying among inner-city junior high school students: Defensive behavior vs. aggressive delinquency. *American Journal of Public Health, 83,* 1604–1608.

Weiss, B., Dodge, K., Bates, J., & Pettit, G. (1992). Some consequences of early harsh discipline: Child aggression and a maladaptive social information processing style. *Child Development, 63,* 1321–1335.

Yung, B., & Hammond, R. (1993). *Evaluation and activity report: Positive Adolescent Choices Training program.* Final grant report to the Ohio Governor's Office of Criminal Justice Services. 92-DG-B01-7138.

Yung, B., & Hammond, R. (1995). *PACT. Positive Adolescent Choices Training: A model for violence prevention groups with African-American youth. Program guide.* Champaign, IL: Research Press.

Yung, B., & Hammond, R. (1997). Antisocial behavior in minority groups: Epidemiological and cultural perspectives. In D. Stoff, J. Breiling, & J. Maser, *Handbook of antisocial behavior* (pp. 474–495). New York: Wiley.

14

Prevention during Adolescence
The Youth Relationships Project

ANNA-LEE PITTMAN, DAVID A. WOLFE, and CHRISTINE WEKERLE

VIOLENCE IN THE LIVES OF CHILDREN AND ADOLESCENTS

The pervasiveness of domestic violence, coupled with the limitations of attempting to treat offenders after the fact (Dutton, 1994; Wolfe & Wekerle, 1993), point to the need for theory-based prevention strategies. Many children and youth—close to one-third, according to a national survey (Boney-McCoy & Finkelhor, 1995)—are assaulted by a family member. In addition, many are subjected to marital violence: according to the national survey on violence against women and children in Canada, 3 in 10 women currently or previously married have experienced at least one incident of physical or sexual violence at the hands of a marital partner (Statistics Canada, 1993).

The significance of such family dynamics is finally being recognized, but the solutions are difficult. Children in these families will witness repeated episodes of wife assault during their formative years (Sinclair, 1985). Disturbingly, such exposure increases the likelihood that they will repeat similar relationship patterns as they begin dating in adolescence (Wolfe, Wekerle, & Scott, 1997). Young women are more accepting of threats and violence from boyfriends, and young men handle their frustration by using the behavior that has been modeled by their fathers (Jaffe, Wolfe, & Wilson, 1990). To no one's surprise, relationships, especially those formed in childhood and adolescence with caregivers, peers, and intimate partners, are both the training ground and the mode of expression of much personal violence.

Dating violence is becoming an issue of greater awareness and concern among teenagers. Approximately one-fifth of high school women have experienced at least one form of sexual or physical abuse in a dating relationship (Bergmann,

ANNA-LEE PITTMAN and DAVID A. WOLFE • Department of Psychology, University of Western Ontario, London, Ontario, Canada N6A 5C2.   CHRISTINE WEKERLE • Department of Psychology, York University, North York, Ontario, Canada M3J 1P3.

Handbook of Child Abuse Research and Treatment, edited by Lutzker. Plenum Press, New York, 1998.

1992; Sudermann & Jaffe, 1993). Consequently, a greater tolerance for and acceptance of abusive, controlling interaction patterns with dating partners emerges from some youth, especially in the context of steady dating relationships (Bethke & Deloy, 1993).

Adolescence is a critical point in the development of intimate relationships; therefore, educating youths about relationships and nonviolent problem resolution methods holds promise as a viable prevention strategy. Prevention entails both an "escape" from a negative life course (Rutter, 1987), as well as an enhancement of competency and knowledge that leads to desired life outcomes. The development of interpersonal adjustment problems among youths who were child victims of maltreatment is readily explained by a number of prominent developmental theories, such as attachment theory (e.g., Crittenden & Ainsworth, 1989), social information processing theory (e.g., Strassberg & Dodge, 1995), and developmental psychopathology (Cicchetti, Toth, & Bush, 1988). Each of these explanations articulates the importance of relationships as an organizer of social experiences, which is reflected in the conceptual model underlying the intervention components described here.

The Role of Prevention with Youth

Prevention programs have been developed for a variety of health problems and social behavior problems, such as smoking, substance/alcohol abuse, teenage pregnancy, eating disorders, family violence, and child abuse (Pransky, 1991). Because treatment alone cannot solve these social problems, something else needs to be done to prevent them from occurring. Most social behavior problems such as smoking, alcohol abuse, and violence have strong learning components which point to the necessity to provide skills and alternative attitudes and behaviors that will prevent the behavior problems from appearing.

However, few prevention programs for adolescents deal with the issues of dating violence (Dryfoos, 1990; Pransky, 1991; Lavoie, Vezina, Piche, & Boivin, 1995). Most prevention efforts with youth are aimed at such health problems as eating disorders, sexual behavior, and substance abuse, whereas violence prevention has generally focused on gang violence or sexual abuse (Pransky, 1991). Therapeutic interventions designed specifically for adolescents are also a relatively recent development. Individual, family, and group therapy programs have all been utilized with different approaches and philosophies in order to curb the violent or victimized behaviors of adolescents. In general, group programs for adolescents from violent families address three skill areas in which victims and perpetrators are both deficient: interpersonal skills, problem-solving skills, and cognitive-coping skills (Straus, 1994). Bringing youth together in a group program helps those from violent backgrounds find peer connection, support, and empowerment.

The American Psychological Association (1993) has also identified important characteristics of effective prevention programs:

- Begin as early as possible in the child's life.
- Address violence as one of many problems that the adolescent and family have.

- Include multiple components that reinforce each other across the child's everyday social contexts such as family, school, peer groups, media, and community.
- Take advantage of developmental "windows of opportunity"—points at which programs are especially needed or likely to make a difference.

Core Themes Related to Prevention of Relationship Violence

We have identified several themes related to the expression and prevention of violence in relationships, themes that set the stage for a health promotion effort aimed at building healthy, nonviolent relationships among youth (adapted from Wolfe et al., 1997):

1. *The expression of violence is most commonly seen in the context of relationships.* We define violence as an issue of power over another, rather than physical injury alone, and thus the relationship itself becomes an important area of concern.
2. *Current policies to address personal violence are outdated and superficial.* We believe that in order to make a significant dent in the incidence of violent and abusive acts, alternative messages, models, and principles for developing healthy, nonviolent relationships must occur systematically. Current policies aimed at preventing violence continue to focus on the most visible and personally frightening forms, especially street and school violence among youth. The more pervasive and systemic forms of violence in the home are ignored, and it is these forms that establish pathways to the next generation.
3. *Violence does not affect everyone equally—it is ingrained in cultural expressions of power and inequality, and affects women, children, and minorities most significantly.* Women's longstanding inequality has a powerful impact on their life experiences, and especially their male–female relationships. To be effective, prevention efforts must reflect the reality of women's lives in terms of inequality and relative imbalance of power, as well as the nature of adolescent relationships in general.
4. *Prevention of violence entails building on the positive (through empowerment) in the context of relationships, not just focusing on individual weaknesses or deviance.* Empowerment plays a very important role in redressing the inequalities and imbalances that contribute to the abuse of power (Amaro, 1995). Through connection with others, youth share their common experiences and concerns, which in turn generates personal power and important resources for change.
5. *Youth are important resources and are part of the solution.* Adolescence marks the stage where primary affective ties are being moved from the family to the peer network and romantic partnerships. This developmental period thus affords an ideal opportunity to influence negative relationship themes from the past as well as the present, such as male entitlement, dominance, and aggression, and female passivity and deference.

THE YOUTH RELATIONSHIPS PROGRAM

The themes and organizing principles just discussed helped to shape the Youth Relationships Project (YRP), a program developed for youth with their prominent input and involvement. The YRP targets the prevention of violence in dating relationships as a way of interrupting the cycle of child abuse and woman abuse in future relationships. Accordingly, it was designed to provide awareness and interpersonal skills development through education, problem solving, and social action opportunities for adolescents who are at risk of becoming victims or perpetrators of violence. The underlying goal is to provide them with the requisite skills before problems emerge, rather than treating problems after they have become entrenched in their personal relationships.

The "window of opportunity" we have chosen for successful prevention and intervention is midadolescence, ages 14–16 years. At this age, adolescents are beginning to look more and more toward their peers for confirmation, acceptance, and support (Furman & Buhrmester, 1992). Dating relationships are also becoming significant for both males and females. Because adolescents are beginning to consider dating relationships and peer groups highly significant, this is an excellent opportunity to educate them about violence as well as help them develop communication, competency, and coping skills.

YRP Goals and Objectives

Based on the themes noted above, we identified four primary goals that formed the foundations for an 18-week group program (Wolfe et al., 1996). These goals are (1) to help youth develop an understanding of the foundations of abusive behavior, including an examination of their own attitudes and beliefs about relationship violence; (2) to develop and enhance skills needed to build healthy relationships, and to recognize and respond to abuse in their own relationships and in relationships of their peers; (3) to understand the societal influences and pressures that can lead to violence and to develop skills to respond to these influences; and (4) to increase their social competencies through community involvement and social action.

To accomplish these goals, youth examine the role of media in enhancing and glamorizing violence, and explore issues of power and control in familial, societal, and relationship contexts. Community agencies and persons are introduced as sources of help and assistance. Social action offers youth a vehicle for empowerment and opportunities for them to make a difference through their social action efforts. The program involves people from their own communities, including former victims and perpetrators of violence, who provide perspectives and awareness regarding the impact of violence in the home and in the community.

The aspects of relationship dynamics which we have identified as suitable targets for prevention of violence and promotion of healthy relationships are outlined in Table 1. We assume that the risk factors identified will have a strong influence on the formation of abusive relationships. By focusing on these risk factors we intend to provide skills and attitudes to counteract these behaviors and prevent abuse from developing in interpersonal relationships. Rather than attempting to address historical factors, such as their own histories of maltreatment, this strat-

Table 1. Moving from Theory to Practice: The Youth Relationships Project's (YRP) Intervention Model

---

YRP prevention goals

1. To prevent violence in close relationships (peer, dating) with respect to both "offender" and "victim" behaviors.
2. To promote positive, egalitarian relationships.

YRP target population

Risk status: History of child maltreatment, including one or more of the following experiences:
    a) witnessing domestic violence
    b) physical abuse
    c) sexual abuse
    d) emotional abuse
    e) physical or emotional neglect

YRP intervention concerns

Cognitive/attentive dimension	Current risk factors
I. Victim/victimizer relationship models	—Current insecure attachment models
	—High interpersonal sensitivity/hostility
II. Power-abusive relationship views and values	—Gender role rigidity
	—Sexist, pro-violent relationship expectations
Behavioral dimension	
III. Conflict resolution and communication skills	—High power assertion in relationships
	—High conflict avoidance
	—Limited problem-solving ability
	—Low positive verbal assertion in relationships
	—High risk-taking/low safety and protection skills

Source: Wolfe, Wekerle, & Scott, 1996.

egy focuses on building on current strengths and exposing youths to healthy role models at a time when they are motivated to learn (Wolfe et al., 1997).

Participants

Our intervention model presumes that relationship violence begins with "initiation" behaviors prior to age 15 (e.g., teasing, pushing, throwing things), and escalates over the next few years of adolescence and young adulthood among those at risk. Support for this model is found in studies of high school students indicating that both males and females engage in low-level coercion and abuse during mid-adolescence (Mercer, 1987; Suderman & Jaffe, 1993; Wolfe, Wekerle, Reitzel-Jaffe, & Lefebvre, in press-b). Young men and young women participate together in the weekly groups; this affords greater opportunity to learn from one another about healthy relationships and to role-play problem-solving skills.

"Risk" of violence in teen and future relationships is defined on the basis of prior maltreatment in childhood, largely because both direct and indirect experiences of family violence increase the probability of violence in future relationships. Although many prevention studies with adolescents concentrate on 15- to

19-year-olds (Dryfoos, 1990), prevention of relationship violence must take place earlier. The 14- to 16-year age range encompasses a transition period for may adolescents who are beginning to date socially. Their interest and motivation to learn about relationships is approaching its peak, and they are also likely to imitate many different relationship patterns—both healthy and unhealthy—that they are exposed to at home, school, and in the media.

The program is appropriate for youth from all types of backgrounds, even though it is particularly aimed at those who experienced violence and abuse while growing up. By this age many youths have been involved in some degree of relationship conflict and abuse, either while going up or in dating situations, yet the patterns are still quite malleable. For research purposes, additional selection criteria have been developed to provide uniformity among group participants, but generally the program has been equally effective with and well-received by youth who are receiving child protective services (due to severe histories of maltreatment), and by a random sample of high school students who report above-average experiences of child maltreatment or domestic violence while growing up.

Description of Program Activities

The YRP operates as an 18-week program. Adolescents meet in small groups for two hours per week with a male and a female facilitator. This is a multifaceted program incorporating a number of learning and educational aids such as videos, print material, discussions, exercises, guest speakers, and action projects. The program is divided into four sections as identified in Table 2. Each section provides

Table 2. The Youth Relationships Project: Program Sections and Weekly Session[a]

Section A: Violence in Close Relationships: It's All about Power
    Session 1   Introduction to Group
    Session 2   Power in Relationships: Explosions and Assertions
    Session 3   Defining Relationship Violence: Power Abuses

Section B: Breaking the Cycle of Violence: What We Can Choose to Do and What We Can Choose Not to Do
    Session 4   Defining Powerful Relationships: Equality, Empathy, and Emotional Expressiveness
    Session 5   Defining Power Relationships: Assertiveness instead of Aggressiveness
    Session 6   Date Rape: Being Clear, Being Safe

Section C: The Contexts of Relationship Violence
    Session 7   Date Rape and Learning How to Handle Dating Pressure
    Session 8   Gender Socialization and Societal Pressure
    Session 9   Choosing Partners and Sex-role Stereotypes
    Session 10 Sexism
    Session 11 Media and Sexism

Section D: Making a Difference: Working towards Breaking the Cycle of Violence
    Session 12 Confronting Sexism and Violence Against Women
    Session 13 Getting to Know Community Helpers for Relationship Violence
    Session 14 Getting Out and About in the Community: Social Service Agencies
    Session 15 Getting Out and About in the Community: Social Service Agencies
    Session 16 Getting Out and About in the Community: Social Action to End Relationship Violence
    Session 17 Getting Out and About in the Community: Social Action to End Relationship Violence
    Session 18 Celebration!

---

[a]From the table of contents of the Youth Relationships Project Manual (Wolfe et al., 1996).

opportunities to gain information regarding issues of violence in relationships, as well as opportunities to develop skills for healthy interpersonal relationships. There are five stages to be incorporated into each lesson when teaching new skills: teach, show, practice, reinforce, and apply (McWhirter, McWhirter, McWhirter, & McWhirter, 1993). These stages are incorporated throughout the program when developing healthy relationship and problem-solving skills. All skills are role-modeled by the co-facilitators, opportunities are given for rehearsal, and ways to practice outside the group are suggested. Prevention of relationship violence, therefore, is achieved through education and information, skill development, and a opportunity for social action—the chance to make a difference and educate others.

Section A: Violence in Close Relationships: It's All about Power

The first three sessions of the program provide a opportunity for the youth and the facilitators to get to know each other and to develop a relationship on which to build in the following weeks. To establish guidelines regarding what is acceptable and what is not acceptable behavior during the group program, youths are asked to develop group agreement with some guidance from the facilitators. This agreement usually involves guidelines regarding attendance, punctuality, smoking, alcohol/drug use, use of foul language, and so on. The group agreement is hung in a prominent location for all to view each session. By the end of the third session, participants are asked to initial the agreement, indicating their willingness to abide by the guidelines established. This exercise provides the youths with a opportunity to attain ownership for their behavior within the group setting. It empowers the youth to speak up when inappropriate behavior occurs among members of the group. This agreement also reduces (but does not eliminate) the responsibility of the co-facilitators to police inappropriate behavior. Each session begins with a check-in, which provides participants with a opportunity to share with the others what has been happening in their lives in the past week. A recap of the previous session follows the check-in, providing everyone with a few moments to review what was discussed and learned and to ask any questions that may have arisen since the last session.

Power dynamics in interpersonal male–female relationships are examined throughout these early sessions. To discuss what makes a person powerful, teens identify their own situations or privileges, such as access to resources, jobs, education, family income, race/ethnicity, gender, and so forth. The "Myths and Facts of Woman Abuse" are explored through the use of a questionnaire allowing youths to test their knowledge regarding violence and abuse. The Power and Control Wheel, developed by the Domestic Abuse Intervention Project of Minneapolis–St. Paul, is used to distinguish how power is abused in male–female interpersonal relationships. Tactics include using coercion and threats, intimidation, emotional abuse, isolation, minimizing, economic abuse, and using male privilege.

Assertiveness skills such as positive communication, active listening, empathy, and emotional expressiveness are developed in these sessions, as well as an exploration of feelings. Youths are encouraged to identify feelings of happiness and anger, as well as more subtle feelings which are not always easily expressed. Participants are challenged to discuss the premise of the program, which focuses on men's violence toward women. Male and female adolescents have difficulty acknowledging that even though both males and females can be abusive, their expressions of anger and violence cannot be considered equal because of the imbalance of power and the ability of men to evoke fear (Jacobson et al., 1994).

Section B: Breaking the Cycle of Violence: What We Can Choose to Do and What We Can Choose Not to Do

The next three sessions continue to build on the first three by exploring power dynamics in relationships as well as aspects of healthy and unhealthy relationships, and comparing these elements. Woman abuse is further explained through the use of a video ("Break the Cycle") and guest speakers, who provide their own personal accounts of the effects of woman abuse in their lives (a strict protocol for selecting and obtaining these speakers is provided in the YRP manual). The male speaker must be a person who has been through counseling, has been nonviolent for a period of two years, and can openly accept that he has been abusive to his partner. He must be able to own his power and admit to how he exploited it in the context of his relationship with his partner. Our experience with this aspect of the program and the response from group participants indicates that this is an interesting and informative part of the program.

Further healthy relationship skills are explored during these sessions, which include exercises that develop attending skills, empathy skills, and listening skills. The DESC protocol developed by Bower and Bower (1976) is used to practice the four-step breakdown of an assertive statement: Describe, Express, Specify, Consequences. This is a assertiveness script which includes statements such as When you . . . (describes the problem), I feel . . . (expresses how this behavior affects me). I want you to . . . (specify the behavior I want the other person to do), then I would, and you would. . . . (the consequences, what I would be prepared to do in return). Opportunity is provided to practice these steps based on recent conflicts as well as using them as a means of providing compliments.

Section C: The Contexts of Relationship Violence

This section is composed of five sessions which expand the issue of intimate violence to a broader setting, including societal, cultural, and media contexts. Videos are used to explain and portray issues of date rape, marital violence, power in relationships, and the portrayal of sexism in the media. These sessions inform youths about how society encourages, accepts, and condones violence and sex role stereotypes. Information regarding sexual assault is presented, including a video entitled "Date Rape," which depicts not only the situation, but, more important, how it is reported and handled by the court. Discussion then ensues regarding the impact of the situation on the victim, offender, family members, and friends, and youth problem-solve ways to prevent such situations in their own schools and communities.

While exploring gender socialization and societal pressure, youths are encouraged to role-play scenarios using the listening skills they have developed to date. The "Power to Choose" video depicts four scenes involving different power relationships, followed by ways of rehearsing healthy communication skills. An opportunity to practice giving compliments is provided in this section, because it is also important for teens to learn that healthy communication skills do not focus only on listening and being assertive. The "Warm Fuzzies" exercise provides all the group participants with an opportunity to express anonymously things that they like, respect, or admire about each person in the group, by having each group member write a compliment or a positive statement anonymously to the others. Each group participant is then able to read the positive comments and compliments they have received.

Another helpful exercise in this section is "How We Choose Partners." Participants, divided into groups by gender, are asked to develop lists of characteristics they would look for when choosing a best friend, a dating partner, and a husband or wife. Once the lists have been completed the groups come together to compare lists and discuss how they differ or are the same. They are also asked to examine critically the differences in characteristics they list when choosing a best friend versus a dating partner and determine why, and if, such differences may exist.

To examine sexism, participants engage in an exercise entitled "Act Like a Man or Act Like a Lady." Developed by Creighton and Kivel (1990), the purpose of this exercise is to increase awareness of gender stereotypes. Women are stereotyped as pretty, quiet, demure, caregivers, while men are characterized as strong, providers, and protectors. The participants read through a scenario between a father and son, and then between a mother and daughter. In both instances the parent admonishes the child for his or her behavior and tells him or her to act like a man/lady. This provides the participants with an opportunity to explore exactly what is meant by these phrases: What is expected when somebody tells you to act like a man? Are there acceptable ways of speaking, behaving, expressing emotions that are meant by this phrase? Does this confine ourselves as individuals to expressing ourselves in specific ways? This exercise allows the teens to examine which characteristics and attributes of males and females are valued and which are not.

Session 11 provides a dynamic opportunity for youths to test what they have learned in the group to date and their ability to make a point in an argument in a responsible pro-social manner. They create a mock TV talk show incorporating the character of a talk show host, similar to many of the talk show hosts who may be found on television today. The host is looking for the controversial aspects of woman abuse and family violence, and tries to direct the topic toward victim-blaming. The guest for the talk show, "Dr. Brutal," is an opinionated "expert" who relies on myths and misconceptions regarding woman abuse to answer the host's questions. The teens, serving as audience participants or panel experts, are given the opportunity to challenge Dr. Brutal about what is being said. They become the pro-social panel of experts who give the appropriate responses to the stereotypes that are being communicated by Dr. Brutal. When possible this exercise is videotaped, partly to simulate a live talk show, and partly to allow participants to review their performance and answers.

To examine the influence of media in defining sex role stereotypes, teens view and discuss the video "Dreamworlds." This video explores the many sexist images, particularly of women, that are built into rock videos. The ways in which women are objectified and portrayed in rock videos are examined thoroughly, followed by ample discussion of sexism in the media. Magazines are also examined for their sexist portrayal of men and women. Youths decode magazines to find sexist images of men and women in photographs, advertisements, headlines, captions, and they cut them out for display on poster board. Participants share with the rest of the group what it is about these items that are sexist, and how they enforce or encourage stereotypes. These sessions help to put the issues of violence and sexism in a cultural context, and help the youth to recognize the many overt and covert societal forces that encourage people to condone violence and sexism.

Section D: Making a Difference:
Working toward Breaking the Cycle of Violence

The final section gets youths out and about in the community and provides them with skills and opportunities to confront sexist attitudes, stereotypes, and myths about violence. Ways of dealing with these issues are discussed and practiced, and they explore firsthand how difficult it is to confront discrimination and abuse among members of their own peer groups as well as society in general. Specifically, youths are given opportunities to access and learn about social agencies in their community that provide assistance if relationship problems, including violence and abuse, become issues in their lives. Scenarios are provided, some from personal experiences and some from videos, where the actors are in trouble—pregnancy, date rape, and similar situations. For each scenario, group participants have to determine what the problems are and the best ways to solve them. Initial steps are taken, such as consulting a telephone book to find out what kinds of services are available in the community. Then, follow-up is made with these agencies by way of an appointment. Youths go to the agency to learn about the services offered and perhaps take a tour in pairs or small groups. Afterwards, they share with other members what they learned at the agency.

These exercises require the knowledge and support of the social agencies in the community. Facilitators contact the social agencies in advance to introduce the program, and to prepare staff for the phone calls they will receive from the youth. Youths are empowered by these visits because they realize there are places to go if violence is a problem, and they learn how to make choices and use skills to help themselves and others if necessary.

In the last few sessions, youths plan a social action event of their choice to raise awareness and/or money for an antiviolence cause or services. This event can be a fund-raiser, such as a carwash, bake sale, raffle, or march/walk-a-thon, or an awareness activity, such as a poster display, a letter to the local newspaper regarding issues of violence, or a community service event (such as organizing a game day for children in the local shelter). We encourage youths to "go public" about their attitudes and beliefs toward violence, and to take responsibility for and make commitments to positive change regarding violence in their lives and in their communities. Through these activities a sense of group cohesion and individual growth is attained. Finally, the program ends with a group celebration of the work they have accomplished, and opportunities to continue meeting informally are explored. Graduates of the program are often invited to return as assistant facilitators for the next program, or to act as spokespersons for the program.

Co-Facilitators

The co-facilitators for the YRP are usually social workers from the community who are familiar with issues of violence and adolescent behavior. Facilitators receive a two-day training program conducted by YRP staff. This includes education about the goals and philosophy of the program, an exploration of the roots of violence in our society, the choices we make when faced with conflict, the contexts of relationship violence, and personal and social options we have available in order to help break a cycle of violence. Practical issues regarding how to implement the exercises in the manual and how to deal with problem behavior, personal disclosures of violence, and safety issues are also explained. Because it is important for youths to be exposed to adults who share respectful, egalitarian relationships, facilitators also serve as powerful role-models of appropriate male–female interactions, communication, and so on. They must be aware of the ways in which their verbal and nonverbal behaviors can be interpreted by youths and be honest about the power and privilege they hold in society and in the group context.

Referral Activities

To evaluate the effectiveness of the YRP program with at-risk adolescents we have developed a referral system which enables us to identify those adolescents who are at risk and would therefore be suitable for the program. Currently, referrals are obtained from Child Protective Service agencies and from high schools. Social workers at the agencies review their caseloads and complete a brief questionnaire for any person who falls in the age category of 14–16 years. The questionnaire determines whether the adolescent has had a history of witnessing or experiencing violence during their childhood prior to age 12. If the adolescent is determined to be at risk based on their history of maltreatment, and meets the other eligibility criteria mentioned earlier, he or she is contacted and asked to participate in the program.

At high schools we use a general screening procedure. Several questionnaires are administered concerning family experiences and background, current adjustment, and dating experiences. These questionnairs are administered to all youth in the school, which avoids a "referral" process and the labeling or identification of students. In both cases adolescents who meet the broad eligibility criteria noted previously are asked to participate voluntarily in a group program regarding developing healthy relationships. The emphasis is placed on health promotion rather than violence prevention, which again avoids stigmatization and accurately reflects the approach of the program. At high schools as well as community agencies the response rate of youth has been high (more than 75% express interest, once contacted), and the subsequent dropout rate is approximately 20% on average. Table 3 presents the number of youths to date who have participated in the research evaluation of YRP groups, the average attendance rates among group members, and dropout rate once group has begun (based on failure to attend 5 or more of the 18 sessions).

Table 3. Attendance and Dropout Rates of Seven Recent YRP Groups[a]

	Number of youths per group	Attendance (%)	Dropout (%)
	11	95	0
	9	83	11
	10	84	30
	11	80	36
	12	80	16
	8	85	25
	14	75	28
Total N:	75	$\bar{x} = 83\%$	$\bar{x} = 20\%$

[a]Participants selected from five child protective service agencies in different communities.

Evaluation Progress

We are currently in the preliminary stages of evaluation of the long-term effects of the program on high-risk individuals. One of our first efforts in this regard was to develop a useful self-report measure of relationship conflict and abuse. The Conflict in Relationships (CIR) questionnaire was developed for this purpose, because existing instruments were not designed to assess the wide-ranging nature of conflict experienced by adolescents. This self-report measure is identical for males and females except for pronoun changes and the elimination of two items concerning sexual coercion that would not apply to females.

Items on the CIR are repeated in two sections: Part A reflects behaviors the respondent has shown *toward a dating partner* (i.e., offending behaviors, such as "did something to make her feel jealous"), whereas Part B reflects behaviors a dating partner has shown *toward the respondent* (i.e., victimization experiences). The measure was constructed to reflect aspects of physical and sexual coercion, psychological abuse, and positive communication strategies. Factor analyses produced three similar factors for Part A (offender experiences) and Part B (victim experiences) for both genders, labeled *Coercion, Emotional Abuse*, and *Positive Communication*. A validity study of the CIR was also conducted to determine its ability to discriminate relationship problems between adolescents with and without backgrounds of maltreatment. The two principal violence scales of the CIR (coercion and emotional abuse) discriminated between youths with backgrounds of maltreatment and those with no history of maltreatment, for both males' and females' reports of offender and victim experiences. Notably, high-risk males (compared to low-risk males) reported significantly more coercion and emotional abuse toward a dating partner, and also perceived their partner as exhibiting more coercion and emotional abuse toward them. In contrast, high-risk females reported more coercion (but not emotional abuse) toward their partners, and saw their partner as more coercive and emotionally abusive toward them, compared to low-risk females (Wolfe et al., in press-b).

Our initial evaluation involved a sample of 58 youth who were receiving services from a child protective service agency because of histories of abuse and neglect. First, Hierarchical Linear Modeling (HLM; Bryk & Raudenbush, 1987) growth analysis was used to explore the degree of interest, motivation, and understanding shown by youth at risk of relationship violence across the weeks of their involvement in our program. Based on weekly co-facilitator ratings, we found considerable growth occurring across the 18 weeks of the program, especially in terms of youth interest and support given and received (Wolfe et al., 1997). These within-group findings showed that the intervention is of interest to youth and results in observable changes in their knowledge of and involvement with the topic.

In the next aspect of the evaluation, we looked at the different emerging rates of growth between subjects randomly assigned to intervention or control conditions, using the CIR across 4 waves of data from pre- to 6-month follow-up (Wolfe & Wekerle, 1996). Controls continued to receive the normal services of the child agency, and by and large did not participate in any documented form of intervention. Level-two HLM analyses were conducted; these involved a comparison of growth curves for participants in each condition. The pilot outcomes are presented in terms of HLM analyses (Table 4), followed by a more traditional analysis of covariance (Table 5), for comparison of these two methods. Gender differences could not be taken into account with this small sample, but will be examined in future studies.

Table 4 indicates a trend ($p < .20$) for the mean growth rate for the intervention group to exceed that of controls, on the use of coercive tactics with a dating partner. The significant X^2 for variance in growth rate (Table 4) also suggests significant variation in the participants' changes in coercive behavior; as expected, some changed at a faster rate than others. Finally, 12.5% of the variance in rate of change on the CIR measure of coercion was accounted for by intervention status. With a greater number of waves and more subjects, these analyses will have more power to detect growth across conditions. Because the richness of HLM analysis is beyond the scope of this chapter, interested readers are encouraged to review

Table 4. HLM Linear Model of Change (Decline) on the CIR for Coercion

Final estimation of fixed effects				
Fixed effect	Coefficient	SE	t Ratio	p Value
Mean initial status, β0				
Intercept, G00	0.78	0.26	3.00	<.01
Exp. condition, G01	−0.15	0.11	−1.31	<.20
Mean growth rate, (slope, β1)				
Intercept, G10	0.00	0.10	0.03	<.40
Exp. condition, G11	0.06	0.04	1.32	<.20

Final estimation of variance components				
Random effect	Variance component	df	X²	p Value
Initial status, U0	0.05	47	61.38	<.10
Growth rate, U₁	0.01	47	64.64	<.05
Level-1 error R	0.05			
Variance explained by experimental condition:		Initial status 47.5%		Growth 12.5%

Table 5. Analysis of Covariance (with Pre-Test Scores) Comparing Treatment (N = 30) and Control (N = 28) Subjects on the CIR (N = 58) at Six-Month Follow-up

	Treatment		Control			
	M	SD	M	SD	F (1, 57)	p <
Conflict in Relationships subscales						
Coercion	.91	.45	1.17	.22	4.62	.05
Emotional Abuse	1.24	.50	1.39	.26	1.15	.30
Positive Communication	1.98	.66	2.20	.53	1.04	.32

Note: Subscale scores are averaged across all items, which can rage from 0 (did not occur) to 3 (occurred very often). The Positive Communication scale is inversed scored to be consistent with the other two; i.e., a higher score equals worse adjustment.

recent discussions (e.g., Bryk & Raudenbush, 1987; Osgood & Smith, 1995; Raudenbush, 1993; Willett, Ayoub, & Robinson, 1991).

The traditional way to look at these data above is to compare groups at follow-up, using analysis of covariance (covarying on the pre-test score), as shown in Table 5. Again, we see a significant difference on the coercion scale favoring the treatment condition, indicating less use of this strategy at 6-month follow-up. Again, with adequate sample size and power, additional effects would likely be demonstrated.

For the full evaluation of the YRP, additional measures regarding peer relations, trauma experiences, dating background, and conflict experiences during dating relationships are also completed by participants at the beginning of the group program, at midpoint, at the end of the program, and every 6 months thereafter for a period of two years. Brief telephone interviews are held with the subjects on a bimonthly basis to maintain contact, and to determine whether the subjects are dating and how the relationship is progressing. When subjects are engaged in a dating relationship, a video interaction is obtained of the couple attempting to solve a problem that exists in their relationship. Dating partners complete questionnaires about each other regarding social competence and conflicts they experience in their relationships. Results of this longer-term evaluation, involving approximately 400 youths across both conditions, will be available in 1999. We look forward to continuing to work with the youth involved in the program, to find new ways to stop the cycle of violence before the behaviors and attitudes become well established in adulthood.

REFERENCES

Amaro, H. (1995). Love, sex, and power: Considering women's realities in HIV prevention. *American Psychologist, 50,* 437–447.

American Psychological Association. (1993). *Commission on youth and violence summary report. Volume 1: Violence and youth: Psychology's response.* Washington, DC: Author.

Bergman, L. (1992). Dating violence among high school students. *Social Work, 37*(1), 21–27.

Bethke, T. M, & Deloy, D. M. (1993). An experimental study of factors influencing the acceptability of dating violence. *Journal of Interpersonal Violence, 8(1),* 36–51.

Boney-McCoy, S., & Finkelhor, D. (1995). Psychosocial sequelae of violent victimization in a national youth sample. *Journal of Consulting and Clinical Psychology, 63*(5), 726–736.

Bower, S. A., & Bower, G. H. (1976). *Asserting yourself: A practical guide for positive change.* Reading, MA: Addison-Wesley.

Bryk, A. S., & Raudenbush, S. W. (1987). Application of hierarchical linear models to assessing change. *Psychological Bulletin, 101,* 147–158.

Cicchetti, D., Toth, S., & Bush, M. (1988). Developmental psychopathology and incompetence in childhood: Suggestions for intervention. In B. B. Lahey & A. E. Kazdin (Eds.), *Advances in clinical child psychology* (Vol. 11, pp. 1–77). New York: Plenum Press.

Creighton, A., & Kivel, P. (1990). *Teens need teens: A manual for adults helping teens to stop violence.* Concord, CA: Battered Women's Alternatives.

Crittenden, P. M., & Ainsworth, M. D. S. (1989). Child maltreatment and attachment theory. In D. Cicchetti & V. Carlson (Eds.), *Child maltreatment: Theory and research on the* causes and *consequences of child abuse and neglect* (pp. 432–463). Cambridge, England: Cambridge University Press.

Dryfoos, J. G. (1990). *Adolescents at risk: Prevalence and prevention.* New York: Oxford University Press.

Dutton, D. G. (1994). *The domestic assault of women: Psychological and criminal justice perspectives.* Vancouver, BC: UBC Press.

Furman, W., & Buhrmester, D. (1992). Age and sex differences in perceptions of networks of personal relationships. *Child Development, 63,* 103–115.

Jacobson, N. S., Gottman, J. M., Waltz, J., Rushe, R., Babcock, J., & Holtzworth-Munroe, A. (1994). Affect, verbal content, and psychophysiology in the arguments of couples with a violent husband. *Journal of Consulting and Clinical Psychology, 62,* 982–988.

Jaffe, P. G., Wolfe, D. A., & Wilson, S. K. (1990). *Children of battered women.* Newbury Park, CA: Sage.

Lavoie, F., Vezina, L., Piche, C., & Boivin, M. (1995). Evaluation of a prevention program for violence in teen dating relationships. *Journal of Interpersonal Violence, 10*(4), 516–524.

McWhirter, J. J., McWhirter, B. T., McWhirter, A. M., & McWhirter, E. H. (1993). *At-risk youth: A comprehensive approach.* Pacific Grove, CA: Brook/Cole.

Mercer, S. L. (1987). *Not a pretty picture: An exploratory study of violence against women in high school dating relationships.* Toronto: Education Wife Assault.

Osgood, D. W., & Smith, G. L. (1995). Applying hierarchical linear modeling to extended longitudinal evaluations. *Evaluation Review, 19,* 3–38.

Pransky, J. (1991). *Prevention: The critical need.* Springfield, MO: Burrell Foundation.

Raudenbush, S. W. (1993). Hierarchical linear models and experimental design. In L. K. Edwards (Ed.), *Applied analysis of variance in behavioral science* (pp. 459–495). New York: Marcel Dekker.

Rutter, M. (1987). Psychosocial resilience and protective mechanisms. *American Journal of Orthopsychiatry 57,* 316–333.

Sinclair, D. (1985). *Understanding wife assault: A training manual for counsellors and advocates.* Toronto: Ontario Government Bookstore.

Statistics Canada. (1993). *Violence against women survey.* Ottawa, Ontario: Author.

Strassberg, Z., & Dodge, K. A. (1995). Maternal physical abuse of the child: A social information processing perspective. Unpublished manuscript, Vanderbilt University.

Straus, M. B. (1994). *Violence in the lives of adolescents.* New York: Norton.

Suderman, M., & Jaffe, P. (1993, August). *Dating violence among a sample of 1567 high school students.* Paper presented in a symposium entitled "Violence in adolescent relationships: Identifying risk factors and prevention methods" (D. Wolfe, Chair), at the annual convention of the American Psychological Association, Toronto.

Willett, J. B., Ayoub, C. C., & Robinson, D. (1991). Using growth modeling to examine systematic differences in growth: An example of change in the functioning of families at risk of maladaptive parenting, child abuse, or neglect. *Journal of Consulting and Clinical Psychology, 59,* 38–47.

Woke, D. A., & Wekerle, C. (1993). Treatment strategies for child physical abuse and neglect: A critical progress report. *Clinical Psychology Reviews, 13,* 473–500.

Wolfe, D. A., Wekerle, C. (1996, August). *Youth Relationship Project: Empowering youth to promote nonviolence.* Paper presented in a symposium titled "Beyond parenting skills: Parent–child relationships and child maltreatment" (L. Peterson, Chair), at the Annual Convention of the American Psychological Association, Toronto.

Wolfe, D. A., Wekerle, C., Gough, R., Reitsel-Jaffe, D., Grasley, C., Pittman, A. L., Lefebvre, L., & Stumpf, J. (1996). *The Youth Relationships manual: A group approach with adolescents for the prevention of woman abuse and the promotion of healthy relationships.* Thousand Oaks, CA: Sage.

Wolfe, D. A., Wekerle, C., Reitzel-Jaffe, D., Grasley, C., Pittman, A., & McEachran, A. (1997). Interrupting the cycle of violence: Empowering youth to promote healthy relationships. In D. Wolfe, R. McMahon, & R. Dev. Peters (Eds.), *Child abuse: New directions in prevention and treatment across the lifespan*. Thousand Oaks, CA: Sage.

Wolfe, D. A., Wekerle, C., Reitzel-Jaffe, D., & Lefebvre, L. (in press). Factors associated with abusive relationships among maltreated and non-maltreated youth. *Development and Psychopathology*.

Wolfe, D. A., Wekerle, C., Scott, K. (1997). *Alternatives to violence: Empowering youth to develop healthy relationships*. Thousand Oaks, CA: Sage.

15

Parenting Issues and Interventions with Adolescent Mothers

KAREN S. BUDD, KRISTIN D. STOCKMAN, and ELIZABETH N. MILLER

INTRODUCTION

The Intersection of Adolescent Motherhood and Child Maltreatment

Adolescent parenthood and child maltreatment rank as two of this country's leading contemporary social problems. Both problems seem, thus far, to be impervious to effective control, despite formidable efforts at prevention and intervention over the past quarter-century (Children's Defense Fund, 1996; National Research Council, 1993; Weatherley, 1991). In addition to their shared status as social morbidities, the two conditions converge in some families. Because few adolescents are ready to independently assume the responsibilities of childrearing, teen mothers, particularly those with limited social and economic resources, are vulnerable to conditions that can escalate into child maltreatment. Thus, a chapter focusing on disadvantaged adolescent mothers is appropriate in a volume on child abuse.

Teenage mothers are presumed to be more likely than older mothers to maltreat their children, in part because they experience the stress of being at once adolescents and parents (McAnarney, 1988; Werkerle & Wolfe, 1993). Many of the characteristics associated with perpetrators of child maltreatment (e.g., poverty, lack of education, childhood history of maltreatment, single parenthood) are true of adolescent mothers as well (Bolton, Laner, & Kane, 1980; Kinard & Klerman, 1980; Zuravin, 1988). However, research investigating a direct link between early parenthood and child maltreatment is scant, contradictory, and complicated by methodological difficulties.

KAREN S. BUDD and KRISTIN D. STOCKMAN • Department of Psychology, DePaul University, Chicago, Illinois 60614.   ELIZABETH N. MILLER • Graduate School of Applied and Preventive Psychology, Rutgers University, Piscataway, New Jersey 08855.

Handbook of Child Abuse Research and Treatment, edited by Lutzker. Plenum Press, New York, 1998.

These difficulties include low base rates, definitional inconsistencies, and problems separating out effects of various adverse conditions associated with both phenomena (Gelles, 1986; Kinard & Klerman, 1980). Mothers' ages may be useful mainly as a convenient but crude index of general readiness and resources for parenting.

Purpose of This Chapter

This chapter examines the parent training needs of adolescent mothers and reviews empirically based parenting interventions designed to address these needs. The first section provides a brief overview of the prevalence, correlates, and developmental implications of adolescent parenthood. The next section summaries findings of a parent training survey (Stockman & Budd, in press) conducted with service providers of teen mothers in the child protective system, in order to highlight priority areas of concern and common parenting intervention approaches in a sample of applied programs. The third section reviews empirically evaluated interventions targeting parenting competence in adolescent mothers, with the goal of identifying effective training approaches and documented areas of positive impact. A concluding section summarizes current knowledge and recommends future directions for parenting interventions with teenage mothers. The overall aim of the chapter is to review parenting programs for adolescent mothers and their children within the broader context of child abuse prevention efforts.

ANTECEDENTS AND CONSEQUENCES OF ADOLESCENT MOTHERHOOD

Prevalence and Predisposing Factors

National attention to adolescent pregnancy and parenting surfaced in the mid 1970s, in reaction to a number of changing demographic trends (Alan Guttmacher Institute, 1981; Furstenberg, 1976; Furstenberg, Brooks-Gunn, & Chase-Lansdale, 1989; Hayes, 1987; Hofferth & Hayes, 1987; Weatherley, 1991). Although the annual rate of teen births had declined steadily from over 90 births per 1,000 females in the 1950s to just under 60 births per 1,000 females by the mid 1970s, teens increasingly gave birth out of wedlock and chose to keep their children rather than place them for adoption. Earlier initiation of sexual activity among adolescents, together with lower rates of teen marriage, resulted in an increased prevalence of single teen mothers. By the mid 1980s, three-fourths of African-American and almost one-half of Caucasian adolescent females reported that they had intercourse by age 18 (Brooks-Gunn & Chase-Lansdale, 1995). The proportion of all teen births by unmarried women climbed from 18% in 1963 to 72% in 1993 (Children's Defense Fund, 1996). In 1993, there were 59.6 births per 1,000 female teens; 44.5 births per 1,000 were to unmarried teens (Children's Defense Fund, 1996).

Teenage pregnancy and childbearing are markedly higher, and contraceptive use is lower, in the United States compared to other industrialized countries (Jones et al., 1985). These figures suggest that national attitudes and practices regarding birth control contribute to the prevalence of teenage childbirth. According to a recent report by the Institute of Medicine (Brown & Eisenberg, 1995), 57% of all pregnancies to U.S. women, and 82% of pregnancies to teenagers, are unintended.

What accounts for the persistence of unplanned pregnancy and parenthood among U.S. adolescents, despite 25 years of concerted social attention toward prevention? Furstenberg (1991), in discussing the discrepancy between teens' intentions and actions regarding sex, listed several possible reasons: the unpredictable and sporadic nature of sexual activity, teens' distortion or misjudgment of the likelihood of becoming pregnant, involuntary or coerced nature of some intercourse, negative views of birth control options, youthful attraction to risky or "underground" behavior, limited sex education in schools, and proliferation of positive images of sex in the media (see also Adler, 1995; Brown & Eisenberg, 1995). Based on his analysis, Furstenberg concluded that teen parents regard unplanned pregnancy (and subsequent parenthood) as a "default option" (p. 134). In other words, parenthood happens because adolescents have sex without using birth control and then fail to take active steps toward abortion or adoption.

A different perspective of adolescent motherhood suggests that it is a reasonable, adaptive response to the social and cultural realities of urban life, particularly for poor African-American teens. For example, Williams (1991) conducted detailed interviews with African-American women in Boston who raised children as teens. Her findings indicated that early, out-of-wedlock births mirrored the experiences of their own mothers, peers, and female relatives. Most of the women had poor academic records at inner-city schools and foresaw little chance of educational or vocational success. Given the dearth of educated, employable black men in their communities, the women generally viewed marriage as an unlikely or even undesirable event. Thus, rather than representing a default option, early childbearing appeared as an accepted "career" option. This rationale echoes the views of other scholars from sociological, child welfare, and public policy perspectives (Hamburg & Dixon, 1992; Ladner, 1987; Wilson, 1987).

The ecological and cultural factors predisposing some teens to view early parenthood as acceptable, in combination with evidence that a majority of teens engage in sexual activity with irregular birth control, reveal reasons for the continued prevalence of adolescent motherhood. As Furstenberg (1991) stated, "Early childbearing owes its persistence to the fact that many women—not just disadvantaged black youth—have relatively little to lose by having a first birth in their teens or early 20s" (p. 136). However, the fact remains that early childbearing exacts a toll on families, as described next.

Consequences for Mother and Child

Consistent evidence indicates negative effects of early childbearing on women and their children (Furstenberg et al., 1989; Hayes, 1987; Hofferth & Hayes, 1987). For example, teenage mothers are less likely than are older mothers of similar backgrounds to complete their education, obtain marketable job skills, enter into stable partner relationships, and achieve economic self-sufficiency. Teen mothers and their children are more likely to experience health problems, many of which are attributed to the lack of adequate prenatal care and nutrition. In addition, as a group, children of adolescent mothers have poorer academic achievement, greater difficulties in peer relationships, and more behavioral and developmental problems than do children of older mothers. Small but consistent adverse effects become evident as children reach preschool years, and they generally persist into adolescence (Brooks-Gunn & Chase-Lansdale, 1995).

The negative outcomes documented for the offspring of teenage mothers are presumed to be mediated by the quality of mother–child interactions. The consensus of reviewers (e. g., Brooks-Gunn & Furstenberg, 1986; Hans, Bernstein, & Percansky, 1991; Osofsky, Hann, Peebles, 1993; Panzarine, 1988) is that teenage mothers, in comparison to older mothers, generally are less effective in interactions with their children and less knowledgeable about childrearing. Emotional immaturity is one factor cited as affecting teenagers' parenting behavior (Reis & Herz, 1987). Younger mothers have been found to exhibit less eye contact and smiling with their infants (Teberg, Howell, & Wingert, 1983), to be less verbal and positively expressive, (Culp, Culp, Osofsky, & Osofsky, 1991; Levine, Garcia Coll, & Oh, 1985; Teberg et al., 1983), and less likely to modify their own behavior in response to their child's behavior (McAnarney, Lawrence, Ricciuti, Polley, & Szilagyi, 1986). Further, teen mothers are more likely than are older mothers to have unrealistic expectations of children's developmental difficulties and to provide less stimulating learning environments for their children (Field, 1981; Parks & Arndt, 1990). However, individual differences exist, and some mothers overcome their initial disadvantages, as do their children.

Developmental Implications

To understand the challenges facing adolescent mothers, it is helpful to consider them within a developmental context. Hill (1983) described five main developmental issues of the teenage years: (1) discovering and understanding oneself as an individual (identity), (2) forming close and caring relationships with others (intimacy), (3) establishing a healthy sense of independence (autonomy), (4) coming to terms with puberty and expressing sexual feelings (sexuality), and (5) becoming a successful and competent member of society (achievement). In addition, cognitively oriented theorists cite a sixth issue: thinking hypothetically about future options, alternatives, and consequences (abstraction) (Inhelder & Piaget, 1964).

From a developmental perspective, the responsibility of caring for a child is likely to interfere with an adolescent's opportunities to concentrate on her own psychosocial changes (Catrone & Sadler, 1984; McAnarney, 1988; Musick, 1993; Trad, 1993). For example, actions directed toward establishing the teen's identity (e.g., experimenting with different ideas, values, and roles) may be hampered by caregiving responsibilities. Similarly, motherhood can interfere with a teen's achievement of personal goals (e.g., academic or vocational interests) or pursuit of intimate relationships. A young mother may need to rely heavily on her family or surrogate family members to obtain basic caregiving assistance, when otherwise she would be developmentally ready to become more independent of her family. As with other adolescents, her problem-solving skills are still developing, so she may fail to anticipate the consequences of her actions. Yet when the young mother's problem-solving attempts involve caring for her infant, her decisions may have negative implications for the child.

To date, little research has tied specific developmental conceptualizations to the circumstances of adolescent parenting (Brooks-Gunn & Chase-Lansdale, 1995). Nevertheless, developmental experts speculate that the stresses of early parenting arise from a conflict between age-appropriate and parent-mandated roles that may engender negative feelings in the teen toward her child. Further, some writers (Osofsky et al., 1993; Trad, 1993) suspect that a subset of adolescents become pregnant as a source of identity, and thus may become resentful of the child if their expectations are not met. The complexity of developmental issues suggests that teens vary considerably in their adaptation to the life changes surrounding motherhood.

The preceding section on antecedents and consequences of adolescent motherhood suggests two patterns that are likely to continue over the next decade. First, demographic trends indicate that a substantial proportion of adolescent females, especially those with fewer economic, social, and interpersonal resources, will continue to become single teen mothers. Second, the combination of environmental disadvantage, parenting gaps, and developmental asynchrony associated with adolescent childbearing poses significant challenges to families. These trends provide a framework for considering interventions to address the needs of adolescent mothers.

SURVEY OF SERVICE PROVIDERS IN ADOLESCENT PARENT PROGRAMS

Purpose and Participants

In the past two decades, numerous community-based programs have been established to provide supportive and educational services to pregnant adolescents and those who are already parents. Although most programs include strengthening parenting and the parent–child relationship among their goals, in fact, the services provided usually concentrate more on the mother's personal functioning than on her child's development or on the parent–child dyad (Hans, Bernstein, & Percansky, 1991; Musick, Bernstein, Percansky, & Stott, 1987). Typically, programs offer services such as prenatal and well-baby care, psychosocial support, resources to keep mothers in school, vocational training, and family planning education (Hofferth, 1991). Less is known about intervention components directed at parenting and the parent–child relationship. To address this issue, the survey described in the following discussion sought information on parenting-specific interventions within service programs for a high-risk subgroup of adolescent mothers.

The first author collaborated with the Illinois Department of Children and Family Services (DCFS) over a 5-year period (1991–1996) to provide assessment and consultation regarding community services to teen mothers who are wards of the state's child protective system (Budd, Heilman, & Kane, 1994; Budd, Holdsworth, & HoganBruen, 1996). The mothers are in substitute care because of abuse, neglect, dependency, abandonment, or other significant problems in their families of origin. They are single, economically dependent, and often emotionally, socially, and educationally disadvantaged. A consistent concern expressed informally by service providers in this project is that adolescent mothers lack crucial knowledge about safe and effective child care, yet the teens often reject traditional parenting education programs. Teen wards themselves acknowledge the need for parenting supports, but informally they often complain that existing training programs are rigid, irrelevant, inconvenient, or boring.

As part of the DCFS collaborative project, Stockman and Budd (in press) conducted a survey of service providers' views, based on their firsthand experiences with wards. This survey solicited information on priority topics in which teen mothers need parent training, methods of delivering training, strategies for engaging adolescents in training, screening and assessment methods used, and impact evaluation procedures. Highlights of the survey are presented below (cf. Stockman & Budd, in press, for a more comprehensive account).

All programs in the state of Illinois with a DCFS contract focused specifically on serving pregnant and/or parenting teen wards were invited to participate in the survey. Twenty-eight of the 30 agencies responded, including 19 agencies (68%) in the Chicago area and 9 (32%) in the remainder of the state. Agencies served between 1 and 39 female adolescent wards, and many also served non-wards. They represented a variety of program types, including group residential facilities, cooperative or independent living programs, high-risk pregnancy intervention programs, transitional living arrangements, shelters or emergency placements, and foster care. Programs offered a variety of substitute care services (e. g., living arrangements, health care, counseling, educational support) in addition to parent training. Agency representatives (1–4 per site) were interviewed during a site visit, lasting approximately 2 hours.

Survey Instrument and Administration Procedures

The Parent Training Survey was specifically developed for this study through a review of common components in existing parent training programs for adolescents. Information also was drawn from sources which address the needs of teen wards specifically (Children's Defense Fund, 1987; Child Welfare League of America, 1993). The survey consists of five main sections: (1) parent training topics, (2) methods of delivery, (3) methods of engaging teen wards in parent training activities, (4) assessment of parenting, and (5) impact evaluation.

The first section of the Parent Training Survey inquired about the topics on which teen mothers need training. Service providers were presented with several parenting-related areas and asked to indicate whether or not their agency provided some education or training in each of these areas. They were then asked to rank the top four most important areas of training for teen wards. The structured questions provided an opportunity to gather systematic information across different agencies and to obtain qualitative information on specific programs. A similar format was followed to gather information in the remaining four sections of the Parent Training Survey. To summarize survey findings, the ratings for each service provider at an agency were averaged into a composite agency rating for each of the areas assessed.

Considering that the survey findings are based on self-reports rather than on objective documentation of parent training activities, they should be interpreted with caution. In an effort to cast their agency in a positive light, responders may have made comments that were overly optimistic or that describe training that occurs occasionally rather than consistently and systematically. However, despite their inherent limitations, the survey findings offer an initial perspective on parent training practices and priorities for adolescent mothers who are wards.

Survey Results and Discussion

Table 1 presents a summary of the survey responses regarding parent training topics covered by agencies serving adolescent mothers. (The far right column of Tables 1–3 pertains to data from a review of parent training studies, which is discussed in the next section.) Overall, providers indicated that virtually all of the listed topics were included in their training agendas. These findings suggest that the providers perceive a need to address a wide range of parenting, child care, and developmental issues with adolescent mothers who are wards. Many providers commented that it seemed essential for the teen to address her own emotional and developmental needs (i.e., Teen Parent Factors) before being in a position to nurture the development of her child(ren).

Table 2 displays the methods of parent training delivery reported by the surveyed agencies, organized from the most frequently reported method (modeling and feedback; 100%) to the least frequently reported method (mentoring programs with experienced parents or role models; 14%). Providers ranked the two most frequently used methods, modeling and feedback and didactic parent training, as high in effectiveness. However, three other methods that providers ranked among the top five in effectiveness (home visiting, peer support groups, and mentoring programs) were reportedly used less frequently than several other methods. This discrepancy may relate to the fact that home visiting, peer support groups, and mentoring programs all require staff with specialized skills to organize the programs, as well as coordination with outside resources and special travel arrangements. Thus, they may be more difficult to implement. Also, the nature of the program affects the methods used. For example, although home visiting is feasible for independent living and high-risk pregnancy programs, it is not an option for group residential programs.

Table 3 displays a summary of the survey findings on strategies used to engage teens in parent training activities. Engagement was defined as a mother's active

Table 1. Parent Training Topics Covered in Programs for Adolescent Mothers

Parent training topic	Examples of content	% of 28 Agencies	% of 20 Studies
Teen parent factors (T)	Anger management, building self-esteem	93	70
Basic caregiving routines (B)	Feeding, bathing, regular sleep times	93	60
Emotional needs of infant (E)	Soothing, handling child fears, showing affection	93	50
Health and medical needs (H)	Parental and well-baby care, general first aid	89	55
Safety (S)	Correcting home hazards, protecting against danger	89	15
Language and communication (L)	Talking to child, labeling objects, reading to child	89	45
Discipline (D)	Setting limits, non-violent punishment	86	25
Child development (C)	Stimulating cognitive, social, or motor skills	86	95

Table 2. Methods of Parent Training Delivery across Programs for Adolescent Mothers

Method of delivery	% of 28 Agencies	Ranking of 28 agencies[a]	% of 20 Studies
Modeling and feedback	100	1	50
Didactic parenting classes	79	3	30
Encourage use of supportive friends or family	75		20
Videotapes on parenting	75		15
Books or readings on parenting	72		50
Home visiting	61	2	55
Homework exercises to practice skills	61		15
Peer support groups	32	4	35
Parent involvement in nursery/daycare	21		5
Mentoring programs with experienced parents or role models	14	5	30
Counseling services	—[b]	—	20
Use of videotapes of parent–child interactions as teaching tool	—	—	5
Connect with other service providers	—	—	40

[a] 1 = Highest ranked in effectiveness.
[b] Delivery methods assessed only in review of parent training literature.

Table 3. Strategies Used to Engage Teens in Parent Training Activities

Strategy	% of 28 Agencies	Ranking of 28 agencies[a]	% of 20 Studies
Serving snacks or food at sessions	68	1	5
Providing transportation to sessions	64	2	20
Providing free babysitting at sessions	57	3	10
Awarding certificates of participation	43		5
Removing privileges for nonattendance	39		0
Awarding special activities	29		20
Releasing checks at sessions	25		0
Giving gifts to baby	21		25
Raffles/lottery at sessions	11		5
Awarding money for attendance	7	4	15
Providing high school credits	—[b]	—	10
Providing paid job training	—	—	5

[a] 1 = Highest ranked in effectiveness.
[b] Strategies assessed only in review of parent training literature.

participation in training toward positive goals (Kanfer & Schefft, 1988). Overall, there was much variability in the methods used by different agencies. The three strategies used by more than 50% of surveyed agencies include serving snacks or food at sessions, providing transportation to sessions, and providing free babysitting at sessions. These same strategies were ranked overall by providers as the most effective means of motivating mothers' participation in parent training activities. Interestingly, the technique used the least frequently, awarding money for attendance (7%), was nevertheless ranked as the fourth most effective strategy by survey respondents.

To obtain more information about engagement issues, service providers were presented with the open-ended question, "What do you believe are the main obstacles in engaging teen wards to participate in parenting education/training programs?" The majority of provider responses can be grouped into five general content areas: (1) logistics (e.g., transportation, scheduling, facility limitations, weather), (2) teens' emotional adjustment (e.g., depression, lack of self-esteem, sense of shame), (3) difficulties in making the topic or presentation interesting for teens, (4) extended-family dynamics (e.g., relatives giving teen conflicting parenting information), and (5) difficulty establishing a trusting relationship with the teen ward. Another engagement question dealt with extending parenting services to male companions of the teen mothers. Two-thirds of the agencies reported that they attempted to include the mother's boyfriend or the child's father in parent training activities. However, all agencies said that their attempts to engage these males were generally unsuccessful, citing the instability of many of the relationships between the teen mothers and their male companions, as well as the teen mother's ambivalence about including the males in parenting.

With regard to the agencies' methods of client assessment and/or program evaluation, few agencies reported that formal assessments were conducted in their programs. Most agencies said they relied on informal staff impressions to estimate parenting skills and needs. The initial intake assessment was cited as a source of general parenting information, such as history of any parent–child difficulties or prior parent training activities. One-quarter of the agencies reported that they conducted child development assessments in their programs, whereas the other agencies reported using community resources to assess child development when concerns arose. With regard to evaluation of program impact, most agencies reported no consistent procedures. The most frequently reported indices were case staffings, teen attendance records at training sessions, and teen satisfaction ratings. In addition, some agencies reported using the goals and objectives from teens' Individual Treatment Plans as a way of evaluating progress in parenting.

Summary and Implications of Survey

The survey findings suggest that a wide array of parenting topics is addressed, at least nominally, within service programs for adolescent mothers in substitute care. However, providers' comments about the difficulties they encounter in engaging teens in training imply that these efforts often are unsuccessful. Also, the lack of formal assessment or evaluation mechanisms within agencies means that parent and child outcomes are not being documented.

The survey results are consistent with Musick and colleagues' (1987) comments about the challenges involved in influencing parent–child relationships in the Ounce of Prevention program for teen mothers. These writers contend that a parent–child focus is difficult for community programs, given the predominant use of paraprofessional staff and other persons without direct training in parenting and child development. In addition, they note that parenting curricula developed for use in adolescent programs often are unsuccessful in achieving meaningful changes in staff or parent performance. To address these difficulties, the Ounce of Prevention adopted a screening protocol involving focused assessments of child development as well as structured observation of parent–child interactions to guide parenting interventions (Musick et al., 1987).

In terms of the methods of delivering parent training, what survey respondents reported as using most frequently did not correspond closely with what they identified as most effective with parenting teen wards. The methods of parent training that were used most often were modeling and feedback, didactic parenting classes, supportive relatives or friends, videotapes, and books. Whereas the first two of these methods were ranked as highly effective, service providers also ranked home visiting, peer support groups, and mentoring among the top five most effective methods of training. The discrepancy between methods used often and those perceived as effective may relate to limitations in the staff and resources available in community programs.

The current survey findings underscore the serious challenges entailed in providing parenting-focused interventions to adolescent mothers in substitute care. Many of these same difficulties are likely to exist in programs serving adolescent mothers who are not clients in the child protective system. However, the "substitute parent" role involved in serving wards means that agencies are obligated to actively promote the teen's welfare, even when the mother may not be responsive to offered services. This dilemma complicates services to adolescent parent wards.

EMPIRICALLY EVALUATED INTERVENTIONS FOR TEEN MOTHERS

Purpose and Method of Parent Training Review

Whereas the survey findings point to commonly reported characteristics of parenting programs for adolescent mothers in substitute care, the extent to which the interventions resemble established parenting programs for other teen mothers is unclear. We reviewed the parent training literature to identify studies focusing on teen mothers. One objective of this review was to compare features of empirically evaluated programs with the features self-reported by surveyed agencies. A second objective was to determine the positive outcomes of the empirically evaluated programs.

Three criteria were used to select studies for this review: (1) the target population for intervention was teenage mothers; (2) part or all of the intervention was directed at facilitating parenting skills and/or the parent–child relationship; and (3) intervention effects were measured by assessing parenting skills, attitudes, or knowledge, parent–child interactions, and/or child development scores. Programs that targeted other subgroups of parents (e.g., older mothers who were poor or had premature infants) in addition to adolescent mothers were excluded, because the review sought programmatic information specific to teen parents.

Using these criteria, 20 studies were identified, as listed in Table 4. Studies varied in number of participants, methodological sophistication, adequacy of experimental design, level of information presented to substantiate results, and programmatic specificity; however, a relatively wide latitude was applied to provide a broad perspective on the outcomes reported across the programs. None of the interventions specifically targeted adolescent wards; however, most participants were economically and socially disadvantaged.

Table 4. Empirically Evaluated Parent Training Programs for Adolescent Mothers

Reference	Age of child	Training topics[a]	Delivery methods[b]	Positive program impacts
Badger, Burns, & Rhoads (1976)	3–4 wks to 6 mos	B,E,H,L,C	1,2,4	• Parenting classes resulted in increased knowledge of preventive health, nutrition, and child development • After training, participants showed more appropriate responding to infants during observed interactions
Baskin, Umansky, & Sanders (1987)	Birth to 12 mos	T,E,L,C	1,5,6,8,13	• Mothers who participated in both home visits and peer support groups became more responsive to their infants than those who only had peer support groups
Butler, Rickel, Thomas, & Hendren (1993)	Prenatal to early infancy	T,H,D,C	10,13	• Parenting attitudes became more negative after infants' birth (at program completion); however, attitudes worsened less for mothers with peer advocates than for a comparison group of teen mothers
Cappleman, Thompson, DeRemer-Sullivan, King, & Sturm (1982)	Birth to 24 mos	T,B,L,C	5,6,11	• Home visit intervention resulted in marginally better infant development scores at 12 & 30 mos than for the control group • At 30 mos, fewer intervention than control infants were considered at risk on the Binet IQ norms
Causby, Nixon, & Bright (1991)	Infancy to early childhood	T,B,E,D,C	1,2,6	• Intervention including a school curriculum and home visits resulted in more positive interactions during teaching and more stimulating home environments than home visits only
Cherniss & Herzog (1996)	Prenatal and/or parenting mothers	T,B,H	3,6,11,13	• In-home family therapy plus individual treatment was associated with significantly higher parenting quality at 12 mos than individual treatment only; however, this effect disappeared at 24 mos
Dickinson & Cudaback (1992)	Prenatal to 12 mos	B,E,H,L,C	5	• Mothers who received educational booklets regarded the booklets highly and reported improved parenting attitudes and practices over a comparison group
Field, Widmayer, Greenberg, & Stoller (1982)	Birth to 6 mos	B,E,H,S,L,D,C	1,5,6,7,9	• Parent training either via home visits or at a nursery improved infant development, temperament, and mother–child interactions compared to controls • Nursery training was superior to home visits in impact

(continued)

Table 4. (*Continued*)

Reference	Age of child	Training topics[a]	Delivery methods[b]	Positive program impacts
Field, Widmayer, Stringer, & Ignatoff (1980)	Birth through 12 mos	B,E,L,C	1,5,6,7	• Home-based intervention with mothers of pre-term infants led to more optimal infant development, temperament, parenting knowledge, and mother–child interactions than controls
Fulton, Murphy, & Anderson (1991)	Prenatal and infancy	T,H,C	4,5,6,13	• Pre-post measures showed increased knowledge of child development and decreased abuse potential after intervention via home visits and supportive resources
Gutelius, Kirsch, MacDonald, Brooks, & McErlean (1977)	Prenatal through 3 yrs	T,B,E,H,L, D,C	3,5,6,8,11	• Mothers who received a package of home-based, clinic, and counseling services showed positive findings over a control group in several child (i.e., diet, behavioral adjustment) and parenting (attitudes, child-rearing practices) variables
Halpern & Covey (1983)	Infancy	T,C	1,6,8,10,13	• After a program of home visits, peer support, and mentoring, participants responded more appropriately to cues from their infants and gained knowledge of child development
Kissman (1992)	Infancy	T,E,D,C	2,3,5	• Mothers who had group parenting classes and counseling in accessing social networks showed improved parenting attitudes and greater social support compared to control mothers
Koniak-Griffin, Verzemnieks, & Cahill (1992)	4–6 wks old	E,L,C	12	• Following videotape instruction and feedback, intervention dyads scored significantly higher than controls on quality of parent–child interactions
Miller (1992)	Prenatal through infancy	T,B,H,S,C	1,2,4,5,8,10	• After a comprehensive intervention, Atlanta teens reported fewer health problems and Toledo teens were more likely to read to their children than controls • However, young mothers did not attend the program regularly, and few behavior changes were observed
Osofsky, Culp, & Ware (1988)	Prenatal through 30 mos	T,B,L,C	1,5,6,8,13	• Active participants in a clinic-and-home intervention showed greater gains in play and interaction, and their children had higher developmental scores at 13 mos, than inactive participants • However, comparisons of intervention and control mothers indicated little or no overall effect

Table 4. (*Continued*)

Reference	Age of child	Training topics[a]	Delivery methods[b]	Positive program impacts
Polit, Quint, & Riccio (1988); Quint (1991)	Prenatal through early childhood	T,B,H,C	1,2,8,10, 11,13	• After 5 yrs, enrollment in Head Start, quality of home environment, and children's vocabulary and behavioral ratings were significantly better for participants in a comprehensive program than the comparison group
Unger & Wandersman (1985); Study 2	Prenatal through 8 mos	T,H,C	3,6,10,13	• Mothers who received home visits and supportive resources showed more parenting knowledge, infant responsiveness, and parenting satisfaction than controls
Weinman, Schreiber, & Robinson (1992)	Infancy or early childhood	T,B,E,H, S,C	2,8,10	• Mothers who participated actively in parent education classes showed greater increases in parenting knowledge than mothers who did not complete training
Widnayer & Field (1980)	Perinatal through 1 mo	C	1,7	• Mothers' observation and feedback re: neonatal assessment of pre-term infants, plus completion of weekly developmental checklists during the first mo, resulted in more optimal maternal feeding and face-to-face interactions than for comparison groups • Maternal observation of assessment plus completion of checklists was more effective than checklists alone

[a] Refer to Table 1, column 1, for key to abbreviations.
[b] Refer to Table 2, column 1, for key to numbers.

The 20 studies were reviewed with respect to parent training topics covered, methods of delivering parent training, strategies used for motivating teen participation, and positive program outcomes. Coding categories for the first three review topics were similar to those used in the parent training survey reported in the previous section; in addition, a few new categories that emerged from the studies were included in the coding. The fourth area, specific program outcomes, was coded based on findings reported in the studies on relevant parent and child variables. It is possible that some programs included features that were not fully described in the published reports, and thus the review may have underestimated some program components.

Results and Discussion of Parent Training Review

The far right column of Table 1 displays the percentage of reviewed programs covering the listed parent training topics in interventions with adolescent mothers. With the exception of Child Development, which was covered by 95% of the programs, the empirically documented interventions cited fewer parent training topics than were reported by service providers in surveyed agencies. The biggest differences were in the areas of Safety and Discipline, on which only a fraction of the empirically evaluated programs provided training, compared to more than 85% of surveyed agencies. The general impression is that the surveyed agencies emphasize a wider variety of topics in programs for teen wards. However, it is possible that the differences, at least in part, are due to differing methods of data collection (self-report of agencies versus review of published studies).

The far right column of Table 2 displays the methods of parent training delivery described in empirically evaluated interventions. The three most frequently used delivery methods in these programs were home visiting (55%), modeling and feedback (50%), and books or readings on parenting (50%). Overall, far fewer delivery methods were cited in the published intervention studies than were reported by service providers in programs for adolescent wards. The reasons for this difference may relate to the differing methods of data collection (self-report versus review of articles); however, other explanations are plausible. For example, interventions represented in the literature may involve systematic use of a narrower range of techniques, in comparison to intermittent use of many techniques in surveyed agencies. Also, the varied types of programs (e.g., residential, foster home, independent living) serving teen wards may influence the delivery methods used.

The far-right column of Table 3 displays the percentage of empirically documented programs that reported using each of the listed engagement strategies. Again, the most striking finding is the reported use of far fewer engagement strategies in reviewed studies than in surveyed programs. The three most frequently reported motivational strategies in the reviewed studies were giving gifts to baby (25%), providing transportation to sessions (20%), and awarding special activities (20%). Interestingly, the study (Miller, 1992) that cited the largest number (6) of motivational strategies also reported that its intervention was largely unsuccessful in affecting parent or child outcomes. Considering that teen wards in the surveyed programs may not be voluntary recipients of services, agencies may assume or have learned that they need to employ more motivational strategies with clients.

Table 4 summarizes the basic characteristics and outcomes of interventions in each of the reviewed studies, including the target age of infants when training occurred, parent training topics and delivery methods, and positive program impacts reported by the authors. The interventions reviewed here fall into one of three formats: individual (45%), group (15%), or a combination of the two approaches (40%). Interventions varied considerably, from relatively narrow programs providing educational booklets (Dickinson & Cudaback, 1992), one-time videotape instruction and feedback (Koniak-Griffin, Verzemnieks, & Cahill, 1992), or observation of neonatal assessment and completion of weekly developmental checklists (Widmayer & Field, 1980), to comprehensive programs involving home visits, peer support groups, and other services (Baskin, Umansky, & Sanders, 1987; Gutelius, Kirsch, MacDonald, Brooks, & McEarlean, 1977; Halpern & Covey, 1983; Miller, 1992; Osofsky, Culp, & Ware, 1988).

The summary of positive program impacts, in the far right column of Table 4, indicates that all but 3 (Butler, Rickel, Thomas, & Hendren, 1993; Osofsky et al., 1988; Weinman, Schreiber, & Robinson, 1992) of the 20 programs reported positive outcomes for the intervention group(s) on at least one parent or child measure. Two of these programs (Osofsky et al., 1988; Weinman et al., 1992) reported differential outcomes for teens who participated actively in intervention compared with those who did not. Miller (1992) reported the most pessimistic account, citing numerous programmatic complications and areas in which no behavioral changes were observed; however, several programs acknowledged only partial success or short-term improvements (e.g., Cappleman, Thompson, DeRemer-Sullivan, King, & Sturm, 1982; Cherniss & Herzog, 1996). The reported challenges are similar to those articulated elsewhere (Ware, Osofsky, Eberhart-Wright, & Leichtman, 1987) in balancing the often conflicting interests of teens, children, and the service system.

Only two studies reported follow-up data beyond one year after program completion. Both studies (Gutelius et al., 1977; Polit, Quint, & Riccio, 1988) indicated the maintenance of some positive effects on parent or child measures. Field and her colleagues (Field, Widmayer, Stringer, & Ignatoff, 1980; Field, Widmayer, Greenberg, & Stoller, 1982) conducted two of the most well-controlled intervention studies, which showed impressive gains in infant development, temperament, and mother–child interactions following home sites or parenting instruction at a nursery. However, a follow-up study (Stone, Bendell, & Field, 1988) of the children at 5–8 years of age revealed no long-term intervention effects; the authors attribute this result to the overriding impact of extreme poverty on the families' lives.

Summary and Implications of Parent Training Review

The general impression that emerges from a review of empirically documented program outcomes is that, even in established programs for adolescent mothers, positive impacts are hard to achieve. This conclusion should not, however, obscure the fact that almost all of the empirically evaluated programs did show successful outcomes on some parent or child variables. There is some evidence that teens who participated more actively in services showed greater benefits.

Programs involving home visits usually reported changes in the quality of parent–child interactions, and, less often, in child development scores (Baskin et al., 1987; Cappleman et al., 1982; Causby, Nixon, & Bright, 1991; Field et al., 1980, 1982; Halpem & Covey, 1983; Unger & Wandersman, 1985). These measures provide the most direct and impressive evidence of intervention success, and they probably reflect the combined influence of several program components. Interventions employing didactic parenting classes or peer support groups more often measured and documented changes in parenting knowledge or attitudes (Badger, Burns, & Rhoads, 1976; Kissman, 1992). These summary comments are consistent with the conclusions reached by Wekerle and Wolfe (1993) in their review of parent training programs targeting young parents.

Comparison of parent training interventions in empirically evaluated programs and those reported in the survey of providers serving teen wards is limited by the differing methods of data collection and lack of outcome measurement in the surveyed programs. Agencies serving adolescent wards reported offering a wider range of parent training topics, more methods of delivery, and greater use of motivational strategies. Given the identified parenting deficits of teen parent wards (Budd et al., 1994), comprehensive services should be available to enhance their parenting capabilities.

CONCLUSIONS AND FUTURE DIRECTIONS

This chapter opened with a discussion of the presumed overlap between adolescent childbearing and a heightened tendency of teen mothers to maltreat their children. Parenting programs for at-risk mothers have the dual aims of both reducing the likelihood of adverse outcomes and strengthening positive developments (Werkerle & Wolfe, 1993). Based on the current review, what conclusions and recommendations can be drawn regarding the preventive impact of parenting interventions with adolescent mothers? Three aspects of this question are briefly addressed.

First, when considering the success of parenting programs in inoculating teen mothers against child abuse or neglect, very little can be concluded from the programs reviewed in this chapter. This is because only one study (Fulton, Murphy, & Anderson, 1991) included data on child maltreatment incidents as part of the evaluation. None of the 76 participating mothers in this intervention were reported for abuse or neglect during a 10-month period following services. Further, the mothers showed significant reductions in scores on the Child Abuse Potential Inventory (Milner, 1986) from before to after intervention. This study is commendable for evaluating child maltreatment data. Ideally, these findings would be accompanied by data on an appropriate comparison group and would extend for a longer follow-up period.

A second way to evaluate the preventive impact of parenting programs is to consider whether the interventions enhance the teen mother's capacity for parenting, the parent–child relationship, or the child's developmental functioning. Findings from the 20 empirically evaluated programs are modestly encouraging in documenting short-term effects on some parent and/or child measures. The most consistent positive outcomes were reported for programs that combined home visits with peer support groups and additional services. Considering that most programs last only a few months or, at most, for the first 2–3 years of the child's life, the duration of services may be an important limiting factor. Chase-Lansdale, Brooks-Gunn, and Paikoff (1992), in reviewing research findings on parenting interventions for teenage mothers, argue that programs need to be longer to accomplish the far-reaching environmental and personal objectives deemed necessary. These authors propose a reinitiation of services with mothers after their children enter school, when mothers have fewer child care demands. In addition, they recommend that services should be offered to the teens' children during their school years, when the detrimental effects of being raised by a teen parent become more evident.

A third question relating to the preventive impact of parenting programs concerns which mothers benefit from services. Teens who participated more fully in training activities appeared to show greater gains, yet little is known about how to predict, in advance, which mothers will be receptive to services. A disproportionately large number of teen mothers are victims of sexual abuse (Boyer & Fine, 1992), have dysfunctional family relationships (Cherniss & Herzog, 1992), or are socially isolated (Kissman, 1992; Unger & Wandersman, 1985). Young mothers in substitute care often have multiple disadvantages, which vary among them. Programs are most likely to succeed if they take into account these individual differences and tailor services accordingly. Some empirically evaluated programs for teen mothers gathered input in the development of their programs from potential participants (Dickinson & Cudaback, 1992) or collaborated with the teens regarding their specific needs in implementing interventions (Fulton et al., 1991; Osofsky et al., 1988; Polit et al., 1988). These strategies would seem to be wise; however, to date, the impact of including teens in planning parenting interventions has not been evaluated.

It is obvious that much work remains to enhance the palatability and effectiveness of parenting programs for teen mothers. At the same time, data on the persistence and negative consequences of teen parenthood imply that interventions for adolescent mothers will be needed for a long time to come. Schorr (1988), in reviewing intervention programs for disadvantaged populations, advises that service providers aim, not to eliminate all risk factors for bad outcomes, but to *change the odds*. Reducing even one or two risk factors can have a beneficial impact. Schorr highlights some characteristics of more successful interventions with high-risk populations as follows: a broad spectrum of services, high intensity services, flexibility and easy access, community-based services, continuity over time, and inclusion of program recipients as collaborators in planning interventions. These characteristics are in line with many of the views expressed by service providers and documented in the parent training literature review. They provide guidelines for designing services to strengthen the parenting capabilities of young mothers and thereby reduce the likelihood of child maltreatment.

ACKNOWLEDGMENTS

This work was partially supported by a contract from the Illinois Department of Children and Family Services (DCFS). The authors wish to thank the staff of DCFS and several private agencies working with adolescent mothers for their cooperation.

REFERENCES

Adler, N. (1995, July). *Adolescent sexual behavior looks irrational—but looks are deceiving.* Address presented at Federation of Behavioral, Psychological and Cognitive Sciences, Washington, DC.

Alan Guttmacher Institute (1981). *Teenage pregnancy: The problem that hasn't gone away.* New York: Author.

Badger, E., Burns, D., & Rhoads, B. (1976). Education for adolescent mothers in a hospital setting. *American Journal of Public Health, 66,* 469–472.

Baskin, C., Umansky, W., & Sanders, W. (1987). Influencing the responsiveness of adolescent mothers to their infants. *Zero to Three, 8*(2), 7–11.

Bolton, F. G., Jr., Laner, R. H., & Kane, S. P. (1980). Child maltreatment risk among adolescent mothers: A study of reported cases. *American Journal of Orthopsychiatry, 50,* 489–504.

Boyer, D., & Fine, D. (1992). Sexual abuse as a factor in adolescent pregnancy and child maltreatment. *Family Planning Perspectives, 24,* 4–19.

Brooks-Gunn, J., & Chase-Lansdale, P. L. (1995). Adolescent parenthood. In M. H. Bornstein (Ed.), *Handbook of parenting* (Vol. 3) *Status and social conditions of parenting* (pp. 113–149). Mahwah, NJ: Erlbaum.

Brooks-Gunn, J., & Furstenberg, F. F., Jr. (1986). The children of adolescent mothers: Physical, academic, and psychological outcomes. *Developmental Review, 6,* 224–251.

Brown, S. S., & Eisenberg, L. (Eds.). (1995). *The best intentions: Unintended pregnancy and the well-being of children and families.* Washington, DC: National Academy Press.

Budd, K. S., Heilman, N., & Kane, D. (1994, November). *Variables associated with increased risk of child abuse in multiply-disadvantaged adolescent mothers.* Paper presented at the conference of the Association for the Advancement of Behavior Therapy, San Diego, CA.

Budd, K. S., Holdsworth, M., & HoganBruen, K. (1996, March). *Teenage mothers in substitute care: A longitudinal investigation of risks and outcomes.* Paper presented at the meeting of the Society for Research on Adolescence, Boston.

Butler, C., Rickel, A. U., Thomas, E., & Hendren, M. (1993). An intervention program to build competencies in adolescent parents. *Journal of Primary Prevention, 13,* 183–198.

Cappleman, M. W., Thompson, R. T., DeRemer-Sullivan, P. A., King, A. A., & Sturm, J. M. (1982). Effectiveness of a home based early intervention program with infants of adolescent mothers. *Child Psychiatry and Human Development, 13,* 55–65.

Catrone, C., & Sadler, L. S. (1984). A developmental model for teen-age parent education. *Journal of School Health, 54,* 63–67.

Causby, V., Nixon, C., & Bright, J. M. (1991). Influences on adolescent mother–infant interactions. *Adolescence, 26,* 619–630.

Chase-Lansdale, P. L., Brooks-Gunn, J., & Paikoff, R. L. (1992). Research and programs for adolescent mothers: Missing links and future promises. *American Behavioral Scientist, 35,* 290–312.

Cherniss, C., & Herzog, E. (1996). Impact of home-based family therapy on maternal and child outcomes in disadvantaged adolescent mothers. *Family Relations, 45,* 72–79.

Children's Defense Fund. (1987). *Teens in foster care: Prevention pregnancy and buiding self-sufficiency.* Washington, DC: The Adolescent Pregnancy Prevention Clearinghouse.

Children's Defense Fund (1996). *The state of America's children: Yearbook 1996.* Washington, DC: Author.

Child Welfare League of America (1993). *Standards for programs serving pregnant and parenting adolescents.* Washington, DC: CWLA Publications.

Culp, R. E., Culp, A. M., Osofsky, J. D., & Osofsky, H. J. (1991). Adolescent and older mothers' interaction patterns with their six-month-old infants. *Journal of Adolescence, 14,* 195–200.

Dickinson, N. S., & Cudaback, D. J. (1992). Parent education for adolescent mothers. *Journal of Primary Prevention, 13,* 23–35.

Field, T. M. (1981). Early development of the preterm offspring of teenage mothers. In K. G. Scott, T. Field, & E. G. Robertson (Eds.), *Teenage parents and their offspring* (pp. 145–175). New York: Grune & Stratton.

Field, T., Widmayer, S., Greenberg, R., & Stoller, S. (1982). Effects of parent training on teenage mothers and their infants. *Pediatrics, 69,* 703–707.

Field, T. M., Widmayer, S. M., Stringer S.. & Ignatoff, E. (1980). Teenage, lower-class, black mothers and their preterm infants: An intervention and developmental follow-up. *Child Development, 51,* 426–436.

Fulton, A. M., Murphy, K. R., & Anderson, S. L. (1991). Increasing adolescent mothers' knowledge of child development: An intervention program. *Adolescence, 26,* 73–81.

Furstenberg, F. F., Jr. (1976). The social consequences of teenage parenthood. *Family Planning Perspectives, 8,* 148–164.

Furstenberg, F. F., Jr. (1991). As the pendulum swings: Teenage childbearing and social concern. *Family Relations, 40,* 127–138.

Furstenberg, F. F., Jr., Brooks-Gunn, J., & Chase-Lansdale, L. (1989). Teenaged pregacy and childbearing. *American Psychologist, 44,* 313–320.

Gelles, R. J. (1986). School-age parents and child abuse. In J. B. Lancaster & B. A. Hamburg (Eds.), *School age pregnancy and parenthood: Biosocial dimensions* (pp. 347–359). New York: Aldine De Gruyter.

Gutelius, M. F., Kirsch, A. D., MacDonald, S., Brooks, M. R., & McErlean, T. (1977). Controlled study of child health supervision: Behavioral results. *Pediatrics, 60,* 294–304.

Halpern, R., & Covey, L. (1983). Community support for adolescent parents and their children: The parent-to-parent program in Vermont. *Journal of Primary Prevention, 3,* 160–173.

Hamburg, B. A., & Dixon, S. L. (1992). Adolescent pregnancy and parenthood. In M. K. Roserheim & M. F. Testa (Eds.), *Early parenthood and coming of age in the 1990s* (pp. 17–33). New Brunswick, NJ: Rutgers University Press.

Hans, S. L., Bernstein, V. J., & Percansky, C. (1991). Adolescent parenting programs: Assessing parent–infant interaction. *Evaluation and Program Planning, 14,* 87–95.

Hayes, C. D. (Ed.). (1987). *Risking the future: Adolescent sexuality, pregnancy, and childbearing* (Vol. I). Washington, DC: National Academy Press.

Hill, J. (1983). Early adolescence: A research agenda. *Journal of Early Adolescence, 3,* 1–21.

Hofferth, S. L. (1991). Programs for high risk adolescents: What works? *Evaluation and Program Planning, 14,* 3–16.

Hofferth, S., & Hayes, C. D. (Eds.). (1987). *Risking the future: Adolescent sexuality, pregnancy, and childbearing* (Vol. II). Washington, DC: National Academy Press.

Inhelder, B., & Piaget, J. (1964). *The growth of logical thinking from childhood to adolescence.* New York: Wiley.

Jones, E. F., Forrest, J. D., Goldman, N., Henshaw, S. K., Lincoln, R., Rosoff, J. Westoff, C. F., & Wulf, D. (1985). Teenage pregnancy in developed countries: Determinants and policy implications. *Family Planning Perspectives, 17,* 53–63.

Kanfer, F. H., & Schefft, B. K. (1988). *Guiding the process of therapeutic change.* Champaign, IL: Research Press.

Kinard, E. M., & Klerman, L. V. (1980). Teenage parenting and child abuse: Are they related? *American Journal of Orthopsychiatry, 50,* 481–488.

Kissman, K. (1992). Parent skills training: Expanding school-based services for adolescent mothers. *Research on Social Work Practice, 2,* 161–171.

Koniak-Griffin, D., Verzemnieks, I., & Cahill, D. (1992). Using videotape instruction and feedback to improve adolescents' mothering behaviors. *Journal of Adolescent Health, 13,* 570–575.

Ladner, J. A. (1987). *Black teenage pregnancy: The black woman.* Garden City, NY: Doubleday.

Levine, L., Garcia Coll, C. T., & Oh, W. (1985). Determinants of mother–infant interaction in adolescent mothers. *Pediatrics, 75,* 23–29.

McAnarney, E. R. (1988). Early adolescent motherhood: Crisis in the making? In M. D. Levine & E. R. McAnarney (Eds.), *Early adolescent transitions* (pp. 139–147). Lexington, MA: Lexington Books.

McAnarney, E. R., Lawrence, R. A., Riccuiti, H. N., Polley, J., & Szilagyi, M. (1986). Interactions of adolescent mothers and their 1-year-old children. *Pediatrics, 78,* 785–790.

Miller, S. (1992). The adolescent parents project: Sharing the transition. In M. Larner, R. Halpern, & O. Harkavy (Eds.), *Fair start for children: Lessons learned from seven demonstration projects* (pp. 136–158). New Haven: Yale University Press.

Milner, J. S. (1986). *The Child Abuse Potential Inventory Manual* (2nd ed.). DeKalb, IL: Psytec Inc.

Musick, J. S. (1993). *Young, poor, and pregnant: The psychology of teenage motherhood.* New Haven: Yale University Press.

Musick, J. S., Bernstein, V., Percansky, C., & Stott, F. M. (1987). A chain of enablement: Using community-based programs to strengthen relationships between teen parents and their infants. *Zero to Three, 8*(2), 1–6.

National Research Council (1993). *Understanding child abuse and neglect.* Washington, DC: National Academy Press.

Osofsky, J. D., Culp, A. M., & Ware, L. M. (1988). Intervention challenges with adolescent mothers and their infants. *Psychiatry, 51,* 236–241.

Osofsky, J. D., Hann, D. M., & Peebles, C. (1993). Adolescent parenthood: Risks and opportunities for mothers and infants. In C. Hanah, Jr. (Ed.), *Handbook of infant mental health* (pp. 106–119). New York: Guilford Press.

Panzarine, S. (1988). Teen mothering: Behaviors and interventions. *Journal of Adolescent Health Care, 9,* 443–448.

Parks, P. L., & Arndt, E. K. (1990). Differences between adolescent and adult mothers of infants. *Journal of Adolescent Health Care, 11,* 248–253.

Polit, D. F., Quint, J. C., & Riccio, J. A. (1988). *The challenge of serving teenage mothers: Lessons from Project Redirection.* New York: Manpower Demonstration Research Corporation.

Quint, J. (1991). Project Redirection: Making and measuring a difference. *Evaluation and Program Planning, 14,* 75–86.

Reis, J. S., & Herz, E. J. (1987). Correlates of adolescent parenting. *Adolescence, 22,* 599–609.

Schorr, L. B. (1988). *Within our reach: Breaking the cycle of disadvantage.* New York: Doubleday.

Stockman, K. D., & Budd, K. S. (in press). Directions for intervention with adolescent mothers in substitute care. *Families in Society: The Journal of Contemporary Human Services.*

Stone, W. L., Bendell, R. D., & Field, T. M. (1988). The impact of socioeconomic status on teenage mothers and children who received early intervention. *Journal of Applied Developmental Psychology, 9,* 391–408.

Teberg, A. J., Howell, V. V., & Wingert, W. A. (1983). Attachment interaction behavior between young teenage mothers and their infants. *Journal of Adolescent Health Care, 4,* 61–66.

Trad, P. V. (1993). Adolescent pregnancy: An intervention challenge. *Child Psychiatry and Human Development, 24,* 99–113.

Unger, D. G., & Wandersman, L. P. (1985). Social support and adolescent mothers: Action research contributions to theory and application. *Journal of Social Issues, 41,* 29–45.

Ware, L., M., Osofsky, J. D., Eberhert-Wright, A. E., & Leichtman, M. L. (1987). Challenges of home visitor interventions with adolescent mothers and their infants. *Infant Mental Health Journal, 8,* 418–428.

Weatherley, R. A. (1991). Comprehensive services for pregnant and parenting adolescents: Historical and political considerations. *Evaluation and Program Planning, 14,* 17–25.

Weinman, M. L., Schreiber, N. B., & Robinson, M. (1992). Adolescent mothers: Were there any gains in a parent education program? *Family & Community Health, 15*(3), 1–10.

Wekerle, C., & Wolfe, D. A. (1993). Prevention of child physical abuse and neglect: Promising new directions. *Clinical Psychology Review, 13,* 501–540.

Widmayer, S. M., & Field, T. M. (1980). Effects of Brazelton demonstrations on early interactions of preterm infants and their teenage mothers. *Infant Behavior and Development, 3,* 79–89.

Williams, C. W. (1991). *Black teenage mothers: Pregnancy and child rearing from their perspective.* Lexington, MA: Lexington Books.

Wilson, W. J. (1987). *The truly disadvantaged: The inner city, the underclass, and public policy.* Chicago: University of Chicago Pres.

Zuravin, S. J. (1988). Child maltreatment and teenage first births: A relationship mediated by chronic sociodemographic stress? *American Journal of Orthopsychiatry, 58,* 91–103.

16

Contributions of Parent Training to Child Welfare
Early History and Current Thoughts

ELSIE M. PINKSTON and MALCOLM D. SMITH

CONTRIBUTIONS OF PARENT TRAINING TO CHILD WELFARE

Core parent training techniques are useful for developing new skills for parents who abuse or neglect their children. In our view parent training has had five primary functions: (1) to improve the quality of parent–child interaction, (2) to prevent further abuse and neglect by the parents, (3) increase community and family linkage, (4) allow parents to resume the care of their children, and (5) reduce the number of children who renter the system. Families who are considered high-risk frequently fit these criteria and techniques may be borrowed from the general parenting literature; its relevance to this population will always be considered.

Other aims of this chapter are to display sensitive parenting interventions that (1) facilitate the transfer of skills from training class to home, (2) extend the effect of training over time, (3) facilitate community and family linkage, and (4) teach the mother to evaluate her own skills.

Single-Parent Families

Single-parent families constitute a growing amalgamation of family types in the population of the United States (U.S. Bureau of the Census, 1991). By 1970, 15 percent of all families were headed by a single woman (Ross & Sawhill, 1975), and 2.9 percent by a single male parent (Blechman & Manning, 1976). Although parent families headed by males have increased more rapidly than have those headed by

ELSIE M. PINKSTON and MALCOLM D. SMITH • School of Social Service Administration, University of Chicago, Chicago, Illinois 60637.
Handbook of Child Abuse Research and Treatment, edited by Lutzker. Plenum Press, New York, 1998.

females, by 1970, 84 percent of all children in single-parent homes lived with a female parent (Ross & Sawhill, 1975). During the decade of 1960–1970, the number of children residing with one parent increased 12 times as fast as did the number of children living with both parents (U.S. Bureau of the Census, 1960, 1970). The absolute increase in the number of children living with single parents concurrently exceeded the increase of children in two-parent families. From these statistics, it is evident that single-parent families comprise a significant segment of the population whose specific needs require consideration in the planning and allocation of family service resources.

The rapid growth of single-parent families in the previous decade has been accompanied by a crucial shift in approaches to their status and function. Historically, single-parent families have been viewed as deviations from "intact" two-parent family norms and have been associated with "broken" homes, illegitimacy, and other disparaging characterizations denoting incompleteness or inadequacy. As a result of increased attention focused on the family (Dworkin, 1978) and single motherhood (Klein, 1973; Mindey, 1969) by the feminist movement, emphasis on family treatment in the helping professions (Fifth Changing Family Conference, 1976; Haley, 1977; Mash, Handy, & Hamerlynch, 1976; Rossi, Kagan, & Hareven, 1977; Satir, 1967), and awareness of the increase in the number of single parents by state (Oregon Bureau of Labor, 1968) and federal governments (Children's Bureau, 1974), single-parent families have begun to be viewed as a "variant child rearing context" (Kadushin, 1970, p. 263) and not inherently or necessarily pathogenic. Single-parent families do seek help for problems, and, according to Beck and Jones (1973), "are disproportionately heavy users of family services" (p. 17). Blechman and Manning (1976) encourage investigators to "train the parent family to compare their outcomes of idealized two-parent families" (p. 80). Although a focus for developing services for single-parent families has been established by census, agency, and conceptual sources, practically no applied versions have been reported. By discarding the notion that they are inherently aberrant and recognizing their increasing representation in the population of family service recipients, researchers and practitioners have been challenged to develop service delivery systems relevant to the needs of single-parent families.

Treatment of Single-Parent Families

Critical reviews of single-parent family literature (Blechman & Manning, 1976; Herzog & Sudia, 1971; Kadushin, 1970; Selden, 1965; Sprey, 1967; Thomes, 1968) have concurred that investigators have emphasized the detrimental effects of family membership, but "have not encouraged planners of primary prevention or secondary intervention to consider the unique treatment needs of parent families, (Blechman & Manning, 1976, p. 61).

However, a growing body of articles has encouraged further investigations of demographic variables, research methods, and social welfare policies to facilitate a constructive approach to one-parent families. Sprey (1967), in proposing guidelines for single-parent family research, endorsed specification of the "conditional characteristics of the families under consideration" (p. 56) and the comparison of carefully chosen samples of different types of single-parent families in order to explicate the unique aspects of single-parent family functioning. Consideration of special acts of a sample may lead to erroneous generalizations, as in the similarity between one-parent families and two-parent families in which a parent is often absent because of work obligations. Rosenfeld and Rosenstein (1973) developed mapping to standard profiles of single-parent families based on the precipitating causes of single parenthood, degrees of parental absence, and their particular effects on family relationships. Consensus on the existence and expression of feelings of social isolation by single mothers is virtually unanimous (Blechman & Manning, 1976; Bould, 1977; Brandwein, Brown, & Fox, 1974; Burgess, 1970; Glasser & Navarre, 1965; Specific variables associated with social isolation that affect parent functioning have been found to include the stigmatizing effects of welfare (Bould, 1977); negative sanctions on single mothers and the poverty resulting from divorce (Bradwein et al., 1974); and the separate personal, family, and role adjustments often required of single parents (Burgess, 1970; Goode, 1960). Similar behavior has been observed in groups of economically deprived families (Besner, 1965), AFDC mothers (Glasser & Navarre, 1965), and British single parents (Ferri & Robinson, 1974; Schlesinger, 1977). Ross and Sawhill (1975) used the phrase "time of transition" to describe single motherhood as a period between living in one nuclear family and another, and also as symbolic of the changing nature of the family in American society, particularly women's expanding roles in the labor force. They emphasized the need for a social policy in regard to families that would allow mothers to improve their economic independence while maintaining a neutral stance toward support of particular family types via family support mechanisms, such as transfer payments and welfare eligibility requirements. Meyer (1978) also recognize the changing structure of family norms and encouraged social policy and practice to maintain neutrality toward them. However, she advised practitioners to remain cognizant of social policy demands which may affect family functioning, and their implications for treatment effectiveness.

Blechman and Manning's (1976) reward–cost analysis emphasized the influence of classes of variables differentiating single-parent families from one another, as well as from two-parent families, and suggested objectives for services to them. Central to their approach is the behavioral diversity among single-parent families attributable to demographic characteristics, such as the gender of the single parent, causes of parental absence, or allocation of parental roles before marital breakup, which mediate members' behaviors. Crucial in an analysis of the mediating functions of demographic variables are their effects on access to rewarding and punishing consequences of the family members' performances of various classes of behaviors. In examining the contingencies that affect single parents, the authors provided two major contributions to the development of this proposal: (1) a description of the role of behavior analysts in engaging in one-parent family treatment; and (2) guidelines for intervention. Clinically oriented social scientists have disparaged the single-parent family's ability to provide adequate role models for children's development (Freud, 1961) or have suggested that women cannot responsibly manage a family outside of marriage (Decter, 1972; Graves, 1965; Staines, Tauris, & Jayaratne, 1974; and Vilar, 1972). Therefore, Blechman and Manning (1976) concluded that "it is not surprising that many therapists have limited therapeutic strategies for the troubled single-parent family" (p. 63). In moving away from treatment focused on the absence of a normal two-parent family, a behavioral treatment approach was considered to be a viable means to change single-parent family behavior without changing family composition.

The guiding philosophy of experimental behavior analysts seems to involve a readiness to view demographic and ecological characteristics as setting events (Bijou & Baer, 1966; Kantor, 1959) that selectively expose the individual to classes of reinforcers and then selectively reinforce behaviors. Demographic characteristics are not uniformly viewed as causes of irreversible structural change within the individual (Blechman & Manning, 1976). The authors expressed optimism that one-parent families could raise children successfully and proposed that their outcomes should be compared to those of other one-parent families rather than to the outcomes of two-parent families, whose behaviors occur under separate sets of setting events. Blechman and Manning (1976) listed the following primary prevention and secondary intervention approaches to behavior and attitude change in single-parent families: (1) train the new single parent to carry out tasks formerly accomplished by the absent parent and self-reward performance of novel tasks; (2) train the single parent to establish personal and parental priorities and to use limited time, energy, and material resources wisely; (3) train to compare outcomes to those of other single-parent families rather than to the outcomes of their idealized two-parent families; (4) prepare the single parents to overcome obstacles to satisfactory adult social relationships; (5) capitalize on the brief period of increased positive interaction between parent and child that may follow one parent's departure; (6) educate the parent about the imbalanced relationship that exists between single parents and children, provide the parent with cognitions that will interfere with a exploited martyred self-concept; and (7) train the parent and children to avoid a spiral of aversive control and avoidance during adolescent socialization.

Fathers

Parent training has proven to be effective for improving the behaviors of children with a variety of conduct problems. It has also helped educate parents about child development; this in turn reduced the rates of abuse and neglect that occur in many households. Much of the research that is conducted on parent training has looked at mothers more than at fathers. Several studies have examined fathers' experiences with parent training programs. One question is whether or not the presence of fathers influences the results of parent training. Over the years, several researchers have begun examining the different effects that fathers' presence or absence in a family has on the results of parent training programs. May argue that a father's presence in the household has no additional effect on the parent training, whereas others insist that the father can enhance the results of parent training programs, or hinder the results if he is not invested in the success of the program. The following will examine research which has been conducted with the intention of answering the question of the influence of fathers on parent training programs.

Several studies have established that parent training classes do assist in the education of parents and the reduction of conduct problems in children. However, many factors influence a program's success. Children's improved behaviors do not diminish when their surrounding environment continues to provide them with consequences for their actions. Studies have found that the involvement of one parent in a child management program is not as effective as having two. If one parent does not participate, the program's potential may lose its power because the parent, often the father, who has not participated, will act in ways that discount the structure of the child management program (Budd & O'Brien, 1982).

Budd and O'Brien (1982) found that fathers are more actively involved in parent training than has been generally recognized. Additional studies have examined ways in which parents' behaviors have influenced the results of parent training programs. Many issues, such as parents' disagreeing on the methods taught in the program and misunderstandings between parents about the implementation of the treatment methods, have created problems with the results of the program. Once misunderstandings of this nature are clarified, the results have been more successful child treatment. Budd and O'Brien present three studies which look at whether the father's presence in the family has a impact on the changes that occur in a child's behavior after the parents have gone through a parent training class. The first study found that parents reported significantly fewer problems with their children after the parents had completed the program, but no major differences were seen as a result of the father's presence or absence in the family (Budd & O'Brien, 1982). In the few situations where the father was present but not a part of the training, the treatment methods were said to be "sabotaged" by the father.

The second study that Budd and O'Brien discuss is a 1980 study by Firestone, Kelly, & Fike (1980). The results of this study were the same as the first, in that the families who participated in the study saw decreases in the negative behaviors of their children. The families where a father who was involved in the parent training showed significant decrease(s) in problematic behavior in one part of the study. There were no differences between a father's presence and a father's absence on other parts of the study.

Adesso and Lipson (1981) performed the third study that Budd and O'Brien presented. The results of the study were similar to the previous two in that behaviors changed, but no significant differences were discovered when both parents were part of the training.

The basic conclusion of all three of the studies was that fathers' involvement did not have a significant impact on the effectiveness of parent training programs. In her article titled "The effects of father involvement in parent training for conduct problem children," Carolyn Webster-Stratton discusses a study by Strain, Young, and Horowitz (1981) which shows that "fathers' involvement [in parent training programs] is an important factor in the maintenance of treatment effects" (Webster-Stratton, 1985). The apparent lack of impact of the fathers' presence created a desire for more research. Many felt that the studies' reliability was invalid because of the methods of data collection.

Webster-Stratton performed a study with 30 families, 18 in which the father was involved and 12 in which the father was absent, that was geared toward determining whether fathers' presence did have an effect on parent training in families. Webster-Stratton found that men's (fathers' and boyfriends') involvement altered their attitudes toward their conduct-disordered children, and the changes were found in the men one year later. In the families in which mothers and their children maintained an improved relationship one year after the parent training program, the fathers' presence yielded a higher number of relationships between mother and child which were reported to have retained the satisfactory improvements. These results suggest that the father's presence helps maintain the efforts of parent training programs. Webster-Stratton suggested that the results of the study show that the male figure can act as a support system for the mother, to maintain the methods of the parent training program in the family. She also suggests, however, that single-parent mothers may want to go through a parent training program with a close friend or relative in order to create a similar support system when a man is not around to encourage the mother to carry out the parent training techniques. Webster-Stratton concludes that other factors such as income could have created the differences that were found a year later, rather than the presence of a male figure.

There still seems to be a question about the importance of a father's presence in terms of creating the best possible parent training results. One could speculate that any individual who is invested in being trained to assist the child would suffice as a partner to the parent of a conduct-disordered child. One must also consider, however, that the presence of the father in the child's life will most likely have an enormous effect on the effectiveness of a parent training program. Additional research should look at differences among groups in which the mother has a partner other than the husband, has the husband as a partner, or has no partner with whom she can go through the parent training. The results of such a study may help reveal additional information about how to continue and enhance the positive results that come from parent training programs.

In conclusion, one must recognize that we have so far examined what dynamics would influence a parent training program in a way that will enhance the results of the program. The parent training programs which have been discussed have produced desired results when the techniques were correctly followed by the families. The presence of the father only introduced the issue of what can be done to improve the already effective results of such programs. In selecting approaches to use while treating families, parent training should be seen as a highly desirable option to help accomplish the desired goals.

Parents with Substance Abuse Problems

Substance abuse is a problem that has spread throughout the United States. Many children are abused and neglected by their substance abusing parents. Parents often do not understand what types of behaviors or activities are appropriate for children of different ages. This often leads to unrealistic expectations being placed on the child. The following looks at how parent training has been useful in working with families in which a parent is abusing substances.

In an article entitled "Intervention with Cocaine-Abusing Mothers," Haskett, Miller, Whitworth, and Huffman (1992) discuss the issue of parenting classes with substance abusing parents. They report that parents who abuse drugs "feel less adequate in the parenting role; have a more authoritarian, controlling approach to interacting with their infants and children; and are less capable of providing appropriate stimulation" (Haskett et al., 1992, p. 456). In a special program designed to teach cocaine-abusing mothers parenting skills, mothers learn about bow their cocaine-exposed babies are easily stimulated. They are taught how to comfort their children without overstimulating them. The mothers are also taught to look for specific signs that would show that the child was becoming overstimulated. The mothers are further taught such skills as stress management, controlling their anger or frustration, and planning ahead for both their baby's care and their own.

DeMarsh and Kumpfer (1985) note that parent training is now considered a necessary component of any comprehensive prevention plan that can affect a wide range of social and health problems, including child abuse and neglect, juvenile delinquency, childhood mental health problems and behavioral problems, and substance abuse.

They go on to elaborate that practitioners are beginning to use parent training methods in order to enhance the work they do with children. By involving parents in the process, the effectiveness of their therapy improves when the parents are conducting the same therapeutic strategies at home (DeMarsh & Kumpfer, 1985). The parents are taught skills such as attending to children, reinforcing behaviors, using appropriate discipline, behavior management, raising a child's self-esteem, improving the family's communication, and assisting children in performing well at school. They are then given homework assignments to help establish the new skills.

DeMarsh and Kumpfer (1985) report that some see parent training with an individual as less effective than training an entire family. Family training techniques also exist. Behavioral sessions with both the parents and the children enable therapists to observe how the parents interact with their children. This proves to be a strong advantage for therapists working with dysfunctional families. Several studies have found family sessions to be effective alternatives to individual parent training.

Azar (1989) has examined the historical background of child abuse and parent training. She states that parents who are typically labeled as child abusers often "demonstrate low cognitive functioning, are poorly educated, and come from low socioeconomic backgrounds" (p. 420). She states that behavioral therapists had found that parent training proved to be effective over a short period of time with dysfunctional families. In the 1970s, behavioral therapists began to apply parent training techniques with abusive parents. Azar writes of the importance of parent training that addresses not only the abuse of the child, but also the lack of parental responses that guide the child toward alternative behaviors that would be seen as appropriate by the parent. Parents must be taught what responses by children are developmentally appropriate. Many adults expect children to respond in ways that are characteristic of adults. To do so sets the child up to fail, which often leads to their abuse by the parent holding the expectation.

Azar (1989) has observed that abusive parents have been shown to have higher levels of unrealistic expectations of their children, to overgeneralize negative ratings of child behavior, to ascribe more negative intention to children's behavior even in situations where they are not at fault, and to have significantly poorer problem-solving ability. Moreover, the fact that abusive parents have been shown to have significantly lower levels of interaction, especially positive interaction, with their children supports the idea that these parents may find contact with their children more aversive.

Parent training provides abusive parents with alternative, nonabusive ways to discipline their children, methods that can be used to shape the child's environment so that the need to punish is decreased. Parents are taught stress reduction techniques for themselves. This allows them to manage their children when their own stress levels are low. Reinforcement, extinction, time-out, and response-cost procedures are other methods which could be taught during parent training sessions (Azar, Benjet, Fuhrmann, & Cavallero, 1995; Azar, Robinson, Hekimian, & Twentyman, 1984).

Azar (1989) suggests that when working with abusive families it is important for the parent trainer to keep the child's safety as the primary concern at all times. At each treatment, clinicians should ask themselves whether or not they suspect any maltreatment. Azar stresses the importance of therapists receiving consultation and of being aware of clinical biases or denial about families whom they would not suspect of being abusive (e.g., middle- and upper-class families, and families who are not of minority status).

According to Azar (1989), many abusive parents frequently have borderline or retarded cognitive functioning levels, which makes it difficult for them to understand the techniques that are being taught. If parents are high on a substance, the same results would most likely occur. In some situations, the cognitive skills are not so limited; however, the parents often have low levels of education and are therefore unable to read the material they are given in parent training sessions. Parent training can be provided to these individuals, but it may be necessary to treat them individually in order to produce the same results. Many parents have histories of maltreatment by their own parents, and many of the techniques that are introduced to them trigger memories of the earlier abuse. In these situations, it is often necessary to help the parents cope with their own memories before teaching them new techniques with their children. Finally, Azar discusses the importance of teaching parents anger control skills. In many situations, the behaviors they are trying to eliminate, with extinction, for example, will increase before they decrease. The parents must have training that will allow them to cope with this increased behavior and will keep the child safe from lashing out by the parent. When a parent is abusing substances, this process may take longer.

Cognitive restructuring and problem solving are also discussed by Azar (1989). She states that it is important for parents to understand the relationship between their thoughts and their responses. With such an understanding, parents are able to work on cognitive restructuring. This process assists the parents in recognizing their unrealistic expectations of their children, or may help increase their problem-solving skills.

Stress management and anger control training are other areas that Azar (1989) highlights as being important parts of the parent training process. Many parents are able to control their stress, but it is control of their anger that often presents problems that lead to abuse. Training parents to recognize signals that occur before the abuse starts helps to reduce abusive behaviors. Recognizing and pinpointing warning signs is often the most difficult part of this intervention for abusive parents. As Azar writes, parents will often say "it just happened." Such techniques as role-playing, guided imagery, and reading scripts have been used to assist parents with the difficult and confronting process. Again, substance abusing parents may take longer to get through this process. Often they may understand what they are taught in the parent training session; however, their cognitive functioning will be so grossly distorted while under the influence of substances that not all of the information they have learned will not be accessible to them.

Azar (1989) details additional techniques that have been used in parent training. One technique teaches families about the use of rewards, consequences, and modeling. Another—the combination approach—included interventions such as desensitization to children's behaviors, targeting situations which are most likely to lead to stress, and child-proofing homes. The results of the combination treatment were positive, but it was difficult to isolate the relevant treatment variables.

Parent training may be presented in several ways. It is often more effective when the primary caretaker is the only one to receive treatment. For other families, family treatment has been more effective in eliminating some of the abusive behaviors. Regardless of how the parent training is delivered, it has consistently assisted in eliminating abusive behaviors. Parents who are substance abusers may forget the information when they are under the influence of a substance, but the studies have shown that substance abusing families are also positively influenced by parent training techniques. Educating parents about appropriate children's developmental behaviors, as well as the options that exist in terms of responding to their children, will assist in the healthy development of family bonds and relationships. It will also assist in reducing the rate of child abuse in the United States, and will provide positive alternatives to families who incorporate the parent training into their daily lives.

Discontinuance

A potential problem in any parenting program is discontinuance. Baekeland and Lundwall's (1995) exhaustive critical review of disengagement in many types of helping interventions presented three ways to conceptualize attrition: (1) demographic, personality, and clinical factors of the client; (2) variables of the therapist's personality, attitudes toward clients, and therapeutic style; and (3) variables related to environmental factors. Of particular relevance to this program are the setting events which may affect parent participation and family functioning, perceptions of the therapists' roles by the parents, and parent attitudes toward their own roles as therapists, a unique component of the program. Treatment literature includes studies of motivation (Ripple, 1957), predictive factors in the initial interview (Blenkner, 1954), types of social environments that may influence disengagement (Mayer & Rosenblatt, 1964; Rosenblatt & Mayer, 1966), and a description of the process of securing and receiving services from the client's perspective (Mayer & Timms, 1970) that contributed to the form and content of the follow-up interview.

Extensive reviews of continuance-discontinuous (C-D) studies revealed that considerable efforts have been expended on issues in one-to-one psychotherapeutic treatment approaches (Baekeland & Lundwall, 1995; Bostwick, 1977; Garfield, 1978). Bostwick (1977) found only one behavioral article that mentioned C-D in parent–child problems (Thomas & Walters, 1973), and, in five studies that directly examine C-D in parent–child treatment, behavioral approaches were not used and parents were excluded from the samples (Clement, 1964; Lake & Levinger, 1960; McAdoo & Roeske, 1973; Ross & Lacey, 1961; Williams & Pollack, 1964). In discussing the paucity of attrition studies in behavior therapy, Garfield (1978) speculated that "since many . . . are planned investigations of therapy outcome, little attention is focused on dropouts; rather, the emphasis is placed on filling the vacated slots in the different subject groups" (p. 210).

One parent training study (Bernal, North, & Kreutzer, 1974) directly examined C-D with single- and two-parent families, and only a few studies even reported dropout rates (Cohen, 1970; Eyberg & Johnson, 1974; Morrey, 1973; Patterson, 1973a; Rickert & Moore, 1970; Stuart & Tripodi, 1971). Results of two studies of procedures used to identify problem children indicated that excuses were related to dropping out, and cooperation with early procedures predicted continuation (Bernal et al., 1974). Although the program was not designed to teach the parents child management skills, the results are relevant to evaluating participating in training: (1) associations between single- and two-parent family membership and phase completion or completion of the entire identification process were insignificant; (2) parents who did not ask for help were more likely to drop out of the program at its outset; (3) time demands and delays in service delivery may increase attrition; (4) parents are more likely to keep home than office appointments; (5) staff expenditure of effort in soliciting parental cooperation may affect continuance. Measures of client satisfaction, parent perceptions of problem severity, and the extent of the child's problems were recommended for a comprehensive evaluation of services. In conclusion, Bernal and associates (1974) predicted that to recruit 22 families to complete the identification process, workers would have had to send letters to 1800 families, of which 50 would meet entrance criteria, considering the 56 percent dropout rate from the two studies (p. 63): Parent training attrition rates have been reported as high as 70 percent, but these figures are not necessarily higher than those of other types of parent treatment programs (Bernal, 1971), and basically reflect a failure to engage the parent initially.

Parents as Therapists for Special Problems of Their Children

The concept of parents as therapists for their children has been widely used by behavior analysts and has been reviewed for its effectiveness (Berkowitz & Graziano, 1972; Johnson & Katz, 1973; O'Dell, 1974), research methodology (Gelfand & Hartman, 1968; Pawlicki, 1970), generality of treatment effects (Forehand & Atkeson, 1977), and effectiveness compared to other treatment models (Anchor & Thomason, 1977; Tavormina, 1974). Four major areas of experimentation are relevant to the program: (1) investigation of currently accepted treatment procedures and their effects (Christopherson, Arnold, Hill, & Quilitch, 1975; Herbert et al., 1973; Pinkston & Herbert-Jackson, 1975; Wahler, 1969a, b, Wahler, Winkel, Peterson, & Morrison, 1965; Wetzel, Baker, Roney, & Martin, 1966); (2) investigation of parent training in the home (Bernal et al., 1968; Budd, Pinkston & Green, 1973; Hawkins, Peterson, Schweid, & Bijou, 1966; Levenstein, Kochman, & Roth, 1973; O'Leary, O'Leary, & Becker, 1967); (3) treatment of parent–child interaction problems via a clinic approach (Bernal, 1971; Budd et al., 1973; Hanf, 1968; Henderson & Garcia, 1973; Russo, 1964; Zeilberger, Sampen, & Sloane, 1968); and (4) application of parent training research criteria to the treatment of single-parent families (Berkowitz & Graziano, 1972; Bernal et al., 1974; Blechman & Manning, 1976; Forehand & Atkeson, 1977; Johnson & Katz, 1973; Patterson, 1973a, 1974b; Patterson et al., 1975).

Extension of procedures supported by existing two-parent family training data to single-parent families appeared feasible because "in nearly all papers the mothers were the primary objects of training and bore the major responsibility for carrying out the home programs," (Berkowitz & Graziano, 1972, p. 465). A glaring omission in the parent training literature has been concern for the effects of parent demographic characteristics on training (O'Dell, 1974), which severely limits the generalizability of the results. Identification of single parents in training reports has usually been confined to their inclusion as a few members of a larger group of two-parent families (Bernal et al., 1972; Eyberg & Johnson, 1974; Karoly & Rosenthal, 1977; Patterson et al., 1975), and outcomes have rarely been analyzed according to family composition variables (Patterson et al., 1975). The lack of systematic evaluation of variables affecting parent participation and success rates for different types of families may be explained by the primary thrust of parent training to date: the efficacy of change procedures for various classes of child behaviors, such as aggression (Patterson et al., 1975), noncompliance (Forehand, King, Peed, & Yoder, 1975; Peed, Roberts, & Forehand, 1977), and toilet training (Foxx & Azrin, 1973a, b). Family characteristics which may affect participation have been viewed as secondary to recruiting families with children who exhibit the specific behaviors under investigation. O'Dell (1974) ascribed sampling problems in parent training to using volunteers as subjects, which may account for parent diversity but does not preclude consideration of variables affecting differential treatment outcomes. Although the field of parent training is moving toward the study of planned generalization of behavior change (Stokes & Baer, 1977), there is an accompanying emphasis on the differential effects of training procedures for parents whose ability to participate in programs may be affected by a variety of conditions associated with family composition.

Drawing from the basic tenets of social learning theory and parent training research, the Parenting Training Program extends the application of home-based contingency management programs to families. Grounded in learning theory (Skinner, 1953, 1969) and applications of the theory to child development (Bijou & Baer, 1965), the program assumed the primacy of the parent as a source of social and material consequences affecting children's behavior in the home (Patterson, 1973b). Therefore, undesirable child behavior was seen as partially caused by the interaction of the child and parent, and the locus of intervention entailed training the parent as a therapist for his or her child (Berkowitz & Graziano, 1972; Johnson & Katz, 1973; O'Dell, 1974). Three principles are implicit in a social learning, or behavioral, approach to parent training programs: (1) most of a child's behavior (maladaptive and desirable) is maintained by its effects on the natural environment and can be most effectively modified by changing the reinforcing contingencies supplied by the social agents who live with the child (Berkowitz & Graziano, 1972; Peine, 1969); (2) demographic and ecological characteristics are setting events that selectively expose an individual or family to classes of reinforcers and that selectively reinforce behavior, but do not cause irreversible personal or group structural changes (Bijou & Baer, 1966; Blechman & Manning, 1976; Kantor, 1959); and (3) actively training parents to be future problem-solvers rather than future service seekers describes a delivery system based on prevention (Berkowitz & Graziano, 1972; Ojeman, 1967; Walder et al., 1971). A constructional approach to behavior change (Goldiamond, 1974) underscored intervention strategies focused on providing reinforcement for attractive behaviors that are incompatible with undesirable ones.

The parenting literature has shown many practical benefits: reduced child abuse behavior, reduced delinquent behaviors, less mental illness in children, and improved quality of life. We will be discussing good parent training practices that will (1) develop more targeted assessment of parents to determine their deficits and strengths, (2) decide the best point of entry for parents to receive training, (3) replace the "one size fits all" model of parent training with a more focused approach to specific parent problems, and (4) use outcome measures that will be more useful to workers and the juvenile court for making decisions regarding parent fitness. Goals designed to correct existing problems in parent training are to (1) facilitate the transfer of skill from training class to home, (2) extend the effect of training over time, and (3) teach the mother to evaluate her own skills. To accomplish these aims we will institute more structured evaluation during home visits, increase the opportunities for mothers whose children are in foster care to practice parenting skills in supervised visits, and add booster sessions, following termination, at 1 month, 3 months, 7 months, and 12 months.

The guiding philosophy we will use in selecting parent training methods involves a readiness to view demographic and ecological characteristics (Bijou & Baer, 1966; Kantor, 1959) as not causing irreversible pathology within the individual (Blechman & Manning, 1976). Parent training selectively exposes the individual to experiences that support desired behavioral outcomes, that is, improved parenting skills and better child developmental repertoires.

Graziano and Diamet (1992) note that the main thrust of parent training with child abuse and neglect has been to alter aggressive behavior toward the child. They found 17 studies with abusive and neglectful parents that showed promise. They point out, and we agree, that more studies should be conducted on parent training that focuses on the positive skills that are needed to care for their children. For instance, using public school records, George, Van Voorhis, Grant, Casey, & Robinson (1992) discovered that more than six times as many foster children receive special education than reported to Illinois Department of Children and Family Services (IDCFS). We infer from this that it is likely that many parents of developmentally delayed children could benefit from parent training that teaches them to understand their children's problems and how to work with them. In some cases developmental disability rnay be environmentally caused and, therefore, foster parents and biological parents need additional training to learn to work with the children. This is also true in the area of emotional and medical disabilities.

Parent training is a substantial source of innovation that could be incorporated in the child welfare endeavor (see Graziano & Diamet, 1992; Polster, Dangel, & Rasp, 1987).

TRAINING METHODS FOR PARENTS

A few studies teaching counting and recording skills (Cohen, 1970) and behavioral vocabulary rather than contingency management skills (Lindsley, 1970) may influence participation, but the bulk of parent training research concerned with factors involved in discontinuance has concentrated on identifying incentives to encourage parents to complete training programs. Services for the parent contingent on engaging in child-related tasks (Patterson & Reid, 1970; Stein & Gambrill, 1976a, b), payment of a contract deposit refundable upon completion of task assignments and training (Eyberg & Johnson, 1974; Patterson et al., 1975), and group training as a means of multiple reinforcement for attendance (Rose, 1977) have been shown to facilitate participation. Parental cooperation and motivation have also been considered important for successful training (Bernal et al., 1968, 1972; Wagner, 1968), and parents with schizophrenia and mental retardation have usually been excluded from training (Karoly & Rosenthal, 1977; Patterson et al., 1975; Wiltz, 1969). However, the effectiveness of parent training procedures and the specific reasons for discontinuance are often vague. O'Dell (1974) offered limited evidence in drawing two conclusions regarding the efficacy of parent training: (1) verbal learning approaches sometimes require more highly educated parents (Patterson et al., 1973; Saliinger et al., 1970); and (2) programs that emphasize actual behavioral learning, and tailored programs, can produce desired results in a wider range of parents (Bernal et al., 1968). Although Patterson and associates (1975) claimed that "poorer treatment outcomes tended to be obtained with father-absent families," (p. 61), the conditions affecting their results were not fully described. Interactive effects of training techniques and individual parent characteristics may further increase diversity in treatment outcomes (Gelfand & Hartman, 1968), even among ostensibly homogeneous groups, such as single parents. The objectives of this program included collecting not only observational data from participants to assess the effects of child management procedures on the children's behavior, but also follow-up interview data from all program entrants to describe the conditions that may have affected parent participation.

The concept of parents as therapists for their children has been widely used, reviewed for its effectiveness (Berkowitz & Graziano, 1972; Johnson & Katz, 1973; O'Dell, 1974), research methodology (Gelfand & Hartman, 1968; Pawlicki, 1970), generality of treatment effects (Forehand & Atkeson, 1977), and effectiveness compared to other treatment models (Anchor & Thomason, 1977; Tavormina, 1974). Four major areas of experimentation are relevant: (1) investigation of currently accepted treatment procedures and their effects (Christopherson et al., 1975; Herbert et al., 1973; Pinkston & Herbert-Jackson, 1975; Wahler, 1969a b, Wahler et al., 1965; Wetzel et al., 1966); (2) investigation of parent training in the home (Beral et al., 1968; Budd et al., 1973; Hawkins et al., 1966; Levenstein et al., 1973; O'Leary et al., 1967); (3) treatment of parent–child interaction problems via a clinic approach (Bernal, 1971; Budd et al., 1973; Hanf, 1968; Henderson & Garcia, 1973; Russo, 1964; Zeilberger et al., 1968); and (4) application of parent training research criteria to the treatment of single-parent families (Berkowitz & Graziano, 1972;, Bernal et al., 1974; Blechman & Manning, 1976; Forehand & Atkeson, 1977; Johnson & Katz, 1973; Patterson, 1973a, 1974b; Patterson et al., 1975).

TRAINING METHODS FOR WORKERS

We regard staff training and supervision as key to any successful improvement in child protective service delivery. Service workers must be trained to strengthen families to prevent unnecessary out-of-home placement of children and to develop and implement acceptable permanency plans. We endorse and will incorporate the recommendations of the report "Review and Revision of Training Chapters Reform Panel" (April, 1993). As noted in Illinois Department of Children and Family Services' (IDCFS) response to the panel report, "Review and Revision of Training Chapters Reform Panel Recommendations," many of the structural changes suggested are under way. In the panel's report they state that, "Training should always reflect the service needs of the clients, the support needs of the workers and respect for the inclusion of cultural diversity" (p. 15). We also endorse their recommendation that *all* new workers receive Core Training. We intend to use their report, which contains excellent suggestions for the structure of core training that would involve (1) the core would be split into two mandatory components, Core I and Core II; (2) Core would occur immediately upon hiring, take 12 weeks, and cover the broad conceptual areas of assessment, protection, documentation, and cultural competency. Core II would include skill-building more closely related to the workers' specific needs and would be selected by the workers and their supervisors. To the suggested Core I curriculum we would add values and ethics; skills for client and family engagement, especially as related to involuntary clients; task analysis; problem solving; behavior management; and education based on the perspective that children preferably should he maintained in their homes, but that regardless of location they should be provided with stability that will allow education and ongoing relationships.

Skills for Workers

All skills required are beyond the scope of this paper but a preliminary list is provided by Maluccio, Krieger, and Pine (1990):

- Assessing and utilizing family strengths
- Assessing, modifying, and using the environment
- Assessing severe pathology, chronic substance abuse, the potential for violent behavior; goal planning, including setting clear, specific, and limited goals on the basis of careful assessment
- Using time frames and setting time limits
- Decision making; contracting with families
- Combining concrete and clinical services
- Using informal as well as formal helping resources
- Teaching life skills, especially skills in parenting, problem solving, negotiation, communication, behavior management, and mood management
- Collaborating with a variety of service providers
- Understanding and working with the policies, rules, and procedures of a variety of child welfare programs
- Tailoring services to the needs of each family, with flexibility in the use of self on the part of the worker, in accessibility of worker, in location of service, and in selection of strategies
- Offering crisis intervention services
- Providing intensive services
- Responding quickly to a family's direct or indirect request for help
- Engaging families in their home settings
- Using termination as an aid in empowering families, and facilitating networking and referrals to ongoing services when needed

One of the great weaknesses in most child welfare staff training systems is the lack of attention to existing staff training literature. The current training literature describes a number of techniques for transferring skills learned in group sessions to the home and community. The absence of this transfer has been one of the most serious problems in the delivery of this treatment approach. Effective staff training produces staff who are knowledgeable about and competently trained in the application of behavioral procedures. In this chapter, special care is taken to distinguish between initial staff training and procedures for the generalization and maintenance of training knowledge and skills (Hersen & Bellack, 1978). Traditional staff training methods have included lectures, discussions, readings, films, and slides (Hersen & Bellack, 1978). These techniques are often informative about general behavioral principles and the global outline of interventions (Cuff, 1977; Delamater, Conners, & Wells, 1984; Gardner, 1972). However, their effectiveness in promoting the acquisition and employment of intervention skills is, at best, equivocal. For example, a few studies note at least some positive effects on caregiver skills (Cuff, 1977), but many others find that such techniques have little or no effect in developing behavior-management skills (Bernstein, 1982; Delamater et al., 1984). Significantly, however, several studies find it possible to greatly augment the positive impact of such instructional methods by supplementing them with other more experiential techniques (McMahon, Forehand, & Griest, 1981). Among the most notable of these experiential techniques are role-playing (Gardner, 1972), modeling, and feedback. Numerous studies have now tested packages of these methods, for example, role-playing, modeling, and feedback; training manuals, modeling, and feedback; lecture and discussion, modeling, rehearsal, and feedback; lecture, case examples, and role-play; and in-service role-play, modeling, rehearsal, feedback, and reinforcement (Delamater et al., 1984). These studies make it evident that a variety of quite effective methods are now available for teaching behavior-change skills.

In addition to the initial acquisition of knowledge and practice skills, there is the matter of generalization, or transfer of new learning from the convenient settings where it is taught to the problematic settings where it is needed. The procedures that can greatly enhance generalization (and maintenance) may be (and optimally would be) incorporated into the initial training, or, if necessary, could be made part of subsequent maintenance procedures. When that is done well, the resultant generality of behavior-management skills greatly increases the probability that new problems will be solved soon after they arise, that new clients will be effectively included as they enter the setting, and that new skills will be maintained at effective levels over time.

Demonstrations of such generality built into initial training processes include generality across problems, generality across clients, and temporal generality (Griest, Forehand, Rogers, et al., 1982). However, a problem with many of these studies is that their assessment of that generality (especially maintenance) was often done far less rigorously than their assessment of the effectiveness of their teaching techniques. In addition, even when we trust their summary conclusions, we rarely can see which parts of their complex packages were responsible for that very attractive outcome.

In light of that uncertainty, and considering the need for strong maintenance after any initial training, posttraining is a useful additional or complementary process. It may take the forms of public posting, practice, and feedback; modeling; planning activities, feedback, and reinforcement; fading out (Herbert & Baer, 1972); and self-monitoring, self-evaluation, and self-reinforcement. Of the studies just mentioned, those that show desirable maintenance of their newly taught skills also employed multiple techniques—a training/maintenance package. Most of these packages included some form of instruction, guided practice, and immediate feedback. We see the desirability of the multimethod approach, probably with instructions, some form of practice, and some form of feedback about that practice as its major components.

CONTRIBUTIONS OF PARENT TRAINING TO CHILD WELFARE

Our review of parent training in child welfare shows that too often there was little in the way of specific plans regarding training (Wolfe, 1985). Most programs seemed to focus primarily on anger control and child management. In general there were no specific plans for dealing with the problems of parents of special needs children or parents with specific problems such as alcohol or drug abuse. The vast number of cases referred to the Illinois Department of Children and Family Service are for neglect. In addition, many of the children in the child welfare system have developmental disability problems; therefore, it would seem that a different focus is called for in the development of contracts. The current contracts are essentially nonspecific in focus. Even basic requirements for information such as the following are missing in most contracts: number of families, number of classes, curriculum, percentage of attendance, and percentage of completion.

Such basic questions as the following about the parenting groups are not required in most proposals: (1) What assessment is used to determine the lack of parenting skills? (2) Does assignment to parenting class involve an assessment of parents' abilities to participate and learn? (3) What is the mental stability of the parent? (4) Is there drug use or the management of drug use by the parent? It is important to state these issues and to analyze their functional relationship to parenting skills.

Other questions that need to be answered are listed: Is the parenting program problem specific? What are the problems to be addressed in training? How does the parent need to change? Is changing behavior a goal? What behaviors will be changed? What are the interventions that will be used to achieve these changes? Are both the child and the parent involved in the training? Are there provisions for additional services such as mental health services and substance abuse programs? Is there an evaluation component, that is, how does the agency know if it has met its goals? How would specific behavioral improvement on the part of the parent be measured? How would developmental and behavioral progress on the part of the child be measured? Is there a home visit component to the program? If so, describe the visits: frequency, length, tasks to promote generalized training. By and large the contracts are too general and do not foster the development of parent training innovations. More seriously, they do not offer a clue as to whether or not the program has any of the characteristics of parenting programs that have been shown to be effective.

REFERENCES

Adesso, V. J., & Lipson, J. W. (1981). Group training of parents as therapists for their children. *Behavior Therapy, 12,* 625–633.

Anchor, K. N., & Thomason, T. C. (1977). A comparison of two parent-training models with educated parents. *Journal of Community Psychology, 5,* 134–141.

Azar, S. A. (1989). Training parents of abused children. In C. E. Schaefer & J. M. Breismeister (Eds.),

Handbook of parent training: Parents as co-therapists for children's behavior problems (pp. 414–444). New York: Wiley.

Azar, S. T., Benjet, C. L., Fuhrmann, G. S., & Cavallero, L. (1995). Child maltreatment and termination of parental rights: Can behavioral research help Solomon? *Behavior Therapy, 26,* 599–623.

Azar, S. T., Robinson, D. R., Hekimian, E., & Twentyman, C. T. (1984). Unrealistic expectations and problem-solving ability in maltreating and comparison mothers. *Journal of Consulting and Clinical Psychology, 52,* 687–691.

Baekelad, F., & Lundwall, L. (1975). Dropping out of treatment: A critical review. *Psychological Bulletin, 82,* 738–783.

Beck, D. F., & Jones, M. A. (1973). *Progress on family problems: A nationwide study of clients' and counselors' views on family agency services.* New York: Family Service Association of America.

Berkowitz, B. P., & Graziano, A. M. (1972). Training parents as behavior therapists: A review. *Behavior Research and Therapy, 10,* 297–317.

Bernal, M. E. (1971). Training parents in child management. In R. H. Bradfield (Ed.), *Behavior modification of learning disabilities.* San Rafael, CA: Academic Therapy Publications.

Bernal, M. E., North, J. A., & Kreutzer, S. L. (1974). Cross-validation of excuses and cooperation in identifying clinic dropouts. *American Journal of Community Psychology, 2,* 151–163.

Bernal, M. E., Williams, D. E., Miller, W. H., & Reagor, P. A. (1972). The use of videotape feedback and operant learning principles in training parents in management of deviant children. In R. D. Rubin, H. Fensterheim, J. D. Henderson, & L. P. Ullman (Eds.), *Advances in behavior therapy* (pp. 19–31). New York: Academic Press.

Bernal, M. E., Duryee, J. S., Pruett, H. L., & Burns, B. (1968). *Journal of Clinical Child Psychology, 32*(4), 447–455.

Bernstein, G. S. (1982). Training behavior change agents: A conceptual review. *Behavior Therapy, 13,* 1–23.

Besner, A. (1965). Economic deprivation and family patterns. *Welfare in Review, 3,* 20–28.

Bijou, S. W., & Baer, D. M. (1966). Oparent methods in behavior and development. In W. K. Honig (Ed.), *Operant behavior: Areas of research and application* (pp. 718–789). New York: Appleton-Century-Crofts.

Blechman, E. A., & Manning, M. (1976). A reward–cost analysis of the single parent family. In E. J. Mash, L. A. Hamerlynck, & L. C. Handy (Eds.), *Behavior modification and families.* New York: Brunner/Mazel.

Blenkner, M. (1954). Predictive factors in the initial interview in family casework. *Social Service Review, 28,* 65–73.

Bostwick, G. J. (1977). *Factors associated with continuance-discontinuance in family therapy: A multivarigate, multi-component analysis.* Unpublished dissertation proposal, University of Chicago, School of Social Service Administration.

Bould, S. (1977). Female-headed families: Personal fate control and the provider role. *Journal of Marriage and the Family, 37,* 339–349.

Brandwein, R. A., Brown, C.A., & Fox, E. M. (1974). Women and children last: The social situation of divorced mothers and their families. *Journal of Marriage and the Family, 34,* 498–514.

Budd, K. S., & O'Brien, T. P. (1982). Father involvement in behavior parent training: An area in need of research. *Behavior Therapist, 5,* 85–89.

Budd, K. J., Pinkston, E. M., & Green, D. R. (1973). *An analysis of two parent-training packages for remediation of child aggression in laboratory and home settings.* Paper presented at the meeting of the American Psychological Association, Montreal, Canada.

Burgess, J. K. (1970). The single-parent family: A social and sociological problem. *Family Coordinator, 19*(2), 137–144.

Children's Bureau. (1974). *One parent families.* Washington, DC: US Department of Health, Education, and Welfare, DHEW Publication No. OHD. 74-44.

Chistopherson, E. R., Arnold, C. M., Hill, D. W., & Quilitch, H. R. (1995). The home point system: Token reinforcement procedures for application by parents of children with behavior problems. *Journal of Applied Behavior Analysis, 5,* 485–499.

Clement, R. G. (1964). *Factors associated with continuance and discontinuance in cases involving problems in the parent child relationship.* Unpublished doctoral dissertation, University of Chicago, School of Social Service Administration.

Cohen, H. C. (1970). *The P.I.C.A. project. Year two. Project interim report. Programming interpersonal curricula for adolescents.* Silver Spring, MD: Institute for Behavioral Research. (ERIC Document Reproduction Service, ED060 584).

Cuff, G. N. (1977). A strategy for evaluating a short course on behavior modification. *Mental Retardation, 2,* 48.

Dancer, D. D., Braukmann, L. J., Schumaker, J. B., Kirigin, K. A., Willner, A. G., & Wolf, M. M. (1978). The training and validation of behavior observation and description skills. *Behavior Modification, 2,* 113–134.

Decter, M. (1972). *The new chastity and other arguments against women's liberation.* New York: Coward-McCann & Geoghegan.

Delameter, A. M., Conners, C. K., & Wells, K. C. (1984). A comparison of staff training procedures: Behavioral application in the child psychiatric inpatient setting. *Behavior Modification, 8,* 39–58.

DeMarsh, J., & Kumpfer, K. L. (1985). Family-oriented interventions for the prevention of chemical dependency in children and adolescents. *Journal of Children in Contemporary Society, 18,* 117–151.

Dworkin, S. (1978). Notes on Carter's family policy—how it got that way, what happened to his White House Conference, and some warning for the future., *Ms.,* September, 61–63, 94–96.

Eyeberg, S. M., & Johnson, S. M. (1974). Multiple assessment of behavior modification with families: Effects of contingency contracting and order of treated problems. *Journal of Consulting and Child Psychology, 42*(4), 594–606.

Ferri, E., & Robinson, H. (1974). *Coping alone.* Windsor, England: NFER Publishing.

Fifth Changing Family Conference, University of Iowa. (1976). Iowa City: University of Iowa.

Firestone, P., Kelly, M. J., & Fike, S. (1980). Are fathers necessary in parent training groups? *Journal of Clinical Child Psychology.* Spring, 44–47.

Forehand, R., & Atkeson, B. M. (1977). Generality of treatment effects with parents as therapists: A review of assessment and implementation procedures. *Behavior Therapy, 8,* 575–593.

Forhand, R. L., King, H. E., Peed, S., & Yoder, P. (1975). Mother–child interactions: Comparison of a noncompliant clinic group and a nonclinic group. *Behavior Research and Therapy, 13,* 79–84.

Foxx, R. M., & Azrin, N. H. (1973a). Dry pits: A rapid method for toilet training children. *Behavior Research and Therapy, 11,* 435–442.

Foxx, R. M., & Azrin, N. H. (1973b) *Toilet training the retarded:A rapid program for day and nighttime independent training.* Champaign, IL: Research Press.

Freud, S. (1961). A critique of Mill on women. In L. Marcus & S. Marcus (Eds.), Ernest Jones, *The life and work of Sigmund Freud* (pp. 117–118). New York: Basic Books.

Gardner, J. M. (1972). Teaching behavior modification to nonprofessionals. *Journal of Applied Behavior Analysis, 5*(4), 517–521.

Garfield, S. L. (1978). Research on client variables in psychotherapy. In S. L. Garfield & A. E. Bergin (Eds.), *Handbook of psychotherapy and behavior change.* Vol. 2,. pp. 191–232). New York: Wiley.

Gelfand, D. M., & Hartman, D. P. (1968). Behavior therapy with children: A review and evaluation of research methodology. *Psychological Bulletin, 69*(3), 204–215.

George, R. M., Van Voorhis, J., Grant, S., Casey, K., & Robinson, M. (1992). Special education experience of foster children: An empirical study. *Child Welfare, 71*(5), 4l9–437.

Gladstone, B. W., & Spencer, C. J. (1977). The effects of modelling on the contingent praise of mental retardation counsellors. *Journal of Applied Behavior Analysis, 10,* 75–84.

Glasser, P. H., & Navarre, E. L. (1965). The problems of families in the AFDC program. *Children, 12,* 151–156.

Goldiamond, I. (1974). Toward a constructional approach to social problems. Ethical and constitutional issues raised by applied behavior analysis. *Behaviorism, 2,* 1–84.

Goode, W. J. (1960). A theory of role strain. *America Sociological Review, 25,* 483–496.

Graves, R. (1965). *Mannon & the black goddess.* New York: Doubleday.

Graziano, A. M., & Diamet, D. M. (1992). Parent behavior training: An examination of the paradigm. *Behavior Modification, 16,* 3–38.

Griest, D. L., Forehand, R., Rogers, T., Breiner, J., Furey, W., & Williams, C. A. (1982). Effects of parent enhancement therapy on the treatment outcome and generalization of a parent training program. *Behavioral Residential Therapy, 20,* 429–436.

Haley, J. (1977). *Problem-solving therapy.* San Francisco: Jossey-Bass.

Hanf, C. (1968). *Modifying problem behaviors in mother–child interaction: Standardized laboratory situations.* Paper presented at the meeting of the Association of Behavior Therapies, Olympia, Washington.

Haskett, M. E., Miller, J. W., Whitworth, J. M., & Huffman, J. M. (1992). Intervention with cocaine-abusing mothers. *The Journal of Human Services, 73,* 451–461.

Hawkins, R. P., Peterson, R. F., Schweid, E., & Bijou, S. W. (1966). Behavior therapy in the home: Amelioration of problem parent–child relations with the parent in the therapeutic role. *Journal of Experimental Child Psychology, 4,* 99–107.

Henderson, R. W., & Garcia, A. B. (1973). The effects of parent training program on the question-asking behavior of Mexican-American children. *American Educational Research Journal, 10*(3) 193–201.

Herbert, E. W., & Baer, D. M. (1972). Training parents as behavior modifiers: Self-recording of contingent attention. *Journal of Applied Behavior Analysis, 5*(2), 139–150.

Herbert, E. W., Pinkston, E. M., Hayden, M. L., Sajwaj, T. E., Pinkston, S., Cordua, G., & Jackson, C. (1973). Adverse effects of differential parental attention. *Journal of Applied Behavior Analysis, 6,* 15–30.

Hersen, M., & Bellack, A. S. (1978). Staff training and consultation. In M. Hersen & A. S. Bellack (Eds.), *Behavior therapy in a psychiatric setting.* Baltimore: Williams & Wilkins.

Herzog, E., & Sudia, C. (1971). Fatherless homes: A review of research. *Children, 15,* 177–182.

Johnson, C. A., & Katz, R. A. (1973). Using parents as change agents for their children: A review. *Journal of Child Psychology* and *Psychiatry and Allied Disciplines, 14*(3), 181–200.

Johnson, W. E., Jr., (1995). Paternal identity among urban, adolescent males. Occasional Paper in *African American Research Perspectives.*

Johnson, W. E., Jr., (1996). *Work preparation and labor market behavior among urban, poor, non-resident fathers.* Conference sponsored by the University of Michigan Research and Training Program on Poverty, the Underclass and Public Policy.

Kadusin, A. (1970). Single-parent adoptions: An overview and some relevant research. *Social Service Review, 44,* 263–274.

Kantor, J. R. (1959). *Interverba psychology.* IN: Principia.

Karoly, P., & Rosenthal, M. (1977). Training parents in behavior modification: Effects on perceptions of family interaction and deviant child behavior. *Behavior Therapy, 8,* 406–410.

Klein, C. (1973). *The single parent experience.* New York: Walker.

Lake, M., & Levinger, G. (1960). Continuance beyond application interview at a child guidance clinic. *Social Casework, 41,* 303–309.

Levenstein, P., Kochman, A., & Roth, H. (1973). For laboratory to real world: Service delivery of the mother–child home program. *American Journal of Orthopsychiatry, 43,* 72–78.

Lindsley, O. R. (1970). Procedures in common described by a common language. In C. Neuringer & J. L. Michael (Eds.), *Behavior modification in clinical psychology* (pp. 221–236). New York: Appleton-Century-Crofts.

Maluccio, A. N., Krieger, R., & Pine, B. A. (1990). *Reconnecting families: Family reunification competencies for social workers.* West Hartford, CT: Center for the Study of Child Welfare, The University of Connecticut, School of Social Work.

Mash, E. J., Handy, L. C., & Hamerlynck, L. A. (Eds.) (1976). *Behavior modification approaches to parenting.* New York: Brunner Mazel.

Mayer, J. E., & Rosenblatt, A. (1964). The client's social context: Its effect on continuance in treatment. *Social Casework, 45,* 511–518.

Mayer, J. E., & Timms, N. (1970). *The client speaks: Working class impressions of casework.* New York: Atherton.

McAdoo, W. G., & Roeske, N. A. (1973). A comparison of defectors and continuers in a child guidance clinic. *Journal of Consulting & Clinical Psychology, 40,* 328–334.

McDonald, M. R., & Budd, K. S. (1983). "Booster Shoots" following didactic parent training. *Behavior Modification, 7,* 211–223.

McMahon, R. J., Forehand, R., & Griest, D. L. (1981). Effects of knowledge of social learning principles on enhancing treatment outcome and generalization in a parent training program. *Journal of Consulting and Clinical Psychology, 49*(4), 525–532.

McMahon, R. J., Tiedemann, G. L., Forehand, R., & Griest, D. L. (1984). Parental satisfaction with parent training to modify child noncompliance. *Behavior Therapy, 15,* 295–303.

Meyer, C. H. (1978). Practice and policy: A family focus. *Social Casework, 59,* 259–265.

Mindey, C. (1969). *The divorced mother: A guide to readjustment.* New York: McGraw-Hill.

Morrey, J. G. (1973). *Parenting in precise behavior management with mentally retarded children.* Doctoral dissertation, Utah State University. (University Microfilms No. 70-27011)

O'Dell, S. (1974). Training parents in behavior modification: A review. *Psychological Bulletin, 81*(7), 418–433.

Ojeman, R. H. (1967). Incorporating psychological concepts in the school curriculum. *Journal of School Psychology, 3,* 195–204.

O'Leary, K. D., O'Leary,, S., & Becker, W. C. (1967). Modification of a deviant sibling interaction pattern in the home. *Behavior Research and Therapy, 5,* 113–120.

Oregon. Bureau of Labor. (1968). *They carry the burden alone: The socio-economic living pattern of Oregon women with dependents.* Salem, OR: Author.

Patterson, G. R. (1973a). Changes in status of family members as controlling stimuli: A basis for describing treatment process. In Hamerlynck et al. (Eds.), *Behavior change: Methodology, concepts, and practice.* (pp. 169–191). Champaign, IL: Research Press.

Patterson, G. R. (1973b). Reprogramming the families of aggressive boys. In C. Thoresen (Ed.), *Behavior modification in education* (72nd yearbook pp. 154–192). National Society for the Study of Education.

Patterson, G. R. (1974a). A basis for identifying stimuli which control behavior in natural settings. *Child Development, 45,* 700–911.

Patterson, G. R. (1974b). Interventions for boys with conduct problems: Multiple settings, treatment, and criteria. *Journal of Consulting and Clinical Psychology, 42*(4), 471–481.

Patterson, G. R., Cobb, J. A., & Ray, R. S. (1973). A social engineering technology for retraining the families of aggressive boys. In H. E. Adams & I. P. Unikel (Eds.), *Issues and trends in behavior therapy* (pp. 139–210). Springfield, IL: Thomas.

Patterson, G. R., & Reid, J. B. (1970). Reciprocity and coercion: Two facets of social systems. In C. Neuringer & J. L. Michael (Eds.), *Behavior modification in clinical psychology.* New York: Appleton-Century-Crofts.

Patterson, G. R., Reid, J. B., Jones, R. R., & Conger, R. E. (1975). *A social learning approach to family intervention: Families with aggressive children.* Eugene, OR: Castalia.

Pawlicki, R. (1970). Behavior-therapy research with children: A critical review. *Canadian Journal of Behavioral Science/Review of Canadian Scientific Comp., 2*(3), 163–173.

Peed, S., Roberts, M., & Forehand, R. (1977). Evaluation of the effectiveness of a standardized parent training program in altering the interaction of mothers and their noncompliant children. *Behavior Modification, 1,* 323–349.

Peine, H. A. (1969). *Programming the home.* Paper presented at the meeting of the Rocky Mountain Psychological Association, Albuquerque, New Mexico.

Polster, R. A., Dangel, R. F., & Rasp, R. (1986–87). Research in behavioral parent training in social work: A review. *Journal of Social Service Research, 10*(2/3/4), 37–51.

Rickert, D. C., & Moore, J. G. (1970). *Parent training in precise behavior management with mentally retarded children.* US Office of Education Project 9-H-016, Final Report.

Ripple, L. (1957). Factors associated with continuance of casework service. *Social Work, 2,* 87–94.

Rose, S. D. (1977). *Group therapy: A behavioral approach.* Englewood Cliffs, NJ: Prentice-Hall.

Rosenblatt, A., & Mayer, J. E. (1966). Client disengagement and alternative treatment resources. *Social Casework, 47,* 3–12.

Rosenfield, J., & Rosenstein, E. (1973). Towards a conceptual framework for the study of parent-absent families. *Journal of Marriage and the Family, 33,* 131–134.

Ross, A. O., & Lacey, H. M. (1961). Characteristics of terminators and remainers in child guidance treatment. *Journal of Consulting Psychology, 25,* 420–424.

Ross, H. L., & Sawhill, J. V. (1975). *Time of transition: The growth of families headed by women.* Washington, DC: Urban Institute.

Rossi, A. S., Kagan, J., & Hareven, T. K. (1977). *The family.* New York: Norton.

Russo, S. (1964). Adaptation in behavior therapy with children. *Behavior Research and Therapy, 2,* 43–47.

Salzinger, D., Feldman, R. S., & Portnoy, S. (1970). Training parents of brain-injured children in the use of operate conditioning procedures. *Behavior Therapy, 1,* 4–32.

Sanders, M. R. (1982). The effects of instructions, feedback and cueing procedures in behavioral parent training. *Australian Journal of Psychology, 34,* 53–69.

Satir, V. (1967). *Conjoint family therapy.* Palo Alto, CA: Science and Behavior Books.

Schlesinger, B. (1977). One parent families in Great Britain. *The Family Coordinator, 26,* 139–141.

Selden, R. H. (1965). Salutary effects of maternal separation. *Social Work, 39,* 25–29.

Serketich, W. J., & Dumas, J. E. (1996). The effectiveness of behavioral parent training to modify antisocial behavior in children: A meta-analysis. *Behavior Therapy, 27,* 171–186.

Skinner, B. F. (1953). *Science* and *human behavior.* New York: Appleton-Century-Crofts.

Skinner, B. F. (1969). *Contingencies of reinforcement: A theoretical analysis.* New York: Appleton-Century-Crofts.

Sprey, J. (1967). The study of single parenthood: Some methodological considerations. *Family Life Coordinator, 16,* 29–34.

Staines, G., Tauris, C., & Jayaratne, T. E. (1974). The queen bee syndrome. *Psychology Today, 7,* 55–60.

Stein, T. J., & Gambrill, E. D. (1976a). Behavioral techniques in foster care. *Social Work, 21,* 34–39.

Stein, T. J., & Gambrill, E. D. (1976b). Early intervention in foster care. *Public Welfare, 34,* 39–44.

Stokes, T. F., & Baer, D. M. (1977). An implicit technology of generalization. *Journal of Applied Behavior Analysis, 10,* 349–368.

Strain, P. S., Young, C. C., & Horowitz, J. (1981). An examination of child and family demographic variables related to generalized behavior change during oppositional child training. *Behavior Modification, 5,* 15–25.

Stuart, R. B., & Tripodi, T. (1971). *Experimental evolution of three time constrained behavioral treatments for predelinquents and delinquents.* Paper presented at meeting of Association for Advancement of Behavior Therapy, Washington, DC.

Tavormina, J. B. (1974). Basic models of parent counseling: A critical review. *Psychological Bulletin, 8*(11), 827–835.

Thomas, E. J., & Walters, C. L. (1973). Guidelines for behavioral practice in the open community agency: Procedures and evaluation. *Behaviour Research and Therapy, 11,* 193–205.

Thomes, M. M. (1968). Children with absent fathers. *Journal of Marriage and the Family, 30,* 89–96.

US Bureau of the Census. *US census of the population in 1960.* Subject Report "Families," PC (2)-4A, Table 6. Washington, DC: Author.

US Bureau of the Census. *US census of the population in 1970.* Subject Report "Family Composition," PC (2)-4A, Table 8. Washington, DC: Author.

US Bureau of the Census. *US census of the population in 1991.* Subject Report US Women's Bureau. (1973). The economic role of women. Reprinted from the *Economic report of the President,* Chapter 4, 89–112. Washington, DC: Author.

US Women's Bureau. (1973). The economic role of women. Reprinted from the *Economic Report of the President,* Chapter 4, 89–112.

Vilar, E. (1972). *The manipulated man.* New York: Farrar Straus.

Wagner, M. K. (1968). Parent therapists: An operant conditioning method. *Mental Hygiene, 52*(3), 452–455.

Wahler, R. G. (1969a). Oppositional children: A quest for parental reinforcement control. *Journal of Applied Behavior Analysis, 2*(3), 159–170.

Wahler, R. G. (1969b). Setting generality: Some specific and general effects of child behavior therapy. *Journal of Applied Behavior Analysis 2*(4), 239–246.

Wahler, R. G., Winkel, G. H., Peterson, R. F., & Morrison, D. C. (1965). Mothers as behavior therapists for their own children. *Behavior Research and Therapy, 3,* 113–134.

Walder, L. O., Cohen, S. I., Breiter, D. W., Warman, F. C., Orme-Johnson, D., & Pavey, S. (1971). Parents as change agents. In S. E. Golan & C. Eisdorfer (Eds.), *Handbook of community psychology.* New York: Appleton-Century-Crofts.

Webster-Stratton, C. (1985). Predictors of treatment outcome in parent training for conduct disordered children. *Behavior Therapy, 16,* 223–243.

Wetzel, R. J., Baker, J., Roney, M., & Martin, M. (1966). Outpatient treatment of autistic behavior. *Behavior Research and Therapy, 4,* 169–177.

Williams, R., & Pollack, R. H. (1964). Some nonpsychological variables in therapy defection in a child guidance clinic. *The Journal of Psychology, 58,* 145–155.

Wiltz, N. A. (1969). *Modification of behaviors through parent participation in a group technique.* Unpublished doctoral dissertation, University of Oregon. (University Microfilms, No. 70-9482)

Wolfe, D. A. (1985). Child-abusive parents: An empthical review and analysis. *Psychological Bulletin, 97*(3), 462–482.

Zeilberger, J., Sampen, S., & Sloan, H. N. (1968). Modification of child's problem behaviors in the home with the mother as therapist. *Journal of Applied Behavior Analysis, 1,* 47–53.

17

Parents with Intellectual Disabilities
Implications and Interventions

MAURICE A. FELDMAN

One group of parents singled out more than any other for being at risk for child maltreatment are parents with intellectual disabilities. This chapter summarizes the results of our 15 years of research and clinical practice with these families. We
describe (1) the parents, (2) the impact on children raised by parents with intellectual disabilities, and (3) a home-based parent education program designed to increase parenting skills and decrease the risk of child neglect and developmental
problems. Most identified parents with intellectual disabilities have IQs between
60 and 80 and have been labeled as having mental retardation. Some are so labeled
despite having IQs above 75, the accepted cutoff for a diagnosis of mental retardation (American Psychiatric Association, 1994; Luckasson et al., 1992). In this chapter, the term "intellectual disabilities" will be used to describe persons with IQs
less than 80 who are considered by the social service system to have mental retardation (Mercer, 1973). Parents with intellectual disabilities routinely have their
children removed from their care, often without evidence of child maltreatment
(Hayman, 1990). Concerns about parenting by persons with intellectual disabilities
center more on physical and psychological neglect than physical and sexual abuse.
In the United States and Canada, about 80% of these parents have their parenting
rights terminated, primarily because of actual or potential child neglect (Feldman,
Case, & Sparks, 1992; Feldman, Sparks, & Case, 1993; Seagull & Scheurer, 1986;
Taylor et al., 1991). To some extent this high percentage may reflect society's bias
toward these families, but it also likely reveals serious parenting difficulties in the
absence of (and sometimes with) community supports and services.

For various reasons there is likely to be an increase in the number of parents with
intellectual disabilities. Virtually every person with intellectual disabilities now

MAURICE A. FELDMAN • Department of Psychology, Queen's University and Ongwanada Centre,
Kingston, Ontario, Canada K7L 3N6.

Handbook of Child Abuse Research and Treatment, edited by Lutzker. Plenum Press, New York, 1998.

grows up in a family environment; many adults have never been institutionalized, or have been living in the community for many years. Not surprisingly, these individuals have developed a set of status quo family values; they are aware of, and may wish to exercise, their full rights as adult citizens, including the right to be parents (Hayman, 1990; Vogel, 1987). Most jurisdictions have banned involuntary sterilization and repealed discriminatory marriage laws. Judges are beginning to question the presumption of parental incompetence based solely on IQ in the absence of additional evidence of risk to the child and are making more custody decisions in favor of the parents (Hayman, 1990; Vogel, 1987). Because of court challenges and research, the child welfare and social service systems are recognizing that many of these parents may be able to provide adequate child care if provided with specialized services and supports (Feldman, 1994).

CHARACTERISTICS OF FAMILIES WITH PARENTS WHO HAVE INTELLECTUAL DISABILTIES

There have been few studies of the qualities of families in which one or both parents have intellectual disabilities. Research has focused on parents who had already come to the attention of the child welfare and social service systems. Accordingly, we do not know to what extent the findings are representative of the population of parents with intellectual disabilities in general. Identified parents with intellectual disabilities probably have the potential to provide adequate child care (with appropriate supports and training), or have sufficient community awareness and self-advocacy skills to obtain legal representation when their child is taken into custody. Parents with more severe developmental disabilities are not likely to be given the chance to be parents, because of the clear danger to the child. Conversely, parents with intellectual disabilities who have acceptable parenting skills and greater cognitive capacities may never come to the attention of, or be of concern to, the child welfare and social service systems.

Research in this area has concentrated on mothers with intellectual disabilities who are typically the primary child-care providers; much less is known about the fathers. Based on characteristics of samples from existing published reports and our database of about 200 families, it appears that when they were children, many parents with intellectual disabilities were victims of abuse or neglect. Most were labeled as having mental retardation when they were in school and consequently received special education services. Currently, they still are (often inappropriately) considered as having mental retardation, impoverished, stigmatized, unemployed, and live in substandard housing. These families usually receive numerous services and are under the surveillance of child protection agencies (Walton-Allen & Feldman, 1991).

Child-Care Skills

Despite the concerns about the parental incompetency of adults who have cognitive limitations, few studies have objectively evaluated their parenting skills. Using parenting skill observational checklists developed with the input of pediatric health-care professionals, we compared the performance of parents with intellectual disabilities referred to a parenting education program, to parents without intellectual disabilities from both low and middle socioeconomic status (SES) families on a variety of child-care skills. The results are presented in Figure 1. As can be seen, across all skills observed, the parents with intellectual disabilities showed significantly lower performance than parents without intellectual disabilities ($p < .05$). The parents with intellectual disabilities scored significantly less in feeding, washing hair, sleep safety, cleaning baby bottles, and nutrition. However, typically they scored above 50%, signifying that they had partial skills. Notice that for the parents without intellectual disabilities, the overall mean percentage correct was 85%; for no skill observed did the mothers without intellectual disabilities have a mean score of 100%. These findings helped us to establish reasonable guidelines for setting child-care skills training criteria by social comparison (Kazdin, 1977).

Parental Stress and Depression

Given their often considerable and varied adverse historical and contemporary experiences, parents with intellectual disabilities are likely to be under considerable stress and may be depressed. Negative parenting and child outcomes are related to both parental stress (Crnic, Greenberg, Robinson, & Ragozin, 1984; Forehand, Lautenschlager, Faust, & Graziano, 1986; Webster-Stratton, 1988; Weinraub & Wolf, 1983) and depression (Forehand et al., 1986; Hammen et al., 1987; Hops et al., 1987; Seifer, Sameroff, & Jones, 1981). There is reason to believe that parents with intellectual disabilities are under stress related to (among other

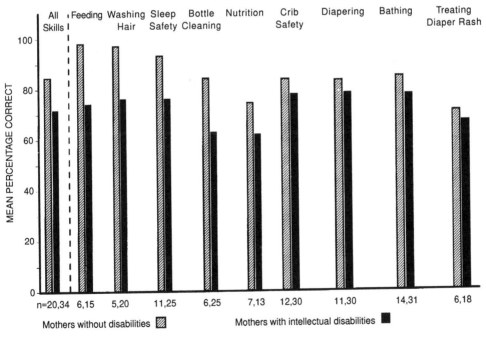

Figure 1. Mean percentage correct child-care skill performance of mothers with and without intellectual disabilities.

things): poverty, inadequate and crowded living conditions, stigmatization, being in an abusive relationship, and threat of child removal.

We (Feldman, Léger, & Walton-Allen, 1997) orally administered the Parenting Stress Index (Abidin, 1990) to 82 mothers with intellectual disabilities (IQ range: 57–80) and found that, compared to the normative sample, they reported experiencing clinically significant stress (≥ 80th percentile). Parenting stress significantly escalated as the child matured from infancy to preschool to school age ($p < .05$). The mean Parenting Stress Index child domain stress score of mothers of infants and preschoolers was in the 90th percentile, but rose to the 99th percentile for mothers with school-age children. With respect to depression, Walton-Allen (1993) found that 62.5% of 40 mothers with intellectual disabilities had clinically significant depressive symptomatology as measured by the Beck Depression Inventory (Beck, Ward, Mendelson, & Erbaugh, 1961). Thus, it is conceivable that many of the problems seen in parents with intellectual disabilities and their children may be related to psychosocial distress that these parents face in addition to parenting deficiencies related to cognitive impairment.

Parental Stress and Social Support

Parents without intellectual disabilities who have children with developmental disabilities or chronic illness may also face considerable stress. In these families social support is negatively correlated with parental stress and may buffer the effects of the strain of raising a child with disabilities (Dunst, Trivette, & Cross, 1986; Minnes, 1994). No study has yet to examine the relationship between stress and social support in parents with cognitive impairments. In another study with 18 mothers with intellectual disabilities, we found a significant negative relationship between overall social support as measured by a modified version of the Interpersonal Support Evaluation List (Cohen & Hoberman, 1983) and the Parenting Stress Index total stress score ($r = -.49$, $p < .05$). The correlations with another measure of social support, the Parenting Social Support Index (Telleen, Herzog, & Kilbane, 1989), revealed that the parent's satisfaction with her support network was negatively correlated with parental stress ($r = -.55$, $p < .05$), but size of the support network was not. The parents' ratings of need for social support were positively correlated with parenting stress ($r = .66$, $p < .01$). Satisfaction with, but not size or need of, social support was correlated with maternal positive interactions ($r = .53$, $p < .05$). Further research is needed to determine to what extent parental stress affects the abilities of parents with intellectual disabilities and whether interventions would be more effective if they included strategies to help these parents cope more adaptively with their seemingly inevitable stressful life events.

CHILDREN OF PARENTS WITH INTELLECTUAL DISABILITIES

Evidence is mounting that children of parents with intellectual disabilities are themselves at risk for developmental delay. Reed and Reed (1965) examined 7,778 children genetically related to 289 Caucasian residents of a Minnesota institution for persons with mental retardation and found the occurrence of mental retardation in children born to two, one, and zero parents with mental retardation to be 40%, 15%, and 1%, respectively. Children of parents with low IQ were found to be at high risk for developmental delay among inner-city African Americans (Garber, 1988), in Sweden (Gillberg & Geijer-Karlsson, 1983), and in Northern Ireland (Scally, 1973). Brandon (1957) did not find a higher incidence of intellectual delay in offspring of parents with mental retardation in England.

Infants

In Canada, we (Feldman, Case, Towns, & Betel, 1985) studied 12, 2-year-olds of Caucasian mothers with intellectual disabilities and found that the children's mean score on Bayley Scales of Infant Development Mental Development Index (Bayley, 1969) was 84, which was significantly lower than the test mean of 100. An item analysis of the Bayley indicated that the most serious delay was in language. Physical development was not significantly below the mean. Child mental development scores were highly correlated with the quality of home environment and maternal interactions as measured by the Caldwell Home Observation for the Measurement of the Environment (HOME) Inventory (Caldwell & Bradley, 1984).

In a recently completed cross-sectional study of 86 infants of parents with intellectual disabilities, we found that not only was the mean Bayley Mental Development Index score significantly below 100, but also there was a significant decrease from a mean of 86.3 to 77.8 from 6 to 23 months of age ($ps < .05$). Unlike the earlier study, the Bayley Psychomotor Index was also significantly delayed in our larger sample ($p < .05$), although the decline in this scale from a mean of 87.3 to 81.7 was not statistically significant. Similar findings were obtained in a longitudinal analysis of 33 children.

School-Age Children

What happens to children of parents with intellectual disabilities during the school years? To begin to answer this question, we (Feldman & Walton-Allen, 1997) attempted to rectify some of the problems of previous research documenting the effects of being raised by parents with intellectual disabilities. First, to control for the possible detrimental effects of poverty, we compared a sample of school-age children ($n = 27$) whose mothers had intellectual disabilities to similarly impoverished children ($n = 25$) whose mothers did not have intellectual disabilities. Second, to ensure that the mothers with intellectual disabilities clearly met the generally accepted intellectual criterion for a diagnosis of mental retardation, we included mothers in this group only if their adult IQ was below 70. Third, to reduce selection bias, we did not approach child welfare agencies for referrals of known child maltreaters. However, if we subsequently found that child welfare was involved, we did not drop the family from the study. Fourth, to take a comprehensive look at the impact on the children, we included not only a measure of intellectual development (i.e., IQ) which had been the focus of most previous studies, but also we investigated academic achievement and behavior disorders.

We found that the children raised by mothers with intellectual disabilities had significantly lower IQs (mean = 80.5) than children raised by parents without intellectual disabilities (mean = 102.9, $p < .001$); both boys and girls were significantly affected. Academic achievement showed similar differences, except that the boys of mothers with intellectual disabilities were affected more than girls. Fifty-nine percent of children of parents with intellectual disabilities were in special education as compared to 12% of children of parents without intellectual disabilities. Overall, children of parents with intellectual disabilities had significantly higher Ontario Child Behavior Checklist (Offord et al., 1987) scores than the low-income children of parents without intellectual disabilities ($p < .03$), and again boys were affected much more than girls. According to the Child Behavior Checklist cutoff scores, more than 40% of the children of mothers with intellectual disabilities had clinically significant behavior disorders, and those children with multiple behavior problems tended to have IQs $\geq$ 85. The quality of the home environment as measured by the Caldwell HOME Inventory was significantly negatively correlated with conduct disorders ($r = -.43$, $p < .05$) and hyperactivity ($r = -.39$, $p < .05$) in the maternal intellectual disabilities group only; Caldwell HOME Inventory total scores were significantly positively correlated with child IQ in the children of parents without intellectual disabilities ($r = .51$, $p < .01$), but not in the children of parents with intellectual disabilities. Not one school-age child of parents with intellectual disabilities in our sample was problem-free: 60% had below average IQs; the remainder had learning disabilities and/or a clinically significant behavior disorder. The adverse effects of poverty cannot fully account for these findings, as similar results were not obtained in impoverished children of parents without intellectual disabilities. Thus, studies, by us and by others, of infants and school-age children strongly suggest that children of parents with intellectual disabilities are at significant early risk for developmental delay that continues, and may worsen, as the child ages. In addition to an increased threat of developmental problems, these children, especially the boys, are at high risk for behavior disorders when they reach school age.

HOME-BASED INTERVENTION

The need for early intervention for families in which the parents have cognitive limitations is clear. It is generally agreed that many of their children's problems reflect inadequate childrearing abilities (Budd & Greenspan, 1984; Tymchuk & Feldman, 1991). Can parenting skills be improved so as to reduce the risk of child neglect, developmental delays, and behavior problems? In this section, we describe our parenting assessment and intervention model, developed over a 15-year period. The intervention occurred in the family home and was provided by specially trained parent education therapists who visited weekly (more often for newborns or family crises). The therapists had B.A. or M.A. degrees in psychology, nursing, or early childhood education. We have found that to work effectively with these families, parent education therapists should have knowledge of both child development and the impact of mild intellectual disabilities on adults. Appreciation and knowledge of behavioral skill training and parent training methods are essential. Also, these therapists must be able to put aside their own (usually middle-class) biases and accept some possible differences in values and practices by adults who have grown up under less optimal conditions.

Referrals were made by child welfare agencies, advocates, hospital social workers, family physicians, family members, and the parents themselves. Often referrals were court-ordered. In about 20% of the cases, the child had already been removed, but could be returned if the parent(s) made demonstrable improvements in skills. Virtually all the referred parents were mothers, about 50% of whom were single. Even when a male assuming the father role was present, it was often difficult to encourage him to participate in the program, as many of them did not accept child-care responsibilities.

Throughout the parents' involvement, we recognized that parenting education was just one part of the continuum of services needed by these multiproblem families. We provided ongoing counseling, stress management, community living and social skills training. We were an integral part of an interagency multidisciplinary team. We worked closely with the family physician, public health nurse, child protection worker, the parents' advocate, and the child's day-care or school staff. When necessary, and with the parents' approval, we referred the families to the failure-to-thrive clinic, psychiatrists, psychotherapists, and women's shelters. We helped the families develop and maintain natural support networks, including family members, friends, neighbors, and organizations.

PARENT EDUCATION CURRICULUM

We were primarily an early intervention program (although we did try to help families with older children who were referred because of child behavior problems). Table 1 presents the typical sequence of parent education for the first 3 years of the child's life. When a family with a newborn or infant entered the parent education program, the first priority was usually remediating basic child-care skill deficiencies affecting child health and safety. Although not true of all referrals, some of the common problems included failure to clean and sterilize baby bottles; this failure resulted in infant gastric distress and infection. Often, formula (or food) preparation

Table 1. Sequence of Training Parenting Skills

0–10 Months
    Basic child-care (e.g., newborn handling, diapering, bathing, feeding)
    Crib and sleep safety
    Infant health and illnesses
    Stimulating child physical development
    Nutrition
10–24 Months
    Home safety
    Handling emergencies
    Positive parent–child interactions
    Stimulating child language and social development
    Nutrition
24–36 Months
    Street safety
    Toilet training
    Parent–child rapport
    Child behavior management
    Cognitive stimulation
    Day care and other community programs
    Parental stress management

and feeding skills were ineffectual; this led to child malnourishment. The parents did not effectively treat diaper rash and other childhood afflictions. Sometimes they placed the child in dangerous situations by using bath water that was too hot, leaving the baby alone on the changing table, using medication incorrectly, or allowing dangerous objects within the child's reach. Once these crucial issues were ameliorated, then we begin to focus more directly on teaching the parents to provide a more stimulating home environment to foster child physical, language, social, and cognitive development. In the second and third years, we expanded upon nutrition, safety, and more sophisticated cognitive stimulation. We also concentrated on maintaining a positive parent–child relationship, as well as preventing and solving child behavior problems. We encouraged the parents to place (or maintain) their child in day care, to access the library and other community resources, and to enroll in programs to upgrade their own academic and vocational skills.

PARENTING ASSESSMENT

General Assessment of Risk Factors

Prior to the child-care skill evaluation, we conducted a variety of standardized assessments, interviews, and observations to identify factors that could facilitate or inhibit the parent's current abilities, their responsiveness to training, and child outcomes (Tymchuk & Keltner, 1991). Consistent with Belsky's (1984) interactional model of parenting, we explored parental, child, and environmental variables that could accumulate and interact to increase risk of inadequate parenting. With respect to parental variables, we examined historical factors (such as parental health and abuse), parenting stress, social support, marital satisfaction, psychopathology, and reading skills. Many of the mothers reported being physically and/or sexually abused when younger; many had chronic physical or mental health problems such as asthma and depression, and reported being highly stressed. Most of the parents had attended special education classes when they were in school and few could read beyond the grade 2 level. Often several agencies were involved, including child protection. To determine the possible role of child variables, we arranged for a standardized developmental assessment of the child (usually with the Bayley Scales of Infant Development) and gathered information about the child's physical health, temperament, behavior problems, skill development, history of abuse, and relationships with siblings and peers. As mentioned earlier, these children often showed problems in development starting in infancy, with language being particularly delayed (Feldman et al., 1985). We looked for adverse environmental factors such as financial constraints, inadequate housing, crowding, unstimulating home environment, and lack of satisfactory natural social supports. Many of the referred parents had several of these risk factors.

Child-Care Skills Assessment

The heart of our parent education assessment was the direct evaluation of child-care skills. We created a variety of task-analysis observational assessments of many important parenting skills. Table 2 illustrates two of these task analyses (a full set is available from the author). The checklists were developed based on the latest available information on child care and were reviewed by pediatric health-care professionals. Our experiences and normative observations showed that sometimes the recommended criterion skills were not always performed by most parents (e.g., washing hands after every diaper change, even when the diaper is not soiled or wet; no toys in the crib). We were faced with a dilemma: Do we teach the parents enrolled in our program to become "superparents" (i.e., perform skills better than the typical parent) or do we set the training criterion such that it resembles the norm, even if the typical parent does not fully follow recommended procedures? We left this decision to the parents themselves, and invariably they chose to learn the ideal set of skills. They said that they wanted to do whatever would be best for their child and to show others (particularly the child protection worker) that they could be good parents. We constantly updated the checklists based on new information and changes in acceptable practice. For example, in our sleep safety checklist we previously advised to lay the baby "on stomach or side" (Feldman, Case, & Sparks, 1992). Given recent evidence on the relationship between Sudden Infant Death Syndrome and sleeping in a prone position, we now recommend laying the baby on *back* or side.

We conducted an extensive series of observations in the home, usually by spending a "day-in-the-life" of the family. We tried not to cue or prompt any child-care skills; we would fill out the appropriate checklist when the parent engaged in the child-care task. If the parent did not perform a task (e.g., bathing, playing) that we wished to observe, then toward the end of our visit we would ask her to do it so that we could evaluate her skill level. The first series of target skills were selected based on these initial observations, concerns expressed by others (especially the child protection worker), and the parent's own preferences.

Table 2. Examples of Child-Care Task Analyses

Sterilizing baby bottles	Feeding solids
1. Puts washed bottles in pot	1. Serves food at room temperature or slightly warmer
2. Puts washed nipples into pot	2. Presents different foods separately on the dish
3. Puts washed caps and rings into pot	
4. Puts can opener (if used) into pot	3. Ties child securely in the high chair
5. Puts washed spoon (if used) in pot	4. Adjusts seat position to allow eye contact with child
6. Puts washed measuring cup and funnel (if used) into pot	5. Uses positive coaxing strategies, if needed
7. Fills pot with tap water until all contents are covered	6. Remains calm if child refuses food
8. Turns on stove and heats water until it boils for 5 minutes	7. Makes four attempts to offer food, but does not force-feed
9. Fills a small pot or kettle with water and boils for 5 minutes	8. Allows child to touch food
10. Pours boiled water from small pot or kettle over tongs	9. Talks to child during the meal
11. Removes contents of pot with tongs	10. Serves vegetables or fruit, protein source, and cereal
12. Puts contents upright on clean surface	11. Does not serve "junk food"
	12. Wipes the child's face after the meal

TEACHING STRATEGIES

For the most part, we used behavioral performance-based training strategies that have been validated in numerous studies teaching community living skills to persons with intellectual disabilities (Matson, 1988). These techniques included simple instructions, task analysis, pictorial prompts, modeling, feedback, role-playing, and positive reinforcement. Many of these strategies have also been used to teach parents without intellectual disabilities child management and skill training techniques (e.g., Hudson, 1982). Thus, it is not surprising that we viewed teaching parenting skills to parents with intellectual disabilities as the *intersection* of training community living skills and parent training.

Training Visits

A typical visit in which training took place usually lasted 1–2 hours depending on the number of skills being observed and other issues that the parent wished to discuss with the parent education therapist. The visit started with a general discussion of the previous week's events, with particular emphasis on the skills being trained (e.g., "Were you able to play every day with Sarah?"). Sometimes, the parents would dwell on an event (e.g., an argument with a family member). Usually, the parent education therapist would ask the parent to hold further discussion of these issues until after the training session, unless the parent's concerns needed to be responded to posthaste. Following the assessment and training portions of the visit, the therapist would discuss or assist on other matters of importance, particularly if raised by the parent (e.g., help in filling out forms, what to do about a nosy neighbor, accessing a community program). Of course, if the parent was in crisis or emotionally distraught, training was canceled for that visit.

Training Probes

Next, the parent would prepare for an observational probe on new target skills (for a baseline score), skills currently being taught or in follow-up. Typically, no more than 2–3 skills were actively taught at any one time. Every attempt was made to accommodate the family schedule so that the training session would occur at a natural time for that task. For example, if the parent was receiving training in increasing positive interactions, then the visit would be scheduled at a time that the parent reported she usually would play with her child. If during the first 15–20 minutes of the visit, the parent did not initiate the child-care routine, this fact was noted and the parent education therapist would ask the parent to perform the activity (e.g., "play with your child the way you usually do," "show me how you clean the baby bottles"). Generalization probes were conducted as necessary (e.g., the observer would record interactions during a meal or a diaper change). No training was provided during these training and generalization probes. These initial observation probes were used to evaluate the parent's retention of training effects from one weekly visit to the next and therefore served as a more conservative measure of the effectiveness of the program than did probes conducted during or immediately after a training session.

Training Strategies

Following the probe, the parent education therapist would go over the results of the probe and highlight several steps of the task analysis that the parent performed correctly and praise the parent (especially for steps previously incorrect or missed). For example, if the target skill was imitating child vocalizations, the parent education therapist may say, "That's great, he said 'mama' and you repeated it; that must make you feel good that he called you 'mama'!" Then the parent education therapist would mention areas that were still missed or needed correction. For example, in training the parent to increase descriptive praise to the child, the therapist may say, "When he built the tower with the blocks, you should say, 'Wow, Jimmy, that's great, you built a tower all by yourself'!" The parent education therapist may play with the child and model some of the skills for the mother; the therapist may exaggerate the skills (e.g., very enthusiastic praise) to try to increase the parent's recognition of the skill being modeled.

After demonstrating the skill, the parent education therapist would take out a blank checklist and ask the mother to try again; unlike the earlier training probe, now the therapist would immediately praise the mother for correct skills and prompt missed opportunities (e.g., "He's climbing on your lap—now's a good time to give him a hug and kiss"; "Don't forget to wipe in the creases before putting the new diaper on"). The therapist would record the parent's performance and prompts required on each step of the child-care checklist. The therapist would calculate the mother's percentage correct (unprompted) performance by dividing the number of steps correct by the total number of steps (for interaction skills; the therapist would divide the number of 10-second observational intervals in which the behavior was observed by the total number of observation intervals).

Training Coupons

The parent would receive parenting coupons based on the score on the (second) checklist filled out during training. When training first commenced, the mother would receive a coupon simply for being home for the training session; from the second training visit on, she could obtain additional coupons for improved unprompted performance, week to week. The training criterion was 80% of steps for child-care skills and 30% of intervals for interaction skills over 2 consecutive visits. These objectives were based on the performance seen in parents without intellectual disabilities (see Figure 1 and Feldman et al., 1986, 1993). When the parent reached criterion, she would receive coupons for maintaining the skill in follow-up visits. Each coupon was worth approximately 50 cents and coupons were exchangeable for small gift items (e.g., children's clothing, toys, accessories; public transit tickets; family photo; movie passes). On a typical visit, a parent usually earned 2–4 coupons, depending on the number and performance of skills being trained or maintained. The parents could cash in their coupons as soon as they earned them (e.g., usually for public transit tickets), but most parents preferred to save them to purchase more expensive items.

During follow-up, observational probes of trained skills were steadily decreased over weeks, then months. Coupon reinforcement also was gradually thinned in follow-up by using a version of a lottery. If the parent met criterion, she selected three numbers from 1 to 6, and then rolled a die; if one of her numbers came up, she won her coupon. Over weeks, the number of guesses she was allowed for maintaining criterion performance was reduced from three to one, then a second die was added, and finally no coupons were distributed. Well before this time, the parent was usually quite proficient and the skill was being maintained by natural (or other) reinforcers (e.g., the child smiling back when the mother praised him or her, the approval of the child protection worker).

EVALUATIONS OF IN-HOME PARENTING EDUCATION

We have completed several evaluations of the child-care training using both single-subject and between-group designs (Feldman, Case, Garrick, et al., 1992; Feldman, Case, Rincover, Towns, & Betel, 1989; Feldman, Case, & Sparks, 1992; Feldman et al., 1993; Feldman et al., 1986). Two studies utilizing between-group designs will be described.

Child-Care Skills Training

The first study evaluated training basic child-care skills for infants and toddlers (age range: 1–23 months) to reduce the risk of child neglect, malnourishment, sickness, and accidents (Feldman, Case, & Sparks, 1992). As we received too many referrals at one time, we randomly assigned mothers with intellectual disabilities to either a training group or a waitlist control group ($ns = 11$). The control group was receiving other services similar to those received by the training group (e.g., visits from public health nurses and advocates). We also included a group of 12 low- and middle-SES mothers without intellectual disabilities to serve as a social comparison group to establish realistic training criteria (Kazdin, 1977). We assessed a wide range of skills in the three groups and then trained the specific skills that had pretraining scores of less than 80% to members of the training group only. Skills trained included treating diaper rash, crib and sleep safety, nutrition, preparing formula, and toilet training. Weekly in-home training continued until each parent met the training criterion of 80% over 2 consecutive visits on each target skill. Mean training duration was 7.7 weeks (range: 2–29 weeks).

As seen in Figure 2, the training group significantly outperformed the control group on the posttest ($p < .001$). Training increased child-care skills in the training group to levels seen in the comparison group of parents without intellectual disabilities. Follow-up results over a 2–76-week period (mean = 28 weeks) showed that original training group parents maintained their skills and that when the control group parents received training, they replicated the training effects. Importantly, parent training had a beneficial impact on the children. After their mothers were trained in skills related to feeding and nutrition, four malnourished, underweight infants showed increases in rate of weight gain. Training in the treatment of diaper rash resulted in elimination of this affliction in six children; another mother successfully toilet trained her child. The training was also associated with increased family preservation. Before participating in the program, 82% of parents with intellectual disabilities (in both the training and control groups) who had a

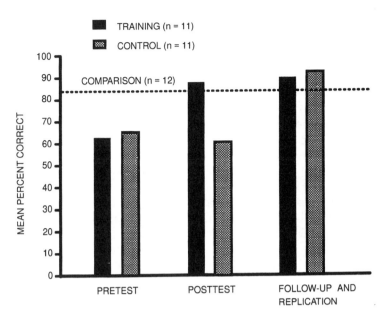

Figure 2. Mean pretest, posttest, and follow-up child-care skill scores for the training and wait-list control groups of parents with intellectual disabilities. The horizontal dotted line represents the performance of mothers without intellectual disabilities. The control group received training during the follow-up period. Reprinted from M. Feldman, L. Case, and B. Sparks. Effectiveness of a child-care training program for parents at-risk for child neglect, *Canadian Journal of Behavioural Science, 24,* p. 23. Copyright 1992. Canadian Psychological Association. Reprinted with permission.

previous child, had lost parenting rights to that child. This percentage is consistent with previous studies of U.S. custody cases involving parents with intellectual disabilities (Seagull & Scheurer, 1986; Taylor et al., 1991). After finishing the parent education program, however, only 19% of the parents forfeited the child who was the target of the intervention. In fact, the four parents who lost custody of their children had dropped out of the program prematurely, against our advice.

Interaction Skills Training

The next study evaluated the effects of teaching parents to be more responsive and reinforcing to their children (Feldman et al., 1993). We were particularly interested in determining if child language development would increase as a function of parent interactional training, as language was found to be particularly deficient in 2-year-old children of parents with intellectual disabilities (Feldman et al., 1985). We had previously conducted several single-subject studies that showed that interaction training rapidly increased the positive interactions of mothers with intellectual disabilities (Feldman et al., 1986, 1989). Given limitations of the research designs, we could not ascertain whether the increases in child language that we observed were due to the parent training or child maturation or experiential effects. Accordingly, we ran a between-groups study to control for expected increases in child language (i.e., any pre- to posttest increases in child language measures in the group of children whose parents did not receive interaction training were thought to represent maturational effects). We also controlled for possible attention-placebo effects of receiving parent education services.

To accomplish these goals, we randomly assigned 28 mothers with intellectual disabilities to either interaction training or emergency and home safety skills training (all mothers needed training in both sets of skills). Mothers in both groups received scheduled weekly visits, training (in either interactions or home safety), and interaction probes during mother–child play. We also collected interaction data from 38 mothers without intellectual disabilities who had children of similar ages (4–44 months) for social comparison (Kazdin, 1977).

As in our previous studies, we trained mothers to increase specific interactional skills known to be strongly related to optimal child language development (Clarke-Stewart & Apfel, 1979). In the child development literature, skills such as praising the child, imitating and expanding child vocalizations, talking and looking at the child when interacting, and providing physical affection would be considered indices of maternal sensitivity and responsivity that foster child development and attachment.

We conducted the training in each parent's home on a weekly basis. To teach all of the interaction skills to criterion (based on the performance of the comparison group of parents without intellectual disabilities) took a mean of 45 weeks (range: 17–89 weeks). Before training, both groups of mothers with intellectual disabilities were scoring significantly below the comparison group mothers on the percentage intervals of total parental interactions ($p < .02$). After training, the training group performance was significantly greater than that of the control group on total interactions and each interaction skill (ps ranged from $< .05$ to $< .001$). On the posttest, the control group, but not the training group, remained significantly below the comparison group in total parental interactions ($p < .05$).

Before parental interaction training, both groups of children whose mothers had cognitive limitations were vocalizing significantly less than the comparison group of age-matched children whose parents did not have intellectual disabilities ($p < .005$). Significantly fewer of the former children were talking compared to the latter children ($p < .01$). Did the improvements in the parents' interaction skills increase the rate of child language development above maturation alone? As seen in Figure 3, the answer is yes. During parent training, child vocalizations and verbalizations increased in both the training and control groups, but the gain was significantly greater in children whose mothers had received interaction training ($p < .01$). The interaction training group children were now in the range of their peers who had mothers without intellectual disabilities. Compared to the children whose mothers received home safety training (attention controls), the children in the interaction training group scored significantly higher on posttest language and social items of the Bayley Scales of Infant Development and they began talking sooner. When the control group parents received interaction training, the children also increased their verbalizations to levels seen in peers of parents without intellectual disabilities. Informal observations and analyses of audiotapes of mother–child interactions suggested that interactional training resulted in qualitative improvements in mother–child interactions. The parents became more affectionate; they were more responsive and reinforcing of child language and other appropri-

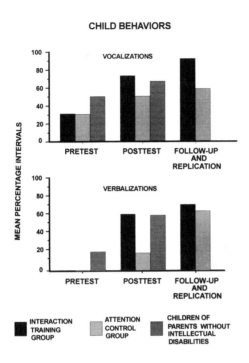

CHILD BEHAVIORS

Figure 3. Mean pretest, posttest, and follow-up percentage intervals of child vocalizations and verbalizations for the children of mothers with intellectual disabilities in the interaction training and attention control groups. Also included is a comparison group of age-matched children whose mothers did not have intellectual disabilities. The control group received training during the follow-up period. Reprinted from M. Feldman, B. Sparks, and L. Case, Effectiveness of home-based early intervention on the language development of children of mothers with mental retardation, *Reseach in Developmental Disabilities, 14*, p. 399, 1993, with kind permission of Elsevier Science Ltd., The Boulevard, Langford Lane, Kidlington OX5 1GB, UK.

ate behaviors. The children began to use language in functionally positive ways and reciprocated affection and play with the mother.

As in the Feldman, Case, and Sparks (1992) research described above, in this study we also found that the rate of child removal dropped considerably from 78% to 20% (up to 3 years after participating in the program). These findings should be interpreted cautiously, because in neither study was there an experimental design to confirm that the reduction in child apprehension could be attributed to program involvement.

Thus, the results of our parent training studies suggest that in-home parent training of parents with intellectual disabilities increased their skills to levels seen in parents without intellectual disabilities. The training appeared to directly bene-fit the children's health and development. This type of intervention, however, is not the only potentially effective strategy. Significant, and perhaps more substantial, im-provements in child intellectual development were found when children of moth-ers with intellectual disabilities were placed in specialized preschools for several years, starting in infancy (Garber, 1988; Ramey & Ramey, 1992). These costly inter-ventions, however, did not specifically attempt to improve parenting skills to reduce the risk of physical neglect or increase stimulation at home. Accordingly, in-home services for at-risk children that produce increases in parenting skills and child de-velopment may be more feasible and cost-effective (Bronfenbrenner, 1974).

FUTURE RESEARCH

We are currently addressing several additional areas related to increasing the effectiveness and scope of parent education.

Self-Instruction

To make parent training more efficient and disseminable, we have designed il-lustrated manuals that depict each step of the task analysis for a variety of child-care skills. Simple text describing the step is placed next to the relevant picture. For those parents who cannot read, we have also made audiotapes that describe the pic-tures while the parents scrutinize them. Preliminary field-testing with more than 30 parents suggests that about 70% of parents with cognitive impairments and low reading levels can improve their child-care skills through self-instruction alone.

Generalization and Maintenance

A recent review of the effectiveness of parenting education for parents with intellectual disabilities (Feldman, 1994) found inconsistent generalization and maintenance of skills within and across studies. Generalization enhancement strategies such as sufficient exemplars, common stimuli, and instructions to gen-eralize (Stokes & Baer, 1977) may promote generalization of parenting skills in these parents (Feldman et al., 1986, 1989). Gradually thinning coupon reinforce-ment may increase maintenance (Feldman et al., 1989; Feldman, Case, Garrick, et al., 1992). We are continuing to evaluate the effects of programmed generalization and maintenance techniques, particularly on parent–child interactions.

Parenting Game

Older children of parents with intellectual disabilities are at risk for behavior problems (Feldman & Walton-Allen, 1997). The parents' own upbringing, ongoing high stress, their lack of positive child behavior management strategies, and other factors, may lead them to use ineffective or potentially abusive discipline. Some parents whom we observed were overly permissive, did not supervise or set lim-its, and allowed their children to run the household. Conversely, other parents were overly restrictive and relied heavily on corporal punishment.

We have developed a "parenting game" to teach parents with intellectual disabilities to use noncorporal, positive-based child management skills. We focused on increasing parent–child cooperation by teaching parents to give clear instructions, reinforce child cooperation, and use noncorporal disciplinary strategies such as taking away privileges and a brief sit-out. We also used the parent game to improve parent–child rapport. We taught the parents to pay more attention to their children, show more interest in their children's lives, allow their children to make reasonable choices and decisions, and increase opportunities for positive engagements. The game is played by two parents at a time (usually two mothers, but sometimes between the spouses) at a clinic. The parents select a card that depicts a typical problem situation (e.g., "you have told your child it is time for bed, but she refuses to go") and must role-play the correct response. The majority of parents reported that they have enjoyed this game and our observations revealed that they readily learned to role-play correct responses. Of course, the crucial issue is whether they would generalize these skills to real-life situations. Preliminary videotaped observations in the homes indicated that the parents generalized most of the skills learned in the game to their natural interactions with their children. Providing consistent consequences for inappropriate child behavior appeared to be the most difficult skill to transfer from the game to home.

Social Support Networks

As mentioned earlier, we found that mothers with intellectual disabilities experienced very high stress levels, but social support was negatively correlated with stress and satisfaction with social support was positively correlated with parental positive interactions. While these results do not indicate causality, future research should examine the possibility that increasing fulfilling natural social support networks in these families may buffer the effects of stressors, increase acceptance of and responsiveness to interventions, and improve parent and child outcomes (Telleen et al., 1989).

CONCLUSION

Although parenting education could be a viable and more humane alternative to the permanent termination of parenting rights, it is not a panacea. These families still have many problems related to parental, child, and contextual factors that can impede adequate parenting and child development (Belsky, 1984). Some of the factors not directly addressed by parent education include (1) parental physical and mental health problems, (2) stigmatization, (3) poverty, and (4) absence of, or dissatisfaction with, family support networks. Future efforts should develop and evaluate expanded services for parents with intellectual disabilities to enhance the effects of parent education in improving parental competencies and reducing the risk for child maltreatment and/or developmental and behavior problems.

ACKNOWLEDGMENTS
Some of the research reported here was supported by grants from the Ontario Mental Health Foundation, the Ontario Ministry of Community and Social Services,

and Queen's University. I would like to thank the following people who served as parent education therapists and/or helped collect, prepare, and analyze the data: Jayne Carnwell, Laurie Case, Amy Cheung, Maria Garrick, Andrea Koster, Michèle Léger, Wanda MacIntyre-Grande, Sylvia Hains, Jennifer Ramsay, Bruce Sparks, Jean Varghese, and Nicole Walton-Allen. I would also like to express my gratitude to the families who participated in the research studies.

REFERENCES

Abidin, R. (1990). *Manual for the Parenting Stress Index.* Charlottesville VA: University of Virginia.

American Psychiatric Association. (1994). *Diagnostic and statistical manual of mental disorders.* 4th ed. Washington, DC: Author.

Bayley, N. (1969). *Bayley Scales of Infant Development: Birth to two years.* New York: Psychological Corporation.

Beck, A. T., Ward, C., Mendelson, M. J., & Erbaugh, J. (1961). An inventory for measuring depression. *Archives of General Psychiatry, 4,* 53–63.

Belsky, J. (1984). The determinants of parenting: A process model. *Child Development, 55,* 83–96.

Brandon, M. W. G. (1957). The intellectual and social status of children of mental defectives. *Journal of Mental Science, 103,* 710–738.

Bronfenbrenner, U. (1974). Is early intervention effective? *Columbia Teachers College Record, 76,* 279–303.

Budd, K., & Greenspan, S. (1984). Mentally retarded mothers. In E. Blechman (Ed.), *Behavior modification with women* (pp. 477–506). New York: Guilford Press.

Caldwell, B., & Bradley, R. (1984). *Home observation for measurement of the environment.* Unpublished manuscript. Little Rock: University of Arkansas.

Clarke-Stewart, K. A., & Apfel, N. (1979). Evaluating parental effects on child development. In L. S. Schulman (Ed.), *Review of research in education* (Vol. 6, pp. 47–119). Itasca, IL: Peacock.

Cohen, S., & Hoberman, H. M. (1983). Positive events and social supports as buffers of life change stress. *Journal of Applied Social Psychology, 13,* 99–125.

Crnic, K., Greenberg, M., Robinson, N., & Ragozin, A. (1984). Maternal stress and social support: Effects on the mother–infant relationship from birth to eighteen months. *American Journal of Orthopsychiatry, 54,* 224–235.

Dunst, C. J., Trivette, C. M., & Cross, A. H. (1986). Mediating influences of social support: Personal, family, and child outcomes. *American Journal on Mental Deficiency, 90,* 403–417.

Feldman, M. A. (1994). Parenting education for parents with intellectual disabilities: A review of outcome studies. *Research in Developmental Disabilities, 15,* 299–332.

Feldman, M. A., Case, L., Garrick, M., MacIntyre-Grande, W., Carnwell, J., & Sparks, B. (1992). Teaching child-care skills to parents with developmental disabilities. *Journal of Applied Behavior Analysis, 25,* 205–215.

Feldman, M. A., Case, L., Rincover, A., Towns, F., & Betel, J. (1989). Parent education project III. Increasing affection and responsivity in developmentally handicapped mothers: Component analysis, generalization, and effects on child language. *Journal of Applied Behavior Analysis, 22,* 211–222.

Feldman, M. A., Case, L., & Sparks, B. (1992). Effectiveness of a child-care training program for parents at-risk for child neglect. *Canadian Journal of Behavioural Science, 24,* 14–28.

Feldman, M. A., Case, L., Towns, F., & Betel, J. (1985). Parent education project I: Development and nurturance of children of mentally retarded parents. *American Journal of Mental Deficiency, 90,* 253–258.

Feldman, M. A., Léger, M., & Walton-Allen, N. (in press). Stress in mothers with intellectual disabilities. *Journal of Child and Family Studies.*

Feldman, M. A., Sparks, B., & Case, L. (1993). Effectiveness of home-based early intervention on the language development of children of mothers with mental retardation. *Research in Developmental Disabilities, 14,* 387–408.

Feldman, M. A., Towns, F., Betel, J., Case, L., Rincover, A., & Rubino, C. A. (1986). Parent education project II: Increasing stimulating interactions of developmentally handicapped mothers. *Journal of Applied Behavior Analysis, 19,* 23–37.

Feldman, M. A., & Walton-Allen, N. (1997). Effects of maternal mental retardation and poverty on intellectual, academic, and behavioral status of school-age children. *American Journal on Mental Retardation, 101,* 352–364.

Forehand, R., Lautenschlager, G., Faust, J., & Graziano, W. (1986). Parent perceptions and parent–child interactions in clinic referred children: A preliminary investigation of the effects of maternal depressive moods. *Behaviour Research and Therapy, 24,* 73–75.

Garber, H. L. (1988). *The Milwaukee Project. Preventing mental retardation in children at risk.* Washington, DC: American Association on Mental Retardation.

Gillberg, C., & Geijer-Karlsson, M. (1983). Children born to mentally retarded women: A 1–21 year follow-up study of 41 cases. *Psychological Medicine 13,* 891–894.

Hammen, C., Adrian, C., Gordon, D., Burge, D., Jaenicke, C., & Hiroto, D. (1987). Children of depressed mothers: Maternal strain and symptom prediction of dysfunction. *Journal of Abnormal Psychology, 96,* 190–198.

Hayman, R. L. (1990). Presumptions of justice: Law, politics, and the mentally retarded parent. *Harvard Law Review, 103,* 1201–1271.

Hops, H., Biglan, A., Sherman, L., Arthur, J., Friedman, L., & Osteen, L. (1987). Home observations of family interactions of depressed women. *Journal of Consulting and Clinical Psychology, 55,* 341–346.

Hudson, A. M. (1982). Training parents of developmentally handicapped children: A component analysis. *Behavior Therapy, 13,* 325–333.

Kazdin, A. E. (1977). Assessing the clinical and applied importance of behavior change through social validation. *Behavior Modification, 1,* 427–452.

Luckasson, R., Coulter, D. L., Polloway, E. A., Reiss, S., Schalock, R. L., Snell, M. E., Spitalnik, D. M., & Stark, J. A. (1992). *Mental retardation: Definition, classification, and systems of supports.* 9th ed. Washington, DC: American Association on Mental Retardation.

Matson, J. L. (1988). Teaching and training relevant community living skills to mentally retarded persons. *Child and Youth Services, 10,* 107–121.

Mercer, J. R. (1973). *Labeling the mentally retarded: Clinical and social system perspectives on mental retardation.* Berkeley: University of California Press.

Minnes, P. M. (1994). Mental retardation: The impact upon the family. In J. A. Burack, R. M. Hodapp, &. E. Zigler (Eds.), *Handbook of mental retardation and development.* New York: Cambridge University Press.

Offord, D. R., Boyle, M. H., Szatmari, P., Rae-Grant, N. I., Links, P. S., Cadman, D. T., Byles, J. A., Crawford, J. W., Blum, H. M., Byrne, C., Thomas, H., & Woodward, C. A. (1987). Ontario child health study. II: Six month prevalence of disorder and rates of service utilization. *Archives of General Psychiatry, 44,* 832–836.

Ramey, C. T., & Ramey, S. L. (1992). Effective early intervention. *Mental Retardation, 30,* 337–345.

Reed, R., & Reed, S. (1965). *Mental retardation: A family study.* New York: Saunders.

Scally, B. G. (1973). Marriage and mental handicap: Some observations in Northern Ireland. In F. F. de la Cruz & G. D. La Veck (Eds.), *Human sexuality and the mentally retarded* (pp. 186–194). New York: Brunner/Mazel.

Seagull, E. A., & Scheurer, S. L. (1986). Neglected and abused children of mentally retarded parents. *Child Abuse & Neglect, 10,* 493–500.

Seifer, R., Sameroff, A. J., & Jones, F. (1981). Adaptive behavior in young children of emotionally disturbed women. *Journal of Applied Developmental Psychology, 1,* 251–276.

Stokes, T. F., & Baer, D. M. (1977). An implicit technology of generalization. *Journal of Applied Behavior Analysis, 10,* 349–367.

Taylor, C. G., Norman, D. K., Murphy, J. M., Jellinek, M., Quinn, D., Poitrast, F. G., & Goshko, M. (1991). Diagnosed intellectual and emotional impairment among parents who seriously mistreat their children: Prevalence, type, and outcome in a court sample. *Child Abuse & Neglect, 15,* 389–401.

Telleen, S., Herzog, A., & Kilbane, T. L. (1989). Impact of a family support program on a mother's social support and parenting stress. *American Journal of Orthopsychiatry, 59,* 410–419.

Tymchuk, A. J., & Feldman, M. A. (1991). Parents with mental retardation and their children: A review of research relevant to professional practice. *Canadian Psychology/Psychologie Canadienne, 32,* 486–496.

Tymchuk, A. J., & Keltner, B. (1991). Advantage profiles: A tool for health care professionals working with parents with mental retardation. *Pediatric Nursing, 14,* 155–161.

Vogel, P. (1987). The right to parent. *Entourage, 2,* 33–39.

Walton-Allen, N. (1993). *Psychological distress and parenting by mothers with mental retardation.* Doctoral dissertation, University of Toronto.

Walton-Allen, N., & Feldman, M. A. (1991). Perception of service needs by parents with mental retardation and their workers. *Comprehensive Mental Health Care, 1,* 137–147.

Webster-Stratton, C. (1988). Mother's and father's perceptions of child deviance: Roles of parent and child behaviors and parent adjustment. *Journal of Consulting and Clinical Psychology, 56,* 909–915.

Weinraub, M., & Wolf, B. (1983). Mother–child interactions in single and two-parent families. *Child Development, 54,* 1297–1311.

18

The Importance of Matching Educational Interventions to Parent Needs in Child Maltreatment

Issues, Methods, and Recommendations

ALEXANDER J. TYMCHUK

In this chapter, a discussion of unresolved definitional, assessment, educational, and policy needs regarding parenting in general and child maltreatment in particular is presented. These unresolved needs are critical to consider when discussing parenting by persons with disabilities. Juxtaposed with the issues surrounding parenting is a presentation of the changing view of disabilities and the adequacy of past, present, and future services and supports available to parents with disabilities. Finally, some of the methods available to professionals who work with parents with disabilities is presented to aid such professionals in preparing their clients for parenting as well as in answering and resolving concerns about their clients' parenting skills.

PARENTING IN A CHANGING SOCIETY

Parents Must Learn to Parent and to Adapt Largely on Their Own

In order to provide for the health and safety of their children, parents must either have extensive knowledge and skills in these areas, or must know how to seek, obtain, and utilize resources that may help them in providing care in these areas. Despite parents' needs for health and safety skills, there has been no systematic

ALEXANDER J. TYMCHUK • Department of Psychiatry, School of Medicine, University of California, Los Angeles, California 90024-1759.

Handbook of Child Abuse Research and Treatment, edited by Lutzker. Plenum Press, New York, 1998.

societal effort to provide education for parenting. The lack of educational services is based in part on the assumption that people will develop the requisite knowledge and skills and will adapt to changing circumstances on their own and/or with whatever resources are currently available. There also has been a general reluctance to intrude into the domain of parenting, which has hitherto been considered a private matter. Parents with higher education, personal abilities, finances, social supports, and other resources will be able to seek, obtain, and acquire parenting knowledge, as well as to adapt to economic and other societal changes. On the other hand, parents who are less educated encounter obstacles in acquiring parenting knowledge. They may have difficulty understanding complex English and have individual learning needs due to a functional or categorical disability, rendering it difficult to access and learn important parent information. In addition, the less educated parents may live in chaotic circumstances with few social supports and face economic impoverishment. In the absence of parent education and supports, the young children of these parents may be at high risk for inadequate health care and for home, personal, and community endangerment (Gaudin, 1993). Such heightened risk status, whether actual or perceived, may place the parents at a higher risk for report for child maltreatment (Gaudin, 1993; West, Richardson, LeConte, Crimi, & Stuart, 1992).

Definitions of Disabilities

Throughout this chapter the word "disability" will be used in a generic sense, although technical use of the word refers to specific characteristics displayed by a person which are categorized and labeled as a disability. There are a number of issues related to the nomenclature of disabilities that confound our understanding and may interfere with the thoughtful development of procedures regarding parents with disabilities within the arena of child abuse and neglect.

The confounding issues include the heavy reliance upon a medical/disease model used to describe behavioral phenomena; historical changes in the terms used; the significant delay between changes in classification and the complete, consistent use of the changes within various societal groups; the variety of terms used to describe a disability or disabilities, as well as the terms' criteria which often differ across discipline or function; the treatment of people to whom such terms were applied; and the basis from which a term is derived and the manner in which the term is used (Nagler, 1993).

Functional versus Categorical Approaches to Disabilities

There are two current perspectives on disabilities: the functional perspective and the categorical perspective. Within a functional perspective, emphasis is on the determination of the person's current knowledge and skills, the learning abilities, and the circumstances under which the person successfully learns or applies what is learned. The advantages of the functional approach are its focus upon abilities, rather than inabilities, and its examination of the circumstances that either encourage or hamper learning. These considerations allow for tailored educational methods that fit the person's specific needs and circumstances.

On the other hand, the primary emphasis of the categorical perspective is on the degree to which the person meets criteria for a particular category. This process is similar to diagnosis and classification. For instance, learning disabilities, mental disabilities, or developmental disabilities are types of diagnoses and classifications. Secondarily, there may be a consideration of ability determination. In the area of child abuse and neglect, a categorical rather than a functional approach has generally been taken.

Current Nomenclature and Epidemiology of Disabilities

Table 1 contains several of the current words and definitions used to describe disabilities. Depending on the circumstances, either a functional approach or a categorical approach is utilized. The inconsistency of the approaches remains even within the recent Americans with Disabilities Act (ADA) (1991). Workers in the field must be aware that different approaches to disabilities exist and must understand the evolution of each approach. Workers should also realize that maintaining both approaches has hindered our understanding of the epidemiology of disabilities.

Although there has not been a systematic epidemiological study of functional or categorical disabilities among parents in any country, it is estimated that between 15% and 25% of Americans have physical or mental impairments that limit their activities (Department of Health and Human Services [DHHS], 1990; Boyle, Decoufle, & Yeargin-Allsopp, 1994). In schools, 43% of the 4.4 million students with "handicaps" who were served had learning disabilities, and high school students with disabilities have an average reading grade 3.5 grades below their actual grade level (e.g., Wagner, 1995). Furthermore, about 20% of adult Americans read at or below a 5th grade level, while another 30% read between a 6th grade and 9th grade reading level (Doak, Doak, & Root, 1996; National Center for Education Statistics, 1993).

What Do We Know about Parents with Individual Learning Needs or Disabilities within the Area of Child Maltreatment?

In the United States, there are no systematically collected data on the number of parents with disabilities who are referred to child protection services, the needs of parents with disabilities, and the ways in which the parents' needs are addressed (National Child Abuse and Neglect Data System [NCANDS], 1994). However, there is a recognition by those who work with parents with disabilities that gross incidence data, more specific needs assessment and intervention data are necessary (NCANDS, 1995; Tymchuk, 1996). The need for such information stems not only from the increasing recognition that these families require more extensive, individualized interventions in order to be successful (Booth, Barnard, Mitchell, & Spieker, 1987; Cohler & Musick, 1984; Tymchuk, 1990a; Tymchuk & Feldman, 1991), but also from the need to find effective strategies for an already overburdened system (Blanch, Nicholson, & Purcell, 1994; Briere, Berliner, Bulkley, Jenny, & Reid, 1996; National Research Council [NRC], 1993). Furthermore, the need for data on parents with disabilities arises from the increased economic costs associated with adjudicating child maltreatment cases involving such parents, the lost economic benefits because of lost productivity of both parents and their children when their lives are disrupted, and an increased recognition of the great potential for a continued cycle of abuse and neglect when the children of parents with disabilities also

Table 1. Disability Terms, Definitions, and Sources

Disabilities

The term "disability" means with respect to an individual:
- (A) A physical[1] or mental impairment[2] that substantially limits one of the major life activities of such individual;
- (B) A record of such impairment; or
- (C) Being regarded as having such an impairment. If an individual meets any one of these three tests, he or she is considered to be an individual with a disability for purposes of coverage under the Americans with Disabilities Act (p. 35699)

[1] Categorical examples include orthopedic, visual, speech and visual impairments, cerebral palsy, multiple sclerosis, cancer, diabetes.
[2] Mental retardation, emotional illness, specific learning disabilities, HIV disease, tuberculosis, drug addiction and alcoholism.

Source: Federal Register, 28 CFR Part 35, July 26, 1991.

Developmental disabilities

The term "developmental disability" means a severe, chronic disability of a person which:
- (A) is attributable to a mental or physical impairment or combination of mental and physical impairments;
- (B) is manifested before the person attains age twenty-two;
- (C) is likely to continue indefinitely;
- (D) results in substantial functional limitations in three or more of the following areas of major life activity: (i) self-care, (ii) receptive and expressive language, (iii) learning, (iv) mobility, (v) self-direction, (vi) capacity for independent living, and (vii) economic self-sufficiency; and
- (E) reflects the person's need for a combination and sequence of special, interdisciplinary, or generic care, treatment, or other services which are lifelong or extended duration and are individually planned and coordinated.

Source: The Developmental Disabilities Assistance and Bill of Rights Act (as amended by P.L. 95–602).

Mental retardation

Mental retardation refers to substantial limitations in present functioning. It is characterized by significantly subaverage intellectual functioning, existing concurrently with related limitations in two or more of the following applicable adaptive skill areas: health and safety, functional academics, leisure, and work. Mental retardation manifests before age 18. (p. 1)

Source: American Association on Mental Retardation. (1993). *Mental retardation definition classification and systems of supports.* Washington, DC: Author.

Specific learning disability

A disorder in one or more of the basic psychological processes involved in understanding or using language, spoken or written, which may manifest itself in an imperfect ability to listen, think, speak, write, spell, or to do mathematical calculations. This category includes perceptual handicaps, brain injury, minimal brain dysfunction, dyslexia, and developmental aphasia, but does not include learning problems resulting from visual, hearing, or motor handicaps, or from mental retardation.

Source: P.L. 94–142 (an act to amend the Education for All Handicapped Children Act of 1975), November 29, 1975.

---

become parents (Barnett, 1993; Bryant & Daro, 1994.; Caldwell, 1992). Juxtaposed against this information, legislation has emerged recognizing the civil rights of persons with disabilities (e.g., ADA, 1991), while other emphases have been placed upon maintaining the integrity of the family unit.

    The actual number of parents with disabilities or individual learning needs who are reported for suspicion of child abuse and/or neglect is not precisely known. However, such parents seem to make up a number of child protective services caseloads that is disproportionate to their actual numbers in society (e.g., Seagull & Scheurer, 1986; Trupin, Tarico, Low, Jemelka, & McClellan, 1993). In other words, the percentage of people with disabilities involved with child protective services appears to be greater than the percentage of people with disabilities in society in general. While this statement must be taken cautiously because of the difficulty of determining the accuracy of diagnosis, description, and reporting across locales, the estimated numbers of parents with disabilities seen in child protective services appear to be substantial.

Because of the variety of disabilities and the different ways in which disabilities are expressed, a person with a disability often requires adaptation of educational methods to their needs in order to learn and apply information (Mercer & Mercer, 1985). Parents with a disability also require adaptations of educational methods in learning parenting skills (e.g., Wells, Ruscavage, Parker, & McArthur, 1994). However, in the absence of a policy for identifying parents with individual needs and the lack of services and education related to those needs, child protective services is often the initial contact agency for reporting possible child maltreatment. It may be found that as the incidence of child maltreatment continues to increase, the numbers of parents with disabilities seen in child protective services will also increase (DHHS, 1988; NRC, 1993). Other factors that may contribute to the increase in child maltreatment by parents with disabilities are (1) the continued deterioration in education, health care, and social services, (2) the lack of integration of service provisions for low-income families, (3) increasing familial disintegration, (4) poverty, (5) homelessness, (6) drug and alcohol abuse, (7) unemployment, and (8) the incidental effect of deinstitutionalization and of full inclusion. In addition, many of those who have a disability are also of low income and therefore especially vulnerable to the problems of society just mentioned.

Needs to Be Addressed in Order to Serve Parents with Specific Learning Needs in Child Maltreatment

Need for Definition of the Components of Parenting: A Focus on Health and Safety

Although there is no agreed-upon definition of parenting, there is a definition of what parenting is not—child abuse and neglect. What constitutes child maltreatment, however, also suffers from inconsistent operationalization (Gaudin, 1993). In the absence of a standard definition of parenting, researchers and practitioners might focus upon the prevention of child maltreatment as a dependent variable, using as a definition whatever appears in case records as indicators of the presence or absence of child maltreatment (e.g., Fink & McCloskey, 1990). However, such an approach could seriously limit the empirical study of parenting.

Need for Empirical Methods of Assessment of Components of Parenting

The absence of a standard definition of parenting also hampers the development of empirical methods for assessing the components of parenting (cf., Saunders, 1995; Runyan, 1991). Lacking such methods, practitioners and researchers are left to either use or adapt methods from related areas of research that may not adhere to basic psychometric criteria (e.g., NCPCA, 1994); they may develop their own methodologies with varying adherence to psychometric criteria. The consequences of uncritical application of methodologies from other areas of research to child maltreatment are unclear.

Need for a Range of Standards for Adequacy of Parenting

The absence of standardized assessment methods also means that there are no recognized standards for the determination of adequacy or inadequacy of parenting other than what the "average" parent does or does not do or what the "normal" parent does or does not do. In order to apply to the wide range of socially acceptable differences in parenting, such established standards must be presented within a range rather than as specific criteria. Most normative data for assessment instruments pertain to the middle socioeconomic class. Applied to parenting, then, the middle-class standard becomes the de facto standard against which the parenting of those in lower socioeconomic classes is compared. In the absence of a range of standards, decision making by caseworkers becomes more subjective, less reliable and more time-consuming. More importantly, the lack of criteria results in the application of more general standards such as "an inability to parent," or "parent places child in danger," or "parent shows an inability to bond," without operationalizing what these mean. Such a lack places parents with disabilities in greater jeopardy of erroneous reporting for child maltreatment, of child removal, and of determinations of parental incompetency.

Need for Empirically Developed Parenting Curricula Materials and Educational Strategies

In addition to the needs for a definition of and range of standards for, parenting, there is a critical need for the development of empirically based parenting curricula and materials. Although there are many parent education programs that detail the topics to be taught, the materials to be used in teaching, and the general strategies to be followed, most of the programs have not been formally developed using empirical criteria.

There are several stages in the design of an empirically based program. The same empirical standards that apply to research also apply to curriculum development in order for confidence to be placed in the information obtained through the program, judgments to be made, theories to be built, policies to be established, and for funding to be given to the program (e.g., Ornstein & Hunkins, 1993; Judd, Smith, & Kidder, 1991).

What We Know about Parenting by Persons with Disabilities

Much of the published research surrounding parents with certain categorical disabilities such as mental illness, alcoholism, learning disabilities, physical disabilities, and visual or hearing impairments have been descriptive in nature and focused upon epidemiology and factors related to child risk status (Quinton, Rutter, & Liddle, 1984; Walker & Emory, 1983). Although there has been an increasing interest in child risk status in cases in which one or both parents have a categorical disability, the descriptions of interventions with parents in these categories suffer from many of the criticisms mentioned earlier (e.g., absence of an operationalized definition of the components of parenting and lack of empirically standardized assessment, instrumentation, educational materials, and educational processes) (Cohler & Musick, 1984). However, there is a growing empirical research base comparing parenting by persons who have developmental disabilities with that by persons who are not seen as disabled, but who exhibit identical levels of parenting knowledge and skills and live in similar environments (Tymchuk, 1992a). In addition, there is extensive literature on early childhood intervention (e.g., Booth, et al., 1987; Martin, Ramey, & Ramey, 1990; Gallagher & Ramey, 1987; Garber, 1988) and parent training (e.g., Helm & Kozloff, 1986) in which assessments and intervention strategies have been developed and evaluated. The foci in these areas, in general, have not included issues related to parents' health and safety skill development or issues related to child maltreatment.

Despite the lack of extensive information on parents with other functional or categorical disabilities, there are definite similarities between the factors that need to be addressed in order to facilitate parenting skill development in these populations, and those factors that need to be addressed with a parent who has a cognitive or developmental disability.

A Systematic Approach to Parenting by Persons with Functional Disabilities

As part of an ongoing, systematic research program studying the adequacy of parenting by persons with individual learning needs, parenting assessment instruments have been developed, evaluated, and refined with large numbers of mothers. Parenting intervention strategies have also been developed, evaluated, and refined with individual mothers or with small groups of mothers referred by health care, education, disability, and child protective service agencies. The environmental, social, and psychological factors that facilitate or inhibit learning have also been identified (e.g., Tymchuk, 1990a; 1992a; Tymchuk & Andron, 1990; Tymchuk, Andron, & Rahbar, 1988; Tymchuk, Hamada, Andron, & Anderson, 1990).

The Need for Specificity in Assessment and Education

A Taxonomy for Parenting: The UCLA Parent/Child Health and Wellness Project

From this empirical base, a model parenting program was developed. This program was created using a multifactorial/multilevel developmental process approach in order to provide criteria for the educational interventions. The goals of the education program are to improve parenting knowledge and skills in persons with individual learning needs and to prevent future child abuse and neglect.

Within the UCLA Parent/Child Health and Wellness Project, four major components of parenting are stressed:

I. Fundamental Knowledge and Skills for Parents
II. Health
III. Safety
IV. Parent and Child Enjoying Each Other

In addition to the development and demonstration of methods and processes, the preparatory work of the Wellness Project demonstrates the need for adaptation and coordination of such community services as health care, education, child protective services, and disability services (Tymchuk, 1990a; 1992a). As can be seen in Table 2, each component contains a number of critical sub-areas.

Table 2. Component Areas Considered to Be Critical
for Parenting Assessments and Education
(from the UCLA Parent/Child Health & Wellness Project)

Component I: Fundamental Knowledge and
Skills for Parents
A. Support Relationships
   1. Social Supports
   2. Service Supports
B. Effective Short and Long-Term Planning
C. Effective Decision-Making
D. Effective Coping
E. Effective Observation Skills
   1. Self-Observer
   2. Child Observer
F. Finances and Budget
G. Meal Planning
H. House Cleanliness
I. Hygiene
   1. Personal Grooming
   2. Child Grooming

Component II: Health
A. Body Works
   1. Understanding Health Comprehension
   2. Parts of the Body
   3. Common Problems Associated with
      Body Parts
   4. Understanding of Sickness and Health
   5. Knowing When You Are Sick
   6. Knowing When Your Child Is Sick
B. Diagnostics
   1. Body Temperature
   2. Pulse
   3. Breathing
   4. Common Health Problems
   5. Diagnosing Common Health Problems
C. Life-threatening Emergencies
   1. Knowledge of Life-threatening
      Emergencies
   2. Causes of Life-threatening Emergencies
   3. Prevention of Life-threatening
      Emergencies
   4. Emergency Planning
   5. When a Life-threatening Emergency
      Occurs
D. Calling the Doctor: Knowing When to Call
   and What to Do
   1. Symptoms to Call the Doctor About

   2. Calling the Doctor
   3. Understanding the Doctor's Directions
E. Medicines
   1. Asking Questions About Prescription
      Medicine
   2. Getting a Prescription Filled
   3. Getting Over-the-Counter Medicine
   4. Using Prescription Medicine
   5. Using Over-the-Counter Medicine

Component III: Safety
A. Partner Safety
B. Safety in the Home or the Apartment
   1. Phone Safety
   2. Door Safety
   3. On Vacation
C. Community Safety
   1. Going Out
      a. Before Going Out
      b. While Out in the Community
      c. Returning Home
   2. Reporting a Crime
D. Home Safety
   1. Home Dangers and Precautions
      Inventory
   2. Fire
   3. Electrical
   4. Danger of Choking From Small Objects
   5. Suffocation
   6. Firearm and Other Projectile Weapons
   7. Poisons
   8. Falling Heavy Objects
   9. Sharp/Pointed Objects
   10. Clutter
   11. Inappropriate Edibles
   12. Dangerous Toys or Animals
   13. Cooking
   14. General Dangers
   15. Yard/Outdoors
   16. Danger & Safety Maps

Component IV: Parent and Child Enjoying
   Each Other
A. ChildSafe
B. Parent & Child Playing
C. Parent Reading and Singing to Child

Making Interventions Work—Areas of Assessment and Intervention

Why Assess?

There are a number of reasons to perform assessments with parents and children: (1) to categorize, diagnose, and label; (2) to describe; (3) to determine strengths and weaknesses in order to design an intervention; and (4) to show change in knowledge (both increases and decreases) as a result of an intervention (Anastasi, 1976; Cronbach, 1970). The majority of studies that assessed parenting in general and child maltreatment specifically have focused upon the first two reasons.

Selecting an Instrument

There are a number of factors that must be considered in the selection of instruments and methods of assessments. These factors include (1) the degree of adherence to psychometric standards (e.g., reliability, validity, and suitability of normative data for the population to be assessed), (2) the appropriateness of the assessment (i.e., can an intervention be designed based on the instrument or would this be an indirect measure of efficacy?), (3) the time it takes to administer (e.g., when combined into a battery of instruments does fatigue affect the results? Are all the data going to be used?), (4) the format (e.g., can the person see, hear, and/or discriminate the information?), (5) the complexity of items (e.g., are the items written at a level so that the person being assessed can understand the questions?), and (6) the training that is required in order to administer the instrument. Consideration to these factors either in the development of new assessments or in the use of existing assessment methods becomes of greater importance in ensuring fairness when a parent has a disability. In the absence of adherence to parts of any or all of the instrumentation standardization (and of curricula) criteria, any deficits in performance may be erroneously attributed to the parent rather than to such absence. Unfortunately, such misattribution has occurred regularly with parents with developmental disabilities (e.g., Hayman, 1990; Miller, 1994; Whitman & Accardo, 1990).

Available Methods and Instruments

Several authors have described the types of instruments that are available and that have been used in the assessment of parenting. Few of these instruments were developed for use in the area of child maltreatment and none was developed for use with individuals who have limited reading or speech comprehension abilities. Virtually all available assessments are meant for descriptive (i.e., description of characteristics and related factors) rather than for prescriptive (i.e., identification of areas of strengths and needs in order to develop educational interventions) purposes (Family Preservation Evaluation Project, 1995; Lubeck & Chandler, 1990; Zill & Coiro, 1992). Thus, most available instruments currently used in child maltreatment have limited value in response to specific parenting needs (NRC, 1993). There are, however, a number of alternative assessment strategies such as the use of direct behavioral observation (e.g., Tymchuk & Andron, 1992) and task analysis (e.g., Williams & Cuvo, 1986) of parenting components (Lubeck & Chandler, 1990; Lutzker & Campbell, 1994; Tertinger, Greene, & Lutzker, 1984). These alternative assessment strategies hold the greatest promise for work with parents with disabilities, and still require adherence to psychometric standards (Bellack, Hersen, & Kazdin, 1982) and training in their application (Bloom & Fischer, 1982). In addition, individuals can develop their own assessment devices for the areas in which they are interested (e.g., Glik, Greaves, Kronenfeld, & Jackson, 1993; Peterson, Harbeck, & Moreno, 1993; Speltz, Gonzales, Sulzbacher, & Quan, 1990).

How to Assess

Demographics

Formal assessment of a parent reported for child maltreatment is used for descriptive or predictive purposes or both rather than for prescriptive purposes. Although prescriptive assessment should be done for all parents associated with child maltreatment, this type of assessment is especially important when a parent has specific learning needs associated with a disability. Since many parents with a disability have limited experiences, their current abilities may be falsely depressed and are not indicative of their capabilities. Prescriptive assessment coupled with studying the effects of education matched to specific needs can help identify those capabilities. In addition to such prescriptive assessments, there are other factors identified during the determination of advantage and risk factor that need to be examined further.

Chief among the specific factors that should be identified are the parent's physical abilities such as vision, hearing, general motility and coordination, and strength of the limbs. Often this information can be gathered by asking the parent. However, some parents may be unwilling to admit that they cannot read information that is in small print, that they cannot recognize information presented at a distance, or that they do not understand information imbedded in other information. Similarly, parents may be unable to hear information, to discriminate noises, or both, from one ear or at certain distances when masked by other noises. In addition, they may be unable to lift or extend their arms or hands without severe involuntary shaking. Each of these may impair current parenting or the learning of new skills. Educational adaptations can be made to overcome the impacts of these impairments. Adaptations include larger print, illustrations, single sets of information, louder speech, and an uncluttered environment (e.g., Berger, Inkelas, Myre, & Mishler, 1994; Tymchuk, Andron, & Tymchuk, 1990).

Cognitive Ability

Few studies in child maltreatment have formally assessed the intellectual abilities of the parents or report the IQ recorded in case records. Assessment of cognitive ability may be seen as unnecessary or inappropriate given the sensitive issues surrounding the meaning of IQ. Nonetheless, IQ can provide useful information particularly regarding learning ability. In general, the lower the IQ is below average, the lower and flatter the learning curve. That is, it takes these individuals longer to learn material and they may not learn it completely. This means that any intervention will take a long time, and this probably will increase costs.

Reading ability instruments. There is an increasing awareness that the level of a person's reading recognition and comprehension abilities can influence their knowledge and skill levels, as well as their learning abilities (Lynn, 1989). Despite this recognition, in the area of child maltreatment there has been virtually no determination of parents' reading abilities in order to match educational materials to these abilities. This is particularly problematic because large-scale studies have reported that about 40% of the general population read at or below a 10th-grade level, whereas 73% of the parents of pediatric patients actually read at less than a 9th-grade level and 31% read at or below a 4th-grade level (Davis et al., 1994). At the same time, the reading complexity of parent education materials is several grades higher. For example, 80% of 129 sampled written parent materials from various professional organizations or available commercially required at least a 10th-grade reading level (Davis et al., 1994). Since these reading formulas measure only reading recognition, there is no determination of level of reading comprehension. At the same time, these formulas do not take into account the fact that information is presented in small, cluttered print using technical terms (Tymchuk, 1990b). Misuse of products such as over-the-counter medications, high-risk household products, or prescription medications is a significant contributing factor in child neglect. Emphasizing the importance of matching information to the intended population's reading level, one study found that when pediatric information materials provided to parents were simplified to the reading grade levels of parents, there was a significant improvement in understanding (Chacon, Kissoon, & Rich, 1994).

Reading recognition.   There are several formal tests to measure reading recognition in English. A widely used one is the Reading Recognition subscale of the Wide Range Achievement Test–Revised (WRAT–R) (Jastak & Wilkinson, 1984), in which the person looks at a list of letters and words of increasing difficulty and states what those letters and words are. This test takes 5 minutes and yields a reader's grade equivalent. There is no Reading Comprehension subscale on the WRAT–R. Norms represent the general population, although there is no comparison for socioeconomic status. The WRAT–R is widely used, reliable, valid, and is easily administered with minimal training. In order to interpret the results, however, training is necessary. Another quick, easily used instrument is the Diagnostic Screening Test (DST) (Gnagey & Gnagey, 1982) which has several subtests, including both reading recognition and reading comprehension. One potential drawback of the DST is that reading comprehension relies heavily on immediate memory typical of many such instruments. However, the DST is well standardized, with a representative sample in norms and provides grade scores. A major drawback for both the DST and the WRAT is the small print of the words. Enlarging and separating the words may be helpful; the effects of this adaptation on the norms is unclear, but they appear to be minimal. Since the words in neither instrument are directly related to parenting issues, neither is useful for prescriptive purposes.

In response to this need, the UCLA Parenting Reading Recognition List (UPRRL) was developed to assess a person's ability to recognize words. The words that comprise the UPRRL represent the areas of parenting within the Wellness Project. There are two equivalent forms of about 50 words each, in increasing syllabic complexity presented in 16-point, Times New Roman (see Table 3). Words were selected from those presented as critical by health care professionals, from those

Table 3. Items in Form One of the Parenting Reading Recognition List

1. 1	14. O.K.	27. warning	40. precaution
2. hot	15. 13	28. violent	41. consequence
3. two	16. practice	29. overdose	42. expiration
4. dose	17. danger	30. resistant	43. immediate
5. sharp	18. patience	31. suffocate	44. vaccination
6. help	19. symptom	32. one hundred	45. prescription
7. fire	20. physician	33. instructions	46. penicillin
8. fever	21. pregnant	34. alcohol	47. appropriate
9. laugh	22. children	35. °F.	48. limitation
10. praise	23. swelling	36. temperature	49. authoritarian
11. side effect	24. poison	37. punishment	50. emetic
12. high risk	25. swallow	38. diarrhea	51. flammable
13. language	26. reward	39. 911	52. nutritious

used on labels of products commonly used by parents, including prescription and over-the-counter medications and high-risk household products. Performance on the UPRR List is highly correlated with performance on the Reading Recognition subscale of the WRAT–R and can be used in the design of parent education.

Reading comprehension. There are several reading scales with reading comprehension subtests including the DST (Gnagey & Gnagey, 1982), which is valid for screening purposes, and the Passage Comprehension subtest of the Woodcock (1987), which samples a broader range of information and is widely used in schools for diagnostic purposes. The latter requires extensive training to administer and takes at least 10 minutes to give.

As with reading recognition, a drawback of all formal reading comprehension assessment devices is the fact that none contain information related to areas of parenting. In response to needs of parents to understand common words used in critical areas of parenting, the UCLA Parenting Reading Comprehension List (UP-RCL) was developed to accompany the UCLA Parenting Reading Recognition List. A single form with 30 items selected as representative of the words are included in the two forms of the UCLA Parenting Reading Recognition List. Each item has three choices written at a 5th-grade level of comprehension and printed in 16-point type for ease of reading. Sample items include:

1. What does *suffocate* mean?
   a. to get tired
   b. to die from not being able to breathe
   c. to run away
2. What does *diarrhea* mean?
   a. a book to write in
   b. a type of medicine
   c. watery poop
3. What does *child abuse* mean?
   a. hurting your child so you could go to jail
   b. not having sex with your child
   c. that you are proud of yourself

Fundamental Knowledge and Skills for Parents

There are certain areas of parenting in which all parents must have sufficient knowledge and skill themselves, or in which they are able to obtain support, in order to ensure the provision for the adequate health and safety of their children. Within the Wellness Project, these have been termed fundamental areas because they form the basis for parenting in other areas or may influence the health and safety of parents and of their children. As listed in Table 2, some of these areas include social and service support, planning for aspects of parenting through the development of their child, following an effective decision-making process as well as making the best decision possible, and coping with problems for which they did not plan. Those areas that influence adequacy of health and safety provided by parents include being able to handle finances, meal planning, home cleanliness, and personal and child hygiene. Although there are a number of devices used to determine social and service support availability and utilization (e.g., Coohey, 1995; Llewellyn, McConnell, & Bye, 1995), there are few devices available to assess the other components. Table 4 contains an example of an assessment used to

---

Table 4. Example of Assessment Regarding Fundamental Parenting Behaviors

Effective Decision-Making

INSTRUCTIONS: Below is a situation in which a parent would have to make a decision on how to act. Following the scenario is a list of good decision-making steps. Read the scenario to the parent and then ask questions 1–7 (#3 does not have a question). Each question is followed by sample responses. For each step, record a *1* if the parent correctly identifies it and a *0* if the parent incorrectly identifies it or no answer is given. Add up the number of points and record this number where it says "Total Points." Using the score guide, determine the parent's final score (0–3) and record the number in the space provided.

SCENARIO—"Your baby has been irritable all morning and will not stop crying."

___ 1. DECISION/PROBLEM: "What is happening in this situation?" "What decision do you have to make?"
  • My baby won't stop crying.
  • Something is wrong with my baby.

___ 2. GOAL: "What would you do? *Why?*"
  • Call the doctor because s/he can tell me what's wrong with the baby.
  • Change her diaper because she might be wet.

___ 3. WHO CAN HELP
  • Call the doctor.

___ 4. ALTERNATIVES: "You said you would _____. Is there anything else you might do?"
  • Call the doctor.
  • Change her diaper.
  • Give her a bottle.
  • Hold her.

___ 5. CONSEQUENCES: "What will happen if you do these things?"
  • The baby may stop crying.
  • I can find out what's wrong.

___ 6. DECISION/CHOOSING AN ALTERNATIVE: "What would your final decision be?"
  • Call the doctor.
  • Call the doctor if the other things don't work.

___ 7. EVALUATION OF DECISION: "Now I am going to tell you the end of this 'story.' It turns out the baby was sick and the doctor says he had a virus. Knowing this, do you think you made a good decision? Why?"   Yes, because the baby didn't get sicker.   No, because the baby could have gotten worse.

---

measure effective decision making (Tymchuk, Andron, & Rahbar, 1988; Tymchuk, Yokota, & Rahbar, 1990). This assessment was in turn used as a basis for a curriculum on effective decision making.

Assessment of the Child

Unlike assessment of parenting, there are many standardized instruments used with children, across various areas of assessment and for various purposes. As with tests of parenting, there are additional issues practitioners and researchers must consider in the selection of assessment methodology when testing children, including duration of the assessment and the qualifications and training required for administration. Some of the more widely used instruments to assess children's general development, such as the Bayley Scales (Bayley, 1969), the Denver II (Frankenburg et al., 1990), and the Wechsler Scales (Wechsler, 1989), require certain qualifications and extensive training and supervision of the assessor. In addition, each takes a long time to administer, ranging from 45 to 60 minutes, depending upon the child. Because these scales were designed to evaluate a child for categorization purposes, for examining the effects of programmatic intervention, or for predictive purposes, rather than for the design of specific education for the child, the time and expense for their use in child maltreatment may be questionable. Unlike many of the assessment devices for children mentioned earlier, the Developmental Profile (Alpern, Boll, & Shearer, 1986) can be used for all of the purposes of those devices as well as for the design of specific child-oriented interventions. It is composed of five subscales, each of which contains individual task-referenced items ranging from birth to age 12 years, 6 months.

Evaluation of the Home and Community Environment

Perhaps the most widely used standardized measure to assess the quality of the home environment is the HOME (Caldwell & Bradley, 1984). The HOME has three roughly equivalent forms (Infant and Toddler, Preschool, and Elementary) which make it useful as the child develops. There also is a Spanish language Infant and Toddler form. The advantages of the HOME are that it is useful over time and with different groups of families. It is also standardized with normative data across the three major socioeconomic groups, with a primary emphasis on impoverished households. The HOME is easily administered, but does require certain qualifications as well as training; it provides both a cumulative score and individual subscale scores. The HOME was originally designed as a dependent measure of the effectiveness of early intervention programs; therefore, it has certain limitations. Care must be used in adapting it directly as a measure of the quality of parenting or the efficacy of parent education, or in using it as a measure for prescriptive purposes either by the parent or by educators, including those addressing issues in child maltreatment.

Functional Assessments

In addition to the assessment devices described thus far, there are a number of valid instruments available that focus upon specific functional components of parenting. Each of these was developed for prescriptive purposes after careful task analysis and validation and each is useful in parenting in child maltreatment. All require training for implementation. Lutzker and his colleagues developed and used the Home Accident Prevention Inventory (HAPI) as a means of identifying home dangers with families in child maltreatment (Tertinger, et al., 1984). An accompanying manual provides instruction on how to successfully implement interventions after assessment with the HAPI. Tymchuk and colleagues (1990; 1992b) developed a series of instruments and curricula that have been revalidated for the Wellness Project. One assessment is the Home Danger and Safety Precaution Checklist; a sample is presented in Table 5. Other functional assessment devices were developed for each of the remaining components within the Wellness Project listed in Table 2. The illustration in Figure 1 is used along with a doll to assess a parent's awareness of parts of a child's body and where specific symptoms of illness can occur.

Table 5. One Portion of Home Danger and Safety Precaution (from the UCLA Parent/Child Health & Wellness Project and the SHARE/UCLA Center for Healthy Families)

Danger	Prevention/precaution	
I. FIRE		
☐ Matches/Lighter	☐ Removes items ☐ Locked drawer/cabinet	☐ Stored out of reach of child
☐ Candles/gas lanterns	☐ Removes items	☐ Uses flashlight
☐ Lighter fluids (e.g. gas)	☐ Removes items ☐ Stored out of reach of child	☐ Stored in own container ☐ Locked drawer/cabinet
☐ Missing fireplace screen	☐ Fireplace screen in place	
☐ Flammable items near heater/stove/oven	☐ Flammable materials stored in cabinets away from heater/stove/oven	
☐ Flamable children's clothing	☐ Buys fire resistant clothing for child	
☐ Oily rags	☐ Always disposes oily rags after use	
☐ Sawdust in a pile	☐ Removes items	☐ Uses sand/cat litter to absorb oil in garage
General Fire Danger	☐ Baking soda available ☐ Fire extinguisher present and knows how to operate ☐ Smoke detectors present and working outside each sleeping area/each floor	☐ Fire drill posted and practiced ☐ Sleeps with doors closed
☐ Other		

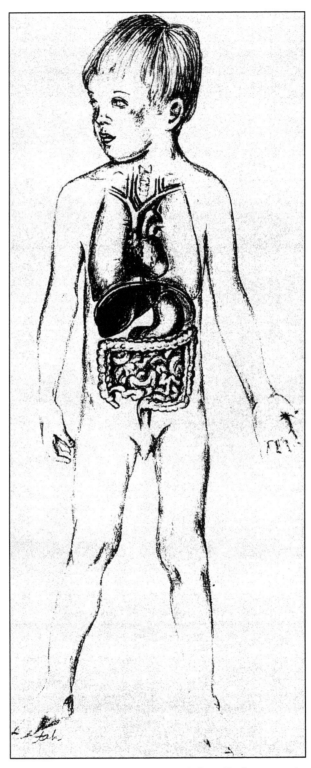

Figure 1. Illustration used in assessment of knowledge of body parts and symptom sites.

Parenting Curriculum and Material Development in Child Maltreatment: The Science of Curriculum and Material Development

Although the NRC report (1993) has recognized the great need for the systematic development of instrumentation in parenting, the even greater need for the systematic development of parenting curricula and materials was not addressed. At present, there are few parenting education curricula and materials that were designed to adhere to the necessary empirical criteria for standardization for any parents, but especially for parents with special leaning needs. Since curricula as well as accompanying materials for teaching purposes in any area of behavior must adhere to the same standardization criteria as does assessment, the development of curricula is time-consuming. However, such curricula must be developed in order to determine whether parents with the characteristics at issue can learn (e.g., Berger et al., 1994; Ornstein & Hunkins, 1993; Rosenblum, 1994; Wells et al., 1994). In child abuse and neglect it is unclear what curricula are used for teaching purposes. This serious deficiency may have occurred as a result of the interest in descriptive studies in the field; however, this lack of standardized curricula also may be a result of the absence of educators in the field and the focus of federal funding. In such other fields as special education, medical patient education, management, policing, and nursing, this need has been met (e.g., American Red Cross, 1989; Kinzie, Schorling, & Siegel, 1993; Tymchuk, Andron, Bavolek, et al., 1990).

As in the area of parenting assessment, service providers in the field of child abuse and neglect must obtain and learn how to apply curricula from related areas to the development of parenting skills.

Interventions for Functional Abilities

Understanding Alternative Learning Styles and Matching Interventions to Those Styles: There Is No Normal or Set Way in Which People Learn

Although it should be self-evident, sometimes we forget that there are many different ways in which people learn. It may seem that most, if not all, people learn all their information and skills on their own, by observing others, by reading books, in classes, or training program continually; this is false. Although it may seem that learning occurs in this manner, one has to look carefully at how much individuals have learned in these circumstances. We need to know what level of information or skills the individual has attained, and determine whether the levels are optimal for the stated purpose. Unfortunately, without more attention to individual learning style, these levels invariably are insufficient, whatever the content area. Some people learn better when they see information printed or clearly written; others do better when information is heard. Still others learn optimally when they see as well as hear information. Some learn when small chunks of information are set at their own pace, whereas others can learn more rapidly. Also, people learn different information and skills in varying ways and at different times in their lives. As people age or become ill, they will even learn new information and skills or maintain previously learned information and skills using strategies that are different from those used earlier in life. In addition, not everyone is capable of learning how to do everything. When a person learns optimally in a manner different from others, this does not devalue that person.

Influences on Learning

In order to examine how people learn, the following framework was adopted. Having a consistent framework that is empirically based allows for familiarization with, and continued use of, terms or phrases. This framework includes three phases:

1. The presentation or input phase refers to how people become prepared for new information and skills and how they obtain or are presented with information and skills.
2. The assimilation or learning phase refers to how people take the new information and assimilate it with their current knowledge or skill bases.
3. The use or output phase, which includes both immediate and delayed use. It includes how people make immediate use of new information and skills and how they maintain the knowledge/skill for use at a later time. Such use can occur in a testing or contrived situation in which the person, in this case the parent, is asked questions on a test, is asked to demonstrate how to do something, or is observed while in the home. A situation that is set up is termed an *in vitro* situation; a real-life situation is referred to as *in vivo*.

Parental Factors that Influence Each Phase of Learning

Each of these individual phases is influenced both by parental factors and by environmental factors. The following are parental factors that influence how well a parent does in each phase: (1) physical functioning (with or without any corrective devices that may be needed), such as vision, hearing, motility, and coordination; (2) previous experience and background, such as familiarity with the components of parenting and societal expectations (e.g., whether the parent ever had a model for parenting from whom to learn parenting and societal expectations, or familiarity with the circumstances of assessment or education being done); (3) current environment, including availability of social supports (e.g., whether learning is valued by those with whom the parent is currently involved; (4) personal values, interest, and motivation (do they want to be parents, do they want to learn, are they doing it all just for the love of parenting, or would they learn better if they received recognition for accomplishments, however small those accomplishments); (5) processing capacity (how much information can parents be given comfortably); (6) memory capacity (how much information can parents remember over the short or long term); (7) reading recognition and reading comprehension ability in English or in their primary language, speech recognition and speech comprehension in English or in their primary language.

Environmental Factors that Influence Each Phase of Parent Learning and Application

Structural environmental elements. For phase I, these can be divided into structural and process elements. Structural elements refer to the content of the education and include such elements as the order, structure and complexity of information, the method of presentation of the information (e.g., written or printed, size or loudness, with or without illustrations, read to or read by a parent), and the amount of information or number of items to be given at one time and whether these items are to be grouped by conceptual category.

Process environmental elements. This refers to where the education occurs (e.g., at home, in class, at a facility, at work); with whom—that is, individually or in a small or large group; time and date of education (e.g., in the morning, afternoon, early evening, or evening, and on which days); duration of each session and length and number of all sessions; whether the parent realistically can accomplish his or her educational responsibilities; and who provides the education and the qualifications and personality of that individual.

Importance of Identifying These Factors

Identifying either parental or environmental factors that influence learning and use is important because the service provider then can provide modifications in order to improve learning and use. Although it is not possible to change historical events that influenced the parent's current learning style, it is very feasible to change current environmental factors that do so. It is straightforward to make such changes, but service providers may be unfamiliar with various options or may consider such changes too time-consuming for the improvement that may result. As in any case presented for adjudication, the extent to which such modification in education does not occur but could benefit the parent and by extension the health, safety, and wellness of their child, must be considered. Table 6 identifies those factors that are related to adequacy of parenting and learning and those that are related to inadequacy of parenting and learning.

Which Factors Are Most Relevant?

There are certain factors that can be changed with minimal cost and time and that provide substantial benefit not only for the parent's learning and care for his or her child, but also for other children and for society over the long term. Table 7 contains a list of these factors.

Putting It All Together: Steps in Setting Up an Optimal Parent Learning Program

The optimal learning program for any parent will vary according to what is expected, that is, knowledge, skill, or both, and according to curriculum area. For some tasks, the parent may need to work one-on-one with the educator, whereas for others the parent may be able to work on his or her own, in small groups or with periodic feedback, recognition and correction. In addition, the success of any education will depend upon some of the factors listed in the previous section as well as on the issues related to the circumstances under which the parent comes to the program. Here, we will go through the steps in setting up, implementing, and evaluating the success of an educational program which we term the Specific

Table 6. Factors Known to Benefit or Hinder Parental/Maternal Care and Learning

Factors known to benefit the adequacy of childcare and to facilitate learning	Factors known to interfere with the adequacy of childcare and to inhibit learning
a. Maternal Historical Advantage Factors	a. Maternal Historical Risk Factors
i. Lived at home	i. Ever institutionalized
ii. Parental approval of marriage or partner/child	ii. Abused as child/incest
iii. Older than 18 when first child born	iii. Younger than 18 when first child born
iv. Parenting education	iv. No parenting education
v. Self healthcare education	v. No self healthcare education
vi. Own parents problem free	vi. Own problem parents (crime/drugs/emotional disturbance
vii. Completed high school	vii. Limited formal education
viii. Stable partner relationships	
b. Maternal Current State Advantage Factors	b. Maternal Current State Risk Factors
i. Healthy physically	i. IQ < 60
ii. Emotionally healthy	ii. Medical distorder
iii. Limited stress	iii. Emotional disorder (depression, mental illness)
iv. Adequate self-esteem	iv. High stress
v. Reading/speech comprehension > grade 5	v. Low self-esteem
vi. No or limited substance intake including alcohol (if so, is actively participating in substance abuse program	vi. Reading Comprehension < grade 4
vii. IQ > 60	vii. Untreated substance abuser
c. Maternal Current Process Advantage Factors	c. Maternal Current Process Risk Factors
i. Good planning	i. Poor coping style
ii. Good decision making	ii. Poor decision making
iii. Good coping style	iii. Punitive child interaction
iv. Nonpunitive child interaction with some positive interaction	iv. Authoritarian child interaction
v. Strict child interaction but not idiosyncratic	v. Unwilling to use supports
vi. Reinforces	vi. Perpetrates abuse
vii. Smiles/empathetic	vii. Rarely reinforces child
viii. Willing to learn/motivated	viii. Rarely smiles/nonempathetic
ix. Learns readily/generalizes	ix. Poor motivation to learn
x. Recognizes own needs	x. Learns slowly/unable to generalize
xi. Has done well in other programs	xi. Does not recognize own needs
xii. Has good adaptive skills	
d. Environmental Advantage Factors	d. Environmental Risk Factors
i. Supports in	i. No or limited supports
1. Healthcare	ii. Supports with prejudicial attitudes
2. Education	iii. Professionals untrained
3. Friend	iv. Any supports some distance away
4. Psychological	v. Multiple agencies with multiple contacts
5. Vocational	
6. Legal	
7. Financial aid	
ii. Available	
iii. Comprehensive	
iv. Frequent as needed	
v. Duration as needed	
vi. Long as needed	
vii. Supports with fair view of capabilities	
viii. Professionals trained	

Table 6. (*Continued*)

Factors known to benefit the adequacy of childcare and to facilitate learning	Factors known to interfere with the adequacy of childcare and to inhibit learning
ix. Supports/interventions match learning ability	
x. Parental agency contacts through single individual	
e. Family Advantage Factors	e. Family Risk Factors
i. Only one child	i. More than one child
ii. Younger child	ii. Older child
iii. Adequate income	iii. Income below poverty level for community
iv. Adequate/safe/stable housing	
v. Infrequent moves	
f. Husband/Partner Advantage Factors	f. Husband/Partner Risk Factors
i. Current partner supportive	i. Current partner abusive
ii. Current partner emotionally healthy	ii. Current partner emotionally disturbed
iii. Current partner involved in vocation	iii. Current partner in criminal activity
iv. Current partner involved in civics	iv. Current partner not in vocation (supported or nonsupported work)
v. Relatively stable relationship	
g. Child Advantage Factors	g. Child Risk Factors
i. IQ > 70	i. IQ < 70
ii. Adequate health	ii. Health problems
iii. Pleasant temperament	iii. Difficult temperament
iv. Few accidents	iv. Frequent accidents
v. Child < age 6	v. Child > age 6
vi. Adequate behavior	vi. Male?
	vii. Child with behavior problems

Parenting Plan (SPP). While the format of the SPP is not presented here because of space issues, the actual contents include the following:

1. Identification of factors that might influence the success of the SPP implementation, a determination of ways to increase the influence of those factors that might be facilitating, and to decrease the influence of those factors that are inhibiting or interfering (see Tables 6 and 7). Since motivation may be an issue in the success of the educational program (e.g., Danoff, Kemper & Sherry, 1994; Saylor, Elksnin, Farah, & Pope, 1990), the +PAS (Positive Parenting Attention System) has been devised in which those materials and processes that are most rewarding to the parent have been identified. Specific behaviors are targeted for acquisition and maintenance, including attendance, timeliness, and actual improvement in knowledge and skills. A schedule of contingencies is developed for providing the materials to the parent. The parent may be overwhelmed when asked or required to make their home safe, for example, and the probability of failure increases. To prevent this, actual materials may be provided for the parent: a home safety kit (e.g., a fire extinguisher, door-handle covers, electrical outlet covers) and a health kit (e.g., thermometer, Ipecac, Band-Aids). In the Wellness Project, these cost in total about $50 per family.
2. Determination of where the needs are within a parenting area (see Table 2), the priority level of each, the parent's current level of functioning in

Table 7. Potential Influences on Learning

I. Parental factors
   A. Physical functioning with or without any corrective devices that may be needed (vision, hearing, motility, coordination)
   B. Previous experience and background (familiarity with components of parenting and societal expectations; e.g., did parent ever have a model for parenting from whom to learn parenting and societal expectations? or familiarity with the circumstances of assessment or education being done)
   C. Current environment (e.g., is learning valued by those with whom the parent is currently involved? availability of social supports)
   D. Personal values, interest, and motivation (do they want to be parents? do they want to learn? are they doing it all just for the love of parenting or would they learn better if they received recognition for accomplishments, however small those accomplishments?)
   E. Processing capacity (how much information can they be given comfortably?)
   F. Memory capacity (how much information can they remember over the short or long term?)
   G. Reading recognition and reading comprehension ability in English or in their primary language if not English, speech recognition and speech comprehension in English or in their primary language if not English.
II. Environmental factors that influence each phase of parent learning and application
   A. Structural environmental elements
      1. Content aspects of the education—include such things as what is to be taught
      2. Order
      3. Structure
         a. Level of difficulty or complexity
         b. Written or printed
         c. Size/loudness
         d. Illustrations
         e. Conceptual groupings
         f. Number of items
   B. Process environmental elements
      1. Circumstances
         a. Place—refer to the circumstances in which education occurs (at home, in class)
         b. Individual, small or large group
         c. Attendance required/mandated
         d. Date, time of day, ease of access
         e. Number, length, duration of sessions
         f. Criteria for changing from one level to another
      2. Educator
         a. Experience, education
            i. Training in parenting by anyone including parenting by persons with special learning needs
            ii. Attitudes regarding individual differences in general but specifically in race/ethnicity, culture, abilities, appearance and parenting
            iii. Knowledge regarding poverty, culture, science of assessment, and know parenting assessments and interventions
            iv. Values such that belief that a certain type of family is best or type of parent is best or parenting style is best and if so, on what basis do you base that/those values?
         b. Other

---

that area, and the degree of support required to fulfill that need. Such assessment may be formal or informal.

   3. This specifies the curriculum that would be used in order to address the specific parenting needs and the steps in that curriculum at which the parent would begin. In Table 8 an example of the topics that are included

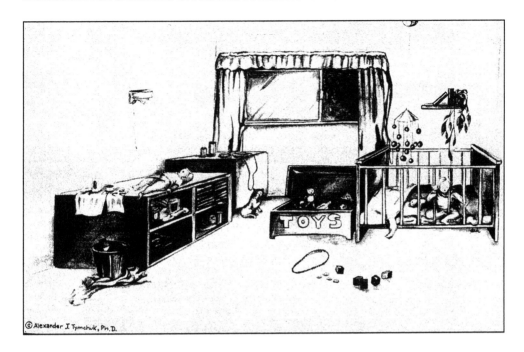

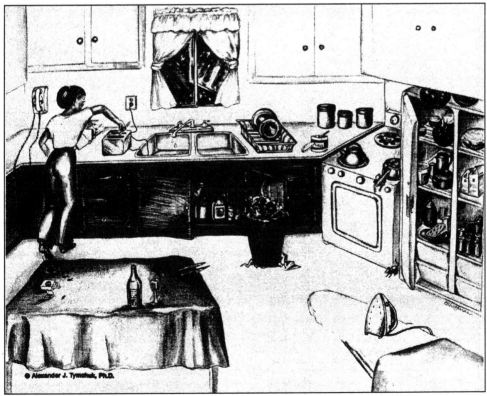

Figures 2 and 3. Illustrations used to help parent identify dangers in the home and implement precautions.

Table 8. Parent Education Topics and Sample Order of Presentation within the UCLA
Parent/Child Health & Wellness Project

Safety and Learning	Knowledge, Causes & Prevention of Life Threatening Emergencies
Health	Planning for Emergencies
Effective Planning	Partner Safety & Safer Sex
Understanding Health	Emergency vs. Common Problems
Support & Service Relations	Home/Apartment Safety
Parts of the Body & Common Problems	Knowing When to Call Dr. & What to Do
Effective Decision Making	Following the Doctor's Directions
Effective Coping	Phone Safety
Understanding Sickness & Health	Prescription Medications
Effective Self Observer	Stranger at the Door Safety
Knowing When You Are Ill	Going Out Safely–Before, While Out, & Returning Home
Handling Finances & Budgeting	Over-the-Counter Medications
Temperature	Infectious Diseases
Effective Child Observer	Outside the Home Safety
Knowing When Your Child Is Ill	On Vacation Safety
Meal Planning	ChildSafe
Pulse	Reporting a Crime
Personal & Child Grooming	Parent & Child Enjoying Each Other
Breathing	Reading & Singing
House Cleanliness	Anticipating Child Behavior
Common Health Problems & Diagnosis	

in the Wellness Project is presented. Each topic has a lesson plan with specific goals and objectives, along with ways to meet those goals and objectives individually or in small groups. Materials written in large print and illustrated are used in each, accompanied by booklets to be used by the parents.

4. Specifies the materials for teaching that would be used in conjunction with the curriculum. This might include such materials as illustrations and actual objects. Figure 2 contains an example of one out of the six illustrations, each in its own parent booklet, that are used to identify dangers and ways to implement precautions. Figure 3 contains another used for teaching purposes. Although these are shown in this text as black and white, color illustrations are used.

5. Determines which learning environment would be optimal for the parent, including who will provide the education.

6. Establishes the parent's motivation and his or her level of individual responsibility so that the consequences of the parent's actions are understood. This might entail a more formal consenting process and may include actual questions to determine the parent's understanding of what is expected and his or her agreement to what the education will entail.

7. Prepares the person for education by familiarizing him or her with the program while keeping in mind the goal of parental success as well as ensuring the safety of the child.

8. Starts easy and in small chunks for initial success.

9. Coaches and congratulates.

10. Continues to measure and provide constructive feedback. If difficulties occur, the learning situation is reexamined and the parent is asked for help in identifying the reasons that the difficulties may be occurring and in making appropriate modifications.
11. Moves to the next level in the curriculum or has the parent assume greater responsibility for self-learning, or both.

SUMMARY AND IMPLICATIONS FOR FUTURE DIRECTIONS

As presented in this chapter, major questions relate to the fact that many parents with any form of functional or categorical disability are reported to child protective services and cases are opened for them. Of concern are the educational needs of the parents and how they can best be addressed while fulfilling society's responsibilities to protect the child as well as the rights of the parent. Currently, there has not been a systematic response to these questions in the area of child maltreatment, but in the absence of such a response, strategies have been described here that may be beneficial to workers in the field.

ACKNOWLEDGMENTS
UCLA Parent/Child Health & Wellness, dedicated to the health and wellness of *all* parents and children, is supported by a grant from the California Wellness Foundation. Support for the earlier empirical work within the SHARE/UCLA Parenting Project was provided by a series of grants from SHARE, Inc. This support continues within the SHARE/UCLA Center for Family Health, Wellness & Safety, dedicated to healthy families. The author expresses his sincere gratitude for this support. All materials including printed materials, illustrations, and processes referred to are copyrighted by Alexander J. Tymchuk, Ph.D. and are included solely for demonstration purposes within this chapter. Some project illustrations were drawn by Teri Hoffman from materials and concepts provided by project staff. The author also wishes to thank staff who have contributed to the success of the Wellness Project including Karen Berney-Ficklin, Rebecca Spitz, Jill Spivak, Elana Evan, Deborah Kanegsberg, Cathy Lang, and Alice West, as well as Annette Groen for her critique of an earlier draft of this chapter, and Dr. John Lutzker for the invitation to contribute a chapter and his continued sharing of information and ready consultation. It is also important to recognize the contributions of the staffs of the agencies with which we are involved as well as the participating families.

REFERENCES

Alpern, G., Boll, T., & Shearer, M. (1986). *Developmental Profile II Manual.* Los Angeles: Western Psychological Services.
American Association on Mental Retardation. (1993). *Mental retardation definition, classification and systems of supports.* Washington, DC: Author.
Americans With Disabilities Act (*Federal Register,* 28 CFR Part 35, July 26, 1991).
American Red Cross. (1989). *Parenting for people with special learning needs.* Los Angeles: Author.
Anastasi, A. (1976). *Psychological testing.* New York: Macmillan.

Barnett, W. (1993). Economic evaluation of home visiting programs. *The Future of Children, 3*, 93–112.

Bayley, N. (1969). *Bayley Scales of Infant Development.* New York: Psychological Corporation.

Bellack, A., Hersen, M., & Kazdin, A. (1982). *International handbook of behavior modification and therapy.* New York: Plenum Press.

Berger, D., Inkelas, M., Myre, S., & Mishler, A. (1994). Developing health education materials for inner-city low literacy parents. *Public Health Reports, 109,* 168–172.

Blanch, A., Nicholson, J., & Purcell, J. (1994). Parents with severe mental illness and their children: The need for human services integration. *The Journal of Mental Health Administration, 21,* 388–396.

Bloom, M., & Fischer, J. (1982). *Evaluating practice: Guidelines for the accountable professional.* Englewood Cliffs, NJ: Prentice Hall.

Booth, C., Barnard, K., Mitchell, S., & Spieker, S. (1987). Successful intervention with multi-problem mothers: Effects on the mother–infant relationship. *Infant Mental Health Journal, 8,* 288–306.

Boyle, C., Decoufle, P., & Yeargin-Allsopp, M. (1994). Prevalence and health impact of developmental disabilities in U.S. children. *Pediatrics, 93,* 399–403.

Briere, J., Berliner, L., Bulkley, J., Jenny, C., & Reid, T. (Eds.). (1996). *The APSAC handbook on child maltreatment.* Thousand Oaks, CA: Sage.

Bryant, P., & Daro, D. (1994). *A comparison of the cost of child maltreatment to the cost of providing all new parents parent education and support.* Chicago: National Committee to Prevent Child Abuse.

Caldwell, B., & Bradley, R. (1984). *The Home Observation for Measurement of the Environment.* Little Rock: University of Arkansas.

Caldwell, R. (1992). *The costs of child abuse vs. child abuse prevention. Michigan's experience.* East Lansing: Michigan State University.

Chacon, D., Kissoon, N., & Rich, S. (1994). Education attainment level of caregivers versus readability level of written instructions in a pediatric emergency department. *Pediatric Emergency, 10,* 144–149.

Cohler, B., & Musick, J. (1984). *Intervention among psychiatrically-impaired parents and their children.* San Francisco: Jossey-Bass.

Coohey, C. (1995). Neglectful mothers, their mothers, and partners: The significance of mutual aid. *Child Abuse & Neglect, 19,* 885–895.

Cronbach, L. (1970). *Essentials of psychological testing.* New York: Harper & Row.

Danoff, N., Kemper, K., & Sherry, B. (1994). Risk factors for dropping out of a parenting education program. *Child Abuse & Neglect, 18,* 599–606.

Davis, T., Mayeaux, E., Fredrickson, D., Bocchini, J., Jackson, R., & Murphy, P. (1994). Reading ability of parents compared with reading level of pediatric patient education materials. *Pediatrics, 93,* 460–468.

Department of Health and Human Services. (1988). *Study of national incidence and prevalence of child abuse and neglect.* Washington, DC: Author.

Department of Health and Human Services. (1990). *Healthy people 2000 national health promotion and disease prevention objectives.* Washington, DC: Author.

Doak, C., Doak, L., & Root, J. (1996). *Teaching patients with low literacy skills.* Philadelphia: Lippincott.

Family Preservation Evaluation Project. (1995). *Instruments used to measure child and family functioning service utilization and client satisfaction in family preservation services.* Department of Child Study, Tufts University: Author.

Feldman, M. (1994). Parenting education for parents with intellectual disabilities: A review of outcome studies. *Research in Developmental Disabilities, 15,* 299–332.

Fink, A., & McCloskey, L. (1990). Moving child abuse and neglect prevention programs forward: Improving program evaluations. *Child Abuse & Neglect, 14,* 187–206.

Frankenburg, W., Dodds, J., Archer, P., Bresnick, B., Maschka, P., Edelman, N., & Shapiro, H. (1990). *Denver II.* Denver, CO: Denver Developmental Materials.

Gallagher, J., & Ramey, C. (Eds.) (1987). *The malleability of children.* Baltimore: Brookes.

Garber, H. (1988). *The Milwaukee Project: Preventing mental retardation in children at risk.* Washington, DC: American Association on Mental Retardation.

Gaudin, J. (1993). *Child neglect: A guide for intervention.* Washington, DC: National Center on Child Abuse and Neglect.

Glik, D., Greaves, P., Kronenfeld, J., & Jackson, K. (1993). Safety hazards in households with young children. *Journal of Pediatric Psychology, 18,* 115–131.

Gnagey, T., & Gnagey, P. (1982). *DST: Reading Diagnostic Screening Test.* East Aurora, NY: Slosson.

Hayman, R. (1990). Presumptions of justice: Law, politics and the mentally retarded parent. *Harvard Law Review, 103,* 1201–1271.

Helm, D., & Kozloff, M. (1986). Research on parent training: Shortcomings and remedies. *Journal of Autism and Developmental Disorders, 16*, 1–22.

Jastak, S., & Wilkinson, G. (1984). *Wide Range Achievement Test-Revised.* Wilmington, DE: Jastak Associates.

Judd, C., Smith, E., & Kidder, L. (1991). *Research methods in social relations.* San Francisco: Holt, Rinehart and Winston.

Kinzie, M., Schorling, J., & Siegel, M. (1993). Prenatal alcohol education for low-income women with interactive multimedia. *Patient Education and Counseling, 21*, 51–60.

Llewellyn G., McConnell, D., & Bye, R. (1995). *Parents with intellectual disability. Support and services required by parents with intellectual disability.* Sydney: University of Sydney.

Lubeck, R., & Chandler, L. (1990). Organizing the home caregiving environment for infants. *Education and Treatment of Children, 13*, 347–363.

Lutzker, J., & Campbell, R. (1994). *Ecobehavioral family interventions in developmental disabilities.* Pacific Grove, CA: Brooks Cole.

Lynn, M. (1989). Readability: A critical instrumentation consideration. *Journal of Pediatric Nursing, 4*, 295–297.

Martin, S., Ramey, C., & Ramey, S. (1990). The prevention of intellectual impairment in children of impoverished families: Findings of a randomized trial of educational day care. *American Journal of Public Health, 80*, 844–847.

Mercer, C., & Mercer, A. (1985). *Teaching students with learning problems.* Columbus, OH: Merrill.

Miller, W. (1944, April 10, 11, 12). State of neglect. Judged unfit before they try. Mentally retarded rarely allowed to raise their babies. *The Spokesman Review,* Spokane, WA, pp. H1, H4.

Nagler, M. (Ed.). (1993). *Perspectives on disability.* Palo Alto, CA: Health Markets Research.

National Center for Education Statistics. (1993). *Adult literacy in America.* Princeton, NJ: Educational Testing Service.

National Child Abuse and Neglect Data System (NCANDS). (1994, 1995). *Detailed case data component.* Gaithersburg, MD: Walter R. McDonald.

National Committee to Prevent Child Abuse (NCPCA). (1994). *Healthy Families America: Standardized measures to assess client outcomes.* Chicago: Author.

National Research Council (NRC). (1993). *Understanding child abuse and neglect.* Washington, DC: Author.

Nelson, D., Walsh, K., & Fleisher, G. (1992). Spectrum and frequency of pediatric illness presenting to a general community emergency department. *Pediatrics, 90*, 5–10.

Olds, D., Henderson, C., & Kitzman, H. (1994). Does prenatal and infancy nurse home visitation have enduring effects on qualities of parental caregiving and child health at 25 to 50 months of life? *Pediatrics, 93*, 89–98.

Ornstein, A., & Hunkins, F. (1993). *Curriculum foundations, principles, and theory.* Boston: Allyn and Bacon.

Peterson, L., Harbeck, C., & Moreno, A. (1993). Measures of children's injuries: Self-reported versus maternal-reported events with temporally proximal versus delayed reporting. *Journal of Pediatric Psychology, 18*, 133–147.

Quinton, D., Rutter, M., & Liddle, C. (1984). Institutional rearing, parenting difficulties and marital support. *Psychological Medicine, 14*, 107–124.

Rosenblum, R. (1994). Developing a pediatric patient-family education program. *Pediatric Nursing, 20*, 359–362.

Runyan, D. (1991). *LONGSCAN Consortium of longitudinal studies in child abuse and neglect.* Chapel Hill: University of North Carolina.

Sarvela, P., & McDermott, R. (1993). *Health education evaluation and measurement: A practitioner's perspective.* Madison, WI: William C. Brown.

Saunders, B. (1995). *Measurement in child abuse and neglect research grantees meeting status report.* Charleston, SC: National Crime Victims Research and Treatment Center.

Saylor, C., Elksnin, N., Farah, B., & Pope, J. (1990). Depends on who you ask: What maximizes participation of families in early intervention programs. *Journal of Pediatric Psychology, 15*, 557–569.

Seagull, E., & Scheurer, S. (1986). Neglected and abused children of mentally retarded parents. *Child Abuse & Neglect, 10*, 493–500.

Speltz, M., Gonzales, N., Sulzbacher, S., & Quan, L. (1990). Assessment of injury risk in young children: A preliminary study of the Injury Behavior Checklist. *Journal of Pediatric Psychology, 15*, 373–383.

Tertinger, D., Greene, B., & Lutzker, J. (1984). Home safety: Development and validation of one component of an eco-behavioral treatment program for abused and neglected children. *Journal of Applied Behavior Analysis, 17*, 159–174.

Trupin, E., Tarico, V., Low, B., Jemelka, R., & McClellan, J. (1993). Children on child protective service caseloads: Prevalence and nature of serious emotional disturbance. *Child Abuse & Neglect, 17*, 345–355.

Tymchuk, A. (1990a). Parents with mental retardation: A national strategy. *Journal of Disability Policy Studies, 1*, 43–55. Also, *Parents with mental retardation: A national strategy White Paper for the President's Committee on Mental Retardation.* Los Angeles: Department of Psychiatry, University of California.

Tymchuk, A. (1990b). What information is actually found on the labels of commonly-used childrens' over-the-counter drugs. *Children's Health, 19*, 174–177.

Tymchuk, A. (1992a). Predicting adequacy and inadequacy of parenting by persons with mental retardation. *Child Abuse & Neglect, 16*, 165–178.

Tymchuk, A. (1992b). Do mothers with or without mental retardation know what to report when they think their child is ill? *Children's Health Care, 21*, 53–57.

Tymchuk, A. (1996). *Parents with "functional or categorical" disabilities: Risk assessment case management and techniques for improving parenting skills. A training program for child protective workers.* Los Angeles. Center on Child Welfare, Department of Social Work, University of Southern California.

Tymchuk, A., & Andron, L. (1990). Mothers with mental retardation who do or do not abuse or neglect their children. *Child Abuse & Neglect, 14*, 313–323.

Tymchuk, A., & Andron, L. (1992). Project Parenting: Child interactional training with mothers who are mentally handicapped. *Mental Handicap Research, 5*, 4–32.

Tymchuk, A., Andron, L., Bavolek, S., Quattrociocchi, A., & Henderson, H. (1990). *Nurturing program for parents with special learning needs and their children.* Park City, UT: Family Development Resources.

Tymchuk, A., Andron, L., & Rahbar, B. (1988). Effective decision-making problem-solving training with mothers who have mental retardation. *American Journal on Mental Retardation, 92*, 510–516.

Tymchuk, A., Andron, L., & Tymchuk, M. (1990). Training mothers with mental handicaps to understand behavioural and developmental principles. *Mental Handicap Research, 3*, 51–59.

Tymchuk, A., & Feldman, M. (1991). Parents with mental retardation and their children: Review of research relevant to professional practice. *Canadian Psychology, 32*, 486–496.

Tymchuk, A., Hamada, D., Andron, L., & Anderson, S. (1990). Home safety training with mothers who are mentally retarded. *Education and Training in Mental Retardation*, June, 142–l49.

Tymchuk, A., Yokota, A., & Rahbar, B. (1990). Decision making abilities of mothers with mental retardation. *Research in Developmental Disabilities, 11*, 97–109.

Wagner, M. (1995). Outcomes for youths with serious emotional disturbance in secondary school and early adulthood. In R. Behrman (Ed.). *The Future of Children, vol. 5* (pp. 90–112). Los Altos: Center for the Future of Children.

Walker, E., & Emory, E. (1983). Infants at risk for psychopathology: Offspring of schizophrenic parents. *Child Development, 54*, 1269–1283.

Wechsler, D. (1989). *Wechsler Preschool and Primary Scale of Intelligence-Revised (WPPSI-R).* San Antonio: The Psychological Corporation.

Wells, J., Ruscavage, D., Parker, B., & McArthur, L. (1994). Literacy of women attending family planning clinics in Virginia and reading levels of brochures on HIV prevention. *Family Planning Perspectives, 26*, 113–115, 131.

West, M., Richardson, M., LeConte, J., Crimi, C., & Stuart, S. (1992). Identification of developmental disabilities and health problems among individuals under child protective services. *Mental Retardation. 30*, 221–225.

Whitman, B., & Accardo, P. (1990). *When a parent is mentally retarded.* Baltimore: Brookes.

Williams, G., & Cuvo, A. (1986). Training apartment upkeep skills to rehabilitation clients: A comparison of task analytic strategies. *Journal of Applied Behavior Analysis, 19*, 39–51.

Woodcock, R. (1987). *Woodcock Reading Mastery Tests–Revised.* Circle Pines,: AGS.

Zill, N., & Coiro, M. (1992). Assessing the condition of children. *Children and Youth Services Review, 14*, 119–135.

19

Enhancing Treatment Adherence, Social Validity, and Generalization of Parent-Training Interventions with Physically Abusive and Neglectful Families

LORI M. LUNDQUIST and DAVID J. HANSEN

The literature on the assessment and treatment of child abuse and neglect has been steadily growing in recent decades. A consistent theme in the literature is that maltreating families generally present with a variety of problems and multiple possible targets for intervention, including many parent and child issues. The treatment picture is also complicated by the diversity of parents, children, problems, personal resources (e.g., financial, social, intellectual), and motivation for change. Unfortunately, due to their challenging circumstances, maltreating families may be among the least likely to succeed with psychological intervention (Wolfe, Edwards, Manion, & Koverola, 1988).

Clinicians and researchers view child abuse and neglect as the result of complex maladaptive interactions or lack of basic caretaking behaviors that are influenced by parental skill or knowledge deficits and other stress factors (Azar & Wolfe, 1989; Hansen & MacMillan, 1990; Hansen & Warner, 1992; Wolfe, 1988). Provision

LORI M. LUNDQUIST and DAVID J. HANSEN • Department of Psychology, University of Nebraska, Lincoln, Nebraska 68588.

Handbook of Child Abuse Research and Treatment, edited by Lutzker. Plenum Press, New York, 1998.

of treatment to these families is complicated by a variety of issues. Problems include, but certainly are not limited to, restricted financial and social resources, marital problems, limited cognitive abilities, substance abuse problems, and multiple personal demands (e.g., variety of appointments with therapists, attorneys) (Lutzker & Newman, 1986; National Center on Child Abuse and Neglect, 1988). In addition, maltreating families are often referred for psychological services under duress or involuntarily (Hansen & Warner, 1994). This makes it difficult to elicit necessary and accurate information from the parents and to establish the credibility and rapport that will likely increase their motivation to modify their parenting style (Wolfe, 1988). Also, the assessment of an abusive act is limited by its relative low frequency, privacy, and illegality.

The potential consequences of abuse vary considerably in type and severity, including emotional, behavioral, social, developmental, and physical sequelae (cf. Ammerman, Cassisi, Hersen, & Van Hasselt, 1986; Azar & Wolfe, 1989; Conaway & Hansen, 1989; Hansen, Conaway, & Christopher, 1990; Malinosky-Rummell & Hansen, 1993). Given the impact of abuse on children, the complex and challenging treatment picture, and the likely recurrence of maltreatment, clinicians and researchers need to learn more about how to enhance treatment adherence, social validity, and generalization of interventions with maltreating families. If parents do not actively participate in treatment, if the effects are not at socially relevant or functional levels, or if the effects of intervention do not maintain over time or generalize across settings, then maltreatment and other dysfunction will continue.

This chapter examines issues regarding the concepts of treatment adherence, social validity, and generalization as related to parent training with maltreating parents. There is significant overlap among the three concepts. For example, the more socially valid the goals and procedures, the more likely the client will adhere to treatment. The more likely the client is to participate in treatment, the more likely the effects will generalize and maintain. Finally, the more the effects generalize and maintain, the more socially valid and functional the effects.

Systematic consideration of treatment adherence, social validity, and generalization is needed from the outset in planning research and treatment to facilitate the development of informative and effective interventions. The information provided in this chapter is drawn from research on parent training and from research on treating abusive and neglectful families, as well as literature on adherence, social validity, and generalization. Given the diversity of literature covered, it will be noted when particular studies or articles focused specifically on maltreating parents. Specific recommendations are made regarding how to enhance adherence, social validity, and generalization to achieve lasting and meaningful impact on parent-training efforts with maltreating families.

TREATMENT ADHERENCE

Treatment adherence has been defined as the "active, collaborative, voluntary involvement of a client in a mutually-acceptable course of behavior to produce a desired preventative or therapeutic result" (Meichenbaum & Turk, 1987, p. 20). Treatment adherence problems with maltreating families are believed to be more common than with nonmaltreating clients because maltreating parents are frequently mandated to attend therapy and may be reluctant participants (Hansen & Warner, 1994). At least three types of parent behaviors need to occur for parent training to be successful. Parents must (1) attend sessions regularly, (2) participate within sessions, and (3) complete out-of-session assignments (Doepke & Hansen, 1992; Hansen & Warner, 1994). Sutton and Dixon (1986) explained that treatment resistance can be evidenced in treatment at both micro and macro levels. Resistance at the micro level is evidenced by challenges, disagreements, disqualifications, and other negative verbal responses by clients to therapist suggestions. Resistance at the macro level is evidenced by clients not completing homework assignments, missing appointments, and dropping out of treatment.

Session attendance is notoriously poor with maltreating families, and dropout rates are high and range from 20% to 70% (e.g., Hansen & Warner, 1994; Smith & Rachman, 1984; Warner, Malinosky-Rummell, Ellis, & Hansen, 1990). Warner and associates (1990) found an overall attendance rate of 67% for maltreating cases, whereas nonmaltreating cases in the same clinic had a significantly higher attendance rate of 82%. Not surprisingly, for maltreating families rates of attendance for home sessions (72%) were significantly higher than rates for clinic sessions (62%). Smith and Rachman (1984) found that only 10 out of 27 families referred for nonaccidental injury to children completed the full psychological intervention. Eleven families withdrew prior to completing the initial assessment procedures and six withdrew before completing treatment.

Participation within sessions is the most complicated and least understood aspect of adherence (Doepke & Hansen, 1992). Within-session adherence responses include talking about relevant topics, following session goals and procedures, and practicing new skills within the session. Little is known about within-session participation during parent training because only a few studies have been conducted (e.g., Chamberlain, Patterson, Reid, Kavanagh, & Forgatch, 1984; Patterson & Chamberlain, 1994; Patterson & Forgatch, 1985).

In a study of the relationship of therapist behavior and client noncompliance, Patterson and Forgatch (1985) found that therapist efforts to either teach or confront parents during therapy sessions increased the probability of parental resistance. The results also showed that if the therapist adopted a nondirective stance and did not teach, the level of resistance was dramatically reduced relative to resistance obtained with a more directive parent training approach. Thus, while "teach" and "confront" were associated with significant increases in the likelihood of client noncompliance, "facilitate" and "support" were followed by reliable decreases in client noncompliance. As Patterson and Forgatch note, the increased likelihood of the occurrence of noncompliance subsequent to teaching behaviors is somewhat of a paradox for many behavior therapists who regularly use teaching and skills training interventions.

Patterson and Chamberlain (1994) reviewed studies of parental resistance during parent training. They reported that analyses of sequential interactions during treatment found that therapists' efforts to intervene produced immediate parental resistance. Therapist efforts to intervene increased from baseline to mid-treatment phases, and this was accompanied by increases in parental resistance. Contextual variables, such as parent pathology, correlated with higher levels of resistance. Decreases in resistance were associated with improvements in parental discipline practices. Furthermore, parental resistance altered the behavior of the therapists (e.g., confronting, reframing), reducing their effectiveness.

Another parental behavior needed for parent training to succeed is completion of assignments outside of therapy sessions. Adherence to homework assignments encompasses a wide variety of responses (e.g., self-monitoring, completing questionnaires, implementing newly learned skills). A survey of 105 professionals reporting on a total of 303 maltreating clients, randomly selected from their caseloads, indicated that approximately 64% of homework assignments were completed (Hansen & Warner, 1994). Newman (1994) noted that this type of resistance "is especially troublesome in that many opportunities for therapeutic learning and practice in the natural environment are lost when clients neglect to engage in their assignments" (p. 51). The success of any parent training program depends on treatment adherence. When clients fail to follow treatment prescriptions, neither clinical experience nor historical efficacy of the treatment procedure will be sufficient to produce a successful outcome (Doepke & Hansen, 1992).

Consideration of Contextual Factors

There are many reasons for noncompliance, and there is not a simple linear relationship between attendance at parent training sessions and treatment outcome. This relationship is moderated by setting events and contextual factors (cf. Dumas & Albin, 1986). Dunst, Leet, and Trivette (1988), suggesting that "a family's failure to adhere to a professionally prescribed regimen may not be because its members are resistant, uncooperative, or noncompliant, but because the family's circumstances steer behavior in other, more pressing, directions" (p. 110).

Dumas and Albin (1986) stated that despite the well-documented successes of the parent training approach, available evidence indicates that "high-risk" families characterized by adverse social and material conditions (e.g., maltreating families) are unlikely to benefit from treatment, even when they do not drop out of treatment before its completion. Such stress factors or setting events include marital discord, social isolation, low parental education, low socioeconomic status, and so forth. A variety of specific problems can arise, such as transportation problems, illness, forgetting, lack of access to a phone to cancel or reschedule appointments, and parent or family concerns about obtaining mental health services.

Research suggests that there are factors that influence the likelihood of treatment adherence, as well as satisfactory completion of therapy. Johnson (1988) found that parents who failed to complete treatment were more likely to have had prior complaints for abuse, have been previously treated, lived alone or with a parent, and were less likely to have volunteered for a parent–toddler interaction group. Dumas and Albin (1986) examined the relationship between setting events (e.g., mother's psychopathology, father's presence), parental involvement (i.e., attendance at scheduled meetings and compliance with program instructions), and parent training outcome. Results indicated that the two measures of parental involvement were significantly related to one another, and attendance at scheduled meetings was related to the father's presence. Compliance with program instructions was negatively correlated with previous services and positively correlated with the father's presence and with income.

In their review of the literature, Patterson and Chamberlain (1994) found that families with older children were significantly more likely to drop out of treatment, and that social disadvantage was significantly related to negative outcomes in parent training (e.g., early dropout, poor outcome at treatment termination). Parental traits such as being depressed or having an antisocial history were related to in-session resistance at all phases of treatment. The socially disadvantaged, depressed, stressed, and antisocial parent was most at risk for disrupted discipline and monitoring practices.

Wolfe et al. (1988) found that when clinicians provided behavioral parent training for young parents and children who had been identified as being at risk of child maltreatment, the parents with very young children (less than 15 months old) often were less committed than parents of toddlers and preschoolers. The researchers suggested this was because there were fewer problems shown during this preambulatory stage of child development. Wolfe, Aragona, Kaufman, and Sandler (1980) found that the most salient indicators of successful outcome were the age of the child (78% were between the ages of 2.5 and 5 years old) and the court status of the family (74% of the successes were court-ordered).

There have been conflicting findings in the literature regarding the effects of court orders on treatment with maltreating families (Hansen & Warner, 1994). As noted previously, Wolfe et al. (1980) found that court orders appeared to be positively related to treatment success. In contrast, Irueste-Montes and Montes (1988) found that families in voluntary and court-ordered treatment participated at comparable levels in a comprehensive child abuse and neglect treatment program. They reported that court-ordered families appeared to benefit particularly when the court specified the nature of the therapy they were to receive, by whom, how frequently, and for what period. They also noted that it was helpful when the therapeutic program articulated expected behavior changes and termination conditions. Warner and colleagues (1990) found that court involvement was positively related to session attendance in the clinic, but not to sessions in the home. This suggests that the extra effort needed to attend sessions outside of the home may be facilitated by the presence of a court order.

Assessment Issues

Adherence responses are likely to be under the control of multiple contingencies operating simultaneously. In light of such contextual considerations, Dunst and colleagues (1988) presented the following recommendations for assessment and treatment: (1) assess family needs as a basis for determining the probability of parents having time and energy to carry out child-level interventions; (2) if certain family needs are found to be unmet, efforts must be made to provide or mediate the types of support that ensure that a family has adequate resources; and (3) adopt a proactive as opposed to a deficit perspective of parents who do not adhere to professionally prescribed regimens.

Newman (1994) suggested that when therapists are frustrated by resistant attitudes and behaviors, they need to curb their exasperation and tendency to arrive at general, but perhaps ill-informed, attributions for the client's behaviors. He also stated that therapists must take an idiographic approach to the assessment of each client's resistance and must examine the unique etiologic and maintaining factors for each client. Each family requires a uniquely tailored assessment and treatment strategy that is sensitive to the family's particular concerns. A functional analysis of the conditions that elicit, maintain, and prevent adherence responses is essential.

Newman suggested that therapists consider the following assessment questions: (1) "What is the function of the client's resistant behaviors?"; (2) "How does the client's current resistance fit into his or her developmental/historical pattern of resistance?"; (3) "What might be some of the client's idiosyncratic beliefs that are feeding into his or her resistance?"; (4) "What might the client fear will happen if he or she complies?"; (5) "How might the client be characteristically misunderstanding or misinterpreting the therapist's suggestions, methods, and intentions?"; (6) "What skills does the client lack that might make it practically difficult or impossible at this point for him or her to actively collaborate with treatment?"; (7) "What factors in the client's natural environment may be punishing the client's attempts to change?"; (8) "Does my conceptualization of this case need to be revised or amended?"; and (9) "What do I still need to understand about this client in order to make sense of his or her resistance?" (pp. 51–55). These questions were written from the perspective of working with an individual client, but one could easily apply them to families.

Antecedent and Consequent Strategies

In addition to a specific functional analysis of each client's adherence, there are general antecedent and consequent strategies that may facilitate treatment adherence (Hansen & Warner, 1992, 1994). The following strategies have some support in the parent training and related research literature, but the research conducted thus far has largely included middle-income clients (Azar & Wolfe, 1989). The effectiveness of compliance enhancement procedures has not yet been fully evaluated with maltreating families. Although some strategies may be appropriate for all types of adherence (e.g., attendance, within-session participation, homework), some may have more specific or limited use. Use of strategies to enhance adherence should begin in the early phases of contact, before any problems are readily apparent.

There are a variety of antecedent strategies that may facilitate adherence. For example, Dush and Stacy (1987) investigated the impact of pretreatment assessments on low socioeconomic status families involved in a prevention program for improving parenting skills. Subjects not pretested demonstrated three times the attrition rate relative to the pretested subjects. Thus, pretesting may be a useful strategy for promoting treatment adherence, possibly because the pretesting provides additional information about what to expect and/or the families may have felt as if they were more a part of the treatment program if they received pretesting.

Cox, Tisdelle, and Culbert (1988) compared the effects of verbal versus written behavioral prescriptions on recall of self-reported adherence to therapeutic homework assignments. Results with 30 adult clients indicated that written prescriptions led to significantly better recall of, and adherence to, homework assignments. Researchers concluded that writing the instructions may have decreased the ambiguity and complexity of the verbal information by structuring assignments into discrete tasks. Furthermore, tasks were easier and more salient to follow, and such structure may have enhanced the congruity of expectations between the therapist and clients. Written prescriptions may also have increased the perceived importance of homework assignments. Finally, written prescriptions can serve as a prompt in the natural environment.

Newman (1994) stated that a method for addressing client resistance is for the therapist to inquire about the client's thoughts that precede or accompany their negative reactions to the therapists' suggestions. For example, the therapist may state, "You rolled your eyes as I was explaining my point of view just now. I'm wondering what went through your mind?" (p. 53).

Adherence can be enhanced when therapists tell families what to expect. For example, Hobbs, Walle, and Hammersly (1990) specifically suggested that therapists tell parents to expect an initial increase in children's acting out when time-out is introduced, and that therapists should train parents to respond to the anticipated behaviors. Precautionary efforts of this type may enhance treatment acceptability and may increase compliance with therapeutic procedures in other environments.

There are several additional antecedent strategies which may be helpful in facilitating adherence (Doepke & Hansen, 1992; Shelton & Levy, 1981): having an empathic and skilled therapist; involving the client in goal and procedure selection; obtaining a private or public commitment from clients; providing additional stimuli such as reminder cards; beginning with small homework requests and gradually increasing assignments; ensuring that assignments contain specific details relevant to the desired behavior; and providing specific training for tasks to be implemented.

Along with antecedent strategies, there are several consequent strategies which may facilitate adherence. Watson-Perczel, Lutzker, Greene, and McGimpsey (1988) used behavioral techniques including feedback, shaping, and positive reinforcement as effective strategies for improving home conditions of families adjudicated for child neglect. A study by Hansen and Warner (1994) indicated that mental health service providers reported that praise and tangible rewards were the most effective techniques for facilitating attendance with maltreating families, while in-session practice was reported to be the most effective technique for enhancing homework completion. Hansen and Warner also found that attendance policies (e.g., termination after a criterion number of sessions are missed by the client) were reported to be used in a small percentage of cases, but they questioned the ethics and utility of such practices.

Wolfe et al. (1988) used financial incentives to facilitate adherence for 30 parent training participants who had been identified as being at risk for child maltreatment. Parents received $10 for completing the initial screening procedures and an additional $10 for each of the posttreatment and follow-up sessions.

Therapists use shaping to promote parent compliance and understanding (Lutzker, 1994). For example, if it is too burdensome for a mother to collect a week's worth of data (e.g., frequency of scolding), the therapist might ask the mother to collect data only for part of a particular day. If the mother complies, the therapist praises her and asks her to collect two days' worth of data, and so on. Another strategy for addressing parental noncompliance can be to hold out preferred training activities (e.g., toileting) until the parent performs less preferred activities (e.g., positive play) (Lutzker, 1994). Providing direct attention to nonadherence responses (e.g., having open discussions, eliciting disagreements, and presenting alternative viewpoints) may also be valuable (Doepke & Hansen, 1992).

Several approaches use both antecedent and consequent strategies, such as working with referral sources (e.g., schools, court, child protective services), advocating for the client (e.g., providing support for interactions with child protective service agencies), using procedures that are acceptable to the client and to significant others, using cognitive rehearsal strategies (e.g., self-management and self-reinforcement), and anticipating and reducing the negative effects of compliance. If the client's environment undermines compliance, the therapist should frequently reinforce compliance, assist the client with integrating self-reinforcement, provide cuing when possible, and closely monitor compliance with as many sources as possible.

In an excellent review on understanding client resistance, Newman (1994) suggested that therapists should do the following to facilitate treatment adherence: (1) assess for client skill deficits that may interfere with adherence, (2) provide the client with choices and an "active say," (3) collaborate and compromise, (4) thoroughly explain homework assignments, (5) review pros and cons of continuing with the status quo and of changing, (6) discuss the conceptualization of the case with the client, (7) speak the client's "language," and (8) be persistent when a client is "stuck." Also, adherence can be increased when specific efforts are made to solicit ongoing feedback from clients about the acceptability of goals, procedures, and effects.

In Project 12-Ways, a well-known ecobehavioral approach, many setting and contextual variables are addressed and treated (e.g., Lutzker, 1984; Lutzker, Wesch, & Rice, 1984; Wesch & Lutzker, 1991). In addition to parent training, parents receive other services that appear to be related to their particular difficulties (e.g., marital counseling, basic skills training). The success of Project 12-Ways suggests that clients demonstrated relatively high levels of compliance with treatment regimens. Several factors may facilitate treatment adherence, including individual attention paid to families, in-home intervention, benefits such as transportation to other service agencies, and casual dress of service providers (i.e., may reduce the distinction between service providers and clients). Furthermore, adherence is facilitated when service providers represent themselves to clients as people who might help families become more independent and less involved with state agencies (i.e., compliance may facilitate termination of protective services' involvement).

Proactive problem solving for potential obstacles to adherence can be valuable to increase the likelihood of adherence. In addition, providing stress-management training to address excessive arousal that may interfere with adherence is also useful (Doepke & Hansen, 1992). Helping the family reframe their problems (i.e., maltreatment) in terms of day-to-day difficulties that the parent can identify with (e.g., child noncompliance, difficulty dealing with stress) can be useful (Azar & Wolfe, 1989). This explanation may be more easily accepted by parents and may reduce their fears of being evaluated and labeled as "bad" parents.

A situation that can affect the therapeutic relationship and subsequent adherence is one in which a therapist encounters recurrences of abuse (Hansen & Warner, 1992). If therapists have any doubts that newly discovered or potential abuse should be reported, they should first inquire unofficially with protective services to ascertain if the report should be submitted (Hansen & Warner, 1992; MacKinnon & James, 1992). This inquiry can help maintain good rapport between the family and clinician by avoiding unnecessary reporting. Furthermore, therapists should take a number of steps to lessen the parent's sense of betrayal and to facilitate the parent's cooperation. Thus, they can provide support and choices before actually reporting (e.g., the parent chooses whether the therapist or the parent makes the notification), and they can prepare the parent for the investigation procedure. Some argue that not informing parents of suspicion or intent to report is deceptive and may be unethical (Racusin & Felsman, 1986).

SOCIAL VALIDITY

Social validity, according to Schwartz and Baer (1991), refers to the acceptability and viability of an intervention both to individuals and to groups (e.g., subcultures). Kazdin (1977) described three general social validity targets: goals, procedures, and outcomes.

In order to facilitate the social validity of interventions, therapists need to consider whether the treatment goals are what the family and/or society wants and whether achieving the goals would actually improve the adjustment and effectiveness of the individual. Most interventions have consisted of teaching behaviors to clients that therapists assumed were important, to levels that therapists assumed were appropriate. As mentioned previously, therapists must consistently consider contextual factors (e.g., financial difficulties) which may take precedence as priorities for clients. The goals of the therapist (e.g., increasing the frequency of positive family interactions) may not match those of the family (e.g., because of different priorities for the family). When the goals of the therapist do not seem socially valid in the view of the family, the likelihood of treatment adherence will be decreased. Considering specific family goals can enhance social validity because family members are much more likely to be satisfied with the results of therapy when treatment is targeted toward areas of their lives they deem important.

Therapists also need to assess whether the maltreating parents and family members consider the assessment and treatment procedures acceptable (Hansen & MacMillan, 1990). According to Kelley, Grace, and Elliott (1990) "poor long-term treatment outcome may be due to abusive parents' lack of acceptance of the child management techniques offered to them. Although the skills may be effective, if parents view the techniques as unacceptable (e.g., unreasonable or unfair), they may not be used consistently and appropriately" (p. 220). From a pragmatic perspective, offering clients an acceptable treatment may increase the likelihood that the intervention will be used correctly (Kazdin, 1980). Frentz and Kelley (1986) demonstrated that parents evaluated taking away privileges when children misbehave as a highly acceptable intervention. Time-out, time-out with spanking, and spanking were significantly less acceptable to parents than taking away privileges. In a similar study, Heffer and Kelley (1987) found that parents generally favored positive reinforcement (e.g., attention and praise) and response cost (e.g., loss of a privilege) over other treatments. Low- and middle- to upper-income parents, however, differed in their acceptance of several child management methods. For example, low-income parents viewed spanking as more acceptable than did middle-income mothers. Thus, therapists must be sensitive to the fact that commonly used parenting techniques may differ in acceptability among parents.

Finally, therapists need to consider whether clients and relevant others are satisfied with all the effects of treatment (e.g., Hansen, Warner-Rogers, & Hecht, Chapter 6, this volume; MacMillan, Olson, & Hansen, 1991). Essentially, evaluation is needed regarding whether behavior changes of individual, clinical, social, or applied importance have been achieved. An important question to address is whether treatment benefits clients to functional (i.e., useful) levels.

Social Validity Assessment

Strategies to enhance social validity are dependent on assessing social validity targets, including goals, methods, and outcomes. Hansen, Watson-Perczel, and Christopher (1989) suggested that investigations sensitive to social validity should include (1) selection of socially valid behaviors, (2) documentation of the need for and criterion levels for training, (3) demonstration of socially valid improvements in performance, and (4) evaluation of the acceptability of treatment goals, procedures, and effects by the clients and others.

The typical ways to assess social validity are either via an idiographic or a nomothetic approach. With the nomothetic approach, researchers and therapists compare client performance with some social standard to evaluate outcome effectiveness (e.g., scores on a normed measure such as the Child Behavior Checklist; Achenbach, 1991). Comparing parents' ratings of children's behavior to national norms can help generate realistic expectations and therefore facilitate social validity. With an idiographic approach, professionals consider whether clients' rates of target behaviors showed significant (e.g., functional) improvements following intervention. They also consider how individual clients rate a variety of factors related to the intervention (e.g., satisfaction with goals, procedures, and effects). In general, when addressing social validity, therapists must consider nomothetic and idiographic approaches and contextual factors in order to maximally facilitate appropriate and effective interventions.

Although it is difficult to imagine a broad-based definition or standard for adequate child care, we may draw some ideas from the literature regarding approaches to assessing child care. Such investigators as Feldman, Case, and Sparks (1992) have developed task analyses and then obtained criterion or "normative" data from parents for many child-care skills (e.g., cleaning baby bottles, toilet training) in which maltreating parents may be lacking. For example, the checklist for bathing includes 24 steps (e.g., gathering necessary supplies, checking water temperature). There are many advantages to such an approach, including the important fact that the parent's performance on the task analytic assessment provides information relevant to goals, methods, and outcomes compared to their own and to others' performances.

Watson-Perczel et al. (1988) surveyed caseworkers to help discern standards for adequate child care and subsequently developed a reliable and valid home observational code called the CLEAN (Checklist for Living Environments to Assess Neglect). The CLEAN provides specific and detailed information regarding goals (e.g., specific target problems). In addition to examining pre/post improvements on the CLEAN, scores have been compared with families who maintain a sufficiently clean home (e.g., a social validation sample of families identified by caseworkers as maintaining acceptably clean homes).

Therapists can utilize interview methods or questionnaires with clients and/or significant others (e.g., spouses, peers, caseworkers) to examine social validity. Examples include asking clients to (1) rate the degree to which problems in assessments and interventions represent home problems, (2) estimate how effective strategies will likely be at home, (3) rate their confidence in their abilities, and (4) indicate whether they would recommend the program to friends or relatives (MacMillan et al., 1991). Therapists can also obtain client predictions of specified functions of behaviors (e.g., desirable and undesirable effects), and they can obtain client judgments of methods such as "acceptable" and "unacceptable." In addition, it is important for therapists to solicit feedback posttreatment (e.g., "To what degree have expectations/therapy goals been met?"). Schwartz and Baer (1991) suggested additional techniques relevant for assessing and facilitating social validity, including the following: (1) allowing the client to choose from one or more interventions, (2) having significant others evaluate target behaviors prior to and following intervention, and (3) evaluating behaviors which are correlated with reported acceptability of intervention (e.g., regular attendance, assignment completion).

Treatment Issues and Examples

A factor that complicates assessment and social validity is that parent training efforts are often too simplistic to address the complexities of parenting, especially for maltreating families. Most research interventions focus on a discrete set of target behaviors which may or may not significantly impact daily functioning with these multichallenged families. An exception to this narrow focus is the ecobehavioral approach, as exemplified by Project 12-Ways (cf. Lutzker, 1984; Lutzker, Wesch, et al., 1984; Wesch & Lutzker, 1991), which was mentioned previously in regard to treatment adherence. Within the ecobehavioral approach, many "setting event" variables are addressed and treated, thereby facilitating client acceptance of treatment goals and methods, which ultimately leads to treatment success.

Although evaluation of social validity should be a vital component to any intervention study, few research projects and clinical interventions consistently assess for social validity (e.g., acceptability of treatment goals). The few studies that have assessed for social validity have typically assessed it postintervention. Some studies have employed subjective evaluation of treatment procedures and effects by having either participants or significant others report on the acceptability and/or effectiveness of the intervention (e.g., Barone, Greene, & Lutzker, 1986; Dachman, Halasz, Bickett, & Lutzker, 1984; Rosenfield-Schlichter, Sarber, Bueno, Greene, & Lutzker, 1983; Tertinger, Greene, & Lutzker, 1984).

Three months after a parent training intervention, Wolfe et al. (1988) had mothers complete a modified version of the Parent's Consumer Satisfaction Questionnaire (Forehand & McMahon, 1981). Of the total comments received, 85% indicated that the parent training groups were enjoyable and had helped the subjects to be better parents, not feel alone in their situations, and acquire information on child care. In addition, the participants rated their treatment satisfaction on a 7-point Likert-type scale. Furthermore, at one year postintervention, researchers solicited feedback from relevant others (i.e., caseworkers) regarding families' progress (e.g., rated how well clients were managing the children and the degree to which children were at maltreatment risk).

MacMillan et al. (1991) examined the utility of a parent training program which included facilitating generalization of skills to high-demand child management situations and employing structured analogue assessments of parent discipline performance in high-demand situations. Postintervention, researchers assessed social validity by soliciting parental responses to the intervention, asking them to rate the following kinds of items: effectiveness in managing the problem scenarios, the degree to which practice would improve their ability to manage home problems, how skillfully they handled similar problem situations prior to treatment, level of stress experienced during assessments, level of anger experienced during assessments, and so forth.

Barone et al. (1986) conducted home interventions with three families being treated for child abuse and neglect. A multiple-baseline design across safety hazards within families and across each family was used to evaluate the effects of the treatment program. When the intervention was completed, participants were given a consumer evaluation questionnaire designed to further assess the usefulness of the safety program. It consisted of 11 questions that required each parent to provide feedback regarding satisfaction with the program, its utility, and so on.

Dachman et al. (1984) found that significant others provided positive reports of intervention effects. The researchers examined the effects of a home-based ecobehavioral parent training package with a low-income single parent referred for child neglect of her 7-year-old son. Subsequent to the end of the intervention, the social significance of the treatment goals, strategies, and outcomes was assessed using a modified form of the Parents' Consumer Satisfaction Questionnaire (Forehand & McMahon, 1981) and a scale evaluating perceptions of change. For example, researchers asked the respondents to rate the mother's ability to handle parenting concerns. One of the mother's close friends and three protective service workers acquainted with the case completed the form. In general, the results indicated respondents were enthusiastic about treatment effects.

Social validation was evidenced in several studies that compared pre- and posttreatment performance of target mothers with the performance of a comparison group of mothers (e.g., Feldman, Case, Rincover, Towns, & Betel, 1989; Feldman et al., 1992; Lutzker, Megson, Webb, & Dachman, 1985). Feldman and colleagues (1992) intervened with 11 mothers with mental retardation to improve child-care skills crucial for children under 2 years old (e.g., diapering, bathing). Posttest scores did not differ significantly from those of a group of middle-class mothers, providing social validation of mothers' improvements in caring for their infants. Furthermore, after the termination of training, researchers interviewed several of the mothers and solicited their opinions regarding participation in the program. All of the mothers reported that what they learned was good for their child, that they were better parents because of having been in the program, that they liked the treatment program, and that they would recommend this program to others.

GENERALIZATION

Generalization was traditionally viewed as a passive phenomenon until Stokes and Baer (1977) published a classic paper that emphasized the need for actively programming for generalization of treatment effects. In a subsequent paper, Stokes and Osnes (1989) defined generalization as "the outcome of behavior change and therapy programs, resulting in effects extraneous to the original targeted changes" (p. 338). Although there are some conceptual disagreements about the use of the term (Edelstein, 1989), generalization is sometimes discussed as three distinct types: stimulus, response, and temporal generalization. Stimulus generalization refers to demonstration of behavior gains in settings other than the therapy setting, or with people other than the therapist. Response generalization refers to changes in behaviors that have not been targets of intervention, and temporal generalization refers to maintenance of treatment effects over time and post-treatment.

Although knowledge of recidivism rates of abuse or neglect following treatment is limited, the available evidence suggests that recurrence of maltreatment is a problem for many parents (Kolko, 1996; Oates & Bross, 1995), and that programming for generalization and maintenance of treatment effects is essential. If effects of intervention do not maintain over time, or if they do not generalize across settings or behaviors, maltreatment and other dysfunction will continue to occur.

Stokes and Osnes (1989) stated "generalization should not be automatically expected unless there are specific procedures implemented in order to facilitate its occurrence" (p. 351). Categories of programming strategies suggested by Stokes and Osnes included the following: (1) exploit current functional contingencies, (2) train diversely, and (3) incorporate functional mediators. There are several subcategories subsumed within these three general categories. We believe a fourth type of strategy is to target contextual factors.

The literature certainly provides guidance on enhancing generalization in clinical populations (e.g., Stokes & Baer, 1977; Stokes & Osnes, 1989), but not specifically with maltreating families. A number of generalization and maintenance strategies have been mentioned in the parent training literature; however, not all authors have designated their research procedures as generalization strategies per se. We will note some strategies that we and others have employed, although their utility and effectiveness have yet to be fully evaluated.

Exploit Current Functional Contingencies

Functional contingencies refer to the arrangement of antecedents, behaviors, and consequences that affect frequency, magnitude, and duration of relevant behavior (Stokes & Osnes, 1989). Strategies for exploiting current functional contingencies include the following: contacting and recruiting natural consequences, modifying maladaptive consequences, and reinforcing occurrences of generalization (Stokes & Osnes, 1989).

Contacting natural consequences is helpful because "[g]eneralization programming seems to be well served by providing the least artificial, least cumbersome, and most natural positive consequences in programming interventions. Such programming most closely matches naturally occurring consequences and their entrapment potential" (Stokes & Osnes, 1989, p. 341). Thus, it is important that therapists identify and teach behaviors that are likely to come into contact with powerful reinforcing consequences that do not need to be programmed by a therapist. For example, therapists can prompt parents to identify existing maltreatment consequences that are unpleasant (e.g., increased parental frustration, CPS involvement) and positive consequences of providing nonpunitive discipline (e.g., improved child behavior, better parent–child relationship).

Another strategy is recruiting natural consequences. For example, parents can expect an increased child compliance rate (eventually) when behavior management is appropriately and consistently implemented. Therapists can have parents systematically self-monitor and record how they feel when appropriately provided discipline is effective. Also, therapists can draw upon family members (e.g., older children) to provide assistance and reinforcement when the targeted parent demonstrates anger control and appropriate behavior management strategies (e.g., Doepke, Watson-Perczel, & Hansen, 1988). Rosenfield-Schlichter and colleagues (1983) provided services for a mother referred because of neglect by recruiting the assistance of an older sibling to improve the cleanliness of two siblings.

Exploiting current functional contingencies can also be done by modifying maladaptive consequences so that more appropriate behavior can be developed and maintained through natural or temporarily artificial consequences. For example, therapists can assist parents in modifying consequences by teaching them to provide immediate, appropriate, and effective discipline strategies (e.g., time-out). With effective provision of time-out, parents will likely feel efficacious, potential anger escalation will be inhibited, and (potential) physical punishment will subsequently be curtailed. Another example of modifying maladaptive consequences is pairing positive events with previously difficult situations. We saw a mother and child who were referred due to the child's nonorganic failure to thrive. The initial assessment suggested that feeding time almost always led to the mother's physically forcing her daughter to eat. By implementing routines and pairing pleasant events such as play periods with feeding, the maladaptive consequences of the previous struggle between mother and child were extinguished, the child's compliance increased, and the mother's harsh interactions and frustration decreased.

A final strategy for exploiting functional contingencies is reinforcing occurrences of generalization. Parents can record occurrences of skill generalization to the home and community. This event should be self-reinforcing, and therapists can provide additional reinforcement. Also, we frequently accompany families on walks in the hallways, outside on the sidewalk, and to the local playground. Therapists provide intermittent reinforcement for a parent's use of skills taught during therapy sessions (e.g., parent reinforcement of children's appropriate behaviors). Therapist prompts in these settings are gradually faded over time to facilitate generalization and maintenance.

Train Diversely

One strategy offered by Stokes and Osnes (1989) that is particularly relevant for parent training is training diversely. When the goals and procedures of training are more widespread, so are the outcomes. Training diversely includes using sufficient stimulus and response exemplars, a relatively common practice in parent training and other skills training efforts. Making antecedents and consequences less discriminable are other approaches in the category of training diversely.

Therapists often use multiple stimulus exemplars to facilitate generalization. For example, a therapist may observe such activities as feeding and toy clean-up to ascertain a parent's current use of prompts, such as warnings and questioning, and ways of attending to the child, such as attention and rewards (Forehand & McMahon, 1981). The therapist can subsequently assist parents in generating multiple effective examples to provide prompts or commands for their children (e.g., "Please put the toys on the shelf" versus "Can you put away all of the toys after you put on your shoes?"). Effective commands are stated in a straightforward, non-questioning manner and are provided in simple, single units versus a series of commands chained together (e.g., Forehand, 1993; MacMillan et al., 1991; Wolfe et al., 1982).

Although clinic observations of behavior may demonstrate value for pin-pointing specific problem areas, such observations may be insufficient by themselves to reveal the range and significance of contextual events that may dramatically be influencing parent and child behavior. Home interventions are not always feasible, but they can be invaluable for programming generalization. Assessment and intervention in the home facilitates identification of relevant stimuli associated with target behaviors and inclusion of relevant stimuli in rehearsal activities.

If home interventions are not feasible, creating high-demand practice situations is helpful (e.g., MacMillan et al., 1991). We have used assessments with assistants acting as children to place the parent in low- and high-demand conditions that require use of skills taught (such as use of praise, commands, and time-out). Also, we have attempted to simulate existing conditions by having families eat a meal during therapy sessions, during which they practice behavior management strategies (e.g., following established meal routines, providing table time-out). The therapist participates initially and gradually withdraws from the meal and the interactions. Also, we have families play at a nearby playground and go for walks around the facility to address safety issues (e.g., praise for appropriate behavior, sidewalk time-out for off-task behavior). Assessment and training in other settings where parenting problems can occur, such as the grocery store or a fast food restaurant, are not common practice but should be considered to facilitate generalization of skills. Finally, clinicians can ask parents to bring videotapes of problems occurring at home (e.g., bedtime transition) and problem-solve during sessions about ways to provide different types of commands, environmental control, and so forth.

Videotaped assessments can also be helpful for assisting parents in generating and using sufficient response exemplars. For example, videotape recordings of parent–child interactions in the home or the clinic are useful in providing feedback regarding child-management skills (e.g., MacMillan, Olson, & Hansen, 1987; Wolfe et al., 1988). Parents can evaluate their behavior and therapists can provide multiple exemplars of skills via instruction, modeling, rehearsal, and feedback.

Golub, Espinosa, Damon, and Card (1987) described a program which offered parent education for abusive and high-risk-for-abuse parents. The program provided videotaped segments of 13 episodes showing common problem situations between parents and their preschool children (e.g., sibling rivalry, bed refusal) along with three or four alternative ways the situation could be resolved. Parents met in a group and discussed one episode per week. The authors stated that parents who completed the program demonstrated increased knowledge of alternatives to physical punishment and understanding of normal child development as well as changed attitudes toward children's misbehavior. The method of Golub and associates is particularly good for facilitating generalization because the problem-solving strategy can generalize to many other situations. Furthermore, the tape was used as a basis for discussion rather than for instruction, and the aim was to generate insight and information from group discussion rather than from presentation by an "expert." Finally, the videotape can be used with several groups of people in many settings. A group intervention procedure may facilitate generalization through exposure to increased stimulus and response exemplars (Hansen et al., 1989), as there is increased opportunity for modeling and rehearsal with several individuals.

Another approach to training diversely involves therapists making antecedents less discriminable. For example, fading prompts and using the bug-in-the ear technique, so that the therapist's presence is less salient, can be useful strategies (Crimmins, Bradlyn, St. Lawrence, & Kelly, 1984; Dachman et al., 1984; Wolfe et al., 1982). Also, as mentioned previously, sessions should occur in a variety of contexts and training conditions so that clients will not readily discriminate performance to a particular setting. The final aspect of training diversely is to make consequences less discriminable. Therapists should employ an intermittent reinforcement schedule and should fade contingencies as parents become more active in providing behavior management (Crimmins et al., 1984).

Incorporate Functional Mediators

Another strategy to enhance generalization is to incorporate functional mediators. A mediator acts as a discriminative stimulus and facilitates or mediates generalization. This category includes use of common salient physical and social stimuli as well as self-mediated physical and verbal stimuli.

Incorporating common salient physical stimuli involves making the training and generalization settings as physically similar as possible, including the transfer of physical object(s) between the training and generalization settings. For example, clinicians may attempt to enhance generalization by asking parents to bring the child's time-out chair or other relevant stimuli (e.g., toys or games) to the therapy session and back home afterward. It may also involve provision of training in naturalistic settings, including the home (e.g., MacMillan, Guevremont, & Hansen, 1988; Watson-Perczel et al., 1988).

Incorporating common salient social stimuli can help facilitate generalization. For example, it can be valuable to involve the entire family in assessment and treatment as much as possible, as the nonabusive spouse or the children can provide ongoing assessment and prompting functions for the abusive parent (Hansen & MacMillan, 1990). There are a variety of examples in the literature of studies incorporating other significant people (e.g., siblings, fathers, teachers) to do such things as prompt, support, or record information about the abusive parent or child (e.g., Doepke et al., 1988; Lutzker, Campbell, & Watson-Perczel, 1984; Rosenfield-Schlichter et al., 1983). In some circumstances, when children are removed from the home, a family support provider accompanies the children to therapy and to home visits. This person can be invaluable for facilitating generalization of treatment effects to the home by reminding the parents about issues and techniques addressed in therapy. Also, when therapists make home visits, naturally occurring events (e.g., television turned on) should not only be tolerated but encouraged during therapy sessions to provide training in the most natural environment possible.

Another strategy for incorporating functional mediators is to incorporate self-mediated physical stimuli. This involves physical stimuli that are beyond those that occur naturally in the environment. Therapists can instruct parents to place prompts such as charts or photos in the home or other appropriate settings (e.g., Watson-Perczel et al., 1988). Also, therapists can prompt families to maintain such things as journals and home record cards.

Therapists may also teach families to incorporate self-mediated verbal and covert stimuli. Parents can be taught cognitive anger control strategies. We frequently ask parents to verbalize their thoughts during therapy sessions when children are presenting challenging behaviors. Parents are prompted to make self-statements such as, "I am calm. I am under control." Wolfe and associates (1988) taught parents in vivo desensitization with their children. Thus, the parents had opportunities to practice relaxation and similar coping responses in the presence of realistic child behaviors. Therapists can also train parents to engage in self-monitoring and self-reinforcement.

Sanders and Glynn (1981) examined the effect of self-management training (e.g., self-monitoring, goal setting) on both parent and child behavior in a home setting and two additional generalization settings. They found that self-management produced generalization of effects to all settings, and the effects were maintained at a 3-month follow-up. Teaching parents self-management skills appeared to facilitate accurate program implementation by parents in nontraining settings.

Finally, research has begun to address the use of problem solving with parents, including maltreating parents. Problem-solving training may be an important initial intervention for dealing with the varied and complex problems of maltreating parents (e.g., Hansen, Pallotta, Christopher, Conaway, & Lundquist, 1995; MacMillan et al., 1988; Spaccarelli, Cotler, & Penman, 1992). Problem-solving training has been shown to facilitate a maltreating parent's ability to generate multiple solutions for problems and to formulate more sophisticated plans for implementing chosen solutions (e.g., Dawson, de Armas, McGrath, & Kelly, 1986; MacMillan et al., 1988).

Target Contextual Factors

A fourth overall strategy that can be added to the Stokes and Osnes (1989) classification is to target contextual factors (e.g., marital problems, social isolation) that interfere with skill acquisition or that limit use of newly acquired skills. As mentioned previously, contextual factors may limit treatment adherence and social validity in addition to limiting generalization of skill acquisition and use. Many of the interventions provided for maltreating families focus on discrete sets of behaviors and have discounted the importance of contextual factors. For example, Lutzker, McGimsey, McRae, and Campbell (1983) reviewed parent training articles in 13 journals and concluded that behavioral parent training had been of such a narrow focus that its interest and utility in promoting significant, durable behavior change in deviant families were limited. Also, Forehand (1993) discussed the importance of focusing on issues other than parenting interventions, for example, marital dissatisfaction and parental depression. Forehand noted that when additional family factors are considered, interventions are more effective in terms of assisting parents in the generalization and maintenance of parenting skills and improvements in child behavior.

Wahler (1980) questioned the long-term efficacy of parent training with certain subtypes of parents. He found that "insular" mothers (i.e., those who have infrequent positive and frequent unpleasant social interactions) often discontinued using positive parenting methods at 1-year follow-up. These findings may be particularly applicable to abusive parents, as insularity is commonly observed in them. Wahler hypothesized that the lack of maintenance of intervention effects may have resulted from mothers being coerced into modifying their parenting by social agency personnel. Once the external control was removed, treatment compliance stopped. Therefore, contextual variables such as insularity should always be considered by therapists concerned with generalization and maintenance of therapy gains.

There are several examples of studies wherein researchers assessed generalization and maintenance of skills (e.g., Feldman et al., 1992; MacMillan et al., 1988; MacMillan et al., 1991); however, there is a paucity of research projects which systematically considered contextual issues or actively programmed for generalization of skills. Some studies that have assessed generalization or maintenance have found that treatment effects did not generalize to other settings, situations, times, or behaviors (e.g., Dachman et al., 1984; Tertinger et al., 1984).

CONCLUSION

In this chapter, treatment adherence, social validity, and generalization have generally been discussed as separate concepts, but it is important to note once again that there is significant overlap among the concepts. For example, the more socially valid the goals and the procedures, the more likely the client is to adhere to treatment; the more likely the client is to participate in treatment, the more likely the effects will generalize and maintain, the more the effects generalize and maintain, the more socially valid and functional the effects. Therapists must actively program for treatment adherence, social validity, and generalization to ensure efficacy of interventions. Figure 1 displays the interrelationships of the three concepts and example strategies.

There are a limited number of published intervention studies that attempt to address the issues of adherence, social validity, and generalization with abusive and neglectful families. A few studies have systematically programmed for treatment adherence, social validity, and/or generalization to facilitate efficacy of parent training interventions (e.g., MacMillan et al., 1988; MacMillan et al., 1991; Watson-Perczel et al., 1988; Wolfe et al., 1982), and there are treatment programs well suited for addressing these issues (e.g., Lutzker, 1984; Lutzker, Wesch, et al., 1984; Wesch & Lutzker, 1991). In one of the most extensive studies to date, Wolfe and colleagues (1988) evaluated an early intervention program for young parents and their children who had been identified as being at risk of child maltreatment. Thirty mother–child dyads were randomly assigned to one of two conditions: (1) a parenting information group offered by the child protection agency (served as a control condition) or (2) a special program of behavioral parent training in addition to the agency group. Significant decreases occurred in the areas of parenting risk and child behavior problems at posttest and at 3-month follow-up for mothers who received parent training in addition to information groups. Caseworker rat-

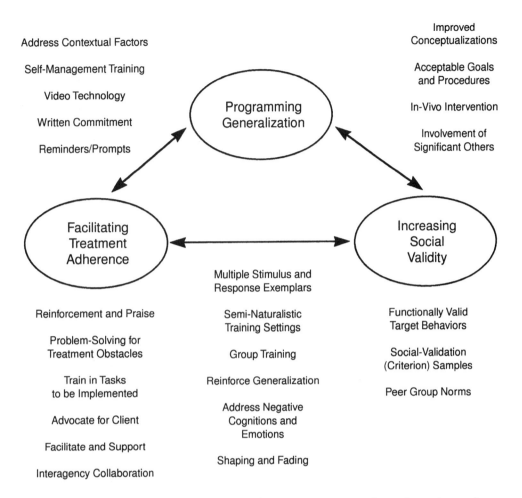

Address Contextual Factors

Self-Management Training

Video Technology

Written Commitment

Reminders/Prompts

Improved
Conceptualizations

Acceptable Goals
and Procedures

In-Vivo Intervention

Involvement of
Significant Others

Programming
Generalization

Facilitating
Treatment
Adherence

Increasing
Social
Validity

Multiple Stimulus and
Response Exemplars

Reinforcement and Praise

Problem-Solving for
Treatment Obstacles

Train in Tasks
to be Implemented

Advocate for Client

Facilitate and Support

Interagency Collaboration

Semi-Naturalistic
Training Settings

Group Training

Reinforce Generalization

Address Negative
Cognitions and
Emotions

Shaping and Fading

Functionally Valid
Target Behaviors

Social-Validation
(Criterion) Samples

Peer Group Norms

Figure 1. Treatment adherence, generalizations, and social validity: interrelationship and example enhancement strategies.

ings of clients' risks of maltreatment and abilities to manage their families at 1-year follow-up significantly favored the families who received parent training in addition to information. Wolfe and associates (1988) utilized a variety of procedures that would facilitate treatment adherence, increase social validity, and enhance generalization. Such procedures included (1) providing training via a bug-in-the-ear radio transmitter, (2) viewing of videotapes of parent–child interactions with mothers critiquing their own behavior, (3) teaching parents in vivo desensitization, (4) making home visits, (5) fading to biweekly sessions, (6) soliciting caseworkers' feedback, and (7) having parents complete a consumer satisfaction questionnaire after treatment. They also utilized an impressive variety of assessment tools pre- and posttreatment to gather information about family-specific issues and to assess efficacy of treatment effects.

Several directions for future research on parent training with maltreating families are apparent from the present review. There is a need for further study of the following issues for maltreating parents: (1) factors that account for enhanced adherence, (2) the social validity of parenting skill component behaviors, (3) the social validity of parent training procedures and child management techniques, (4) the accuracy and validity of current generalization assessment procedures, as well as the development of methods to assess generalization of training effects, (5) methods to enhance the generalization and maintenance of training effects, and (6) the influence of the many contextual factors that impact treatment participation and outcome. Further research on these issues will aid our efforts to facilitate treatment adherence, social validity, and generalization, and therefore promote intervention efficacy with these multichallenged families.

REFERENCES

Acbenbach, T. M. (1991). *Manual for the Child Behavior Checklist/4-18 and 1991 Profile.* Burlington: University of Vermont.

Ammerman, R. T., Cassissi, J. E., Hersen, M., & Van Hasselt, V. B. (1986). Consequences of physical abuse and neglect in children. *Clinical Psychology Review, 6,* 291–310.

Azar, S. T., & Wolfe, D. A. (1989). Child abuse and neglect. In E. J. Mash & R. Barkley (Eds.), *Treatment of childhood disorders* (pp. 451–489). New York: Guilford Press.

Barone, V. J., Greene, B. F., & Lutzker, J. R. (1986). Home safety with families being treated for child abuse and neglect. *Behavior Modification, 10,* 93–114.

Chamberlain, P., Patterson, G. R., Reid, J. B., Kavanagh, K., & Forgatch, M. S. (1984). Observation of client resistance. *Behavior Therapy, 15,* 144–155.

Conaway, L. P., & Hansen, D. J. (1989). Social behavior of physically abused and neglected children: A critical review. *Clinical Psychology Review, 9,* 627–652.

Cox, D. J., Tisdelle, D. A., & Culbert, J. P. (1988). Increasing adherence to behavioral homework assignments. *Journal of Behavioral Medicine, 11,* 519–522.

Crimmins, D. B., Bradlyn, A. S., St. Lawrence, J. S., & Kelly, J. A. (1984). A training technique for improving the parent–child interaction skills of an abusive-neglectful mother. *Child Abuse & Neglect, 8,* 533–539.

Dachman, R. S., Halasz, R. M., Bickett, A. D., & Lutzker, J. R. (1984). A home-based ecobehavioral parent-training and generalization package with a neglectful mother. *Education and Treatment of Children, 7,* 183–202.

Dawson, B., de Armas, A., McGrath, M. L., & Kelly, J. A. (1986). Cognitive problem-solving training to improve the child-care judgment of child neglectful parents. *Journal of Family Violence, 1,* 209–221.

Doepke, K. J., & Hansen, D. J. (1992). *Facilitating treatment adherence with maltreating families: Conceptualization and review.* Unpublished manuscript.

Doepke, K. J., Watson-Perczel, M., & Hansen, D. J. (1988, November). *Modification of an abusive and neglectful home environment: Children as behavior change agents.* Presented at the meeting of the Association for the Advancement of Behavior Therapy, New York.

Dumas, J. E., & Albin, J. B. (1986). Parent training outcome: Does active parental involvement matter? *Behaviour Research and Therapy, 24,* 227–230.

Dunst, C. J., Leet, H. E., & Trivette, C. M. (1988). Family resources, personal well-being, and early intervention. *The Journal of Special Education, 22,* 108–116.

Dush, D. M., & Stacy, E. W. (1987). Pretesting enhancement of parent compliance in a prevention program for high-risk children. *Evaluation & the Health Professions, 10,* 201–205.

Edelstein, B. A. (1989). Generalization: Terminological, methodological and conceptual issues. *Behavior Therapy, 20,* 311–324.

Feldman, M. A., Case, L., Rincover, A., Towns, F., & Betel, J. (1989). Parent education project III: Increasing affection and responsivity in developmentally handicapped mothers: Component analysis, generalization, and effects on child language. *Journal of Applied Behavior Analysis, 22,* 211–222.

Feldman, M. A., Case, L., & Sparks, B. (1992). Effectiveness of a child-care training program for parents at-risk for child neglect. *Canadian Journal of Behavioral Science, 24,* 14–28.

Forehand, R. (1993). Twenty years of research on parenting: Does it have practical implications for clinicians working with parents and children? *The Clinical Psychologist, 46,* 169–176.

Forehand, R., & McMahon, R. (1981). *Helping the noncompliant child: A clinician's guide to parent training.* New York: Guilford Press.

Frentz, C., & Kelley, M. L. (1986). Parents, acceptance of reductive treatment methods: The influence of problem severity and perception of child behavior. *Behavior Therapy, 17,* 75–81.

Golub, J. S., Espinosa, M., Damon, L., & Card, J. (1987). A videotape parent education program for abusive parents. *Child Abuse & Neglect, 11,* 255–265.

Hansen, D. J., Conaway, L. P., & Christopher, J. S. (1990). Victims of child physical abuse. In R. T. Ammerman & M. Hersen (Eds.), *Treatment of family violence: A sourcebook* (pp. 17–49). New York: Wiley.

Hansen, D. J., & MacMillan, V. M. (1990). Behavioral assessment of child abusive and neglectful families: Recent developments and current issues. *Behavior Modification, 14,* 255–278.

Hansen, D. J., Pallotta, G. M., Christopher, J. S., Conaway, R. L., & Lundquist, L. M. (1995). The Parental Problem-Solving Measure: Further evaluation with maltreating and nonmaltreating parents. *Journal of Family Violence, 10,* 319–336.

Hansen, D. J., & Warner, J. E. (1992). Child physical abuse and neglect. In R. T. Ammerman & M. Hersen (Eds.), *Assessment of family violence: A clinical and legal sourcebook* (pp. 123–147). New York: Wiley.

Hansen, D. J., & Warner, J. E. (1994). Treatment adherence of maltreating families: A survey of professionals regarding prevalence and enhancement strategies. *Journal of Family Violence, 9,* 1–19.

Hansen, D. J., Watson-Perczel, M., & Christopher, J. S. (1989). Clinical issues in social-skills training with adolescents. *Clinical Psychology Review, 9,* 365–391.

Heffer, R., & Kelley, M. L. (1987). Mother's acceptance of behavioral interventions for children: The influence of parent race and income. *Behavior Therapy, 18,* 153–163.

Hobbs, S. A., Walle, D. L., & Hammersly, G. A. (1990). The relationship between child behavior and acceptability of contingency management procedures. *Child & Family Behavior Therapy, 12,* 95–102.

Irueste-Montes, A. M., & Montes, F. (1988). Court-ordered versus voluntary treatment of abusive and neglectful parents. *Child Abuse & Neglect, 12,* 33–39.

Johnson, W. B. (1988). Child-abusing parents: Factors associated with successful completion of treatment. *Psychological Reports, 63,* 434.

Kazdin, A. E. (1977). Assessing the clinical or applied importance of behavior change through social validation. *Behavior Modification, 1,* 427–452.

Kazdin, A. E. (1980). Acceptability of alternate treatments for deviant child behavior. *Journal of Applied Behavior Analysis, 13,* 259–273.

Kelley, M. L., Grace, N., & Elliott, S. N. (1990). Acceptability of positive and punitive discipline methods: Comparisons among abusive, potentially abusive, and nonabusive parents. *Child Abuse & Neglect, 14,* 219–226.

Kolko, D. (1996). Child physical abuse. In J. Briere, L. Berliner, J. A. Bulkley, C. Jenny, & T. Reid (Eds.), *The APSAC handbook on child maltreatment* (pp. 21–50). Thousand Oaks, CA: Sage.

Lutzker, J. R (1984). Project 12-Ways: Treating child abuse and neglect from an ecobehavioral perspective. In R. F. Dangel and R. A. Polster (Eds.), *Parent training* (pp. 260–297). New York: Guilford Press.

Lutzker, J. R. (1994). Practical issues in delivering broad-based ecobehavioral services to families. *Revista Mexicana De Psicologia, 11,* 87–96.

Lutzker, J. R., Campbell, R. V., & Watson-Perczel, M. (1984). Using the case study method to treat several problems in a family indicated for child neglect. *Education and Treatment of Children, 7,* 315–333.

Lutzker, J. R., McGimsey, J. F., McRae, S., & Campbell, R. V. (1983). Behavioral parent training: There's so much more to do. *The Behavior Therapist, 6,* 110–112.

Lutzker, J. R., Megson, D. A., Webb, M. E., & Dachman, R. S. (1985). Validating and training adulthood interaction skills to professionals and to parents indicated for child abuse and neglect. *Journal of Child and Adolescent Psychotherapy, 2,* 91–104.

Lutzker, J. R., & Newman, M. R. (1986). Child abuse and neglect: Community problem, community solutions. *Education and Treatment of Children, 9,* 344–354.

Lutzker, J. R., Wesch, D., & Rice, J. M. (1984). A review of Project 12-Ways: An ecobehavioral approach to the treatment and prevention of child abuse and neglect. *Advances in Behavior Research and Therapy, 6,* 63–74.

MacKinnon, L., & James, K. (1992). Raising the stakes in child-at-risk cases: Eliciting and maintaining parents' motivation. *The Australian and New Zealand Journal of Family Therapy, 13,* 59–71.

MacMillan, V. R., Guevremont, D. C., & Hansen, D. J. (1988). Problem-solving training with a multiply distressed abusive and neglectful mother: Effects on social insularity, negative affect, and stress. *Journal of Family Violence, 3,* 313–326.

MacMillan, V. M., Olson, R. L., & Hansen, D. J. (1987). Facilitating the maintenance of relationship building skills in a parent training program for a physically abusive and her husband. Paper presented at the Rivendell Conference of Clinical Practitioners, Memphis, TN.

MacMillan, V. M., Olson, R. L., & Hansen, D. J. (1991). Low and high deviance analogue assessment of parent-training with physically abusive parents. *Journal of Family Violence, 6,* 279–301.

Malinosky-Rummell, R., & Hansen, D. J. (1993). Long-term consequences of childhood physical abuse. *Psychological Bulletin, 114,* 68–79.

Meichenbaum, D., & Turk, D. C. (1987). *Facilitating treatment adherence: A practitioner's guidebook.* New York: Plenum Press.

National Center on Child Abuse and Neglect (1988). *Study of national incidence and prevalence of child abuse and neglect: 1988.* Washington, DC: U.S. Department of Health and Human Services.

Newman, C. (1994). Understanding client resistance: Methods for enhancing motivation to change. *Cognitive and Behavioral Practice, 1,* 47–69.

Oates, R. K., & Bross, D. C. (1995). What have we learned about treating child physical abuse? A literature review of the last decade. *Child Abuse & Neglect, 19,* 463–473.

Patterson, G. R., & Chamberlain, P. (1994). A functional analysis of resistance during parent training therapy. *Clinical Psychology: Science and Practice, 1,* 53–70.

Patterson, G. R., & Forgatch, M, S. (1985). Therapist behavior as a determinant for client noncompliance: A paradox for the behavior modifier. *Journal of Consulting and Clinical Psychology, 53,* 846–851.

Racusin, R. J., & Felsman, J. K. (1986). Reporting child abuse: The ethical obligation to inform parents. *Journal of the American Academy of Child Psychiatry, 25,* 485–489.

Rosenfield-Schlichter, M. D., Sarber, R. E., Bueno, G., Greene, B. F., & Lutzker, J. R. (1983). Maintaining accountability for an ecobehavioral treatment of one aspect of child neglect: Personal cleanliness. *Education and Treatment of Children, 6,* 153–164.

Sanders, M. R., & Glynn, T. (1981). Training parents in behavioral self-management: An analysis of generalization and maintenance. *Journal of Applied Behavior Analysis, 14,* 223–237.

Schwartz, I. S., & Baer, D. M. (1991). Social validity assessments: Is current practice state of the art? *Journal of Applied Behavior Analysis, 24,* 189–204.

Shelton, J. L., & Levy, R. L. (1981). *Behavioral assignments and treatment compliance.* Champaign, IL: Research Press.

Smith, J. E., & Rachman, S. J. (1984). Non-accidental injury to children—II: A controlled evaluation of a behavioral management programme. *Behaviour Research and Therapy, 22,* 349–366.

Spaccarelli, S., Cotler, S., & Penman, D. (1992). Problem-solving skills training as a supplement to behavioral parent training. *Cognitive Therapy and Research, 16,* 1–18.

Stokes, T. F., & Baer, D. M. (1977). An implicit technology of generalization. *Journal of Applied Behavior Analysis, 10,* 349–367.

Stokes, T. F., & Osnes, P. G. (1989). An operant pursuit of generalization. *Behavior Therapy, 20,* 337–355.

Sutton, C. S., & Dixon, D. (1986). Resistance in parent training: A study of social influence. *Journal of Social and Clinical Psychology, 4,* 133–144.

Tertinger, D. A., Greene, B. F., & Lutzker, J. R. (1984). Home safety: Development and validation of one component of an ecobehavioral treatment for abused and neglected children. *Journal of Applied Behavior Analysis, 17,* 159–174.

Wahler, R. (1980). The insular mother: Her problems in parent child treatment. *Journal of Applied Behavior Analysis, 13,* 207–219.

Warner, J. E., Malinosky-Rummell, R., Ellis, J. T., & Hansen, D. J. (1990, November). An examination of demographic and treatment variables associated with session attendance of maltreating families. Paper presented at the annual conference of the Association for the Advancement of Behavior Therapy, San Francisco.

Watson-Perczel, M., Lutzker, J. R., Greene, B. F., & McGimpsey, B. J. (1988). Assessment and modification of home cleanliness among families adjudicated for child neglect. *Behavior Modification, 12,* 57–81.

Wesch, D., & Lutzker, J. R. (1991). A comprehensive 5-year evaluation of Project 12-Ways: An ecobehavioral program for treating and preventing child abuse and neglect. *Journal of Family Violence, 6,* 17–35.

Wolfe, D. A. (1988). Child abuse and neglect. In E. J. Mash & L. G. Terdal (Eds.), *Behavioral assessment of childhood disorders* (2nd ed., pp. 627–669). New York: Guilford Press.

Wolfe, D. A., Aragona, J., Kaufman, K., & Sandler, J. (1980). The importance of adjudication in the treatment of child abusers: Some preliminary findings. *Child Abuse & Neglect, 4,* 127–135.

Wolfe, D. A., Edwards, B. E., Manion, I., & Koverola, C. (1988). Early intervention for parents at risk for child abuse and neglect: A preliminary investigation. *Journal of Consulting and Clinical Psychology, 56,* 40–47.

Wolfe, D. A., St. Lawrence, J., Graves, K., Brehony, K., Bradlyn, D., & Kelly, J. A. (1982). Intensive behavioral parenting training for a child abusive mother. *Behavior Therapy, 13,* 438–451.

Part IV

Sex Abuse

Although the bulk of this book is dedicated to physical child abuse and neglect, it would seem incomplete to have no mention of the assessment, treatment, and prevention of child sexual abuse, a most serious problem. Chapters by Swenson and Hanson and by Wurtele exemplify both sensitivity for the problem and an empirical approach to it.

Swenson and Hanson take note of the attention-grabbing issue that child sexual abuse represents, but again stress the need for empirically based research so that we can see through emotion and truly begin to learn how to deal with the serious nature of this kind of child maltreatment. In their chapter they review research-based methods of assessment and treatment and examine the mental health consequences of child sexual abuse and its prevalence.

Wurtele takes a tack similar to that of Swenson and Hanson, but her focus is on school-based education programs aimed at the prevention of child sexual abuse. The "bottom line" of Wurtele's presentation is that children must learn avoidance and recognition *behaviors* as opposed to feelings or strictly verbal behavior. This theme echoes the general theme of all of the contributors to this volume, the need for direct assessment and training.

20

Sexual Abuse of Children
Assessment, Research, and Treatment

CYNTHIA CUPIT SWENSON and
ROCHELLE F. HANSON

Child sexual abuse (CSA) has been the focus of considerable attention among researchers, clinicians, the courts, and, recently, the news media. In many cases assessment and treatment techniques have been under close scrutiny and professionals have been challenged to demonstrate the effectiveness of their work. More than ever, research-based methods are needed. This chapter presents research on assessment and treatment of sexually abused children. First, the prevalence of child sexual abuse is discussed. Second, mental health consequences related to CSA are summarized. Third, clinical assessment of sexually abused children and their families is reviewed. Finally, treatment of sexually abused children and their families is examined.

PREVALENCE OF CHILD SEXUAL ABUSE

Despite the attention that child sexual abuse has received in recent years, the victimization of children has not declined. Just how prevalent sexual abuse is has been difficult to determine. Methods of prevalence data collection and characteristics of child disclosure have contributed to a likely underestimate of CSA rates. For example, some prevalence rates are based on reported cases, and only a small percentage of sexual abuse crimes are ever reported (Kilpatrick, Edmunds, & Seymour, 1992). Further, some child protection agencies report rates based on number of families rather than number of children in the family who experienced CSA, yielding a lower rate (McCurdy & Daro, 1994). Moreover, the nature of child disclosure can

CYNTHIA CUPIT SWENSON • Department of Psychiatry and Behavioral Science, Family Services Research Center, Medical University of South Carolina, Charleston, South Carolina 29425. ROCHELLE F. HANSON • Center for Sexual Assault/Abuse Recovery and Education, University of Florida, Gainesville, Florida 32607.

Handbook of Child Abuse Research and Treatment, edited by Lutzker. Plenum Press, New York, 1998.

sometimes lead to false negatives in substantiation of abuse. According to Sorenson and Snow (1991), children rarely give a full disclosure the first time they talk about the abuse. Instead, for many children the disclosure process involves initial denial, tentative disclosure, then full disclosure, and recantation of the report of abuse is not unusual (Sorenson & Snow, 1991). These characteristics of disclosure may lead agencies to unfound cases, resulting in lowered prevalence rates.

Although subject to the problems noted above regarding child disclosure, national surveys probably provide a more accurate picture of prevalence because they capture abuse cases that may not have been reported to authorities or other agencies. Finkelhor and Dziuba-Leatherman (1994) conducted telephone interviews assessing multiple traumatic events with 2000 children who were 10- to 16-years-old. They found that 15.3% of girls and 5.9% of boys reported having experienced attempted and completed sexual abuse. Of interest, 1.7% of girls and 16.2% of boys reported attempted and completed violence to genitals that was separate from sexual abuse reports. In a national telephone survey of more than 4000 women, Kilpatrick, Edmunds, and Seymour (1992) found that one out of every eight women had been raped in her lifetime and more than 70% of those rapes occurred before age 18. These studies underscore the great number of children who experience sexual abuse and who may be at risk for mental health difficulties in their lifetime.

EFFECTS OF CHILD SEXUAL ABUSE

Two major conclusions can be drawn from the extant research on the effects of CSA: (1) findings are inconsistent and show considerable variability across studies, and (2) there are a wide range and array of outcomes associated with childhood sexual victimization, meaning that no single symptom characterizes the majority of sexually abused children. The sequelae associated with CSA include the entire array of mental health, emotional, familial, and social problems, including depression, sexual dysfunction, sexual acting out behaviors, anxiety, dissociation, posttraumatic stress disorder (PTSD), and relationship difficulties. However, it is also important to recognize that sexually abused children may not evince symptoms at the time of assessment. In their review of the research, Kendall-Tackett, Williams, and Finklelhor (1993) found that between one-fourth and one-half of children were asymptomatic at the time of assessment. These findings may be the result of the use of insensitive measures or of the fact that the children had not yet developed any symptoms. This suggests that the response to sexual abuse may be gradual or delayed.

The variability in response to CSA highlights the need to use developmentally appropriate measures for assessment. As discussed by Kendall-Tackett et al. (1993), there appear to be developmental differences in children's response to sexual abuse. For example, preschoolers are more likely to show anxiety symptoms, nightmares, PTSD, internalizing and externalizing behaviors, and sexual acting out; school-age children are more likely to experience fears, aggression, and school problems. Adolescents are more prone toward depression, withdrawal, suicidal or self-injurious behaviors, somatic complaints, illegal acts, substance abuse, and running away. These age differences mean that different assessment measures will be appropriate depending upon the age or developmental level of the child.

Another important component to understanding the effects of CSA is to recognize that certain assault characteristics increase the risk of negative mental health outcomes (Kendall-Tackett et al., 1993). For example, studies have been fairly consistent in finding that threats, the use of force, weapons, and penetration increased the risk for problems, such as PTSD (Wolfe, Sas, & Wekerle, 1994). The relationship of the offender to the victim also affects outcome, with increased symptoms found in victims who were abused by a close family member (Beitchman et al., 1992). A greater frequency and longer duration of abuse, lack of maternal support at the time of disclosure, and the victim's negative outlook or coping style were other variables found to be associated with increased symptomatology (Kendall-Tackett et al., 1993).

In sum, there does not appear to be a definitive pattern of symptoms associated with CSA. Symptoms differ across age groups, and data suggest that the response to sexual abuse may be gradual and/or delayed. The findings on the effects of CSA also indicate the importance of examining specific assault characteristics, because these appear to be related to the development and severity of symptoms. Before beginning any treatment program with abused children and their families it is important to conduct a comprehensive assessment. The next section discusses a multifaceted assessment approach for use with sexually abused children.

MULTIFACETED ASSESSMENT

Forensic versus Clinical Assessment

When an allegation of sexual abuse is made, two types of assessments are typically conducted: forensic and clinical (Lutzker, Bigelow, Swenson, Doctor, & Kessler, in press). A forensic assessment includes a determination of whether the child was sexually abused, specifics of the incident, current safety of the child, risk for future maltreatment (i.e., whether the alleged offender still resides in the home and/or current placement of the child), and the ability of the nonoffending caregiver to be supportive and protective. Details of the index abuse event that may be assessed include the relationship of the child to the offender, the onset, frequency, and duration of the abuse, the use of physical force, threats or coercion, and contextual information, such as where the abuse occurred and time of day. Formal psychological testing for the purpose of substantiating an abuse allegation is typically not included in the forensic assessment (APSAC, 1990). Forensic assessments may be conducted by law enforcement officials, child protection workers, and/or mental health professionals. Regardless of the evaluator's discipline, the APSAC guidelines (1990) recommend that the evaluator have a minimum of two years professional experience with children, including specialized training in child development and child sexual abuse. Furthermore, the guidelines state the necessity of previous experience in conducting court evaluations and testifying in court on child abuse cases.

A clinical assessment involves a comprehensive evaluation of the impact of the CSA on the child and family. Obtaining a clear picture of the child's and family's symptom pattern aids in individual treatment planning and provides a means of evaluating treatment effectiveness. The clinical assessment typically includes the use of standardized measures. As such, the evaluator should have training and experience in test administration, scoring, and interpretation. If specific training is not obtained through a graduate program, formal assessment skills may be obtained through supervised on-the-job training and workshops.

In some instances, the forensic and clinical assessment may be conducted together, but this generally depends on the standard method of assessment in a given community and the availability of a multidisciplinary team. The focus of the next section will be on clinical assessment, as this is within the role of the therapist who treats the child and family.

Clinical Assessment

The purpose of the clinical assessment is to obtain an accurate picture of the child's and family's current functioning. A comprehensive, multifaceted assessment includes multiple methods (e.g., direct observation, interview, self-report questionnaires) and multiple respondents, such as the nonoffending parent, child victim, siblings, and extrafamilial reporters (i.e., teachers, day-care workers, previous therapists, child protection workers). Multiple respondents help to determine how generalized a child's problems are (e.g., at home vs. at school) (Friederich, 1995), and minimize reliance on the parent's report. A parent whose child has been abused is, in all likelihood, experiencing distress which could bias the parent's reports of problems in the child, either by minimizing the child's difficulties, or exaggerating symptoms, perhaps as a cry for help. In addition to interviews, the use of standardized instruments is becoming increasingly important. As discussed by Letourneau and Saunders (1996), standardized measures provide consistency, generalizability, reliability, and validity. They enable the evaluator to compare the child's responses to normative data, thus permitting meaningful conclusions. Despite the importance of standardized measures, obtaining information about available instruments and assessment procedures is often difficult. In a project funded by the National Center on Child Abuse and Neglect, the National Crime Victims Research and Treatment Center at the Medical University of South Carolina recently developed the Child Abuse and Neglect Database Instrument System (CANDIS). This system consists of a personal computer (PC)-based data base that provides information about standardized instruments used in the field of child abuse and neglect, and a text-based comprehensive reference guide that provides detailed information about each measure. CANDIS provides descriptive information about each measure, including author, construct measured, psychometric properties, method of administration (e.g., interview, self-report), number of items, cost, and availability (Letourneau & Saunders, 1996). Clearly, this data base system provides many advantages to professionals in the area of child abuse, particularly because it enables professionals to rapidly find and use the best tools available when conducting assessments.

Table 1 presents interview and standardized assessment procedures used in CSA. Several domains are assessed using multiple respondents. The areas to assess include (1) trauma history, (2) mental health symptoms and behavior problems, and (3) family history and relationships. One caveat for the ensuing discussion is the importance of including developmentally appropriate measures in assessment procedures.

Table 1. Multifacted Assessment

Respondent	Trauma history	Mental health/ behavior problems	Family history/ family relationships
		Area of assessment	
Victim/siblings	Clinical interview, BATE	CDI, RCMAS, STAIC, Piers-Harris, TSC–C, CITES, CAPS	CAM, CAF
Parent/guardian/ caregiver	Clinical interview, Parent Impact Questionnaire	SCL-90–R (self), TSI (self) CBCL, PEDS, CSBI	IPA, FES, FOS
Extrafamilial sources	History of Victimization Form	CBCL, PEDS, CSBI	

Trauma History: Child/Victims and Sibling(s) Report

As stated previously, specific characteristics of the abuse incident may be obtained during the forensic assessment and passed on to the therapist. However, if important details are missing, particularly those related to the child's symptomatology, it may be necessary for the primary therapist to interview the child directly regarding case characteristics. For example, research has suggested that certain incident characteristics may be associated with an increased risk for the development of Posttraumatic Stress Disorder (PTSD). These include physical injury, perception of life threat, whether penetration occurred, and the response of others to the abuse disclosure (Lipovsky, 1991). A clinical interview with the child may yield this important information. However, when conducting interviews with children (sexually abused children, in particular), it is essential for the interviewer to take time to develop rapport and to be sensitive to the child's readiness to talk about the abuse and trauma and to the child's developmental level. If children appear uncomfortable discussing their abuse history, it may be necessary to incorporate other mediums, such as puppets, drawings, or dolls, into the interview process (Lutzker et al., in press; Wolfe & Gentile, 1992).

In addition to interviewing the child about the index abuse incident, questions regarding other traumatic experiences, including physical abuse, natural disaster, fire, car accidents, life-threatening illnesses, or violence witnessed should be asked (Lutzker et al., in press). The Brief Assessment of Traumatic Events (BATE; Lipovsky & Hanson, 1992a,b; Lipovsky, Hanson, & Hand, 1993) is a structured interview designed to assess history of traumatic events, which include physical abuse, sexual abuse, and witnessing violence. This instrument has been used clinically with outpatient and inpatient populations, but, to date, lacks empirical validation.

Siblings can also be administered the BATE and a clinical interview. This combination provides a more comprehensive picture of the family's trauma history.

Trauma History: Parent/Caregiver Report

A clinical interview with the parent or primary caregiver is an essential component of the assessment process. The caregiver can provide information about the index abuse incident that the child may be unable or unwilling to disclose. For example, the caregiver may have knowledge of the legal status of the case and may also be able to provide useful information concerning the child's current safety (i.e., the child's accessibility to the offender). The caregiver can also provide historical information about the child that may be relevant to the presenting symptoms or problems. The child's educational, medical, mental health, developmental and family history prior to and following the abuse are important in assessing the child's current functioning.

In addition to assessing the child's history, it is important to obtain information concerning the parent's or caregiver's own trauma history. Unresolved issues concerning the parent's or caregiver's own victimization may surface after a parent learns about the child's abuse. This can have an adverse impact on the child's recovery because unresolved parental abuse issues may interfere with the parent's capacity to believe, support, and protect the child (Wolfe & Gentile, 1992). A clinical interview with the parent should include questions to assess childhood history of physical or sexual abuse, problems in the family of origin (e.g., alcoholic parent, poverty, neglect), as well as adult victimization experiences (e.g., rape, battery, and spousal violence). The Parent Impact Questionnaire (Wolfe & Gentile, 1992) is a structured interview designed to obtain historical information as well as specific abuse related experiences. It is composed of four sections, two of which focus on problems in the family of origin and history of physical or sexual abuse. Family-related problems include parental separations or divorce, excessive parental arguing or physical fighting, inadequate housing, parental mental health problems, alcohol or drug abuse, neglect, and excessive physical punishment. Problems during adulthood include marital separations or divorce, physical violence from a partner, drug or alcohol dependence, and mental health problems. This type of structured interview enables the evaluator to collect basic historical information from the parent directly and then employ follow-up questions to further explore specific areas.

Trauma History: Extrafamilial Sources of Information

Extrafamilial sources, such as teachers, former therapists, and child protection workers, may also provide information concerning both the abuse itself and the child's functioning in different contexts. Wolfe and Gentile (1992) developed the History of Victimization Form to obtain detailed information from social workers regarding the child's history of maltreatment and to obviate the need to interview the child directly. The measure has five scales: sexual abuse, physical abuse, neglect, exposure to family violence, and psychological abuse. Social workers provide information about the specific types of maltreatment and also rate the severity of the abuse incidents on a scale from 1 to 5. Additional questions are asked to assess factors related to the severity of the abuse, including physical sequelae to the abuse, the relationship between the offender and child, the emotional closeness of the offender to the child, and the time frame, duration, and frequency of the abuse. For the Sexual Abuse Scale, the respondent is also asked to provide information on the use of force or coercion during the abuse, and whether he/she believes the sexual abuse "eventually elicited the child's sexual response resulting in eroticism" (p. 6).

Mental Health Symptoms/Behavior Problems: Child-Completed Measures

Because a parent may be unaware of certain difficulties experienced by a child, it is important to obtain information from the source itself, that is, the child. Self-report measures completed by the child provide an additional dimension to assess current functioning. It is useful to assess a child's general mental health symptoms as well as trauma-specific symptoms. A widely used self-report measure of depression is the Children's Depression Inventory (CDI; Kovacs, 1992). This 27-item inventory assesses affective, cognitive, and behavioral dimensions of depression in children ages 7–17. Each item presents three statements which range from mild to severe symptomatology for a specific symptom of depression. The respondent must choose the statement that best describes him or her over the past two weeks. Normative scores based on age and grade have been reported by Finch, Saylor, and Edwards (1985). The Revised Children's Manifest Anxiety Scale (RCMAS; Reynolds & Richmond, 1978) has been used as a child self-report measure of anxiety symptoms. Each of the 37 items is a statement that reflects a symptom of anxiety (e.g., "I worry a lot of the time") to which the child answers "yes" or "no." In addition to the total anxiety score, three factor scores can be assessed: Physiological Anxiety, Worry and Oversensitivity, and Concentration Anxiety. Finally, two Lie factors (combined for scoring purposes) are designed to detect a social desirability response bias (Reynolds & Paget, 1981). Studies using the RCMAS indicate internal consistency and test–retest reliability coefficients greater than .80 (Finch & Rogers, 1984). Another measure used to assess anxiety symptoms in children is the State–Trait Anxiety Inventory for Children (STAIC; Spielberger, 1973). The two separate scales of the STAIC, State Anxiety and Trait Anxiety, assess how the child is feeling at the moment (State Anxiety) and how the child usually feels (Trait Anxiety).

Another area that may be important to assess is the child's self-concept. The Piers-Harris Self-Concept Scale (Piers-Harris; Piers, 1984) is an 80-item measure that assesses how children feel about themselves. Dimensions assessed include behavior, intellectual and school status, physical appearance and attributes, anxiety, popularity, happiness, and satisfaction. Higher scores reflect more positive self-esteem. Reliability and validity of the instrument have been demonstrated.

Research has been equivocal in demonstrating whether sexually abused children differ from nonabused children on mental health symptoms. For example, Lipovsky, Saunders, and Murphy (1989) found no significant differences on the RCMAS between sexually abused children and their nonabused siblings. Similarly, in studies conducted by Cohen and Mannarino (1988), using the Piers-Harris, and Wolfe, Gentile, and Wolfe (1989) using the RCMAS, sexually abused children did not significantly differ from normative samples on either measure. However, Tong, Oakes, and McDowell (1987) found significant elevations on the Piers-Harris for sexually abused girls compared to a control group. It should be noted that Tong et al. (1987) administered the Piers-Harris an average of 2.6 years after the abuse. Further, Lipovsky and associates (1989) found higher rates of depression among incest victims compared to their nonabused siblings. In contrast, Cohen and Mannarino (1988) found no significant differences on depression scores between sexually abused girls and a nonclinical sample. Overall, these data suggest that the development of mental health symptoms may be gradual and/or delayed (Wolfe & Gentile, 1992). Despite the mixed findings, these instruments may still be useful in providing reports of children's perceptions of their own distress, as well as assessing the potential development of problems over time.

For trauma-specific symptoms, such as PTSD, dissociation, and sexual concerns, the Trauma Symptom Checklist–Children (TSC–C; Briere, 1989) can be used. This instrument consists of six subscales: Anxiety, Depression, Posttraumatic Stress, Sexual Concerns, Dissociation, and Anger. It is used with children ages 8–15. The scale has been found to have relatively high internal consistency (total α = .96) and construct validity, as demonstrated by its correlations with the CBCL and CDI, its association with characteristics of the abuse incidents (e.g., age at first abuse, penetration), and decreases in TSC–C scores over the course of abuse-focused treatment (Lanktree, Briere, & Hernandez, 1991). Another measure of PTSD symptoms is the Children's Inventory of Traumatic Events Scale–Revised (CITES–R; Wolfe, Gentile, Michienczi, Sas, & Wolfe, 1991). The revised scale is composed of 78 statements to assess children's perceptions and attributions about their sexual abuse, as well as PTSD symptoms. The instrument, appropriate for children ages 8–16, is administered as a standardized interview with objective response options. The 11 subscales are Intrusive Thoughts, Avoidance, Hyperarousal, Sexual Anxiety, Negative Reactions from Others, Social Support, Self Blame/Guilt, Dangerous World, Empowerment, Vulnerability, and Eroticism. The subscales form four dimensions, PTSD (Intrusive Thoughts, Avoidance, Sexual Anxiety, and Hyperarousal), Social Reactions (Negative Reactions from Others, and Social Support), Abuse Attributions (Self Blame/Guilt, Dangerous World, Empowerment, and Vulnerability) and Eroticism. Reliability for the overall scale was .89, with alpha values for the four dimensions ranging from .57 for Eroticism to .88 for PTSD. Significant convergent and discriminant validity have been demonstrated (Wolfe et al., 1991). Studies using this scale indicate that sexually abused children report a variety of symptoms following disclosure (Wolfe & Gentile, 1992).

The Children's Attributions and Perceptions Scale (CAPS; Mannarino, Cohen, & Berman, 1994) is a newly developed measure designed to assess cognitive sequelae of child sexual abuse. The instrument has 18 items which comprise four subscales: Feeling Different from Peers, Personal Attributions for Negative Events, Perceived Credibility, and Interpersonal Trust. Internal consistency for the subscales ranges from .64 to .73 and 2-week test–retest reliabilities were found to range from .60 to .82. The CAPS is administered in an interview format, with response options raging from (1) never to (5) always. In their study of sexually abused females ages 7–12 and a nonabused control group, Mannarino and colleagues (1994) found that the sexually abused group scored significantly higher than the nonabused controls on the total CAPS score and three subscales. For the sexually abused group, significant correlations were obtained between the CAPS and self-report measures of depression, anxiety, and self-esteem.

All of the measures described in this section can be administered to siblings to provide information on their functioning in the assessed areas. However, based on the child protection investigation, if there is no reason to suspect that the siblings have been abused, the trauma-specific measures (i.e., CITES and TSC–C) do not need to be included in the assessment protocol.

Mental Health Symptoms/Behavior Problems: Parent-Completed Measures

Parent functioning. Parents who discover that their child has been abused will undoubtedly experience symptoms of distress, which may have an adverse effect on the child. In addition, the way the parent responds to the abuse disclosure can have a profound impact on the child's recovery (Everson, Hunter, Runyon, Edelsohn, & Coulter, 1989; Wolfe & Gentile, 1992). As a cousequence, it is important to include a measure that specifically assesses the parent's degree of distress. The resulting information can be integrated into the treatment process. The Symptom Checklist-90–Revised (SCL-90–R; Derogatis, 1983) is one measure used to assess the parent's or guardian's current symptomatology. This is a 90-item self-report questionnaire that assesses a variety of symptoms and problems experienced by the respondent over the past week. The respondent rates each item on a 5-point scale (0 = no discomfort to 4 = extreme discomfort) to reflect the level of symptoms experienced during the past week. The measure includes 9 symptom scales: Somatization, Obsessive–Compulsive, Interpersonal Sensitivity, Depression, Anxiety, Hostility, Phobic Anxiety, Paranoid Ideation, and Psychoticism, as well as three global stress indices: Global Severity, Positive Symptom Distress, and Positive Total. Previous studies have found test–retest reliability for the 9 factors ranging from .77 to .86 and internal consistency estimates ranging from .78 to .90 (Derogatis, 1977). Adequate concurrent and discriminant validities have also been demonstrated (Derogatis, 1977).

As stated in the previous section, the Parent Impact Questionnaire (Wolfe & Gentile, 1992) consists of four sections designed to obtain information on a parent's trauma/family history and experiences related to the specific abuse incident. The two sections dealing with the current abuse incident include questions to assess the impact of the child's sexual abuse and disclosure on the individual parent and the family, as well as events surrounding the sexual abuse incident (e.g., the mother's feelings of responsibility and guilt, experiences with legal and investigative agencies, and types of interventions being sought).

If it has been determined that a parent has a history of abuse or other types of traumatic events, it is useful to assess their trauma-related symptoms. The Trauma Symptom Inventory (TSI; Briere, 1995) is a trauma-specific measure composed of 10 scales: Anxious Arousal, Depression, Anger/Irritability, Intrusive Experiences, Defensive Avoidance, Dissociation, Sexual Concerns, Dysfunctional Sexual Behavior, Impaired Self-Reference, and Tension Reduction Behavior. The TSI has demonstrated acceptable psychometric properties in both clinical (Briere, Elliott, Harris, & Cotman, 1995) and nonclinical samples (Briere, 1995; Smiljanich & Briere, 1993).

Child functioning. The nonoffending parent or caregiver provides a primary source of information on the child's current level of functioning. Several parent-completed measures have been used to assess children's mental health symptoms and behavior problems. One of the most widely used instruments is the Child Behavior Checklist (CBCL; Achenbach, 1991), a scale composed of 118 items assessing social skills and internalizing and externalizing behavior problems in children ages 4–16. Extensive psychometric data are available on the CBCL (Achenbach, 1991). It has also been used in studies of sexually abused children, with findings that sexually abused children are rated as having significantly more behavior problems than nonabused children, but fewer problems than nonabused clinical samples; these differences are maintained at 6- and 12-month follow-ups (Mannarino, Cohen, Smith, & Moore-Motily, 1991). The Pediatric Emotional Distress Scale (PEDS; Saylor, Swenson, Stokes, Wertlieb, & Casto, 1994; Swenson et al., 1994) is another parent-completed measure consisting of 25 items that assess general behavior problems and trauma-related symptoms in young children. The scale items were theoretically derived; however, factor analysis yields three reliable factors: Anxious/Withdrawn, Acting Out, and Fearful (Saylor et al., 1994). Psychometric properties of the scale have been demonstrated with an overall internal consistency of $\alpha = .85$, and good concurrent validity with the Eyberg Child Behavior Inventory (Eyberg & Ross, 1978) and the Reaction Index (Frederick, 1985). In addition, construct validity has been demonstrated, in that PEDS scores significantly differentiate between traumatized and nontraumatized children (Swenson et al., 1994).

A measure used to assess parent perceptions of child sexual behavior problems is the Children's Sexual Behavior Inventory (CSBI; Friedrich, Grambsch, Broughton, Kuiper, & Beilke, 1991; Friedrich et al., 1992). This is a 35-item parent-completed scale that assesses the frequency of a wide variety of sexual behaviors related to self-stimulation, sexual aggression, gender role behavior, and personal boundary violations in 2–12 year old children during the past six months. Reliability and validity of the scale have been demonstrated (Friedrich et al., 1991, 1992). Specifically, the scale has been found to differentiate between sexually abused and nonabused children, and is also related to sexual abuse variables, such as abuse severity, number of offenders, and the use of force or threat of death (Friedrich et al., 1992).

Mental Health Symptoms/Behavior Problems: Extrafamilial Sources of Information

In addition to obtaining information from the parent, the multifaceted assessment approach identifies the importance of including multiple respondents. Teachers, child protection workers, and previous therapists, for example, can provide useful information about the child. Instruments such as the CBCL, PEDS, and CSBI can also be administered to these extrafamilial sources. The information obtained from these data enable the evaluator to examine similarities and differences in the child's behavior across settings, thus providing a more comprehensive picture of the child's functioning. In addition, these data can aid in treatment planning. For example, if the assessment indicates that the child is experiencing specific problems in the classroom setting, the therapist can work with the teacher to design individually tailored interventions.

Family History/Family Relationships: Child-Completed Measures

The relationship between child and parent appears to be an important variable in recovery. Positive relationships with a caregiver facilitate disclosure, enhance feelings of safety, and generally help the child cope with the victimization experience (Wolfe & Gentile, 1992). In contrast, child victims whose relationship with the mother is emotionally distant may be at greater risk for the development of mental health difficulties (Finkelhor, 1984). Several reports (e.g., Adams-Tucker, 1982; Everson et al., 1989) have found a significant relationship between low maternal support and psychological disturbance in victims of sexual abuse. To assess the child's perception of his or her relationship with his or her parents, the Child's Attitude towards Mother/Father Scales (CAM/CAF; Guili & Hudson, 1977) can be used. The scale is composed of 25 items measuring the degree, severity, and magnitude of problems children report in their relationships with their parents. The 2 scales are identical, with the exception that on the CAF the word "mother" is replaced with "father." The score ranges from 0–100, with higher scores reflecting a more severe parent-relationship problem (Saunders & Schucts, 1987). Both scales have demonstrated good internal consistency reliability (α = .93–.96), test–retest reliability (r = .89–.96), and discriminant validity (r = .86–.87). They have a validated clinical cutting score and a useful set of normal comparison scores (Saunders & Schuchts, 1987).

Family History/Family Relationships: Parent/Guardian Completed Measures

The Index of Parental Attitudes (IPA; Giuli & Hudson, 1977; Hudson, Wung, & Borges, 1980) is a scale parallel to the CAM and CAF that assesses the parent–child relationship from the caregiver's perspective. Similar to the CAM and CAF, the IPA consists of 25 brief statements about family relationships. The internal consistency reliability of the IPA is excellent (α = .96) and it possesses good discriminant validity (r = .89) for clinically rated relationships. The scale also has a validated clinical cutting score.

To obtain a complete assessment of parent–child relationships within the family, it is important to include the siblings in the completion of these measures. Siblings can complete the CAM/CAF and parents can complete the IPA for each child in the family. There have been some data to suggest that relationships between the victim and parents differs from that between nonabused siblings and parents. For example, in their study of incest families, Lipovsky, Saunders, and Hanson (1992) found that victims reported greater relationship difficulties with fathers who were offenders than did siblings.

In addition to assessing the parent–child relationship, it is useful to obtain information on patterns of family interactions. Studies comparing individuals from abusive versus nonabusive families have indicated that incest families are more socially isolated, less cohesive, more disorganized and chaotic as compared with controls (Alexander & Lupfer, 1987; Harter, Alexander, & Neimeyer, 1988; Saunders, McClure & Murphy, 1986, 1987; Williams & Finkelhor, 1990). The Family Environment Scale (FES; Moos & Moos, 1981, 1983, 1990) is a 90-item true-false scale that yields 10 scales on dimensions of family interactions: Cohesion, Expressiveness, Conflict, Independence, Organization, Control, Achievement Orientation, Intellectual–Cultural Orientation, Moral–Religious Emphasis, and, Active–Recreational Orientation. Discriminant validity has been found for the Cohesion, Independence, Expressiveness, Conflict, and Control subscales. In addition, the scales have been found to reflect changes in family interaction patterns as a consequence of therapy.

In addition to information concerning parental levels of distress and relationship dynamics within the current family, it may be important to assess the parents' perceptions of their family of origin. Clinical accounts of incest families have revealed that the parents (both father/offenders and mothers) report chaotic, dysfunctional families of origin (e.g., Alexander, 1985; Araji & Finkelhor, 1986; Sgroi, 1982). The few empirical studies that have examined families of origin have generally supported these clinical accounts (Lipovsky & Saunders, 1989; Parker & Parker, 1986). Inclusion of a measure that assesses functioning within the parents' family of origin would provide useful information to use in treatment planning. The Family of Origin Scale (FOS) (Hovestadt, Anderson, Piercy, Cochran, & Fine, 1985) is a self-report instrument consisting of 40 questions designed to measure self-perceived levels of health in one's family of origin. The 10 core constructs measured are clarity of expression, responsibility, respect for others, openness to others, acceptance of separation and loss, range of feelings, mood and tone, conflict resolution, empathy, and trust. The scale also has two second-order factors, intimacy and autonomy, and an overall family health factor. Previous studies have demonstrated good test–retest reliability for the family health factor ($r = .97$), autonomy ($r = .77$), and intimacy ($r = .73$).

In summary, a comprehensive assessment is a key tool for guiding the treatment process. Formal assessment measures may be administered prior to, during, and upon completion of treatment to evaluate the course of symptoms and the effectiveness of treatment.

TREATMENT OF SEXUALLY ABUSED CHILDREN AND THEIR FAMILIES

The impact of sexual abuse is a family problem, not solely a child problem. Even in cases of extrafamilial abuse, the support of family is important to child adjustment (Everson et al., 1989). In intrafamilial abuse cases the family must participate to increase child safety and parental support, and to reduce the risk of re-abuse (Giarretto, 1982; Ribordy, 1990). The primary focus of this section is on intrafamilial abuse, although some treatment components discussed are appropriate for extrafamilial abuse cases. The components presented include child treatment, sibling treatment, nonoffending parent treatment, offender treatment, and family treatment. These components are provided to families in the order listed. Individual therapy and dyadic work with the nonoffending parent are recommended prior to family treatment because beginning with family therapy may be traumatizing to the child who initially may not have sufficient support from the parents (Silovsky & Hembree-Kigin, 1994).

Child Treatment

Abuse-Specific Treatment Preconditions

Four preconditions should be met before beginning trauma-specific treatment with children: assessment, child safety, crisis stabilization, and support. If these preconditions are not met, doing so must be the first priority. As described earlier, a forensic and clinical assessment should be conducted. Treatment of the effects of a trauma cannot begin until confirmation of the abuse allegations has been established and certain incident characteristics are obtained. Moreover, a comprehensive treatment plan cannot be developed until the functioning of the child and family is assessed. The child must also be in a safe environment. If the child is living with an untreated or nonacknowledging offender, the risk for reabuse may be high. Discussion of the abuse in treatment sessions under these conditions may increase the child's anxiety or the likelihood of recantation (Lipovsky & Elliott, 1993). If the child is currently in crisis; that is, if the child is suicidal, homicidal, or psychotic, then the crisis should be stabilized before beginning trauma-specific work. Finally, the child needs a supportive caregiver. If the child is not believed and supported by the caregiver, the focus of treatment should then be on helping the caregiver become more supportive of the child.

Factors that Facilitate Treatment

In addition to meeting these preconditions for treatment, several factors facilitate individual work with the child. First, therapists should let the child know that they are aware of the CSA and that treatment will focus on this experience. Second, the child should be fully informed of confidentiality limits and should understand that discussions of previously reported abuse will not mean that a new report to child protection is needed. Third, the therapist should avoid loyalty conflicts. For example, the offender can be referred to as someone who broke the rules or the law, rather than using criticisms or other derogatory statements about that person. Fourth, therapists should be aware of cultural/ethnic differences between themselves and the child and family and should strive to learn how the family's beliefs influence their view of the abuse and treatment. Fifth, although therapy should be viewed as teamwork, rules for appropriate behavior and boundaries around the therapeutic relationship should be fully explained and followed. Finally, therapy should be perceived by the child as a safe place. Children should not be forced to have contact in the therapeutic context with someone who sexually, physically, or emotionally abused them until it is in the child's best interest to have this contact. Each of these factors is important to the therapeutic process and is implemented along with specific therapeutic techniques.

Abuse-Specific Treatment Components

Treatment of sexually abused children from a number of theoretical orientations has been described in the research literature (see Finkelhor & Berliner, 1995; O'Donohue & Elliott, 1992, for reviews). It should be noted that few of the CSA studies used adequate controls and many included small sample sizes. Thus, firm conclusions have not been reached regarding the most effective techniques for treating sexually abused children.

Cognitive–behavioral therapy enjoys a history of empirical support regarding its efficacy with impulsive disorders (Kendall & Braswell, 1993) and anxiety disorders (Kendall, 1994) in children. Recent group (Stauffer & Deblinger, 1996) and individual treatment research (Cohen & Mannarino, 1996; Deblinger, McLeer, & Henry, 1990) shows promise for the efficacy of cognitive–behavioral treatment with sexually abused children. Thus, the focus of this section will be cognitive–behavioral treatment. The treatment components discussed are used when sexually abused children are experiencing trauma-related emotional symptoms (e.g., fear, anxiety, depression), and the goal is to reduce those symptoms. It should be noted that sexually abused children may experience other behavioral problems (e.g., aggression, sexual acting out) that may require specific interventions. These interventions will not be discussed here.

Cognitive–behavioral techniques. Within a cognitive–behavioral framework, three channels within which children experience anxiety and fears are explored, including thinking, feeling, and doing (Lang, 1979; Ribbe, Lipovsky, & Freedy, 1995). The primary focus is on changing thinking and doing, which hypothetically changes feelings. In this section techniques that teach skills for changing thinking, doing, and feeling are described. It should be noted that, even though the theoretical basis for treatment will be consistent across children, specific techniques will vary according to the child's developmental level. For example, for a preschooler, play may be incorporated into cognitive–behavioral techniques, whereas for adolescents, play may inappropriate.

Psychoeducation. The main purpose of psychoeducation is to help children normalize their feelings about the sexual abuse experience by addressing beliefs about the event and how their feelings and beliefs are similar to those of other children. Psychoeducation activities include defining the various types of sexual abuse (e.g., fondling, oral, penetration, peeping), and directly discussing the child's affective experience and cognitions related to their experience.

Anxiety management. Prior to beginning exposure work, skills training on coping with anxiety and fears is conducted. Anxiety management training gives children tools to aid in coping when they begin to talk in treatment about the sexual abuse. This training also helps the child deal with anxiety and fears that may accompany posttraumatic symptoms, such as nightmares or intrusive thoughts. A number of techniques have been developed for managing anxiety and have been applied to children. These include breathing retraining (Craske & Barlow, 1990; Kolko & Swenson, 1996; Swenson, 1996), deep muscle relaxation (Ollendick & Cerny, 1981), and guided imagery (Berliner & Wheeler, 1988). Simplified forms of deep muscle relaxation have been described for use with young children. For example, teaching the child to act like a tin soldier emphasizes muscle tension and having the child act like a wet noodle emphasizes muscle relaxation (Deblinger,

1995). Anxiety management techniques taught early in therapy are used through-out the treatment process.

Graduated exposure. The purpose of graduated exposure is to break the link between anxiety and cues that serve as reminders of the sexual abuse. For exam-ple, if a offender was wearing a certain cologne during the CSA, the smell of the cologne is paired with anxiety and fear the child feels. Later, when the child is no longer in the abuse situation, the smell of the cologne or a similar cologne may elicit anxiety. Graduated exposure is used to break such links so that the child re-duces experiences of conditioned anxiety.

Prior to beginning exposure work, children are given a rationale for doing this very difficult task. For example, Deblinger (1992) compared exposure work to a child's experience of turning on the light at night and discovering that what looked like a monster was not really a monster at all. Thus, in therapy children are encouraged to face their fears about the abuse so that they will gradually feel less distress. During graduated exposure the child recapitulates the abusive incident(s) by beginning with situations provoking less anxiety (e.g., where they were during the abuse) and eventually talking about those situations provoking greater anxiety. During the recapitulation, the child is asked to talk about specific sights, sounds, or smells remembered from the abuse. Anxiety is countered with performing re-laxation techniques. Telling about the abusive experience may be done by talking, drawing, through the use of puppets, and through any other modalities, depend-ing on the child's developmental level and choice. For some children, talking about their abusive experience is highly anxiety provoking, and this anxiety may be paired with treatment resulting in the child's attempting to avoid coming to treatment. Predicting the avoidance experience for parents and children may as-sist them in normalizing this tendency and enable them to work through it.

Cognitive treatment. Throughout the individual work with the child, cogni-tive approaches are used to challenge faulty beliefs children may have as a result of the CSA. For example, some children may attribute the abuse to something they did or wore; other children may believe that they have contracted a physical illness such as AIDS. Countering these beliefs may help reduce unnecessary anxiety. In some cases children are fearful of the offender and need cognitive treatment to un-derstand their current level of safety. Sometimes children are not believed or sup-ported by their families. Cognitive treatment can help them explore why their family has this difficulty and to see that there are other people who do believe and support them. Techniques used to correct thinking errors include cognitive re-structuring, guided self-dialogue, and thought stopping (Deblinger et al., 1990).

Sexual abuse education/prevention. To help clarify inappropriate sexual information children may have obtained directly from the offender or on their own, and to clarify safety issues, sexual abuse education/prevention is provided. This part of training addresses (1) the right to say no, (2) facts on AIDS and sexually transmitted diseases, (3) facts on functions of sexual body organs and pregnancy, (4) recognition of danger cues that may indicate heightened risk for reabuse, (5) development of a safety plan, and (6) sexualized feelings and behaviors (Deblinger et al., 1990). Prior to talking about sexual abuse education, nonoffending parents should be informed of this topic. They may be able to help counter any of the child's faulty beliefs about sex or the child's concern over medical conditions.

Clarification. A common task in sexual abuse treatment of the child is addressing responsibility for the abuse, with absolving the child of blame as one of the components (Berliner, 1987). Some debate has taken place in the literature regarding whether attributing sole blame to the offender is adaptive or whether an external attribution leaves the victim with a sense of helplessness (Dalenberg & Jacobs, 1994; Shapiro, 1989). Shapiro (1989) suggests that therapists may need to consider the distinction between source and solution attributions (Brickman et al., 1982). That is, victims and their families would attribute the source or origin of the abuse to the offender, and the solution to the child, offender, and family.

Abuse responsibility may be addressed in two ways: through individual or group treatment of the child, and through treatment with the offender and family. Clarification of the abuse may be viewed as a precondition to beginning family treatment. It is a process that directly addresses three goals: (1) acceptance of responsibility for the CSA by the offender, (2) presentation of an apology to the victim and family by the offender, and (3) development of a plan by the family for continued child safety and family restructuring. Clarification is typically conducted when the offender is a family member and when the child will derive benefit from this process.

Preparation for clarification is done by the therapist, individually with the child. First, the rationale for clarification is explained. For example, the child can be told that the offender will be apologizing to the child and the family, will hear what the victim would like to say, will answer questions the victim and family may have, and will discuss strategies the family will use to prevent future abuse. Second, the child and therapist make the rules for the clarification meeting. These may include no touching, no emotional outbursts by the offender, and no blaming of the victim or family. Third, if appropriate, the child, along with the therapist and nonoffending parent, develop a list of what they would like to say to the offender, for example, how the CSA made them feel and any questions they have for the offender. The rules, questions, and comments developed by the child may be presented to the nonoffending parent if the child wishes to do so. Each of these will be used in the clarification session with the offender and other family members.

Sibling Treatment

Although sibling treatment has not received attention in the research literature, clearly, in some cases, siblings are indirect victims and should also receive attention in treatment. The victim's sibling may have observed the abuse or may have been negatively affected by incidents that occurred after the abuse was discovered. As a result, they may have questions about the CSA or may be experiencing posttraumatic symptoms. Moreover, in some families the sibling may also have experienced CSA that has not been reported. At the least, all siblings should be interviewed forensically to determine whether they also have experienced sexual abuse. They also may complete a clinical assessment to determine the impact of the CSA on them. Based on the results of the assessment, individual treatment may be appropriate for siblings. Certainly, siblings will be included in the family treatment.

Nonoffending Parent Treatment

Two goals may be accomplished in treatment with nonoffending parents: (1) reduction of their own symptoms (e.g., depression, anxiety, anger) related to their child's sexual abuse and (2) strengthening of their belief and support of the child victim. Following abuse of the child, the nonoffending parent may experience posttraumatic stress symptoms, guilt, and feelings of sadness and betrayal. Overwhelming emotional feelings may lead to compromised parenting. If the offender of abuse is a parent, then disclosure of the abuse also may have severe economic consequences for the family, not to mention a stigmatizing effect. Individual or group treatment may assist the nonoffending parent in reducing emotional symptoms, improving parenting, and increasing both level of independence and support networks. Some assistance may also be needed to pursue services such as housing and other governmental support.

Not only is support of the parent important; support of the child victim has been identified as strongly related to the child's adjustment (Everson et al., 1989). Therefore, treatment of nonoffending parents who are unable to provide belief and support to their child is paramount. Nonoffending parents may have difficulty believing the child victim, especially when the child did not report the abuse to the parent. When the nonoffending parent exhibits belief and support of the child, dyadic treatment may be used to improve their relationship.

Although limited research exists on treatment of the nonoffending parent, three recent studies highlighted the importance of including nonoffending mothers in the child's treatment. Deblinger and colleagues (1990) and Stauffer and Deblinger (1996) provided cognitive–behavioral treatment to nonoffending mothers as a parallel to treatment of the child victim. Components of the treatment included (1) education and coping, (2) behavior management, and (3) communication with the child about the sexual abuse. Following treatment, mothers reported significant reductions in overall distress, avoidance of abuse-related thoughts and feelings (Stauffer & Deblinger, 1996), and reductions in child symptoms (Deblinger et al., 1990; Stauffer & Deblinger, 1996).

Cohen and Mannarino (1996) randomly assigned preschoolers and their mothers to either cognitive–behavioral treatment or nondirective supportive therapy. Issues addressed with the parents included

> ambivalence in belief of the child's abuse, ambivalent feelings toward the offender, attributions regarding the abuse, feeling that the child is "damaged," providing appropriate emotional support to the child, management of inappropriate child behaviors (including regressive and sexual behaviors), management of fear and anxiety symptoms, parental issues related to their own history of abuse (if applicable), and legal issues (p. 45).

Although parent outcomes were not measured, the combination of parent and child cognitive–behavioral treatment resulted in significantly greater improvement in children's symptoms than did nondirective supportive child and parent treatment.

Offender Treatment

Although sex offenders may receive treatment for difficulties other than their offending behavior (e.g., depression, substance abuse), treatment specific to the sexual offending has been described in the research literature. Reviews of sex offender treatment (e.g., Becker & Hunter, 1992; Kelly, 1982) indicate that current treatments are optimistic for some offenders. Nonetheless, guides for matching offender characteristics with the most efficacious treatment have yet to be made. Furthermore, although treatment outcome studies are improving methodologically, few of the existing studies utilized random assignment or controlled conditions, and most were conducted with male offenders. Nonetheless, some cognitive–behavioral and behavioral treatments appear to hold promise for decreasing the risk for reoffending and these will be the focus of this section.

Sex offender treatment is conducted individually or in group formats and focuses on decreasing deviant sexual arousal and increasing age-appropriate sexual activities (Fish & Faynik, 1989). For incest offenders who will remain with or reunite with their family, or visit with their victims, individual or group treatment is only one component of a comprehensive program. Common treatment components of offender-specific treatment include masturbatory satiation and arousal conditioning, covert sensitization, cognitive restructuring, sex education, social skills training, biofeedback, and relapse prevention.

Among published treatment studies, recidivism rates for offenders have varied from 12% (Abel, Mittelman, Becker, Rathner, & Rouleau, 1988) to 31% (Rice, Quinsey, & Harris, 1991). Studies separating recidivism rates of treated incest offenders and other sex offenders have found differences. Lang, Pugh, and Langevin (1988) provided incest offenders and pedophiles with inpatient group treatment that included social skills training, anger management, stress inoculation, and use of psychodrama and films discussing victims for building victim empathy. At a 3-year follow-up, incest offenders had lower recidivism rates than did pedophiles (7% vs. 18%). Marshall and Barbaree (1988) assessed recidivism of incest offenders and molesters of nonfamilial female and male children and found differential rates at a 1–11-year follow-up period (8%, 17.9%, and 13.9%, respectively). The offenders had all received treatment consisting of electrical aversion, masturbatory reconditioning, and conflict resolution. Moreover, in this same program treated offenders had significantly lower recidivism rates than did nontreated offenders (Marshall & Barbaree, 1988).

Overall, offender-specific treatment studies have yielded positive outcomes for some offenders. More research is needed to determine which treatments work best for which offenders. Methodological improvements over current studies (e.g., random assignment, control groups) will be a necessary part of making this determination.

Preparation for Clarification

Although not empirically validated, the process by which offenders prepare for clarification with their victims has been described in the literature (Kahn,

1991). Typically, offenders are asked to work to understand why they sexually abused the child, to take full responsibility for the abuse, and to include this information in a letter to the victim. The letter contains very specific information about the grooming process, what the offender did, and the offender's plan to prevent recurrence of the abuse (Kahn, 1991). Prior to reading the letter to the victim, the offender has the letter approved by the nonoffending parent.

The Abuse Clarification Meeting

The clarification meeting is held when the offender, nonoffending parent, and victim have progressed in treatment to the point that each is ready for this meeting. Several tasks are accomplished in the clarification meeting: (1) clarification of the facts, (2) acceptance of responsibility for the abuse by the offender, (3) agreement by the parents regarding degree of their involvement with the care of the children, (4) discussion of family separations and how this relates to safety, and (5) agreement over visitation and long-term plans for the family (Furniss, 1987). The meeting is generally held at the child therapist's office, and seating may be decided by the child victim prior to the meeting. During the clarification meeting, the therapist explains the rules, and strategies are suggested to the offender to help with managing emotions (e. g., leave the room). The reading of the letter written by the offender takes place in this session. The child victim is given the opportunity to express her or his feelings about the abuse, to make any comments, or to ask any questions of the offender. If the child is unable to do this, then another person may be designated to perform this task. The meeting ends with a plan for risk reduction and family treatment if the family is to reunite.

Completion of the clarification process does not signify the end of treatment for offenders or their families. Subsequent family treatment is important to risk reduction and child safety. Couple and individual treatment may be needed to address relationship issues and reduce symptoms related to the abuse. For offenders, long-term treatment follow-up will be important to the lifelong task of monitoring and reducing the risk for relapse.

Family Treatment

Family therapy is an important component in sexual abuse cases and the definition of family will depend on the goal of treatment. If the offender will not be reuniting with the family, then the nonoffending parent, child victim, and sibling(s) may participate in family treatment to address restructuring the family without the offender. In cases where the offender will rejoin or has remained with the family, therapy focuses on restructuring the family with the offender.

To restructure the family several goals are addressed. First and foremost is the goal of prevention of reabuse. Ultimately, the offender is responsible for relapse prevention, but the family may provide support and help with the prevention plan. The offender's primary responsibility in relapse prevention is to avoid high-risk situations and utilize therapeutic techniques that reduce risk. For example, the offender will not be alone with the children, will avoid inappropriate physical contact that may lead to abuse (e.g., lap sitting), will recognize and stop any grooming behaviors, and will follow all family safety and privacy rules. The nonoffending parent will accept responsibility for helping to protect the children, will work to strengthen his or her relationship with the child victim, and will take on decision making regarding the children. The child victim and siblings are responsible for following the family safety and privacy rules and confronting the offender or letting the nonoffending parent know of any uncomfortable situations or feelings. The parents are responsible for strengthening the marital relationship and for developing relationships outside the family (e.g., church, community) to decrease isolation. The family as a whole is responsible for establishing family rules regarding safety and privacy, strengthening communication, and supporting the autonomy of individual members (Ribordy, 1990). According to Meinig and Bonner (1990), within the new family structure the mother makes the decisions regarding the children, the father is never alone with the children, and the family communicates and solves problems at a higher level and has regular family meetings.

The Child Sexual Abuse Treatment Program of Santa Clara County, California (Giarretto, 1982, 1989), includes individual treatment of all family members, mother–daughter treatment, marital counseling, and father–daughter counseling. Evaluations of this program have shown low recidivism rates for offenders (< 1%), and in 85% of cases offenders returned to the family. According to Giarretto (1982), the focus of the program is restructuring the family around the mother–daughter core.

Meinig and Bonner (1990) describe a family reunification model that specifies how to prepare each of the family members for visitation and full reunification. This model has been applied to more than 300 families and one–third of them were reunited. Recidivism rates have not been reported.

In summary, family therapy is a critical component of treatment for sexually abused children. Several models have been described in the literature. Some have been evaluated, but none with scientific rigor. Extant data indicate that comprehensive models that include family treatment as a component are associated with family reunification and lowered recidivism. Further research is needed to determine the effectiveness of family treatment and when and with whom this treatment should be conducted.

SUMMARY

Child sexual abuse is a complex problem that carries significant mental health consequences for many children and families. A thorough assessment of the child, the offender, and the family will determine the extent of these consequences, guide treatment for the child and family, and provide a tool for determining treatment effectiveness. Research on measures used with traumatized children and their families is growing, and high-tech data bases such as CANDIS (Letourneau & Saunders, 1996) simplify the task of choosing appropriate assessment instruments. Despite this growth, additional measurement development and validation is needed (Hanson, Smith, Saunders, Swenson, & Conrad, 1995).

Over the past 10 years, there have been considerably more treatment outcome studies and clinical case studies that have emphasized the importance of including the children and parents in treatment. Many of the recent models advocate a comprehensive program consisting of individual, dyadic, and family treatment. Moreover, there is some evidence that a comprehensive treatment program is related to lowered recidivism. Nonetheless, we are in the early stages of understanding which techniques are most effective (Giarretto, 1982).

Although sexually abused children and their families are assessed and treated daily, much work is needed to assure that they are receiving effective services. Through additional research on assessment measures, child treatment, sibling treatment, nonoffending parent treatment, offender treatment, and family treatment, we may begin to make a difference for sexually abused children and their families.

REFERENCES

Abel, G. G., Mittelman, M., Becker, J. V., Rathner, J., & Rouleau, J. L. (1988). Predicting child molesters' response to treatment. In R. A. Prentky & V. L. Quinsey (Eds.), *Annals of the New York Academy of Science* (pp. 223–235). New York: New York Academy of Science.

Achenbach, T. M. (1991). *Manual of the Child Behavior Checklist and 1991 Profile.* Burlington: University of Vermont, Department of Psychiatry.

Adams-Tucker, C. (1982). Proximate effects of sexual abuse in childhood: A report on 28 children. *American Journal of Psychiatry, 139,* 1252–1256.

Alexander, P. C. (1985). A systems theory conceptualization of incest. *Family Process, 24,* 79–87.

Alexander, P. C., & Lupfer, S. L. (1987). Family characteristics and long-term consequences associated with sexual abuse. *Archives of Sexual Behavior, 16,* 235–245.

APSAC (American Professional Society on the Abuse of Children). (1990). *Guidelines for psychosocial evaluation of suspected sexual abuse in young children.* Chicago: Author.

Araji, S., & Finkelhor, D. (1986). Abusers: A review of the research. In D. Finkelhor (Ed.), *A sourcebook on child sexual abuse* (pp. 89–118). Newbury Park, CA: Sage.

Becker, J. V., & Hunter, J. A., Jr. (1992). Evaluation of treatment outcome for adult offenders of child sexual abuse. *Criminal Justice and Behavior, 19,* 74–92.

Beitchman, J. H., Zucker, K. J., Hood, J. E., daCosta, G. A., Akman, D., & Cassavia, E. (1992). A review of the long-term effects of child sexual abuse. *Child Abuse & Neglect, 15,* 537–556.

Berliner, L. (1987). Treating the effects of sexual abuse on children. *Journal of Interpersonal Violence, 2,* 415–434.

Berliner, L., & Wheeler, J. R. (1988). Treating the effects of sexual abuse on children, *Journal of Interpersonal Violence, 2,* 415–434.

Brickman, P., Rabinowitz, V. C., Karuza, J., Coates, D., Cohen, E., & Kidder, L. (1982). Models of helping and coping. *American Psychologist, 37,* 368–384.

Briere, J. (1989). *Trauma Symptom Checklist for Children.* Odessa, FL: Psychological Assessment Resources.

Briere, J. (1995). *Trauma Symptom Inventory professional manual.* Odessa, FL: Psychological Assessment Resources.

Briere, J., Elliott, D. M., Harris, K., & Cotman, A. (1995). Trauma Symptom Inventory: Psychometrics and association with childhood and adult victimization in clinical samples. *Journal of Interpersonal Violence, 10,* 387–401.

Cohen, J. A., & Mannarino, A. P. (1988). Psychological symptoms in sexually abused girls. *Child Abuse & Neglect, 12,* 571–577.

Cohen, J. A., & Mannarino, A. P. (1996). A treatment outcome study for sexually abused preschool children: Initial findings. *Journal of the American Academy of Child and Adolescent Psychiatry, 35,* 42–50.

Craske, M. G., & Barlow, D. H. (1990). *Therapist's guide for the mastery of your anxiety and panic (MAP) program.* Albany, NY: Graywind.

Dalenberg, C. J., & Jacobs, D. A. (1994). Attributional analyses of child sexual abuse episodes: Empirical and clinical issues. *Journal of Child Sexual Abuse, 3,* 37–50.

Deblinger, E. (1992). Child sexual abuse. In A. Freeman & F. M. Dattilio (Eds.), *Comprehensive casebook of cognitive therapy* (pp 159–167). New York: Plenum Press.

Deblinger, E. (1995, January). Cognitive behavioral interventions for treating school age sexually abused children. Paper presented at the San Diego Conference on Responding to Child Maltreatment, San Diego, CA.

Deblinger, E., McLeer, S. V., & Henry, D. (1990). Cognitive behavioral treatment for sexually abused children suffering post-traumatic stress: Preliminary findings. *Journal of the American Academy of Child and Adolescent Psychiatry, 29,* 747–752.

Derogatis, L. R. (1977). *SCL-90: Administration, scoring, and procedure manual for the R(revised) version.* Baltimore: Johns Hopkins University School of Medicine.

Derogatis, L. R. (1983). *The SCL-90–R: Administration, scoring, and procedures manual-II.* Townson, MD: Clinical Psychometric Research.

Everson, M. D., Hunter, W. M., Runyon, D. K., Edelsohn, G. A., & Coulter, M. L. (1989). Maternal support following disclosure of incest. *American Journal of Orthopsychiatry, 59,* 197–206.

Eyberg, S. M., & Ross, A. W. (1978). Assessment of child behavior problems: The validation of a new inventory. *Journal of Clinical Child Psychology, 7,* 113–116.

Finch, A. J., & Rogers, T. R. (1984). Self-report instruments. In T. H. Ollendick & M. Hersen (Eds.) *Child behavior assessment: Principles and procedures.* New York: Pergamon.

Finch, A. J., Saylor, C. F., & Edwards G. E. (1985). Children's Depression Inventory: Sex and grade norms for normal children. *Journal of Consulting and Clinical Psychology, 53,* 424–425.

Finkelhor, D. (1984). *Child sexual abuse: New theory and research.* New York: Free Press.

Finkelhor, D., & Berliner, L. (1995). Research on the treatment of sexually abused children: A review and recommendations. *Journal of the American Academy of Child and Adolescent Psychiatry, 34,* 1408–1423.

Finkelhor, D., & Dziuba-Leatherman, J. (1994). Children as victims of violence: A national survey. *Pediatrics, 94,* 413–420.

Fish, V., & Faynik, C. (1989). Treatment of incest families with the father temporarily removed: A structural approach. *Journal of Strategic and Systemic Therapies, 8,* 53–63.

Frederick, C. J. (1985). Children traumatized by catastrophic situations. In S. Eth & R. S. Pynoos (Eds.), *Post-traumatic stress disorders in children* (pp 73–99). Washington, DC: American Psychiatric Press.

Friedrich, W. N. (1995). *Psychotherapy with sexually abused boys: An integrated approach.* Thousand Oaks, CA: Sage.

Friedrich, W. N., Grambsch, P., Broughton, D., Kuiper, J., & Beilke, R. L. (1991). Normative sexual behavior in children. *Pediatrics, 88,* 456–464.

Friedrich, W. N., Grambsch, P., Damon, L., Hewitt, S., Koverola, C., Lang, R., Wolfe, V., & Broughton, D. (1992). The Child Sexual Behavior Inventory: Normative and clinical contrasts. *Psychological Assessment, 4,* 303–311.

Furniss, T. H. (1987). An integrated treatment approach to child sexual abuse in the family. *Children and Society, 2,* 123–135.

Giarretto, H. (1982). A comprehensive child sexual abuse treatment program. *Child Abuse & Neglect, 6,* 263–278.

Giarretto, H. (1989). Community-based treatment of the incest family. *Psychiatric Clinics of North America, 12,* 351–361.

Giuli, C. A., & Hudson, W. W. (1977). Assessing parent–child relationship disorders in clinical practice: The child's point of view. *Journal of Social Service Research, 1,* 77–92.

Hanson, R. F., Smith, D. W., Saunders, B. E., Swenson, C. C., & Conrad, L. (1995). Measurement in child abuse research: A survey of researchers. *The APSAC Advisor, 8,* 7–10.

Harter, S., Alexander, P. C., & Neimeyer, R. A. (1988). Long-term effects of incestuous child abuse in college women: Social adjustment, social cognition, and family characteristics. *Journal of Consulting and Clinical Psychology, 56,* 5–8.

Hovestadt, A. J., Anderson, W. T., Piercy, F. P., Cochran, S. W., & Fine, M. (1985). A Family-of-Origin Scale. *Journal of Marital and Family Therapy, 11*(3), 287–297.

Hudson, W. W., Wung, B., & Borges, M. (1980). Parent–child relationship disorders: The parent's point of view. *Journal of Social Service Research, 3,* 283–294.

Kahn, T. (1991). *Pathways: A guided workbook for youth beginning treatment.* Orwell, VT: Safer Society Press.

Kelly, R. (1982). Behavioral reorientation of pedophiliacs: Can it be done? *Clinical Psychology Review, 2,* 387–408.

Kendall, P. C. (1994). Treating anxiety disorders in children: Results of a randomized clinical trial. *Journal of Consulting and Clinical Psychology, 62,* 100–110.

Kendall, P. C., & Braswell, L. (1993). *Cognitive–behavioral therapy for impulsive children* (2nd ed.). New York: Guilford Press.

Kendall-Tackett, K., Williams, L., & Finkelhor, D. (1993). Impact of sexual abuse on children: A review and synthesis of recent empirical studies. *Psychological Bulletin, 113*, 164–180.

Kilpatrick, D. G., Edmunds, C. N., & Seymour, A. K. (1992). *Rape in America: A report to the nation.* National Victim Center.

Kolko, D. J., & Swenson, C. C. (1996, January). *Psychosocial evaluation and treatment of physically abused children.* Workshop presented at the San Diego Conference on Responding to Child Maltreatment, San Diego, CA.

Kovacs, M. (1992). *The Children's Depression Inventory.* North Tonawanda, NY: Multihealth Systems.

Lang, P. J. (1979). A bio-informational theory of emotional imagery. *Psychophysiology, 16*, 495–511.

Lang, R., Pugh, G., & Langevin, R. (1988). Treatment of incest and pedophilic offenders: A pilot study. *Behavioral Sciences and the Law; 6*, 239–255.

Lanktree, C. B., Briere, J., & Hernandez, P. (1991, August). Further data on the Trauma Symptom Checklist for Children (TSC-C): Reliability; validity and sensitivity to treatment. Paper presented at the annual meeting of the American Psychological Association, San Francisco.

Letourneau, E. J., & Saunders, B. E. (1996). Measurement and assessment tools: New section—introduction. *The APSAC Advisor, 9*, 8–10.

Lipovsky, J. A. (1991). Posttraumatic stress disorder in children. *Family Community Health, 14*, 42–51.

Lipovsky, J. A., & Elliott, A. N. (1993). Individual treatment of the sexually abused child. *The APSAC Advisor, 6*, 1–18.

Lipovsky, J. A., & Hanson, R. F. (1992a, October). Multiple traumas in the histories of child/adolescent psychiatric inpatients. Paper presented at the annual meeting of the International Society for Traumatic Stress Studies, Los Angeles.

Lipovsky, J. A., & Hanson, R. F. (1992b, November). Traumatic event histories of child adolescent psychiatric inpatients: What is being done to our children? Paper presented at the annual meeting of the Association for the Advancement of Behavior Therapy, Boston.

Lipovsky, J. A., Hanson, R. F., & Hand, L. (1993, January). Sexual abuse, physical abuse, and witnessing violence in child/adolescent psychiatric inpatients: Relationship to psychopathology. Paper presented at the San Diego Conference on Responding to Child Maltreatment, San Diego, CA.

Lipovsky, J. A., & Saunders, B. E. (1989, November). Characteristics of incest families and victim emotional responses. Paper presented at the annual meeting of the American Criminology Society, Reno, NV.

Lipovsky, J. A., Saunders, B. E., & Hanson, R. F. (1992). Parent–child relationships of victims and siblings in incest families. *Journal of Child Sexual Abuse, 1*, 35–50.

Lipovsky, J. A., Saunders, B. E., & Murphy, S. M. (1989). Depression, anxiety, and behavior problems among victims of father–child sexual assault and nonabused siblings. *Journal of Interpersonal Violence, 4*, 452–468.

Lutzker, J. R., Bigelow, K. M., Swenson, C. C., Doctor, R. M., & Kessler, M. L. (in press). Problems related to child abuse and neglect. In S. Netherton, D. Holmes, & C. E. Walker (Eds.), *Comprehensive textbook of child and adolescent disorders: A guide to DSM-IV.*

Mannarino, A. P., Cohen, J. A., & Berman, S. R. (1994). *Journal of Clinical Child Psychology, 23*, 204–211.

Mannarino, A. P., Cohen, J. A., Smith, J. A., & Moore-Motily, S. (1991). Six- and twelve-month follow-up of sexually abused girls. *Journal of Interpersonal Violence, 6*, 494–511.

Marshall, W. L., & Barbaree, H. E. (1988). The long-term evaluation of a behavioral treatment program for child molesters. *Behaviour Research and Therapy, 26*, 499–511.

McCurdy, K., & Daro, D. (1994). Child maltreatment: A national survey of reports and fatalities. *Journal of Interpersonal Violence, 9*, 75–94.

Meinig, M. B., & Bonner, B. L. (1990). Returning the treated sex offender to the family. *Violence Update, 1*, 1–11.

Moos, R. H., & Moos, B. S. (1981). Family Environment Scale Manual. Palo Alto: Consulting Psychologists Press.

Moos, R. H., & Moos, B. S. (1983). Adaptation and the quality of life in work and family settings. *Journal of Community Psychology, 11*, 158–170.

Moos, R. H., & Moos, B. S. (1990). Conceptual and empirical approaches to developing family-based assessment procedures: Resolving the case of the Family Environment Scale. *Family Process, 29*, 199–208.

O'Donohue, W. T., & Elliott, A. N. (1992). Treatment of the sexually abused child: A review. *Journal of Clinical Child Psychology, 21*, 218–228.

Ollendick, T. H., & Cerny, J. A. (1981). *Clinical behavior therapy with children.* New York: Plenum Press.

Parker, H., & Parker, S. (1986). Father–daughter sexual abuse: An emerging perspective. *American Journal of Orthopsychiatry, 56,* 531–549.

Piers, E. V. (1984). *Piers-Harris Children's Self-Concept Scale. Revised Manual, 1984.* Los Angeles: Western Psychological Services.

Reynolds, C. R., & Paget, K. D. (1981). Factor analysis of the Revised Children's Manifest Anxiety Scale for blacks, whites, males and females. *Journal of Consulting and Clinical Psychology, 49,* 352–359.

Reynolds, C. R., & Richmond, B. O. (1978). "What I Think and Feel": A revised measure of children's manifest anxiety. *Journal of Abnormal Child Psychology, 6,* 271–280.

Ribbe, D. P., Lipovsky, J. A., & Freedy, J. R. (1995). Posttraumatic stress disorder. In A. R. Eisen, C. A. Kaemey, & C. E. Schaeffer (Eds.), *Clinical Handbook of Anxiety Disorders in Children and Adolescents* (pp. 317–356). Northvale, NJ: Jason Aronson.

Ribordy, S. C. (1990). Treating intrafamilial child sexual abuse from a systemic perspective. *Journal of Psychotherapy and the Family, 6,* 71–88.

Rice, M. E., Quinsey, V. L., & Harris, G. T. (1991). Sexual recidivism among child molesters released from a maximum security psychiatric institution. *Journal of Consulting and Clinical Psychology, 59,* 381–386.

Saunders, B. E., McClure, S. M., & Murphy, S. M. (1986). *Profile of incest offenders indicating treatability—Part I: Final report submitted to the U. S. Department of the Navy.* Unpublished manuscript.

Saunders, B. E., McClure, S. M., & Murphy, S. M. (1987, July). Structure, function, and symptoms in father–daughter sexual abuse families: A multilevel-multirespondent empirical assessment. Paper presented at the Family Violence Research Conference, Durham, NH.

Saunders, B. E., & Schuchts, R. A. (1987). Assessing parent–child relationships: A report of normative scores and revalidation of two clinical scales. *Family Process, 26,* 373–381.

Saylor, C. F., Swenson, C. C., Stokes, S. J., Wertlieb, D., & Casto, Y. (1994, August). The Pediatric Emotional Distress Scale: A brief new screening measure. Paper presented at the annual meeting of the American Psychological Association, Los Angeles.

Sgroi, S. M. (1982). *Handbook of clinical intervention in child sexual abuse.* Lexington, MA: Lexington Books.

Shapiro, J. P. (1989). Self-blame versus helplessness in sexually abused children: An attributional analysis with treatment recommendations. *Journal of Social and Clinical Psychology, 8,* 442–455.

Silovsky, J. F., & Hembree-Kigin, T. L. (1994). Family and group treatment for sexually abused children: A review. *Journal of Child Sexual Abuse, 3,* 1–20.

Smiljanich, K., & Briere, J. (1993, August). Sexual abuse history and trauma symptoms in a university sample. Paper presented at the annual meeting of the American Psychological Association, Toronto, Ontario, Canada.

Sorenson, T., & Snow, B. (1991). How children tell: The process of disclosure in child sexual abuse. *Child Welfare League of America, 70,* 3–15.

Spielberger, C. C. (1973). *Preliminary manual for the State–Trait Anxiety Inventory for Children* ("How I Feel Questionnaire"). Palo Alto, CA: Consulting Psychologists Press.

Stauffer, L. B., & Deblinger, E. (1996). Cognitive behavioral groups for nonoffending mothers and their young sexually abused children: A preliminary treatment outcome study. *Child Maltreatment, 1,* 65–76.

Swenson, C. C. (1996, February). Group treatment for physically abused children. Workshop presented at the second annual Colloquium of the South Carolina Professional Society on the Abuse of Children, Charleston, SC.

Swenson, C. C., Saylor, C. F., Stokes, S., Ralston, M. E., Smith, D. E., Hanson, R. F., & Saunders, B. E. (1994, January). Anxiety and fear in traumatized children: The validity of a new brief screening instrument. Paper presented at the San Diego Conference on Responding to Child Maltreatment, San Diego, CA.

Tong, L., Oakes, K., & McDowell, M. (1987). Personality development following sexual abuse. *Child Abuse & Neglect, 11,* 371–383.

Williams, L. M., & Finkelhor, D. (1990). The characteristics of incestuous fathers: A review of recent studies. In W. L. Marshall, D. R. Laws, & H. E. Barbaree (Eds.). *Handbook of sexual assault: Issues, theories, and treatment of the offender* (pp. 231–255). New York: Plenum Press.

Wolfe, D., Sas, L., & Wekerle, C. (1994). Factors associated with the development of posttraumatic stress disorder among child victims of sexual assault. *Child Abuse & Neglect, 18,* 37–50.

Wolfe, V. V., & Gentile, C. (1992). Psychological assessment of sexually abused children. In W. T. O'Donohue and J. H. Geer (Eds.), *The sexual abuse of children: Theory, research, and therapy* (pp. 143–187). Hillsdale, NJ: Erlbaum.

Wolfe, V. V., Gentile, C., Michienczi, T., Sas, L, & Wolfe, D. A. (1991). The Children's Impact of Traumatic Events Scale: A measure of post-sexual abuse PTSD symptoms. *Behavioral Assessment, 13,* 358–383.

Wolfe, V. V., Gentile, C., & Wolfe, D. A., (1989). The impact of sexual abuse on children: A PTSD formulation. *Behavior Therapy, 20,* 215–228.

21

School-Based Child Sexual Abuse Prevention Programs
Questions, Answers, and More Questions

SANDY K. WURTELE

INTRODUCTION AND OVERVIEW OF CHAPTER

In response to the growing awareness of the extent and consequences of child sexual abuse (CSA: see Chapter 20), many programs to prevent its occurrence have been developed and disseminated since the 1980s. In contrast to efforts to prevent the physical abuse or neglect of children (which attempt to modify adult behavior), the focus of CSA prevention efforts has been primarily to alter the knowledge and skills of children, through group-based instruction on personal safety, usually conducted in educational (preschool or elementary school) settings.

School-based personal safety programs have been widely distributed. In 1989, 36% of states mandated school-based CSA prevention (Kohl, 1993). Surveys of school administrators have found that 48% to 85% of school districts offer CSA prevention programs (Daro, 1994: Helge, 1992). Over 90% of teachers across the country viewed school-based CSA prevention programs as valuable and effective in one survey (Abrahams, Casey, & Daro, 1992), and in another, 96% of elementary school principals rated the provision of CSA prevention education as average to above average in importance (Romano, Casey, & Daro, 1990). Parents have also been in favor of personal safety programs. For example, our local survey of parents of preschool-aged children found them to be supportive of including CSA prevention programs in preschools, and a majority (84%) indicated that they would be either somewhat or very likely to allow their children to participate in a CSA prevention program (Wurtele, Kvaternick, & Franklin, 1992). And children do participate in these programs. Finkelhor and Dziuba-Leatherman (1995) surveyed 2,000 young people between the ages of 10 and 16, finding that 67% of the

SANDY K. WURTELE • Psychology Department, University of Colorado, Colorado Springs, Colorado 80933-7150.

Handbook of Child Abuse Research and Treatment, edited by Lutzker. Plenum Press, New York, 1998.

respondents reported having participated in a school-based antivictimization program at some time in their educational careers.

Clearly, child-focused, group-based CSA prevention programs have become the strategy of choice used by communities to protect children from being sexually abused. This widespread adoption notwithstanding, concerns remain about this approach. The purpose of this chapter is to present and address some of those concerns. The format of the chapter is as follows. A number of questions typical of those asked by both proponents and critics of CSA prevention programs will be posed, followed by responses to each question with reference to the extant literature.

What Are the Objectives of CSA Prevention Programs?

The primary focus of CSA prevention programs is to strengthen a child's ability to recognize and resist assault (primary prevention), although they often have a secondary prevention focus as well (Miller-Perrin & Wurtele, 1988). The secondary prevention objective is to encourage victims to disclose abuse and to improve adults' responses to these disclosures so that children can receive early intervention and protection to reduce the negative consequences of sexual exploitation.

Although the programs vary widely in their length, target group, instructors, and presentation formats (e.g., films/videotapes, theatrical productions, discussions, behavioral skills training), most have these objectives in common: (1) helping children to *recognize* potentially abusive situations, (2) teaching children to try to *resist* by saving "no" and removing themselves from the potential perpetrator, (3) encouraging children to *report* previous or ongoing abuse to an authority figure, and (4) *reassuring* them that abuse is never a child's fault. Thus, classroom-based curricula most likely emphasize training in these four "R's (Recognize, Resist, Report, Reassure). Along with skills, these programs also attempt to enhance children's knowledge about CSA by teaching various concepts (e.g., that both boys and girls can be victims; that familiar adults or relatives can be perpetrators). Another concept taught in many programs is body ownership, that is, teaching children that they are in charge of their bodies. For example, in our program we teach children that their bodies are special, and that each child is the "boss" of his or her body, meaning that they can make the rules about who can touch their bodies.

Have the Programs Been Successful in Teaching Children to Recognize Abuse?

The first major skill objective is to help children recognize potentially abusive situations, so that they will know when to apply the other resistance skills. Achieving this first objective is imperative; warnings can be effective only if children have a clear idea about what they are being warned of. Unfortunately, meeting this first objective has proved to be problematic.

Recognizing or defining CSA is difficult for a number of reasons. All definitions of CSA are time- and culture-bound, as well as direct reflections of the values of communities and societies at large. In some societies, sexualized behavior, such as fondling or kissing genitals, are normative child-rearing practices. In other societies, sexual contact between adults and children occur during religious or ceremonial events (Korbin, 1990). Definitions of CSA also depend on the perception of the observer, including biases of an individual's personal values and professional training and experience. Wurtele and Miller-Perrin (1992) describe how professionals (from medicine, law, mental health, and social work), researchers, members of the general public, developers of prevention programs, and children all have different definitions of CSA.

Given these differing definitions of CSA, it comes as no surprise that programs define sexual abuse in different ways. Some programs teach children that sexual abuse is when children are forced or tricked into sexual contact. Others include information about a perpetrator's motivation or intentions (e.g., "sexual abuse is the use of a child for the sexual gratification of an adult"). The majority of prevention programs use the concepts of "touches" and "feelings" to explain abuse (Tharinger et al., 1988). Here, children are taught about good, bad, and confusing touches, and the feelings resulting from these touches. They are then taught to use their feelings to decide whether a touch is appropriate or inappropriate (e.g., program participants are taught to say "no" to any touch that makes them feel uneasy, uncomfortable, or confused). But, there is concern about young children's abilities to use their feelings to recognize abuse. Wurtele, Kast, Miller-Perrin, and Kondrick (1989) compared the effectiveness of the feelings approach with a rule-based approach, where preschool-aged children were taught to follow a body safety rule: "It is not okay for a bigger person to touch or look at my private parts (unless I need help, like if my private parts are hurt or sick)." Children taught using the feelings approach were less able to distinguish between appropriate and inappropriate touches compared with children who were taught the body safety rule.

Our research also shows that before participating in a personal safety program, few young children are able to recognize inappropriate touch requests. This finding underscores the naïveté of young children and their possible vulnerability to sexual abuse. Following program participation, however, children have improved in their ability to recognize inappropriate touches. Typically, the recognition skill is measured by describing various touch requests to the child, and asking him or her to define the appropriateness of the request. Children's ability to recognize unsafe situations has been demonstrated with both school-aged children (Blumberg, Chadwick, Fogarty, Speth, & Chadwick, 1991; Hazzard, Webb, Kleemeier, Angert, & Pohl, 1991; Swan, Press, & Briggs, 1985), and 3–6-year-old children (Harvey, Forehand, Brown, & Holmes, 1988; Peraino, 1990; Ratto & Bogat, 1990; Sarno & Wurtele, 1997; Stilwell, Lutzker, & Greene, 1988; Wurtele, 1990; Wurtele, 1993b; Wurtele, Currier, Gillispie, & Franklin, 1991; Wurtele, Gillispie, Currier, & Franklin, 1992; Wurtele, Kast, & Melzer, 1992; Wurtele et al., 1989). Thus, the ability to discriminate between appropriate and inappropriate touching of the genitals improves more when young children are taught using a rule-based (as opposed to a feelings-based) approach (Blumberg et al., 1991; Wurtele et al., 1989).

Have the Programs Been Successful in Teaching Children to Resist Abuse?

The second skill objective of a prevention program is to teach some form of self-protection, usually some verbal skill (e.g., saying "no," yelling, or threatening to tell), and some behavioral skill (e.g., trying to get away, or, more rarely, fighting back). To measure these skills, researchers often use written, verbal, or videotaped vignettes in which hypothetical abusive situations are described to the children and their responses to potential perpetrators are solicited. After participating in a personal safety program, school-aged children's scores on these measures (say "no," get away) improve significantly (Kolko, Moser, & Hughes, 1989; Saslawsky & Wurtele, 1986), as do scores for younger children (Harvey et al., 1988; Miltenberger & Thiesse-Duffy, 1988; Nemerofsky, Carran, & Rosenberg, 1994; Nibert, Cooper, Ford, Fitch, & Robinson, 1989; Ratto & Bogat, 1990; Sarno & Wurtele, 1997; Stilwell et al., 1988; Wurtele, 1990; Wurtele, 1993b, Wurtele et al., 1989, 1991; Wurtele, Gillispie, et al., 1992; Wurtele, Kast, et al., 1992; Wurtele, Marrs, & Miller-Perrin, 1987). Resistance skill scores are higher when children participate in active-learning programs that provide multiple opportunities for children to practice the skills during the program (Blumberg et al., 1991; Wurtele et al., 1987).

It must be noted, however, that not all children achieve criterion performances (e.g., Harbeck, Peterson, & Starr, 1992; Kraizer, Witte, & Fryer, 1989; Sarno & Wurtele, 1997; Stilwell et al., 1988: Wurtele et al., 1991). Program impact on resistance skills may be enhanced by employing active learning techniques (e.g., practicing self-protective skills in response to role-plays), extending the training, using multiple trainers in multiple settings, and including periodic reviews (e.g., booster sessions). Research is also needed to determine which skills are learned by which type of student.

Because of practical and ethical considerations, little research has been conducted on whether children actually use the skills in real-life abusive situations. A few researchers have used confederates to role-play inappropriate advances and then measured children's responses (Harbeck et al., 1992; Kraizer et al., 1989; Stilwell et al., 1988). Kraizer and colleagues (1989) found strong effects on their skills measure for young children, whereas children's performances during role-plays were less effective in the other two studies. The discrepancy most likely was due to the heavy emphasis on practicing these skills in the Kraizer and associates (1989) program as opposed to the more passive instruction provided in the others.

Using an alternative strategy to measure resistance skills, Finkelhor and his colleagues telephoned a nationally representative sample of 2,000 young people between the ages of 10 and 16. Youth were asked about their experiences with and responses to actual or threatened sexual assaults. Among their survey respondents, a surprisingly high number (40%) of them reported specific instances where they used the information or skills taught in an antivictimization program to protect themselves (Finkelhor & Dziuba-Leatherman, 1995). Victimized and threatened children were more likely to use self-protection strategies if they had received comprehensive prevention instruction, which included opportunities to practice the skills in class, multiday presentations, and materials to take home to discuss with their parents (Finkelhor, Asdigian, & Dziuba-Leatherman, 1995).

Interestingly, the most frequently used self-protection responses reported by the youth were generally not those taught in prevention programs. Only a minority of children used the strategies taught in prevention programs, such as yelling, threatening to tell, or running away. Instead, boys, especially teenaged boys, used more aggressive forms of resistance (get away, fight back, threaten to harm the perpetrator), and viewed those strategies as being more effective, relative to younger boys and girls (Asdigian & Finkelhor, 1995). Although program developers need to heed these researchers' advice that "prevention messages sent by educators may need to be tailored to specific subgroups of children, such as boys and girls and younger and older children" (p. 413), they are less likely to follow the suggestion to encourage children to fight back. Teaching self-defense skills as part of prevention continues to be controversial. The concern has been that fighting back may put children at greater risk for injury, may make children overly confident, and it may also promote the aggressive and pro-violence orientation to which many prevention advocates are opposed. There is also evidence that children taught self-defense skills may use them in inappropriate circumstances (Nibert, Cooper, Ford, et al., 1989).

Have the Programs Been Successful in Teaching Children to Report Abuse?

The third skill objective of most personal safety programs is to encourage children to report past or ongoing abuse. One method of assessing this skill is to ask children whether they would tell someone if they were involved in an abusive situation. After participating in personal safety programs, preschool- and school-aged children indicate a greater willingness to tell (Binder & McNiel, 1987; Kolko, Moser, Litz, & Hughes, 1987; Sarno & Wurtele, 1997; Swan et al., 1985; Wolfe, MacPherson, Blount, & Wolfe, 1986; Wurtele, 1990, 1993b; Wurtele et al., 1991; Wurtele, Gillispie, et al., 1992). However, preschool-aged children have difficulty describing the abusive situation to the resource person (Ratto & Bogat, 1990; Stilwell et al., 1988; Wurtele, 1990; Wurtele et al., 1991).

Another way to determine whether these programs are facilitating reporting is to present information on unsolicited disclosures. Unfortunately, very few researchers have reported disclosures occurring during or after the program, despite their importance as a secondary prevention method. Published disclosure rates immediately following the program have ranged from a low of 0% (Gilbert, Berrick, Le Prohn, & Nyman, 1989; Hill & Jason, 1987), to over 5% (Hazzard et al., 1991), to a high of 11% (Kolko et al., 1989). The 11% figure is quite impressive, given that sexually abused children rarely disclose purposefully (Sorenson & Snow, 1991). Nevertheless, program evaluators are urged to document the frequency, type, and consequences of disclosures, to better determine the secondary prevention efficacy of these programs.

Do These Programs Enhance Children's Knowledge about CSA?

Although the actual questions included in knowledge measures depend on the content of the program, children are usually queried about their knowledge of what the names of body parts are, who strangers, perpetrators, and victims are, what secrets should or should not be kept, whether children always have to obey grown-ups, what is meant by sexual abuse, whether sexual abuse happens only to girls, and whether abuse is ever the child's fault. Three commonly used knowledge measures with demonstrated psychometric properties include our 13-item Personal Safety Questionnaire (Saslawsky & Wurtele, 1986), Tutty's (1992) 40-item Children's Knowledge of Abuse Questionnaire (and its latest 24-item revision; Tutty, 1995), and the 25-item "What I Know About Touching Scale" (Hazzard et al., 1991).

School-aged and preschool-aged children demonstrate enhanced knowledge about CSA prevention concepts following program participation, with younger children having lower knowledge scores, compared with older children. In their meta-analysis of CSA prevention evaluation studies, Berrick and Barth (1992) reported large effect sizes for both preschool-aged children ($d = .86$) and elementary school-aged children ($d = .98$). Knowledge gains have also been shown to be maintained for periods up to 3 months (Ratto & Bogat, 1990; Saslawsky & Wurtele, 1986; Wurtele, Saslawsky, Miller, Marrs, & Britcher, 1986), 5–6 months (Kolko et al., 1987, 1989: Tutty, 1992; Wurtele, Kast, et al., 1992), and 1 year (Briggs & Hawkins, 1994; Hazzard et al., 1991).

Most of these evaluations utilize average or composite scores. Although composite scores describe the overall effect of a program, they do not tell us the extent to which children understand certain concepts. In order to determine whether there are certain concepts that children at certain ages or after participating in certain programs are not comprehending, researchers are encouraged to also report item analyses (see Tutty, 1992, 1994, for examples).

Have the Programs Been Successful in Reassuring Children that Abuse Is Never the Child's Fault?

Reassuring children that abuse is never the child's fault is a concept taught in most personal safety programs and it has been included in several knowledge questionnaires. As noted above, the use of average or composite scores obscures children's performances on individual items, including those items measuring children's perceptions of fault or blame. In the few published reports where children's responses to this item were analyzed separately, children's postprogram responses indicated an understanding that they are not to be blamed for abuse (e.g., Currier & Wurtele, 1996; Sarno & Wurtele, 1997; Tutty, 1994; Wurtele, 1993b; Wurtele et al., 1991). One exception was the first-grade children in the Tutty (1994) research, who were more likely at the posttest to believe it is a child's fault if abuse occurs. Perhaps the 45-minute play was not potent enough to overcome young children's tendency to employ the concept of immanent justice. Given the importance of the fault/blame concept, researchers are urged to analyze children's responses separately.

Do These Programs Actually Prevent Sexual Victimization?

One way to answer this question is to monitor incidence rates; if programs are effective, then CSA incidence rates should decrease over time. To date, there is no evidence suggesting that these programs are helping to decrease the incidence of CSA. Given the low base rate of sexual abuse, answering this important question would require following very large samples of trained and untrained children and documenting a lower incidence of abuse among the former. At this point, the degree to which programs actually reduce the incidence of CSA is an unanswered empirical question. Rather than mislead the public and raise false hopes about what these programs can do, Wurtele and Miller-Perrin (1992) suggest that these programs be referred to as "personal safety programs," a descriptor that more accurately (and humbly) reflects the content and outcomes of these programs. In reality, these programs teach knowledge and strategies that *may* prevent CSA.

Do These Programs Have Any Negative Side Effects?

A major concern has been whether children can learn about sexual abuse and its prevention without becoming upset, frightened, or suspicious of nurturing touch. Critics also contend that CSA prevention programs might harm children's normal sexual development. The suggestion is that these programs cause more harm than good (Reppucci & Haugaard, 1989). In this section, the evidence concerning possible negative side effects of CSA prevention programs is reviewed.

Anxiety

When researchers have administered anxiety measures to program participants (whether measures of general anxiety or program-specific anxiety), none of them have found significant increases in anxiety (Hazzard et al., 1991; Ratto & Bogat, 1990; Wurtele et al., 1989; Wurtele & Miller-Perrin, 1987). When researchers have asked children whether the program made them feel worried or scared, the percentages of children responding "yes" have ranged from 11% (Hazzard, Kleemeier, & Webb, 1990) to more than half (Finkelhor & Dziuba-Leatherman, 1995; Garbarino, 1987). At first glance, the latter statistic is troubling, but neither study employed pretests or control programs. Thus, we do not know what percentage of nonprogram children would report fear of being abused, but in today's violent world, chances are the percentages would be just as high, if not higher. It is also interesting to note that those children who reported increased levels of fear and anxiety in the study by Finkelhor and Dziuba-Leatherman (1995) were also the ones who rated the programs most positively and were the ones most likely to use the skills taught in the programs. The authors suggested that these higher anxiety ratings reflect that the children were taking the message of the training seriously, and they concluded in urging professionals to refrain "from assuming that reports of increased fear and anxiety are a negative outcome of training programs" (p. 137).

Acting Out

When parents and teachers have been asked to report on adverse reactions among the children, few parents report observing problems (e.g., 3% in Finkelhor & Dziuba-Leatherman, 1995; 5% in Swan et al., 1985 and Hazzard et al., 1991; 7% in Nibert, Cooper, & Ford, 1989). Likewise, teachers and parents noticed few, if any, signs of increased emotional distress in several studies (Binder & McNiel, 1987; Wurtele, 1990, 1993b; Wurtele et al., 1989; Wurtele, Gillispie, et al., 1992; Wurtele, Kast, et al., 1992).

Overgeneralization

Another concern about CSA prevention programs is that program participants will overgeneralize the rules and concepts learned, and will thus become oversensitive to situations involving appropriate touch. The fear is that such overgeneralization could lead to false CSA allegations (Krivacska, 1989). One strategy to address the concern about overgeneralization has been to gather information on children's abilities to recognize appropriate touches, before and after a program. It is reassuring that children's appropriate-touch recognition scores do not decrease significantly, and have, in some instances, even increased significantly (Blumberg et al., 1991; Wurtele, 1993b). Thus, most children do not overgeneralize their recognition skills to hypothetical appropriate-touch requests, suggesting that program participants are not likely to misinterpret nurturing touches or make false accusations of CSA. This conclusion is bolstered by the fact that there are no published accounts of false accusations following a personal safety program.

Negative Effects on Sexual Development

The concern has been expressed that CSA prevention programs might harm children's normal sexual development (e.g., Krivacska, 1990). Unfortunately, few researchers have assessed children's knowledge about and attitudes toward their own sexuality so as to be able to address this concern. There is, however, a growing body of literature showing that personal safety programs may actually enhance young children's sexual development. For example, there is evidence that these programs can teach young children (3- to 5-year-olds) the anatomically correct terminology for their genitals (Wurtele, 1993a; Wurtele, Melzer, & Kast, 1992), and that after participating in the program significantly more children say they like their private parts (suggesting increased body pride) and also say it is acceptable for them to touch their own private parts (Wurtele, 1993a, b; Wurtele et al., 1991; Wurtele, Kast, et al., 1992). It must be recognized, however, that most CSA prevention programs avoid discussion of sexuality of adults or children. This avoidance is often done intentionally—to enhance community acceptance and avert conflict with schools and parents. Clearly, research is needed to determine how these programs affect older children and adolescents in terms of their sexual development.

Do These Programs Have Any Positive Side Effects?

Several researchers have found what might be considered positive side effects. For example, Binder and McNiel (1987) reported that 64% of the children in their study said that the program made them feel much safer (as did 71% of the children in Hazzard et al., 1990), and 72% felt better able to protect themselves. Finkelhor and Dziuba-Leatherman (1995) found that 95% of youth who participated in a school-based antivictimization program said they would recommend it to other children, and those who reported being victimized or threatened perceived themselves as having been more effective in keeping themselves safe and minimizing their harm.

Another positive side effect has been the consistent finding that after participating in a program, children are more likely to discuss the contents of the program with their parents (Binder & McNiel, 1987; Finkelhor et al., 1995; Hazzard et al., 1991; Kolko et al., 1987; Wurtele, 1990; Wurtele et al., 1989; Wurtele & Miller-Perrin, 1987). Increasing parent–child communication about CSA not only reduces the secrecy surrounding this topic, but also increases the effectiveness of school-based personal safety instruction (Finkelhor et al., 1995; Wurtele, Kast, et al., 1992).

Are These Programs Effective with Young Children?

Although young children are at particular risk for sexual abuse, critics of child-focused CSA prevention programs have asserted that preschoolers and kindergartners cannot learn CSA prevention concepts because of their limited cognitive abilities (Gilbert et al., 1989; Reppucci & Haugaard 1989). Krivacska (1990) has claimed that "below the age of 7, instruction in CSA concepts is contraindicated" (p. 67). Granted, early research showed that 3–5-year-old children achieved few, if any, knowledge gains (e.g., Borkin & Frank, 1986; Christian, Dwyer, Schumm, & Coulson, 1988; Conte, Rosen, Saperstein, & Shermack, 1985; Gilbert et al., 1989). However, more recent, methodologically rigorous studies demonstrate that children as young as $3^1/_2$ years do indeed benefit from these programs in terms of both knowledge and skill acquisition (Harvey et al., 1988; Kraizer et al., 1989; Miltenberger & Thiesse-Duffy, 1988; Nemerofsky et al., 1994; Nilbert, Cooper, Ford, et al., 1989; Peraino, 1990; Ratto & Bogat, 1990; Sarno & Wurtele, 1997; Stilwell et al., 1988; Wurtele, 1990, 1993b; Wurtele et al., 1987 1989, 1991; Wurtele, Gillispie, et al., 1992; Wurtele, Kast, et al., 1992). With young children, knowledge and skill gains are more likely to be achieved when programs teach concrete concepts, and include active learning (rehearsal, role-play), repetition, multiple sessions. and teacher/parent education.

Although younger children can benefit from participating in personal safety programs, it must be acknowledged that they generally learn less from these programs compared with older children. In studies that compared responses of children from different age groups, older children knew more initially and learned more of the concepts, compared with younger children (Binder & McNiel, 1987; Blumberg et al., 1991; Borkin & Frank, 1986; Conte et al., 1985; Harbeck et al., 1992; Hazzard et al., 1991; Liang, Bogat, & McGrath, 1993; Nemerofsky et al., 1994; Saslawsky & Wurtele, 1986; Tutty, 1992; Wurtele et al., 1986, 1991). The one exception was a study by Kraizer et al. (1989) in which preschoolers and kindergartners showed greater gains in knowledge compared with first-, second-, and third-graders. Given these consistent effects for age, programs and evaluation instruments must be tailored to the developmental needs of the audience. The same program should not be used in the same manner with children of varying ages.

Are These Programs Successful with Special Needs Children?

It has been proposed that special needs children are at higher risk for sexual abuse because their handicapping conditions (e.g., mental retardation, communication problems) make it difficult for them to protect themselves or to report maltreatment. Their greater dependency on caregivers, inability to differentiate basic assistance with personal care from sexual exploitation, desire to be accepted, and unquestioning compliance may also make them more vulnerable (Brookhauser, Sullivan, Scanlan, & Garbarino, 1986; Cole, 1984–1986; Cruz, Price-Williams, & Andron, 1988; Moglia, 1986; Ryerson, 1984; Sobsey & Mansell, 1990; Tharinger, Horton, & Millea, 1990). Although prevention curricula have been developed for youth with various disabilities (Dreyer & Haseltine, 1986; Krents & Atkins, 1985; LaBarre, Hinkley, & Nelson, 1986; O'Day, 1983; Seattle Rape Relief, 1980), these programs have rarely been evaluated. Haseltine and Miltenberger (1990) demonstrated the effectiveness of a 9-week behavioral skills training curriculum for teaching self-protection skills to young adults with mild to moderate mental retardation. Researchers are urged to evaluate other programs designed for special needs children.

Although not usually considered "special needs" children, there is a concern about how sexually abused children would react to a personal safety program. Evaluating sexually abused children's responses to a personal safety program is important for several reasons. First, given that many children experience sexual abuse, it is quite likely that abused children are in the audience and are being exposed to personal safety programs designed primarily for use with nonsexually abused children. Second, sexually abused children's conceptions of personal safety violations differ from those of their nonsexually abused counterparts due to the former's experience with sexual exploitation (Miller-Perrin, Wurtele, & Kondrick, 1990). Thus, children who have experienced sexual abuse may respond differently to a personal safety program than would nonsexually abused children. Third, prevention programs insensitive to the special needs of victims may be placing such children at risk for developing anxiety, guilt, sexual acting out, or confusion about appropriate touches. And finally, given that victims of sexual abuse are at risk for revictimization (Boney-McCoy & Finkelhor, 1995; Browne & Finkelhor, 1986), there is a need to educate these children about personal safety.

To address this concern, Currier and Wurtele (1996) compared 13 sexually abused and 13 nonsexually abused children's responses to a personal safety program taught by their parents (or caretakers). Both groups of children demonstrated significant increases in skill and knowledge scores following the program. Both groups of children improved significantly in their recognition of inappropriate touches and in all four resisting/reporting skills. Both groups also improved in their recognition that abuse is not a child's fault. More than half (54%) of the sexually abused children disclosed information about their abuse after they had completed the program. No negative reactions to the program were observed by the parents, and sexually abused children exhibited fewer inappropriate sexual behaviors following program participation. Although the small sample size limits the generalizability of the findings, this preliminary investigation suggests that young sexually abused children can learn personal safety concepts and skills, and can do so without exhibiting negative effects.

Should This Topic Be Conveyed to Children by Their Parents?

Absolutely! But the reality is that relatively few parents discuss CSA with their children. Studies indicate that although the majority of parents report teaching their children general safety rules, very few discuss personal safety in particular (Berrick, 1988; Finkelhor, 1984; Porch & Petretic-Jackson, 1986; Wurtele & Miller-Perrin, 1987). Wurtele and Miller-Perrin (1992) review some of the reasons for parents' failure to discuss CSA with their children (e.g., not aware of the need for discussion, difficult subject to discuss, topic might frighten child, and lack of confidence, knowledge, vocabulary, or materials). This research suggests that parents need more information about CSA, as well as guidance in disseminating this information to their children.

Recently, prevention experts have urged that more attention be paid to involving parents as "partners in prevention" (Wurtele & Miller-Perrin, 1992). There are several potential advantages to such collaboration. The impact of a school-based curriculum depends on the support of parents at home. Parent support includes permitting their children to participate in the programs, clarifying concepts and correcting misconceptions, and helping children apply their new knowledge in daily life (Conte & Fogarty, 1989). Furthermore, if parents could be trained to be prevention educators, children would receive repeated exposure to prevention information in their natural environment, thus providing a series of booster sessions to supplement other prevention efforts. Indeed, Finkelhor and colleagues (1995) found that children who had received victimization prevention instruction from their parents (in addition to a school-based curriculum), had substantially more knowledge about CSA, made more use of self-protection strategies, were better able to thwart victimization attempts, and were more likely to disclose victimizations. In addition, we have found in several studies that parents (when provided with a script, materials, and encouragement) can be very effective personal safety instructors for their young children (Wurtele, 1993a, Wurtele et al., 1991; Wurtele, Gillispie, et al., 1992; Wurtele, Kast, et al., 1992; Wurtele, Melzer, et al., 1992). Given the numerous advantages of, and initial successes in, involving parents as "partners in prevention," researchers are urged to focus their efforts on ways to encourage parents (especially fathers) to become more involved.

What Role Should School-Based Programs Play in the Prevention of CSA?

Schools provide an appropriate setting for educating children about sexual abuse, given that their primary function is to inform and educate. Teachers have appeal as instructors, given their expertise as educators. Through their ongoing relationships with students and their families, they also play a key role in identifying and supporting abused children. School-based programs also have appeal because they are able to reach large numbers of children of every racial, ethnic, and socioeconomic group in a relatively cost-efficient fashion. A universal primary prevention strategy likewise eliminates the stigma of identifying specific children or families as being at risk for sexual abuse, and thus avoids costly and intrusive interventions into family privacy (Daro, 1994). The strategy of targeting the general population of children also reflects the fact that we lack clear explanatory models for sexual abuse. Although risk factors (personal and environmental) have been identified for other types of child maltreatment, similar prediction models are not yet available for sexual abuse. Finally, as described here, extant evaluations suggest that personal safety programs can teach children the knowledge and skills thought to be useful in avoiding sexual assault, and they can do so without increasing anxiety, acting out, or confusion about appropriate touch. There is also preliminary evidence that children are able to apply this information in real-life situations. Learning how to value and protect themselves are important lessons; children deserve this instruction. Clearly, child-focused personal safety programs play an important part in the effort to keep children safe from sexual victimization.

At the same time, the responsibility for preventing CSA must be shared. Programs must be developed to focus on audiences other than potential victims. As Plummer (1993) reminds us, "Children were never meant to accomplish [CSA] prevention single handed" (p. 296). There are numerous ways to expand the efforts to prevent CSA, and useful blueprints are available (e.g., Daro, 1994; Finkelhor, 1990; Tutty, 1991; Wurtele & Miller-Perrin, 1992). A variety of prevention strategies have been proposed (e.g., public awareness messages, treatment programs for male and female victims of CSA, comprehensive sexuality education for children and youth, training and education for professionals). The general public, professionals, and parents play important roles in this endeavor, but, unfortunately, these groups have not received as much attention as have children. It is clearly time to extend preventive efforts and target others, especially parents, to play a more active part in preventing CSA. Children should not shoulder the full responsibility for prevention.

CONCLUSION AND MORE QUESTIONS

School-based personal safety programs can teach children to distinguish between abusive and nonabusive situations, increase their knowledge, and enhance their skills. They can do so without producing negative side effects and may actually have positive side effects. But evidence for primary prevention is lacking, and support for secondary prevention efficacy is limited. Should they, therefore, be abolished? Although some critics might answer this question affirmatively, this author shouts a resounding "No!" What we should do, however, is view (and refer) to them more realistically as "personal safety" or "sexual abuse resistance education" programs. The importance of these types of programs is not lessened by a change of name; enhancing children's sense of body importance and personal safety are important goals in their own right.

Even with a more realistic descriptor, several questions about these programs remain unanswered. These questions include:

- How can these programs be more developmentally appropriate? What are the effects of different types of programs on different types of children (e.g., who vary in age, race, gender, socioeconomic status, intelligence, etc.)?
- How can these programs incorporate sexuality education? What are the effects of these programs on children's sexual attitudes and behaviors?
- Would these programs be more effective if they were integrated into a more comprehensive, multiyear curriculum focusing on "human relations training" (e.g., covering decision making, problem solving, empathy, impulse control, social skills, anger management, conflict resolution)?
- Do these programs result in the reporting of abuse? What types of assaults are children reporting? What are their responses to these assaults? Does the system respond sensitively to children's disclosures?
- How can more parents be educated simultaneously with their children? How can they be encouraged to be more involved? What should be included in parent-focused programs, and what are the most effective ways to inform parents? How can parents' abilities to nurture their children's healthy sexual development be strengthened?

These questions are raised not to imply that personal safety programs should be abolished, but are posed to challenge improvement. These questions demand the attention of program developers and evaluators. Children deserve no less!

REFERENCES

Abrahams, N., Casey, K., & Daro, D. (1992). Teachers' knowledge, attitudes, and beliefs about child abuse and its prevention. *Child Abuse & Neglect, 16*, 229–238.

Asdigian, N. L., & Finkelhor, D. (1995). What works for children in resisting assaults? *Journal of Interpersonal Violence, 10*, 402–418.

Berrick J. D. (1988). Parental involvement in child abuse prevention training: What do they learn? *Child Abuse & Neglect, 12*, 543–553.

Berrick, J. D., & Barth, R. P. (1992). Child sexual abuse prevention: Research review and recommendations. *Social Work Research & Abstracts, 28*, 6–15.

Binder, R. L., & McNiel, D. E. (1987). Evaluation of a school-based sexual abuse prevention program: Cognitive and emotional effects. *Child Abuse & Neglect, 11*, 497–506.

Blumberg, E. J., Chadwick, M. W., Fogarty, L. A., Speth, T. W., & Chadwick. D. L. (1991). The touch discrimination component of sexual abuse prevention training: Unanticipated positive consequences. *Journal of Interpersonal Violence, 6*, 12–28.

Boney-McCoy, S., & Finkelhor, D. (1995). Prior victimization: A risk factor for child sexual abuse and for PTSD-related symptomatology among sexually abused youth. *Child Abuse & Neglect, 19*, 1401–1421.

Borkin, J., & Frank, L. (1986). Sexual abuse prevention for preschoolers: A pilot program. *Child Welfare, 65*, 75–82.

Briggs, F., & Hawkins, R. M. F. (1994). Follow-up data on the effectiveness of New Zealand's national school based child protection program. *Child Abuse & Neglect,18*, 635–643.

Brookhouser, P. E., Sullivan, P., Scanlan, J. M., & Garbarino, J. (1986). Identifying the sexually abused deaf child: The otolaryngologist's role. *Laryngoscope, 96*, 152–158.

Brown, A., & Finkelhor, D. (1986). Impact of child sexual abuse: Offenders' attitudes about their efficacy. *Child Abuse & Neglect, 13*, 77–87.

Christian, R., Dwyer, S., Schumm, W. R., & Coulson, L. A. (1988). Prevention of sexual abuse for preschoolers: Evaluation of a pilot program. *Psychological Reports, 62*, 387–396.

Cole, S. S. (1984–1986). Facing the challenges of sexual abuse in persons with disabilities. *Sexuality and Disability, 7*, 71–87.

Conte, J. R., & Fogarty, L. A. (1989). Attitudes on sexual abuse prevention programs: A national survey of parents. (Available from J. R. Conte, School of Social Work, University of Washington, Mailstop 354900, 4101 15th Avenue N. E., Seattle, WA 98195-6299).

Conte, J. R., Rosen, C., Saperstein, L., & Shermack, R. (1985). An evaluation of a program to prevent the sexual victimization of young children. *Child Abuse & Neglect, 9*, 319–328.

Cruz, V. K., Price-Williams. D., & Andron, L. (1988). Developmentally disabled women who were molested as children. *Social Casework, 69*, 411-419.

Currier, L. L., & Wurtele, S. K. (1996). A pilot study of previously abused and non-sexually abused children's responses to a personal safety program. *Journal of Child Sexual Abuse, 5*, 71–87.

Daro, D. (1994). Prevention of child sexual abuse. *The Future of Children, 4*, 198–223.

Dreyer, L. B., & Haseltine, B. A. (1986). *The Woodrow Project: A sexual abuse prevention curriculum for the developmentally disabled.* Fargo, ND: Rape and Abuse Crisis Center.

Finkelhor, D. (1984). *Child sexual abuse: New theory and research.* New York: Free Press.

Finkelhor, D. (1990). New ideas for child sexual abuse prevention. In R. K. Oates (Ed.), *Understanding and managing child sexual abuse* (pp. 385–396). Sydney, Australia: Harcourt Press.

Finkelhor, D., Asdigian, N., & Dziuba-Leatherman, J. (1995). The effectiveness of victimization prevention instruction: An evaluation of children's responses to actual threats and assaults. *Child Abuse & Neglect, 19*, 141–153.

Finkelhor, D., & Dziuba-Leatherman, J. (1995). Victimization prevention programs: A national survey of children's exposure and reactions. *Child Abuse & Neglect, 19*, 129–139.

Gaibarino, J. (1987). Children's response to a sexual abuse prevention program: A study of the Spiderman comic. *Child Abuse & Neglect, 11*, 143–148.

Gilbert, N., Berrick, J. D., Le Prohn, N., & Nyman, N. (1989). *Protecting young children from sexual abuse: Does preschool training work?* Lexington, MA: Lexington.

Harbeck, C., Peterson, L., & Starr, L. (1992). Previously abused child victims response to a sexual abuse prevention program: A matter of measures. *Behavior Therapy, 23*, 375–387.

Harvey, P., Forehand, R., Brown, C., & Holmes, T. (1988). The prevention of sexual abuse: Examination of the effectiveness of a program with kindergarten-age children. *Behavior Therapy, 19*, 429–435.

Haseltine, B., & Miltenberger, R. G. (1990). Teaching self-protection skills to persons with mental retardation. *American Journal on Mental Retardation, 95,* 188–197.

Hazzard, A, Kleemeier, C. P., & Webb, C. (1990). Teacher versus expert presentations of sexual abuse prevention programs. *Journal of Interpersonal Violence, 5,* 23–36.

Hazzard, A, Webb, C., Kleemeier, C., Angert, L., & Pohl, L. (1991). Child sexual abuse prevention: Evaluation and one-year follow-up. *Child Abuse & Neglect, 15,* 123–138.

Helge, D. (1992). *Child sexual abuse in America—A call for school and community action.* Bellingham, WA: National Rural Development Institute.

Hill, J. L., & Jason, L. A. (1987). An evaluation of a school-based child sexual abuse primary prevention program. *Psychotherapy Bulletin, 22,* 36–38.

Kohl, J. (1993). School-based child sexual abuse prevention programs. *Journal of Family Violence, 8,* 137–150.

Kolko, D. J., Moser. J. T., & Hughes, J. (1989). Classroom training in sexual victimization awareness and prevention skills: An extension of the Red Flag/Green Flag people program. *Journal of Family Violence, 4,* 25–45.

Kolko, D. J., Moser, J. T., Litz, J., & Hughes, J. (1987). Promoting awareness and prevention of child sexual victimization using the Red Flag/Green Flag program: An evaluation with follow-up. *Journal of Family Violence, 2,* 11–35.

Korbin, J. E. (1990). Child sexual abuse: A cross-cultural view. In R. K. Oates (Ed.), *Understanding and managing child sexual abuse* (pp. 42–58). Sydney, Australia: Harcourt Brace.

Kraizer, S., Witte, S. S., & Fryer, G. E., Jr. (1989). Child sexual abuse prevention programs: What makes them effective in protecting children? *Children Today, 18,* 23–27.

Krents, E., & Atkins, D. (1985). *No-Go-Tell! A child protection curriculum for very young disabled children.* New York: Lexington Center.

Krivacska, J. J. (1989). Child sexual abuse prevention programs and accusation of child sexual abuse: An analysis. *Issues in Child Abuse Accusations, 1,* 8–13.

Krivacska, J. J. (1990). *Designing child sexual abuse prevention programs: Current approaches and a proposal for the prevention, reduction, and identification of sexual misuse.* Springfield, IL: Thomas.

LaBarre, A., Hinkley, K. R., & Nelson, M. F. (1986). *Sexual abuse! What is it? An informational book for the hearing impaired.* St. Paul, MN. St. Paul-Ramsey Foundation.

Liang, B., Bogat, G. A., & McGrath, M. P. (1993). Differential understanding of sexual abuse prevention concepts among preschoolers. *Child Abuse & Neglect, 17,* 641–650.

Miller-Perrin, C. L., & Wurtele, S. K. (1988). The child sexual abuse prevention movement: A critical analysis of primary and secondary approaches. *Clinical Psychology Review, 8,* 313–329.

Miller-Perrin, C. L., Wurtele, S. K., & Kondrick, P. A. (1990). Sexually abused and nonabused children's conceptions of personal body safety. *Child Abuse & Neglect, 14,* 99–112.

Miltenberger, R. G., & Thiesse-Duffy, E. (1988). Evaluation of home-based programs for teaching personal safety skills to children. *Journal of Applied Behavior Analysis, 21,* 81–87.

Moglia, R. (1986). Sexual abuse and disability. *SIECUS Reports, 14,* 9–10.

Nemerofsky, A. G., Carran, D. T., & Rosenberg, L. A. (1994). Age variation in performance among preschool children in a sexual abuse prevention program. *Journal of Child Sexual Abuse, 31,* 85–102.

Nibert, D., Cooper, S., & Ford, J. (1989). Parents' observations of the effect of a sexual abuse prevention program on preschool children. *Child Welfare, 68,* 539–546.

Nibert, D., Cooper, S., Ford, J., Fitch, L. K., & Robinson, J. (1989). The ability of young children to learn abuse prevention. *Response, 12,* 14–20.

O'Day, B. (1983). *Preventing sexual abuse of persons with disabilities: A curriculum for hearing impaired, physically disabled, blind and mentally retarded students.* Santa Cruz, CA: Network.

Peraino, J. M. (1990). Evaluation of a preschool antivictimization prevention program. *Journal of Interpersonal Violence, 5,* 520–528.

Plummer, C. A (1993). Prevention is appropriate, prevention is successful. In R. J. Gelles and D. R. Loseke (Eds.), *Current controversies on family violence* (pp. 288–305). Newbury Park, CA: Sage.

Porch, T. L., & Petretic-Jackson, P. A. (1986, August). Child sexual assault prevention: Evaluating current education workshops. Paper presented at the convention of the American Psychological Association, Washington, DC.

Ratto, R., & Bogat, G. A. (1990). An evaluation of a preschool curriculum to educate children in the prevention of sexual abuse. *Journal of Community Psychology, 18,* 289–297.

Reppucci, N. D., & Haugaard, J. J. (1989). Prevention of child sexual abuse: Myth or reality? *American Psychologist, 44,* 1266–1275.

Romano, N., Casey, K., & Daro, D. (1990). *Schools and child abuse: A national survey of principals' attitudes, beliefs, and practices.* Chicago: National Committee for the Prevention of Child Abuse.

Ryerson, E. (1984). Sexual abuse and self-protection education for developmentally disabled youth: A priority need. *SIECUS Reports, 13,* 6–7.

Sarno, J. A. & Wurtele, S. K. (1997). Effects of a personal safety program on preschoolers' knowledge, skills, and perceptions of child sexual abuse. *Child Maltreatment, 2,* 35–45.

Saslawsky, D. A., & Wurtele, S. K. (1986). Educating children about sexual abuse: Implications for pediatric intervention and possible prevention. *Journal of Pediatric Psychology, 11,* 235–245.

Seattle Rape Relief. (1980). *Sexual assault of handicapped students.* Seattle, WA: Seattle Rape Relief.

Sobsey, D., & Mansell, S. (1990). The prevention of sexual abuse of people with developmental disabilities. *Developmental Disabilities Bulletin, 18,* 51–66.

Sorenson, T., & Snow, B. (1991). How children tell: The process of disclosure in child sexual abuse. *Child Welfare, 70,* 3–15.

Stilwell, S. L., Lutzker, J. R., & Greene, B. F. (1988). Evaluation of a sexual abuse prevention program for preschoolers. *Journal of Family Violence, 3,* 269–281.

Swan, H. L., Press, A. N., & Briggs, S. L. (1985). Child sexual abuse prevention: Does it work? *Child Welfare, 64,* 395–405.

Tharinger, D. J., Horton, C. B., & Millea, S. (1990). Sexual abuse and exploitation of children and adults with mental retardation and other handicaps. *Child Abuse & Neglect, 14,* 301–312.

Tharinger, D. J., Krivacska, J. J., Laye-McDonough, M., Jamison, L., Vincent, G. G., & Hedlund, A. D. (1988). Prevention of child sexual abuse: An analysis of issues, educational programs, and research findings. *School Psycholology Review, 17,* 614–634.

Tutty, L. M. (1991). Child sexual abuse: A rage of prevention options. In B. Thomlison & C. Bagley (Eds.), *Child sexual abuse: Expanding the research base on program and treatment outcomes. Journal of Child and Youth Care* [Special issue], 23–41.

Tutty, L. M. (1992). The ability of elementary school children to learn child sexual abuse prevention concepts. *Child Abuse & Neglect, 16,* 369–384.

Tutty, L. M. (1994). Developmental issues in young children's learning of sexual abuse prevention concepts. *Child Abuse & Neglect, 18,* 179–192.

Tutty, L. M. (1995). The revised Children's Knowledge of Abuse Questionnaire: Development of a measure of children's understanding of sexual abuse prevention concepts. *Social Work Research, 19,* 112–120.

Wolfe, D. A., McPherson, T., Blount, R., & Wolfe, V. V. (1986). Evaluation of a brief intervention for educating school children in awareness of physical and sexual abuse. *Child Abuse & Neglect, 10,* 85–92.

Wurtele, S. K. (1990). Teaching personal safety skills to four-year-old children: A behavioral approach. *Behavior Therapy, 21,* 25–32.

Wurtele, S. K. (1993a). Enhancing children's sexual development through child sexual abuse prevention programs. *Journal of Sex Education and Therapy, 19,* 37–46.

Wurtele, S. K. (1993b). The role of maintaining telephone contact with parents during the teaching of a personal safety program. *Journal of Child Sexual Abuse, 2,* 65–82.

Wurtele, S. K., Currier, L. L., Gillispie, E. I., & Franklin, C. F. (1991). The efficacy of a parent-implemented program for teaching preschoolers personal safety skills. *Behavior Therapy, 22,* 69–83.

Wurtele, S. K., Gillispie, E. I., Currier, L. L., & Franklin, C. F. (1992). A comparison of teachers vs. parents as instructors of a personal safety program for preschoolers. *Child Abuse & Neglect, 16,* 127–137.

Wurtele, S. K., Kast, L. C., & Melzer, A. M. (1992). Sexual abuse prevention education for young children: A comparison of teachers and parents as instructors. *Child Abuse & Neglect, 16,* 865–876.

Wurtele, S. K., Kast, L. C., Miller-Perrin, C. L., & Kondrick, P. A. (1989). A comparison of programs for teaching personal safety skills to preschoolers. *Journal of Consulting and Clinical Psychology, 57,* 505–511.

Wurtele, S. K., Kvaternick, M., & Franklin, C. F. (1992). Sexual abuse prevention for preschoolers: A survey of parents' behaviors, attitudes, and beliefs. *Journal of Child Sexual Abuse, 1,* 113–128.

Wurtele, S. K., Marrs, S. R., & Miller-Perrin, C. L. (1987). Practice makes perfect? The role of participant modeling in sexual abuse prevention programs. *Journal of Consulting and Clinical Psychology, 55,* 599–602.

Wurtele, S. K., Melzer, A. M., & Kast, L. C. (1992). Preschoolers' knowledge of and ability to learn genital terminology. *Journal of Sex Education and Therapy, 18,* 115–122.

Wurtele, S. K., & Miller-Perrin, C. L. (1987). An evaluation of side effects associated with participation in a child sexual abuse prevention program. *Journal of School Health, 57,* 228–231.

Wurtele, S. K., & Miller-Perrin, C. L. (1992). *Preventing child sexual abuse: Sharing the responsibility.* Lincoln: University of Nebraska Press.

Wurtele, S. K., Saslawsky, D. A., Miller, C. L., Marrs, S. R., & Britcher, J. C. (1986). Teaching personal safety skills for potential prevention of sexual abuse. A comparison of treatments. *Journal of Consulting and Clinical Psychology, 54,* 688–692.

Part V

Early Intervention and Ethics

Poverty itself is a risk factor for children. In Chapter 22, Wasik reviews the problems associated with poverty and early childhood programs aimed at reducing risk factors.

In Chapter 23, Tymchuk provides a critique of the paucity of ethical decision making guidelines in human research in general, and child abuse and neglect research in particular. In two especially helpful tables, Tymchuk lays out a systematic process for ethical decision making.

22

Implications for Child Abuse and Neglect Interventions from Early Educational Interventions

BARBARA HANNA WASIK

Family impoverishment as evidenced by low income, low educational levels, and unemployment is the strongest predictor of poor developmental outcomes for children. Two domains in particular, school failure and abuse and neglect, are highly associated with poverty and have been at the center of many prevention and intervention efforts during the past three decades. Separate groups and organizations, however, have worked independently to address these two concerns about children. Predictably, most of the attention to reducing school failure originated in the fields of education and child development, where the goals are to enhance children's cognitive development and school performance. By contrast, the attention to reducing abuse and neglect derived from social services and health organizations, and aims to protect the child from further abuse and neglect, provide treatment and, more recently, develop prevention strategies. In addition to being influenced by different professions and different objectives for the child, these two areas of concern have also been characterized by different intervention procedures.

During the past few years several events necessitated the examination of the early childhood intervention literature for the implications it holds for work with children at risk for abuse and neglect. First, there is increasing evidence that poverty is a major condition influencing a wide range of poor outcomes for children (Duncan, 1991; Garbarino, 1990; Lazar, Darlington, Murray, Royce, & Snipper, 1982; McLoyd, 1990). Second, there has been an increase in the number of children living in poverty, portending a corresponding increase in both school failure and

BARBARA HANNA WASIK • School of Education, University of North Carolina, Chapel Hill, North Carolina 27599.
Handbook of Child Abuse Research and Treatment, edited by Lutzker. Plenum Press, New York, 1998.

maltreatment. Third, there is increasing evidence that negative parent–child interactions and unresponsive parenting contribute both to poor cognitive outcomes and to neglect (Hart & Risley, 1995; Wolfe, 1987). Fourth, there is increasing congruence among theories and principles identified as guiding best practices across all domains of child development (Wasik, Roberts, & Lam, 1994). And, fifth, the environment is seen as a determinant of developmental vulnerability for both groups (Garbarino, 1990; Ramey & Ramey, 1992).

The existence of common antecedents to cognitive delays and child maltreatment may point to common developmental pathways and common ways of improving outcomes for children in both domains. In this chapter, intervention programs designed to ameliorate cognitive delays for children from low-income families will be reviewed and implications regarding the maltreatment of children will be discussed. Early intervention efforts will first be placed into a historical perspective, identifying the major theoretical beliefs that have influenced practice. Then studies from both the first and second waves of research efforts on early educational interventions for children from families of low socioeconomic status will be described. A conceptual model for evaluating intervention strategies for children and their families will provide a framework for summarizing current research on early educational interventions and implications for programs aimed at preventing child abuse and neglect.

HISTORICAL BACKGROUND

The Progressive Era

Although child services can be traced back for several centuries as society responded to the needs of widows, orphans, the sick, and the poor, the time between the 1890s to the beginning of World War I is particularly relevant to contemporary services. It was during this "progressive era" that almost all human services in use today were developed (Levine & Levine, 1970, 1992; Wasik, Bryant, & Lyons, 1990). This era saw the rise of visiting teachers, school social workers, services for juvenile delinquents, and child guidance clinics, with home visiting serving as the primary method of reaching families. Indeed, the visiting teacher served as a bridge between schools and homes, and social workers and nurses also provided services directly to families. School attendance, poor school performance, neglect, poverty, and delinquency were some of the social concerns addressed. Services for children during this time were viewed more holistically than today, with family and community taken into consideration when addressing the needs of children (Levine & Levine, 1970, 1992; Wasik, Bryant, et al., 1990).

The 1920s to the 1960s

This more holistic and environmental approach started to change during the 1920s when services for children and adults began to reflect a psychoanalytic orientation, focusing on the individual's personality when evaluating and treating problematic situations. Parents were frequently blamed for their child's problems and, as a result, children with difficulties were frequently removed from their parents. Residential or institutional care came to be seen as an effective method for addressing concerns with children.

Two significant experiments conducted between 1930 and 1950 illustrate the influence of major environmental changes on children's long-term intellectual development. Skeels (1966) studied children living in an orphanage who had IQs below 70 and whose mothers were also mentally retarded. As part of the intervention study, 13 of these children were moved from the orphanage to the care of female inmates of a state institution for individuals with mental retardation, one child to each ward, while a control group remained in the orphanage. The results thirty years later showed that of the original 13 experimental children, all had become self-supporting, most had completed high school, and some had attended college. By contrast, adults from the control group either remained institutionalized or had died. In a second study of the effects of early intervention, 100 children whose biological parents were both socioeconomically disadvantaged and had mental retardation were investigated (Skodak & Skeels, 1949). On or before the time they were 6 months of age, the children were placed with foster families whose educational and economic levels were average for their communities. By the time they were 13, the children placed with foster families scored significantly higher on measures of cognitive abilities than children who remained with their birth families. In both these studies very clear effects were obtained for positive cognitive outcomes as a result of dramatic changes in the child's life. In spite of these studies and the lessons they provided for the importance of a child's early interactions with significant adults, it was not until considerably later in this century that children's intelligence came to be seen as influenced by early relational experiences.

SOCIAL, THEORETICAL, AND ECONOMIC INFLUENCES: THE 1960s TO THE 1990s

Social and Theoretical Influences

A number of events converged in the 1960s to generate interest in early interventions that could alter the cognitive development of young children. There was an increased awareness of the intellectual malleability in children, an increased interest in the importance of children's early experiences (Hunt, 1961), and considerable social concern for the low achievement and school failure of children reared in poverty. Spurred on by national concern with the plight of children living in poverty, attention was devoted to initiating programs that could help compensate for what were considered deficits in the home environment of many children. This model of cultural deficiency considered poor children to lack the benefits of middle-class families; consequently, compensatory educational programs were created and implemented to provide remediating opportunities (Bloom, Davis, & Hess, 1965). These political and theoretical influences resulted in the initiation of Project Head Start (Zigler & Freedman, 1987), as well as a large number of model programs designed to evaluate the effects of child- or parent-focused interventions.

Interesting parallels are seen in the early intervention literature and the child abuse and neglect literature of the 1960s. First, both the debilitating effects of poverty on children's later school performance (Bloom et al., 1965) and the prevalence of abuse and neglect of children came to be recognized as serious social issues

(Wolfe, 1987). Second, behavioral views of children's development were gaining prominence (Ullmann & Krasner, 1965), adding to the half century of psychoanalytic orientation. These two prevailing theories emphasized parental influences on the child's development, and thus provided support for interventions initiated early in the child's life

During the 1970s other, broader theories began to gain prominence, including the work of Bell (1974) who emphasized the bidirectionality of effects between parent and child. Systems theory, which emphasized the effect one part of a system has on another, influenced the development of other theories of child development, including the biosocial model (Ramey, MacPhee, & Yeates, 1982) and the transactional model (Sameroff & Chandler, 1975) of development. In both these models, child outcomes are seen as a product of both the individual and his or her experiences; alone, neither the child nor the environment is sufficient to predict child outcomes.

Possibly the most influential contemporary theory related to early interventions for children is the ecological theory posited by Bronfenbrenner (1979, 1986; Bronfenbrenner & Crouter, 1983). Bronfenbrenner's early writings promoted a shift toward recognizing the family itself as a much more appropriate focus of intervention than only the child (Bronfenbrenner, 1974). Based upon a detailed review of existing intervention programs, Bronfenbrenner concluded that "the family seems to be the most effective and economical system for fostering and sustaining the child's development. Without family involvement, intervention is likely to be unsuccessful, and what few effects are achieved are likely to disappear once the intervention is discontinued" (Bronfenbrenner, 1974, p. 300). His ecological theory envisioned the child as nested within a set of increasingly complex environments, beginning with the family, and nesting, in turn, within the neighborhood, the community, and finally the larger social structure. His theory predicts that the most enduring child outcomes occur from interventions that encompass a variety of significant people and settings in the child's life.

By the mid-1980s, there was a convergence of principles of care or "best practices" that include current beliefs about the role of the family in children's physical, mental, and social well-being (Wasik et al., 1994). Writers across all fields of human services, including health (Hutchins & McPherson, 1991; Koop, 1987; Behrman, 1992), mental health (Huxley, 1990; Knitzer, 1982), and education (Johnson, McGonigel, & Kaufmann, 1989), were articulating common principles and concepts important in services for children. The terms "family-centered," "community-based," and "coordinated" were the most commonly articulated. These principles of care have emerged as a result of individuals and groups struggling with the delivery of services to families, the escalation of social problems in spite of numerous intervention programs, the lack of integration and coordination of intervention efforts, and the increase in factors that are strongly associated with the occurrence of many serious social problems, especially poverty, teen parenting and single-parent households.

Poverty and Developmental Outcomes

The evidence that poverty is the single most significant condition predicting developmental difficulties for children is extensive (Garbarino, 1990; Duncan, 1991; Duncan, Brooks-Gunn, & Klebanov, 1994). Although low socioeconomic status or poverty can be defined in several ways, including family income and personal resources, when used to predict child outcomes it might best be used as a marker variable. Poverty is highly associated with low parental education and single or teen parenthood. It is also associated with a higher incidence of depression, stress, fewer social supports and services, unemployment, and low literacy levels. Poverty is predictive of a number of negative child outcomes including low birthweight, infant mortality, lower cognitive functioning, and poor school performance. Strong links exist between poverty and child maltreatment (Garbarino & Crouter, 1978; Garbarino & Sherman, 1980) and negative parenting behavior (McLoyd, 1990).

Poverty has consistently been found to be predictive of poor school outcomes. Its association with school outcomes is seen during infancy and the preschool years as children in low-income families demonstrate poorer language skills and cognitive development than do their more financially advantaged peers (Lazar et al., 1982; Duncan et al., 1994; Ramey, Sparling, Bryant, & Wasik, 1982). Poorer educational status is also seen across the school years, reflected not only in language and achievement (Felner et al., 1995), but also in grade retention and school dropouts (Alexander & Entwisle, 1996).

Socioeconomic status (SES) plays a significant role in child abuse and neglect. In describing this role, Wolfe (1987) wrote that "[l]ow SES, typically defined as family incomes below the poverty mark, underemployment, and less education, has proved to be a powerful aggregate variable associated with negative outcomes at several points in child development. Impoverished pregnant women are prone to be undernourished, to receive poor prenatal care, are exposed to more toxic agents, and consequently suffer more complications at delivery. After delivery, their children are exposed to greater postnatal risks, such as malnutrition, injury, and lack of stimulation, that are commonly associated with ongoing poverty and family disadvantage. Thus, it is widely accepted that lower socioeconomic level can serve as a significant risk factor to child development and child maltreatment, whereas higher SES can serve as an ameliorating, protective factor" (p. 21).

Although not all families living in poverty experience the characteristics or outcomes just described, it was not until the 1980s that investigators began to go beyond definitions of poverty to obtain better predictors of children's risk status. A study by Sameroff, Seifer, Barocas, Zax, and Greenspan (1987) is of value in elucidating the role of poverty. The investigators studied the following correlates of SES in the developmental outcomes of 4-year-old children: mental illness, maternal anxiety, parent perspectives on child development, spontaneous positive maternal interactions, occupation of head of household, maternal education, disadvantaged minority status, family support, stressful life events, and family size. The investigators found major differences in a comparison between those children with low multiple risk scores and those with high scores. In terms of intelligence, children with no environmental risks scored more than 30 points higher than children with eight or nine of the ten risk factors studied. Similar findings were obtained on a measure of social and emotional competencies (Sameroff et al., 1987). Researchers in the 1960s and 1970s did not have such data available to them and as a result they focused almost exclusively on poverty as the defining participant characteristic.

EARLY EDUCATIONAL INTERVENTION PROGRAMS: 1960–1990

The 1960s were a time of considerable optimism regarding the potential of educational interventions to prevent the cognitive deficits of children living in poverty. The optimism driving this first wave of interventions for disadvantaged children was influenced by both theory and empirical findings on the importance of early experiences in the lives of young children, the malleability of intelligence, and the importance of the parent in influencing children's development. The extent of this optimism is reflected in the large number of experimental programs initiated during this time. These early studies asked the simple question "Is early intervention effective?" More complex questions about program effects were raised later (e.g., Guralnick, 1989; Wasik, 1993a, 1993b). The background variable of concern was low family income, the intervention was either directly focused on the child or mediated through interventions with the parent, and cognitive performance was the primary outcome assessed. Programs varied along several dimensions, including location, the age of entry of the child, program intensity and duration, and the comprehensiveness of the intervention procedures. Intervention strategies included attendance at day-care centers, home visiting programs, parent support groups, and job training. Within this framework a variety of intervention efforts were implemented, including specific curricula to enhance children's cognitive development, efforts to enhance parent–child interactions and parenting skills, and the provision of parent support (Ramey et al., 1982).

Critical Reviews

The early educational intervention research literature has captured the attention of numerous writers, resulting in a plethora of reviews. Perhaps the best known of those reviews was conducted by Lazar and his colleagues (Lazar et al., 1982). This study reviewed school-age follow-up data on 11 projects initiated between 1962 and 1972 designed to enhance children's cognitive development. All but three of the projects began when children were 3 years of age or older, 6 used preschool centers, 2 provided home-based services, and 3 used a combination of center and home services. The major findings from this report provided support for positive school outcomes, showing that children participating in preschool programs were less likely to repeat a grade in school or be placed in a special education class than were children in a control group. Although the longitudinal data on intelligence tests and achievement did not distinguish between experimental and control groups, a finding inconsistent with the high expectations of social reform in the 1960s, this report provided important support for the field of early intervention at a time when the benefits were being questioned (Ramey, 1982).

In order to examine previous work for implications for child abuse and neglect, this chapter has drawn on some of the more rigorous research studies to illustrate both the first wave and later research. Reviews of this literature have also been considered, with reviews published since 1990 emphasized because they have the advantage of perspective as well as the ability to present longitudinal data. Specifically excluded were reviews focused on children with disabilities, and large-scale evaluation studies. The eight reviews considered include those by Farran (1990); Benasich, Brooks-Gunn, and Clewell (1992); Ramey and Ramey

(1992); Olds and Kitzman (1993); Wasik and Karweit (1994); Barnett (1995); Yoshikawa (1995); and Bryant and Maxwell (1997). Collectively, these reviews address both outcomes and theoretical issues, compare programs across major dimensions, contrast earlier and later studies, and investigate maternal as well as child outcomes. An analysis of the programs covered in these reviews shows that almost all major early intervention studies for children from low-income families designed to enhance cognitive performance and initiated between 1960 and 1980 have been covered in one or more of these publications.

Farran reviewed 32 studies for disadvantaged children focusing on long-term follow-up data of projects begun in the late 1960s or early 1970s. All of the studies involved children who were at risk for school problems, mild mental retardation, and reading difficulties. The type of interventions varied, but the focus of all these projects was cognitive remediation or support, and low socioeconomic status was the defining criterion for participation.

Benasich and colleagues' review (1992) examined maternal benefits of 27 early intervention programs designed to improve children's social and educational outcomes. These studies were based upon a model that assumes that changes in child outcomes will result from changes in the mother's attitudes or behavior. This review focused on actual maternal outcomes, rather than viewing maternal changes as mediating variables.

Olds and Kitzman (1993) examined the effectiveness of home visiting programs in improving the lives of children and their families. Concentrating on studies with randomized designs, they evaluated programs for low-income families, families at risk for child maltreatment, and programs focused on preventing preterm or low-birthweight infants, or on improving their developmental outcomes.

In a 1992 review of early educational interventions, Ramey and Ramey examined 25 years of research in order to identity major conclusions and political and scientific issues. They used data from the more rigorous research studies as the basis of their review. The authors identified six principles derived from the literature—timing, intensity, direct versus indirect services, breadth, individual differences, and environmental maintenance—and provided empirical support for each of these. Their observation that children within the same intervention program vary in their responses is important because most of the emphasis in this literature is on group outcome data.

The Wasik and Karweit review (1994) considered studies where the primary focus was children from birth to age 3. They divided studies into high-intensity (e.g., Milwaukee Project, Garber & Heber, 1981; the Carolina Abecedarian Project, Ramey, Yeates, & Short, 1984; and Project CARE, Wasik, Ramey, Bryant, & Sparling, 1990), moderate-intensity (e.g., Gordon Parent Education Program, Gordon & Guinagh, 1978), and low-intensity programs (e.g., Verbal Interaction Project, The Mother–Child Home Program, Levenstein, O'Hara & Madden, 1983; and the Family-oriented Home Visiting Program, Gray & Klaus, 1970, Klaus & Gray, 1968). In 8 of these 11 studies, participants were randomly assigned to groups; in two studies, sites, not individuals, were assigned to treatment conditions.

Barnett (1995) reviewed 36 studies, of which 15 were model demonstration projects and 19 were large-scale public programs, to examine the long-term effects on the cognitive development of children from low-income families. All but one model program reviewed had a center-based program for children, and most offered home visiting. Included in Barnett's review were many of the classic studies completed before 1980; all studies showed strong research designs.

Because low SES is one of the factors associated with chronic delinquency and conduct disorders, Yoshikawa (1995) examined data from early intervention studies for children from low-income families to see if there were positive effects on antisocial behavior. He reasoned that early interventions focused on improving the parent–child relationship might also influence children's later social behaviors, given that hostile or rejecting parenting is associated with children's antisocial behavior.

Bryant and Maxwell (1997) reviewed two groups of studies. The first was a set of five long-term studies initiated between 1962 and 1972 that followed children into adolescence or young adulthood, including the Perry Preschool (Schweinhart, Barnes, Weikart, Barnett, & Epstein, 1993), the Chicago Child and Parent Centers (Fuerst & Fuerst, 1993), the Syracuse Family Development Research Project (Honig & Lally, 1982), the Houston Parent Child Development Center (Johnson & Walker, 1991), and the Carolina Abecedarian Project (Ramey et al., 1984). These studies share an emphasis on measuring cognitive and academic outcomes and comparing the intervention program with a comparison group.

The second set of studies considered by Bryant and Maxwell (Project CARE by Wasik, Ramey, et al., 1990; the Portage Program in the Gaza Strip by Oakland & Ghazaleh, in press; the Jamaica home visiting study by Powell & Grantham-McGregor, 1989; the Mother–Child Home Program in Bermuda by Scarr & McCartney, 1988; the Comprehensive Child Development Programs by St. Pierre, Goodson, Layzer, & Bernstein, 1994; and Head Start experiments, for example, Lee, Brooks-Gunn, Schnur, & Liaw, 1990) addressed more complex questions, including the relationship between program variables and outcomes and between child and family characteristics and outcomes. The authors also examined noncognitive outcomes.

Examples of Program Diversity

To illustrate the diversity of these early intervention studies, several will be described in detail. Schaefer and Aaronson's (1977) intervention provided young children between 15 and 36 months of age with in-home tutorial sessions one hour daily, although no parent involvement was initiated. Testing at 36 months showed significant improvement in differences on cognitive measures by the experimental group. At age 5, no long-term effects were observed for intelligence scores, leading the investigators to call for the addition of parental involvement to early intervention programs. Another program focused specifically on the child's needs was the Verbal Interaction Project (The Mother–Child Home Program, Levenstein et al., 1983). Toy demonstrators visited mothers of two- and three-year-old children in the home, providing on each visit a new toy that could be used to stimulate the child's cognitive development. The focus was only on the child's cognitive development, not on more general parenting concerns.

Gutelius and her colleagues recognized the importance of working with the parent as well as the child. Home visits that focused on parent inclusion were provided by a physician and a nurse who focused on the child's health. Follow-up visits by the nurse encouraged children's cognitive development. Children who participated in studies combining home visits and parent intervention outperformed control children on measures of cognitive development at ages one, two, and three, and the experimental mothers outperformed control mothers on education levels and employment rates (Gutelius, Kirsch, MacDonald, Brooks, & McErlean, 1977).

Center-based or educational day-care programs are also characterized by considerable diversity. Children typically began attending programs during the preschool years, either during infancy or when they were ages three, four or five. Two well-known studies initiated in 1962 included home visiting and a preschool program. One was the Early Training Project conducted by Gray and Klaus which started when children were ages four to five. The preschoolers attended a summer program and their families were visited in the home during the intervening nine months. Cognitive measures for the children receiving intervention were significantly higher during preschool and the early school years (Gray & Klaus, 1970; Klaus & Gray, 1968) than for the control children. The High/Scope Perry Preschool Project (Schweinhart et al., 1993), one of the most frequently referenced early intervention programs, combined preschool with home visits. Children were randomly assigned to treatment or control groups. Children in the intervention program entered the preschool classes when they were ages three or four and attended preschool for $2^1/_2$ hours daily for the two years before school entrance. Long-term follow-up has shown higher rates of high-school graduation and college attendance for the treatment children, as well as improved employment and reduced crime and teen pregnancy rates (Schweinhart et al., 1993).

Other more comprehensive programs were the Milwaukee Project (Garber & Heber, 1981), the Abecedarian Project (Ramey et al., 1984; Campbell & Ramey, 1994), and Project CARE (Wasik, Ramey, et al., 1990), all of which employed rigorous experimental designs. The Carolina Abecedarian Program will be used to illustrate these programs. This study was initiated in 1972 for children from impoverished backgrounds, using a high-risk index to determine selection (Ramey et al., 1984). Families were randomly assigned to either a treatment or a comparison group. All children received nutritional supplements and social services. Children in the treatment group began attending a full-day child development center between the ages of six weeks and three months and continued in the program until school entrance. The curriculum focused on cognitive, language, and social development, fine and gross motor skills, and adaptive skills (Sparling & Lewis, 1979; Sparling & Lewis, 1984). Intellectual assessments showed that from 18 months, the children who attended an educational day-care program performed significantly better than the comparison children (Ramey et al., 1984). Longitudinal data on school performance have demonstrated continuing positive effects for the intervention children (Campbell & Ramey, 1994; Ramey & Ramey, 1992).

Summary of First Wave Studies

The first wave of these early intervention studies can be summarized along several dimensions, including participant selection; program variables, including location, intensity, child's age at entrance, mediated versus direct intervention, and comprehensiveness; child outcomes; maternal outcomes; and design issues.

Participants

For almost all studies, family income was seen as a sufficient variable to determine eligibility for participation. Additional parent and child risk variables were rarely considered in the selection process.

Program Variables

To examine what program variables contributed to child outcomes, a number of variables have been studied, including (1) the location of services, usually center-based versus home-based; (2) the child's age at entry into the program; (3) program intensity; (4) whether the intervention was focused on the child (direct) or focused on the parent as a mediator of child outcomes (indirect); and (5) program comprehensivenss. Because investigators did not begin to compare treatments as part of an experimental design to any large degree until the late 1970s (Bryant & Maxwell, 1997), many conclusions drawn about the effects of program variables have been made by comparisons across studies. Consequently, these earlier study conclusions are more tentative than are conclusions from later studies.

Center-based programs, as compared with home-based programs, seem to have stronger and more enduring effects (Wasik & Karweit, 1994), although this conclusion is confounded with program intensity (Ramey, Ramey, Gaines, & Blair, 1995). Children in center programs generally attend on a daily basis (up to 40 or more hours per week), whereas home visits usually occur for 1 hour a week and typically address parenting skills and parent interactions, rather than provide direct child services.

Programs that start earlier tend to have stronger effects than those that begin later, but age of entry is also confounded with duration. The most effective programs not only began in infancy, but also continued throughout the preschool years, providing children with a continuous enriched experience throughout this time (Ramey et al., 1995). Results also show that programs that provide direct experiences for children have direct outcomes and those that provide direct experiences for parents have direct parent outcomes (Barnett, 1995; Gomby, Larner, Stevenson, Lewit, & Behrman, 1995). Furthermore, programs that focus on the role of the parent in helping his or her child tend to have less effects on the child and inconsistent parent effects (Barnett, 1995).

Child Outcomes

The most consistent finding is that children who participated in child-focused programs tended to experience a significant increase in intelligence by the end of the program, typically of the magnitude of 8 to 10 IQ points or one-half a standard deviation, in comparison to control children (Zigler, 1995). School-age gains were reflected more often in reduced grade retention and special class placement. Intelligence scores tended not to be significantly different from control group children at follow-up, except for the more intensive Abecedarian and Milwaukee Projects, primarily because the control children frequently improved their performance once they entered school.

Parent Outcomes

Benesich and her colleagues summarized a wide range of outcomes for mothers in these programs. Their review moved beyond the general assumption in this research that maternal behaviors are a mediating variable for child outcomes, to investigating maternal outcomes as a main issue, a focus particularly relevant when considering implications for abuse and neglect. The authors found a range of positive maternal outcomes, including maternal employment and education, subsequent fertility, and improvement in mother–infant interactions. Few patterns emerged concerning the types of early interventions that best predicted positive maternal outcomes, but it is clear that maternal benefits do occur from many of these early intervention efforts.

Although education and employment were only infrequently evaluated in the first wave of early interventions, the Milwaukee Project, the Yale Child Welfare Program (Seitz, Rosenbaum, & Apfel, 1985) and the Nurse Visitation Program (Olds, Henderson, Tatelbaum, & Chamberlin, 1986; Olds & Kitzman, 1993) were all concerned with parental employment and educational status and found improvements on these parent outcomes as a result of program participation (Barnett, 1995).

Design Issues

These early studies used a wide variety of experimental designs, ranging from highly controlled studies with random assignment of participants to treatment or control conditions to the use of matched control groups, thus tempering the conclusions that can be drawn. Two other factors also temper any conclusions on outcomes: subject recruitment and retention rates. Participants were often referred to the programs by different agencies, and it is not always clear what the initial referral criteria were. Also, for some of the studies, follow-up data were obtained for a reduced sample, potentially introducing bias into the interpretations. Consequently, findings from these initial studies must be accepted with some caution.

CONCEPTUAL MODEL

Beginning in the late 1970s and 1980s, several trends occurred in early intervention programs designed for children in poverty and their families, although each of these trends has roots in the preceding years. In order to facilitate the discussion of these trends, a conceptual model developed by Wasik for evaluating early intervention programs (Wasik, 1993a,b) will be used as an organizing framework. In this conceptual model, background variables are seen as including child, parent, family, and community characteristics. Program characteristics and processes include all components of a program: program intensity, curricula, location, resources, and staff qualifications and training. Outcome variables include child, parent, family, and community changes. Each major variable can be described more specifically. For example, parent variables can include age, gender, education level, literacy level, occupation, income, race and ethnicity, parenting knowledge and skills, physical and emotional health, coping and problem-solving skills, history of child abuse, alcohol and drug abuse, and social supports (Wasik 1993a,b).

This conceptual framework provides an expanded view of important variables and relationships to consider when examining intervention programs. It can be contrasted with a simpler view of background, program, and outcome relationships posited for programs conducted at an earlier time when low family income was seen as predicting low cognitive outcomes for children. Interventions were either directly focused on the child or were mediated through work with the parents. This earlier intervention model did not prompt consideration of other child and parent background variables or of program variables, nor did it promote the consideration of other potential outcomes.

The conceptual model in Figure 1 also can be distinguished from the general models guiding earlier work in that it emphasizes the importance of program processes and characteristics. Early investigators traditionally identified program intervention procedures, but rarely described them in depth or obtained program monitoring data. Only infrequently were any analyses conducted of the relationships between program characteristics and program outcomes. Outcomes focused almost exclusively on children's cognitive abilities, with little attention devoted to other child, parent, family, or community outcomes. This model can also be used to generate more complex hypotheses about potential relationships among variables. In the following section on what has been called the second wave or second generation of early educational intervention, this model will be used as a framework to review trends in research.

RECENT TRENDS IN EARLY EDUCATIONAL INTERVENTIONS

In the late 1970s, investigators began to explore more complex questions related to early educational interventions. Moving beyond questions of "Does it work?" they focused on the relative merits of different programs, the relationship between child and parent characteristics to outcomes, and participation levels and outcomes. Major trends in this work are presented below.

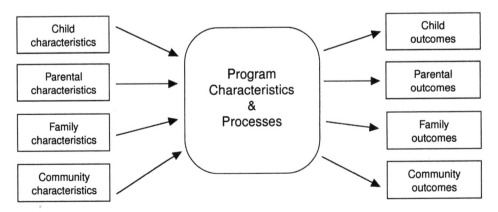

Figure 1. Conceptual model for evaluating early intervention programs.

Background Variables

At least three major trends have become apparent in the category of background variables: (1) there is a shift toward using more specific criteria for selecting participants, such as parental educational level or other parent or child variables, rather than relying upon poverty as the criterion for participation (e.g., IHDP, 1990); (2) there is a call to provide universal services, based upon the assumption that there are times in the lives of all parents when extra support and assistance is needed; (3) the role of community in influencing families has received increased attention and has resulted in an increasing body of research showing that community variables interact with child and family variables to influence child development (Duncan et al., 1994; Garbarino, 1990). Although conflicting opinions exist on the role of community, the inclusion of community variables is a significant departure from the first wave of research. The importance of community is also influenced by calls for services to be community-based and integrated with other community supports (Wasik et al., 1994).

Program Variables

A clear trend has emerged stressing the importance of examining program quality, monitoring program implementation, and relating program characteristics and processes to outcomes (Guralnick, 1989; Ramey et al., 1992). It seemed less important to researchers during the first wave of early intervention studies to document the parameters of implementation, and they rarely published detailed accounts of the actual intervention activities. There is also evidence that programs are becoming more comprehensive, with a variety of services being offered to families, encompassing education, health, and social services (IHDP, 1990). This shift is consistent with calls for services for children and their families to be comprehensive, integrated, and continuous (e.g., Johnson et al., 1989). Another very significant trend is the development of two-generation programs; that is, programs specifically designed to address the needs of both the child and the parent (Smith, 1995; Smith & Zaslow, 1995; St. Pierre, Layzer, & Barnes, 1995; St. Pierre & Swartz, 1995). This trend has resulted from beliefs in the importance of improving parental education, employment, and income, although the effects on children's development from such changes is not clear.

Program Outcomes

There is a strong trend toward broadening the measures of child outcomes to include domains other than cognitive development (e.g., Olds et al., 1986; Olds, Henderson, Tatelbaum, & Chamberlin, 1988). There is considerable interest in obtaining outcome measures on other family members, especially the parents. This latter trend reflects an interest in assessing parent effects as a goal in itself, not simply as mediating child outcomes (Benasich et al., 1992), and increasing interest in two-generation programs. There is also interest in examining social and community outcomes (Roberts & Wasik, 1996).

Experimental Design

Most early research did not use rigorous research designs, nor address more complex questions. Beginning in the late 1970s, interest has increased in examining the effects of different intervention programs and different levels of program intensity through direct comparisons within the same research design. Studies using direct comparisons have been reviewed by Bryant and Maxwell (1997) and Ramey and associates (1995) and include Project CARE, the first planned comparison of a direct intervention (day care) with a mediated intervention (home visiting and family education) (Wasik, Ramey, et al., 1990), and the Jamaica study that compared the intensity of home visiting by varying the intensity of home visits (Powell & McGranthan-McGregor, 1989). The Abecedarian Project implemented a planned comparison of school-age intervention, showing that children in a preschool program performed better than children in a school-age intervention (Campbell & Ramey, 1994). Studies such as these in which direct comparisons of program variation are made for participants in the same study provide stronger support for differential program outcomes.

An Illustrative Model Program

Initiated in 1984 for low-birthweight infants, the Infant Health and Development Program (IHDP, 1990; Ramey et al., 1992) illustrates many of the trends identified previously. Designed as a national, multisite, randomized clinical trial and the largest rigorous experimental test of efficacy of a specific early intervention program, the IHDP was based upon the intervention programs used in two earlier studies, the Abecedarian Program (Ramey et al., 1984) and Project CARE (Wasik, Ramey, et al., 1990). The intervention in IHDP called for weekly home visits and parent groups from the time the infant went home after delivery to the age of one. From ages one to three, a daily, full-time, developmentally appropriate day care was provided with home visits decreasing to once of twice a month. The focus of home visiting was to examine parenting skills and responsiveness, parent–child interactions, and parent coping and problem solving (Wasik, Bryant, Lyons, Sparling, & Ramey, 1997; Wasik, Bryant, Ramey, & Sparling, 1997). Within the IHDP there was an effort to coordinate and integrate services for children and their families. Staff included individuals trained in education, psychology, health, and the social services. In order to assure adherence to the treatment protocol, however, the program was free-standing and not integrated with other community agencies or services.

Going beyond typical analyses of outcome data, Ramey and colleagues (1992) developed a Family Participation Index to examine the relationship between intensity, participation, and outcomes. The index was the sum of the number of home visits, attendance at parent group meetings, and days attended at the child development centers. Intensity of participation was found to be related to children's cognitive development at age 3 with less than 2% of the children of families in the highest tercile of participation scoring in the mentally retarded range compared with 3.5% and 13% of children in the middle and lowest participation levels, respectively. Participation was not found to vary with mother's ethnicity, age, or education or with the child's birth weight, gender, or neonatal health status, leaving unresolved the question of how family background variables contribute to the family's participation, a question that needs further exploration.

An Illustrative Large-Scale Community Program

An evaluation of the Even Start Family Literacy Program illustrates large-scale intervention programs that take place in the community, in contrast to the experimental rigor and adherence to a highly specific program protocol, as exemplified in the IHDP. These large-scale programs are typically ongoing at the time an evaluation is implemented and rarely lend themselves to research designs to compare treatment effects (see Barnett, 1995, for a review of large-scale evaluations; also St. Pierre, Layzer, et al., 1995). The Even Start Family Literacy Programs require that participating adults be eligible for adult basic education programs, live in the attendance area of an elementary school receiving Chapter 1 funds, and have a child younger than age 8. Programs are required to offer three integrated components: early childhood education, adult basic education, and parenting education, which frequently includes a parent–child interaction time in the center setting, Programs are to build on and be integrated with other community activities and thus might have the adults take classes provided by a local community college.

Abt Associates conducted a two-part study of the Even Start Family Literacy Program, one based on an annual survey of all Even Start projects and participating families, and one in-depth study based on data from an experimental study of a subset of five Even Start projects with approximately 200 families, randomly assigned to treatment or control groups. Children who participated in Even Start increased their language scores by more than double the expected rate, but after 18 months control children caught up with their Even Start peers. The nonsignificant follow-up data were attributed to the fact that the control children later enrolled in preschool or kindergarten and the Even Start children no longer participated in the program. Data from the in-depth study showed that four times as many adults attained their GED as adults in the control group (22.4% compared to 5.7%). An investigation of the effects of program intensity showed that positive gains made by children and parents were related to the amount of participation in the program (St. Pierre, Swartz, et al., 1995), a finding consistent with the analysis of participation data in the IHDP (Ramey et al., 1992).

IMPLICATIONS

In drawing conclusions from the literature discussed in this chapter, it is important to keep in mind some of the limitations of this work related to client and community characteristics, program processes, and outcomes. First, it is clear that a much more diverse population of the children being raised in poverty needs to be studied. Almost all earlier studies have limited generalization for today's low-income families, which now include many Hispanic/Latino families, Native American families, and numerous others for whom English is a second language. Furthermore, although the percentage of Caucasian families living in poverty is lower than the percentage for most minority groups, the total number of Caucasian children living in poverty is high and these families deserve much more attention from the research community than they have yet received.

Second, because the early educational research took place in a culture that differs on several important dimensions from our present culture, contemporary studies are needed to determine the efficacy of current interventions. The increased use of drugs, alcohol, and tobacco by young women of childbearing age, the rise in the numbers of single-parent families, and the increase in violence not only point toward an even higher incidence of negative outcomes for children and their families, but also must be assessed for their influence on the effectiveness of early interventions.

As we increasingly move toward community-based programs, we need a more complete understanding of how the unique strengths and weaknesses of those communities can help shape our approaches to providing services to children and their families. Accumulated evidence indicates that children from low-income neighborhoods suffer higher risks for infant mortality, child maltreatment, poor school performance, delinquency, and acts of violence. Unfortunately, we have far too little evidence about how to involve communities in constructive ways.

In order to design more effective interventions, further research comparing alternative intervention approaches and conducting more fine-grain analyses of the effects of program processes and procedures is required. Additional longitudinal studies that examine a variety of child, parent, family, and community outcomes, both short- and long-term, also need to be conducted. Even with these limitations, there remain important implications from this literature to consider. Both theory and data provide strong support for offering programs that begin early, provide both child and parent components, and are intensive and comprehensive.

Child Age at Intervention

Although there exists some controversy over whether programs to promote school success should begin in infancy, preschool, or primary grade school (Farran, 1990; Ramey et al., 1995), the weight of both theoretical and empirical evidence points toward prompt intervention. Three important areas with implications for abuse and neglect are influenced by beginning earlier: parent–child interactions, parent responsiveness, and child language. Helping parents at the time of their first child's birth can help assure that parents develop positive ways of interacting with their child, and this earlier intervention averts the use of inappropriate behavior due to a lack of knowledge or skill. Support for beginning during the child's infancy comes from the compelling data in a recent publication of early language development by Hart and Risley (1995), who conducted in-home observations of early language development and found that, without intervention, by age three children from poor families lag considerably behind children from working class and professional class families. They found positive parent interactions and the amount of interactions to be critical to the development of early language skills. The clear message from Hart and Risley's work is not to wait until children are three years old and significantly behind their peers in language skills. The intensity of interventions required for such children to catch up is too expensive to obtain the level of social support necessary to fund them. Furthermore, delaying intervention with children at risk for maltreatment is unnecessary and potentially fatal.

Parent and Child Focus

Consideration of the effects of a wide range of early intervention studies shows that programs that focus directly on the parent are more likely to have parent effects and those that focus more directly on the child are more likely to have child effects (Barnett, 1995; Gomby et al., 1995). Although this statement may seem self-evident, many of the early educational programs have been guided by assumptions that targeting the parent would be as effective in bringing about specific child gains as would child-focused programs. Though this assumption has strong support from theory, for families living in poverty the support needed for many children to develop often exceeds what their parents can provide. These children frequently derive benefits from significant environmental changes provided by quality day care even for part of the day.

Many programs with significant child outcomes have frequently taken place in day-care or preschool settings, a component not typically considered in most interventions for abused and neglected children. Yet we should not rule out the advantages of attending developmentally appropriate day care for preschool children at risk of maltreatment. Such settings have the advantage of providing a safe and nurturing environment as well as helping to prepare children to function better once they enter school. Further, center-based programs can offer the parent relief from child care for a period of time, and can teach the child skills, especially communication skills and problem-solving skills, that might help buffer him or her from some of the effects of neglect. Because they already include both parent and child components, two-generation early intervention programs may offer the best model for designing programs to prevent abuse and neglect.

Intensity

One of the most consistent findings from interventions designed to enhance children's cognitive development is the importance of intensity in program efficacy. This finding is seen in the most rigorous studies and has been identified by almost all reviewers (e.g., Bryant & Maxwell, 1997; Wasik & Karweit, 1994; Ramey et al., 1995; St. Pierre & Swartz, 1995). Intensity, however, has not been disentangled from program location (i.e., center-based versus home), focus (parent versus child), or duration. For example, intense programs that end a year or two before the child enters public school (e.g. IHDP 1990; Brooks-Gunn et al., 1994) are not predicted to have the same outcomes as a program that continues from birth to school entrance (e.g., Ramey et al., 1984; Wasik, Ramey, et al., 1990). Because preventive programs for abuse and neglect almost always take place in the home, this issue is especially important to our analysis. Although the National Committee to Prevent Abuse and Neglect has recommended home visiting as its treatment of choice, more intense analyses must be conducted on the home visiting experience. As discussed earlier, we know that home visiting programs are not as effective for the child as center-based programs, but we also know that home visiting is less intensive than a center-based program for children. Also, within home visiting programs there is considerable variation in home visitor credentials and training (Wasik & Roberts, 1994). Consequently, practitioners must keep in mind multiple dimensions of programs and how these interact to bring about the most desirable outcomes.

It is also important to remember the distinctions between program protocol and the actual participation by parents and children. Actual participation levels in the program are related to child outcomes as shown from the analysis of the IHDP data (Ramey et al., 1992), but we need to learn considerably more about ways to increase participation levels.

Comprehensiveness

In the area of child outcomes, we know that programs addressing only child cognitive development sometimes overlook other critical needs. One of the most significant conclusions from the early intervention research is that a focus on cognitive development is most likely not a sufficient intervention, given the complex set of variables that contribute to a child's development. Children's development cannot be easily compartmentalized. Service providers need to consider all domains of children's development and make provisions for integrated and comprehensive services. As noted earlier, calls for integrated services are being made across all human services, but much work still has to be done to break down barriers across agencies and disciplines so that child and family needs can be met.

We know that the presence of multiple risk factors considerably increases the likelihood that children from low-income families perform poorly on measures of intelligence and achievement (Sameroff et al., 1987). Assessing for multiple risk factors is seen as the most important method for identifying parents at risk for abuse and neglect (Kempe, 1976). Consequently, it has been argued that interventions designed to reduce risk factors and promote positive parent–child interactions could help prevent maltreatment. Providing quality out-of-home day care could potentially enhance children's development in ways that might buffer them from abuse and neglect. Day-care programs could also include time for parent–child interactions, similar to those in family literacy programs, thus providing parents with a chance to model and practice positive parenting skills.

FUTURE DIRECTIONS

In the future, it would be desirable to study more comprehensive interventions designed to address multiple child and parent outcomes. Currently, two such studies are under way in Hawaii and California. These studies are not only designed to prevent abuse and neglect, but will also include evaluation measures from the early educational interventions. They provide examples of how multiple domains of child development and parent competencies might be addressed. Both studies assess the Hawaii Healthy Families program, which is based on work initiated 20 years ago by Kempe (1976). He helped physicians and other health workers identify warning signs of abuse and neglect before a child's delivery as well as during postpartum checkups. His recommendations and research have served as the basis for the Hawaii Healthy Families Program and its widespread emulation throughout the remaining states as the Healthy Families American Program.

Duggan at Johns Hopkins and her colleagues are conducting an experimental study of the Hawaii Healthy Families Program and Landsverk and his colleagues at San Diego State University are investigating the Healthy Families America program in California. Both of these efforts screen families at or near the time of delivery and provide frequent home visits. Employing rigorous experimental designs, both studies seek data on a range of family background characteristics, program processes, and child and parent outcomes. Using single-subject designs, Lutzker is also conducting a rigorous evaluation of in-home interventions for families at risk of abuse and neglect, described in Chapter 10 in this book. Together these studies should help establish the efficacy of these particular procedures, paving the way for implementation on a larger scale.

CONCLUSIONS

Results from the early education interventions clearly call for an intensity and duration that can make a difference in the lives of families. As concern for abuse and neglect grow, efforts to reduce maltreatment must avoid providing programs of insufficient intensity and scope during this period of rapid expansion. Although such programs may appear to reach large numbers of individuals, they might also fail to provide the kind of individualization and attention required to make a significant difference in the lives of children and their families. Programs that begin early, address multiple domains of child development, include a focus not only on parenting but on parent needs, and are intensive and comprehensive have the most likelihood of being successful. For the children at risk for maltreatment, we cannot afford to provide anything less.

REFERENCES

Alexander, K. L., & Entwisle, D. R. (1996). Schools and children at risk. In A. Booth & J. F. Dunn (Eds.), *Family school links: How do they affect educational outcomes?* (pp. 67–88). Mahwah, NJ: Erlbaum.

Barnett, W. S. (1995). Long-term effects of early childhood programs on cognitive and school outcomes. *Future of Children 5*(3), 25–50.

Behrman, R. E. 1992. (Ed.). (1992). U.S. health care for children. *Future of Children, 3*(2).

Bell, R. Q. (1974). Contributions of human infants to caregiving and social interaction. In M. Lewis & R. A. Rosenblum (Eds.), *The effect of the infant on its caregiver.* New York: Wiley.

Benasich, A. A., Brooks-Gunn, J., & Clewell, B. C. (1992). How do mothers benefit from early intervention programs? *Journal of Applied Developmental Psychology, 13,* 311–362.

Bloom, B. S., Davis A., & Hess R. (1965). *Compensatory education for cultural deprivation.* New York: Holt, Rinehart and Winston.

Bronfenbrenner, U. (1974). Is early intervention effective? *Teacher's College Record, 76,* 279–303.

Bronfenbrenner, U. (1979). *The ecology of human development: Experiments by nature and design.* Cambridge, MA: Harvard University Press.

Bronfenbrenner, U. (1986). Ecology of the family as a context for human development: Research perspectives. *Developmental Psychology, 22,* 723–742.

Bronfenbrenner, U., & Crouter, A. C. (1983). The evolution of environmental models in developmental research. In P. H. Mussen (Series Ed.) & W. Kessen (Vol. Ed.), *Handbook of child psychology: Vol. I. History, theory, and methods* (4th ed., pp. 357–414). New York: Wiley.

Brooks-Gunn, J., McCarton, C. M., Casey, P. H., McCormick, M. C., Bauer, C. R, Bernbaum, J. C., Tyson, J., Swanson, M., Bennett, F. C., Scott, D. T., Tonascia, J., & Meinert, C. L. (1994). Early intervention in low-birth-weight premature infants: Results through age 5 years from the Infant Health and Development Program. *Journal of the American Medical Association, 272*(16), 1257–1262.

Bryant, D. M., & Maxwell, K. (1997). The effectiveness of early intervention for disadvantaged children. In M. Guralnick (Ed.), *The effectiveness of early intervention* (pp. 23–46). Baltimore: Paul H. Brookes.

Campbell, F. A., & Ramey, C. T. (1994). Effects of early intervention on intellectual and academic achievement: A follow-up study of children from low-income families. *Child Development, 65,* 684–98.

Duncan, G. J. (1991). The economic environment of childhood. In A. C. Houston (Ed.), *Children in poverty: Child development and public policy* (pp. 23–50). Cambridge, England: Cambridge University Press.

Duncan, G. J., Brooks-Gunn, J., & Klebanov, P. K. (1994). Economic deprivation and early-childhood development. *Child Development, 65,* 296–318.

Farran, D. C. (1990). Effects of intervention with disadvantaged and disabled children: A decade of review. In S. J. Meisels & J. P. Shonkoff (Eds.), *Handbook of early childhood intervention* (pp. 501–539). New York: Cambridge University Press.

Felner, R. D., Brand, S., DuBois, D. L., Adan, A. M., Mulhall, P. F., & Evans, E. G. (1995). Socioeconomic disadvantage, proximal environmental experiences, and socioemotional and academic adjustment in early adolescence: Investigation of a mediated effects model. *Child Development, 66,* 774–792.

Fuerst, J. S., & Fuerst, D. (1993). Chicago experience with an early childhood program: The special case of the child parent center program. *Urban Education, 28*(1), 69–96.

Garbarino, J. (1990). The human ecology of early risk: In S. J. Meisels & J. P. Shonkoff (Eds.), *Handbook of early childhood intervention* (pp. 78–96). New York: Cambridge University Press.

Garbarino, J., & Crouter, A. (1978). Defining the community context of parent-child relations. *Child Development, 49,* 604–616.

Garbarino, J., & Sherman, D. (1980). High-risk neighborhoods and high-risk families: The human ecology of child maltreatment. *Child Development, 51,* 188–198.

Garber, H. L., & Heber, R. (1981). The efficacy of early intervention with family rehabilitation. In M. Begab, H. C. Haywood, & H. L. Garber (Eds.), *Psychosocial influences in retarded performance* (pp. 71–82). Baltimore: University Park Press.

Gomby, D. S., Larner, M. B., Stevenson, C. S., Lewit, E. M., & Behrman, R. E. (1995). Long-term outcomes of early childhood programs: Analysis and recommendations. *Future of Children, 5*(3), 6–21.

Gordon, I. J., & Guinagh, B. J., (1978). A home learning center approach to early stimulation. *JSAS Catalog of Selected Documents in Psychology, 8*(6), Ms. No. 1634.

Gray, S. W., & Klaus, R. A. (1970). The early training project: A seventh-year report. *Child Development, 41,* 909–924.

Guralnick M. J. (1989). Recent developments in early intervention efficacy research: Implications for family involvement in P. L. 99–457. *Topics in Early Childhood Special Education, 9*(3), 1–17.

Gutelius, M. F., Kirsch, A. D., MacDonald, S., Brooks, M. R., & McErlean, T. (1977). Controlled study of child health supervision: Behavioral results. *Pediatrics, 60,* 294–304.

Hart, B., & Risley, T. R. (1995). *Meaningful differences in the everyday experience of young American children.* Baltimore: Brookes.

Honig, A. S., & Lally, J. R. (1982). The Family Development Research Program: Retrospective review. *Early Child Development and Care, 10,* 41–62.

Hunt, J. M. (1961). *Intelligence and experience.* New York: Ronald Press.

Hutchins, V. L., & McPherson, M. (1991). National agenda for children with special health needs: Social policy for the 1990's through the 21st century. *American Psychologist, 46,* 141–143.

Huxley, P. (1990). *Effective community mental health services.* London: Athenaeum Press.

Infant Health and Development Program Consortium (IHDP). (1990). Enhancing the outcomes of low birth weight, premature infants: A multi-site randomized trial. *Journal of the American Medical Association, 263,* 3035–3042.

Johnson, B. H., McGonigel, M. J., & Kauffman, R. K. (1989). *Guidelines and recommended practices for the individualized family service plan.* Washington, DC: Association for the Care of Children's Health.

Johnson, D. L., & Walker, T. (1991). A follow-up evaluation of the Houston Parent–Child Development Center: School performance. *Journal of Early Intervention, 15*(3), 226–236.

Kempe, H. (1976). Approaches to preventing child abuse: The health visitor concept. *American Journal of Diseases of Children, 130,* 941–947.

Klaus, R. A, & Gray, S. W. (1968). The Early Training Project for Disadvantaged Children: A report after five years. *Monographs of the Society for Research in Child Development, 33*(4, Serial No. 120).

Knitzer, J. (1982). *Unclaimed children: The failure of public responsibility to children and adolescents in need of mental health services.* Washington, DC: Children's Defense Fund.

Koop, C. E. (1987). *Surgeon general's report: Children with special health care needs.* Washington, DC: U.S. Department of Health and Human Services.

Lazar I., Darlington, R., Murray, H., Royce, J., & Snipper, A. (1982). Lasting effects of early education: A report from the consortium for longitudinal studies. *Monographs of the Society for Research in Child Development, 47*(2–3, Serial No. 195).

Lee, V. E., Brooks-Gunn, J. U., Schnur, E., & Liaw, G. (1990). Are Head Start effects sustained? A longitudinal follow-up comparison of disadvantaged children attending Head Start, no preschool, and other preschool programs. *Child Development, 61*(2), 495–507.

Levenstein, P., O'Hara, J., & Madden, J. (1983). The Mother–Child Program of the Verbal Interaction Project. In Consortium for Longitudinal Studies, *As the twig is bent . . . Lasting effects of preschool programs* (pp. 237–263). Hillsdale, NJ: Erlbaum.

Levine M., & Levine, A. (1970). *The social history of the helping services: Clinic, court, school and community.* New York: Appleton-Century-Crofts.

Levine, M., & Levine, A., (1992). *Helping children: A social history.* New York: Oxford University Press.

McLoyd, V. C. (1990). The impact of economic hardship on black families and children: Psychological distress, parenting, and socioemotional development. *Child Development, 61,* 311–346.

Oakland, T., & Ghazaleh, H. A. (in press). *Primary prevention of handicapping conditions among Palestinian children in Gaza.* Cited in D. Bryant & K. Maxwell (1997). The effectiveness of early intervention for disadvantaged children.

Olds, D. L., Henderson, C. R, Tatelbaum, R., & Chamberlin, R. (1986). Improving the delivery of prenatal care and outcomes of pregnancy: A randomized trial of nurse home visitation. *Pediatrics, 77,* 16–28.

Olds, D. L., Henderson, C. R, Tatelbaum, R, & Chamberlin, R. (1988). Improving the life-course development of socially disadvantaged mothers: A randomized trial of nurse home visitation. *American Journal of Public Health, 78*(11), 1436–1445.

Olds, D. L., & Kitzman, H. (1993). Review of research on home visiting for pregnant women and parents of young children. *Future of Children, 3*(3), 53–92.

Powell, C., & Grantham-McGregor, S. (1989). Home visiting of varying frequency and child development. *Pediatrics, 84,* 157–164.

Ramey, C. T. (1982). Commentary. *Monographs of the Society for Research in Child Development, 47*(2–3, Serial No. 195).

Ramey, C. T., Bryant, D. M., Wasik, B. H., Sparling, J. J., Fendt, K. H., & LaVange, L. M. (1992). The Infant Health and Development Program for low birthweigt, premature infants: Program elements, family participation, and child intelligence. *Pediatrics, 3,* 454–465.

Ramey, C. T., MacPhee. D., & Yeates, K. O. (1982). Preventing developmental retardation: A general systems model. In J. M. Joffee & L. A. Bond (Eds.), *Facilitating infant and early childhood development* (pp. 343–401). Hanover, NH: University Press of New England.

Ramey, C. T., Ramey, S. L., Gaines, K. R., & Blair, C. (1995). Two-generation early intervention programs: A child development perspective. In I. E. Sigel (Series Ed.) & S. Smith (Vol. Ed.), *Advances in applied developmental psychology: Vol. 9. Two generation programs for families in poverty: A new intervention strategy* (pp. 199–228). Norwood, NJ: Ablex.

Ramey, C. T., Sparling, J. J., Bryant, D. M., & Wasik, B. H. (1982). Primary prevention of developmental retardation during infancy. *Journal of Prevention and Human Services, 1,* 61–83.

Ramey, C. T., Yeates, K. O., & Short, E. J. (1984). The plasticity of intellectual development: Insights from preventive intervention. *Child Development, 55,* 1913–1925.

Ramey, S. L., & Ramey, C. T., (1992). Early educational intervention with disadvantaged children: To what effect? *Applied & Preventive Psychology, 1,* 131–140.

Roberts, R. N., & Wasik, B. H. (1996). Evaluating the 1992 and 1993 CISS projects. In J. M. Marquart & E. Konrad (Eds.), *New Directions in Program Evaluation (NDPE): Evaluation of human services intention* (pp. 35–49). San Francisco: Jossey-Bass.

Sameroff A. J., & Chandler, M. J. (1975). Reproductive risk and the continuum of caretaking casualty. In F. D. Horowitz, M. Hetherington, S. Scarr-Salapatek, & G. Siegel, (Eds.), *Review of child development research* (Vol. 4, pp. 187–244). Chicago: University of Chicago Press.

Sameroff, A. J., Seifer, R., Barocas, B., Zax, M., & Greenspan, S. (1987). IQ scores of 4-year-old children: Social-environmental risk factors. *Pediatrics, 79*(3), 343–350.

Scarr, S., & McCartney, K. (1988). Far from home: An experimental evaluation of the mother–child home program in Bermuda. *Child Development, 59*(3), 531–543.

Schaefer, E. S., & Aaronson, M. (1977). Infant Education Research Project: Implementation and implications of the home tutoring program. In M. E. Day & R. K. Parker (Eds.), *The preschool in action* (2nd ed., pp. 52–71). Boston: Allyn and Bacon.

Schweinhart, L. J., Barnes, H. V., Weikart, D. P., Barnett, W. S, & Epstein, A. S. (1993). *Significant benefits: The High/Scope Perry Preschool Study through age 27.* Ypsilanti, MI: High/Scope Press.

Seitz, V., Rosenbaum, L. K., & Apfel, N. H. (1985). Effects of family support intervention: A ten year follow-up. *Child Development, 56,* 376–391.

Skeels, H. M. (1966). Adult status of children from contrasting early life experiences. *Monographs of the Society for Research in Child Development, 31*(3, Serial No. 105).

Skodak, M., & Skeels, H. M. (1949). A final follow-up study of one hundred adopted children. *Journal of Genetic Psychology, 75,* 85–125.

Smith, S. (1995). Evaluating two-generation interventions: Current efforts and directions for Future Research. In I. E. Sigel (Series Ed.) & S. Smith (Vol. Ed.), *Advances in applied developmental psychology: Vol. 9. Two generation programs for families in poverty: A new intervention strategy* (pp. 251–270). Norwood, NJ: Ablex.

Smith S., & Zaslow, M. (1995). Rationale and policy context for two-generation interventions. In I. E. Sigel (Series Ed.) & S. Smith (Vol. Ed), *Advances in applied developmental psychology: Vol. 9. Two generation programs for families in poverty: A new intervention strategy* (pp. 1–36). Norwood, NJ: Ablex.

Sparling, J., & Lewis, I. (1979). *Learning for the first three years: A guide to parent–child play.* New York: Walker.

Sparling, J., & Lewis, I. (1984). *Learning for threes and fours: A guide to adult and child play.* New York: Walker.

St. Pierre, R., Goodson, B., Layzer, J., & Bernstein, L. (1994). *National evaluation of the Comprehensive Child Development Program: Report to Congress.* Cambridge, MA: Abt Associates.

St. Pierre, R. G., Layzer, J. L., & Barnes, H. V. (1995). Two-generation programs: Design, cost and short-term effectiveness. *The Future of Children, 5*(3), 51–75.

St. Pierre, R. G., & Swartz, J. P. (1995). The Even Start Family Literacy Program. In I. E. Sigel (Series Ed.) & S. Smith (Vol. Ed.), *Advances in applied developmental psychology: Vol. 9. Two generation programs for families in poverty: A new intervention strategy* (pp. 37–66). Norwood, NJ: Ablex.

St. Pierre, R., Swastz, J. P., Gamse, B., Murray, S., Deck, D., & Nickel, P. (1995). *National evaluation of the Even Start Family Literacy Program: Final Report.* Cambridge, MA: Abt Associates.

Ullmann L. P., & Krasner L. (1965). *Case studies in behavior modification.* New York: Holt, Rinehart and Winston.

Wasik, B. A. & Karweit, N. L. (1994). Off to a good start: Effects of birth to three interventions on early school success. In R. E. Slavin, N. L. Karweit, & B. A. Wasik (Eds.), *Preventing early school failures: Research, policy and practice* (pp. 13–57). Needham, MA: Allyn & Bacon.

Wasik, B. H. (1993a, April). *Research and evaluation strategies for family literacy.* Paper presented at the National Center on Family Literacy Conference, Louisville, KY.

Wasik, B. H. (1993b). *Theoretical and social shifts in early intervention: Implications for researchers and evaluators.* Unpublished manuscript.

Wasik, B. H., Bryant, D. M., & Lyons, C. (1990). *Home visiting: Procedures for helping families.* Newbury Park, CA: Sage.

Wasik, B. H., Bryant, D. M., Lyons, C., Sparling, J. J., & Ramey, C. T. (1997). Home visiting in the Infant Health and Development Program. In R. T. Gross, D. Spiker, & C. Haynes (Eds.), *The Infant Health and Development Program* (pp. 27–41). Palo Alto, CA: Stanford University Press.

Wasik, B. H., Bryant, D. M., Ramey, C. T., & Sparling, J. J. (1997). Maternal problem solving. In R. T. Gross, D. Spiker, & C. Hayes (Eds.), *The Infant Health and Development Program* (pp. 276–289). Palo Alto, CA: Stanford University Press.

Wasik, B. H., Ramey, C. T., Bryant, D. M., & Sparling, J. J. (1990). A longitudinal study of two early intervention strategies: Project CARE. *Child Development, 61*(6), 1682–1696.

Wasik, B. H., & Roberts, R. N. (1994). Survey of home visiting programs for abused and neglected children and their families. *Child Abuse & Neglect, 18*(3), 271–283.

Wasik, B. H., Roberts, R. N., & Lam, W. K. K. (1994, July). *The myths and realities of family-centered community-based, coordinated, cuiturally-competent systems of care.* Paper commissioned for the Maternal and Child Health Bureau Research Priorities Conference, Columbia, MD.

Wolfe, D. A. (1987). *Child abuse: Implications for child development and psychopathology.* Newbury Park, CA: Sage.

Yoshikawa, H. (1995). Long-term effects of early childhood programs on social outcomes and delinquency. *Future of Children, 5*(3), 51–75.

Zigler, E. F. (1995). Can we "cure" mild mental retardation among individuals in the lower socioeconomic stratum? *American Journal of Public Health, 85,* 302–304.

Zigler, E. F., & Freeman, J. (1987). Head Start: A pioneer of family support. In S. L. Kagan, D. R. Powell, B. Weissbourd, & E. F. Zigler (Eds.), *America's family support programs, perspectives, and prospects* (pp. 57–76). New Haven, CT: Yale University Press.

23

Addressing Current and Planning for Future Ethical Issues in Child Maltreatment Research
Professional and Policy Ethical Decision Making

ALEXANDER J. TYMCHUK

INTRODUCTION

Although the ethical challenges facing investigators in planning for and performing child maltreatment research are being recognized, formal discussion is just beginning regarding the complexities of those ethical questions, regarding the methods available to aid investigators in the identification of the issues, and regarding how investigators might learn acceptable ways in which to address those issues. Also, there has been little discussion regarding how investigators can best be informed about past and current ethical issues, about the guides that were available at those times to address the issues and how the results of the application of those guides might be applied to specific circumstances today. Ethics education in professional curricula, for example, has been very limited; this has resulted in inconsistency of interpretation of current ethical guidelines, especially regarding novel or less familiar ethical dilemmas (see, e.g., Rae & Worchel, 1991; Tymchuk, 1985; Tymchuk et al., 1979, 1982).

Child maltreatment, as a relatively new field, however, is evolving and like other new fields, it takes time to begin to develop various procedures, particularly

ALEXANDER J. TYMCHUK • Department of Psychiatry, School of Medicine, University of California, Los Angeles, California 90024-1759.

Handbook of Child Abuse Research and Treatment, edited by Lutzker. Plenum Press, New York, 1998.

those needed to address sensitive ethical issues (Finkelhor, 1996). Specific requirements for the conduct of research funded by the U.S. government are a recent phenomenon. The first regulations were enunciated in the Public Health Service in 1966, expanded in the 1971 Institutional Guide to Department of Health, Education and Welfare (DHEW) Policy of Protection of Human Subjects, with current regulations taking effect August 19, 1991 (45 Code of Federal Regulations [CFR] 46). There also has been variability in the degree to which these regulations were understood and applied, in part because of the absence of formal dissemination.

Further, there has been little discussion regarding the anticipation of future ethical issues and the proactive development of plans in the event of their occurrence. There also has been a marked absence of any research addressing ethics and child maltreatment research (National Research Council, 1993). This absence of a research agenda in ethics is not unique to child maltreatment.

The Complicated Nature of Child Maltreatment Research

Child maltreatment, by its very nature, is complicated, and research in child maltreatment is even more complicated, having to be accomplished at a time when various legal and social service agencies are attempting to fulfill their obligations to resolve reported maltreatment incidents, to protect children and families during and after such resolution, to prevent the occurrence of future incidents, and to develop meaningful policy based on those experiences. Research involving intervention procedures becomes even more difficult because, in order to be able to engage families in their home environments, researchers may be confronted with dangerous situations, perhaps involving police or emergency personnel. And each agency has procedures for the conduct of research in addition to those from the investigator's own agency. As a result, investigators need to be informed of the ethical challenges in child maltreatment research and of the regulations such research must adhere to, as well as the ethical guidelines available to help deal with unresolved dilemmas. They also need to be aware of the legal implications of child abuse and neglect in general (Myers, 1992).

Purpose

Given this cornerstone importance, the purpose of this chapter is to familiarize the reader with requirements for the conduct of research in child maltreatment, with some of the identified ethical dilemmas in the conduct of research in which interpretation of the established regulations is required, and to familiarize the reader with the available guides to facilitate the ethical decision making when the researcher is confronted with a dilemma to which regulations do not apply. Such ethical decision making also can benefit policy makers, administrators, and members of the court.

Child Maltreatment Research Requirements

There are specific federal requirements for the conduct of human research that are applicable to child maltreatment research. These requirements can be found in 45 CFR 46. Additional documents include *The Belmont Report* (National Commission for the Protection of Human Subjects of Biomedical and Behavioral

Research, 1979) and the *Institutional Review Board Guidebook for Protecting Human Research Subjects* (OPRR, 1993). All are available from the federal Office for the Protection from Research Risks (OPRR).

Although the code of federal regulations for the protection of human subjects (Title 45 Code of Federal Regulations, Part 46-45 CFR 46) in biomedical or behavioral research technically is applicable only to research that is federally funded or that which occurs within an agency that receives federal funds, in reality these regulations have become the standards for all human research. They also apply to international research done by U.S. researchers and to collaborative research where regulations differ from those in the United States. All child maltreatment research also must adhere to applicable state law.

While continuing to evolve such that the investigators and various gatekeepers, including administrators, must be aware of the "spirit" of the regulations, these regulations require that key elements are to be addressed before any human research can be attempted by professionals or by students. This includes pilot studies in all situations (e.g., public and private schools, religious institutions, hospitals, government, corrections). The elements in the code include those related to:

1. The *development* of the research such as
   a. adequacy of the basis for the research including an analysis of previous scientific literature directly related to the topic or from adjunct research (e.g., assessment, health, ethics)
   b. overall adequacy of the research design
   c. suitability of the research design for the stated purpose
   d. population to be included and whether "vulnerable," including children, persons with a cognitive impairment (e.g., psychiatric disorder, organic impairment, or developmental disorder such as mental retardation) or who are elderly with potentially diminished capacity; additional issues pertain to inclusion of persons of minority status and women
   e. whether participants are expected to benefit directly, indirectly or not at all from their participation
   f. evidence of a risk and expected benefit analysis
   g. where the population is located and whether in a facility (e.g., hospital) or institution (e.g., jail) where voluntariness of participation could be compromised, and whether in a vulnerable situation such as being homeless or in the military
   h. competency of the investigators
   i. a determination that the information being gathered in fact will be used
   j. method of assignment of participants to group if an intervention
2. The *beginning* of the research, including
   a. appropriate review (expedited, exempt, or full) by a duly constituted institutional review board (IRB) including a community member and, in some instances, a person of the group to be studied
   b. identification of sources for potential participants and how those sources were identified
   c. use of advertisements, payment, and incentives and what is given or lost if there is refusal to participate or if there is withdrawal before the completion of the study

     d. recruitment of participants

     e. determination of competency of participants to consent

     f. adequacy of consent process procedures done in the primary language in order to ensure voluntariness and adherence to all required content

     g. adequacy of initial, as well as delayed, understanding and decision making particularly related to child maltreatment reporting provisions, and freedom to withdraw from the research at any time (note: although understanding is required, there are no set criteria for determination of what is adequate)

3. The *continuation* of the research, including

     a. responding to adverse reactions by participants during the time of the study and directly related to the study procedures (e.g., emotional upset/trauma by child or parent)

     b. reporting of adverse events to the IRB (e.g., safety of personnel threatened or observation of unethical practices by service agencies)

     c. reporting of single-case results to the IRB in the event of high risk

     d. actual IRB monitoring of implementation of study procedures

     e. preliminary reporting of results

     f. follow-up of participants

4. The *completion* of the research, including

     a. use of the data and by whom

     b. protection of the data

     c. use of the data for other than its original purpose

     d. debriefing if necessary

In addition, there are requirements for the composition and functioning of the IRB.

ETHICAL DILEMMAS IN THE APPLICATION OF REGULATIONS TO CHILD MALTREATMENT RESEARCH

Interpreting the Regulations

The developers of the federal regulations recognize the fact that, like all regulations, current regulations do not cover all circumstances that will arise, particularly when research involves multiple agencies serving multiple-problem families. Institutional review boards thus encourage investigators to seek the advice of their IRB when a circumstance arises to which the regulations do not seem to apply. IRB members, too, are required to make judgments when regulations do not fit. Although such intra-IRB decision making has not been described, the process is similar to that described in the following discussion of ethical decision making. Such *fluidity* (author's italics) of interpretation of regulations occurs with various codes of ethics and even with laws (see, e.g., Dalglish, 1976). Such *fluidity* occurs in part not only because not all circumstances that face the investigator can be completely anticipated, but also because all regulations, codes, and laws are developed in reaction to something in the past rather than in anticipation of something in the future. Thus, the regulations are *reactive* rather than *proactive* and therefore are immediately outdated. Ideally, regulations (and codes of ethics) would have an ethical decision-making process as part of the regulations (and of the codes of ethics) to guide individual investigators when confronted with situations to which the regulations do not apply (note: ideally, they also would contain specific requirements for dissemination). To date, only the Canadian Psychological Association has included an ethical decision-making process (CPA, 1991).

As a result of the need for being informed of regulations and the need to interpret those regulations at times, individual investigators then are placed in a difficult situation and may suffer ethical stress as a result (Raines & Tymchuk, 1993). On the one hand, investigators must adhere to both the fact as well as to the spirit of the regulations; on the other hand, in the absence of such a process, they must interpret the spirit of the regulations so that what they choose to do would coincide with what the IRB (or profession) would want them to do (if the IRB had developed procedures). Without criteria for such interpretation, investigators may be open to criticism. Investigators also may be personally legally liable if adverse events occur during research that has not been approved by the IRB to which they are responsible.

The members of the National Research Council's panel on child abuse (1993) also identified a number of critical ethical dilemmas in child maltreatment research. Although the list is not comprehensive and is based on the members' expertise, it is instructive. The identified dilemmas included (1) ensuring that all elements of informed consent were fulfilled for all affected parties (e.g., parents, child, others); (2) ensuring adequacy of protections for the recruitment of study participants from an identified pool in which people may not be completely free to volunteer, or to refuse to participate, or free to withdraw even after consenting (note: this includes parents who believe that their participation in a research project would ensure or influence the return of their child or the dropping of charges; parents who are so impoverished economically that refusal to participate would mean the loss of a desired commodity, however small, which is punishment; parents who are so impoverished socially that any contact with others, no matter how slight, is desirable, so that refusal to participate, again, would mean punishment that the parent would not wish to endure, and therefore the parent may feel coerced to participate); (3) ensuring equitable assignment of high-need participants to nonintervention contrast or control groups (or families where no other service is available) (note: contrast conditions should never involve no treatment in child maltreatment research); (4) ensuring respect for individual privacy when the investigators are privy to personal information perhaps from observations during home visits or revelations during interviewing (see, e.g., Melton, 1992); (5) maintaining confidentiality of information (e.g., when investigators receive requests from child protective services regarding the parent); (6) respect for individual autonomy by providing information ensuring understanding and respect for the decision that is made; and (7) provision for debriefing after completion of the study if information in the consent was incomplete or superficially presented (e.g., requirement to report) or actually was deceptive (Bok, 1989). Other ethical dilemmas that have been identified for the investigator include the circumstances under which a research participant is to be reported for suspected child maltreatment, what criteria are to be used in making this determination, and what the consequences of such reporting are for continued parental participation (Finkelhor & Strapko, 1992). Investigators also must consider to whom they make their reports, as they may work in a hospital (Joint Council on Accreditation of Healthcare Organizations, 1994) or other institution that is required to have its own child and elder abuse reporting standards. They are required to make reports of adverse incidents to their IRB as well.

The Need for Ethical Decision Making in Child Maltreatment Research

Although the NRC (1993) outlined a preliminary research agenda to address ethical questions they had identified, until such research occurs, investigators must be able to address those as well as other questions independently.

There are a number of guides that are available for investigators to use in their deliberation; these guides cover personal and social values, professional or organizational ethical codes, regulations, laws, research, and clinical findings. Each of these guides has been used as a standard for determination of what is ethical and what is unethical in research; however, because each is open to interpretation and hence to misapplication, strict adherence to one or even to several is problematic. Taken together, however, these guides comprise a process for ethical decision making. One such process or model is presented in Table 1 (Tymchuk, 1981, 1982a, 1983a, 1983b, 1986). This one has been adapted for inclusion in the Canadian Psychological Association's Manual for the Code of Ethics (CPA, 1991) and in various texts (e.g., Keith-Spiegel & Koocher, 1985; Corey, Corey & Callahan, 1984), is used as part of coursework in preparing psychologists, marriage and family counselors, and child counselors for licensure (Association for Advanced Training in the Behavioral Sciences [AATBS], 1991) and has been used in a variety of studies (Gawthrop & Uhlemann, 1992). There are a number of supplemental resources related to ethical decision making and to decision making (cf. Bowie, Higgins & Michaels, 1992; Clemen, 1986; Gonsalves, 1989; Halpern, 1989; and Harron, Burnside & Beauchamp, 1983).

Advantages in the Use of an Ethical Decision Making Process

There are clear advantages in using an ethical decision making (EDM) process such as that outlined here; this process is composed of current recognized guides for ethical decision making (Francoeur, 1983; Janis & Mann, 1977). First, although initially time-consuming to learn and to apply, after similar dilemmas have been analyzed and the deliberations summarized and disseminated, the process becomes relatively easy. The results of the use of the EDM process then can become the basis upon which additional regulations or rules in professional or organizational ethical codes can be developed. But most important, depending on the degree to which the investigator adheres to the EDM process, there can be reasonable satisfaction that not only was the decision ethical, but also the process followed in making that decision was ethical. Second, the results of the EDM analysis, when used in conjunction with a display system (e.g., a form listing each ethical dilemma along with applicable guides and outcomes), allow for documentation of the process that was followed and the information on which decisions were reached; this is helpful to the IRBs (and to the courts hearing expert testimony). Third, the results of the EDM process can point to areas in which additional evidence is critically needed in order to support decisions. Thus, a research agenda can be developed. Fourth, such analysis can be used for educational purposes within university curricula as a means of developing ethical decision making skills in students and as a means to demonstrate where such ethical decision making started and where it is at present.

Table 1. The Ethical Decision Making Process

One: Identify and clarify ethical dilemma.

Two: Identify and consult guidelines that may be available. These guidelines may include:

1. Individual, group or societal values including religious, political, philosophical and economic orientations;
2. Professional standards for all elements of research design and implementation (e.g., for acceptable research design including number of participants, how selected and assigned, standardization of descriptive or measurement devices, of education or intervention methodologies, of curricula used in education or interventions and of materials provided to participants);
3. Ethical codes including those for specific professions, for scientific groups (e.g., American Association for the Advancement of Science, American Psychological Association), or other organizations (e.g., American Professional Society on the Abuse of Children, National Committee to Prevent Child Abuse) that provide guidance to, and govern the behavior of, members of those groups (e.g., competencies of researchers involving procedures and specific populations, research standards, what to do in the absence of applicable standards, research participant complaint procedures);
4. Voluntary or mandatory regulations regarding research procedures and populations (e.g., consent, external review);
5. Federal, state, and local laws including those related to the regulation of the profession of the researchers if applicable or to the functioning of an agency delivering service where the researcher either works or wishes to recruit participants (e.g., private or public healthcare agency or hospital, child protective service agency, court, women's shelter, private or public school);
6. Reports about previous identical or similar research in child maltreatment and how that research was accomplished with what outcomes;
7. Evidence related to procedures to be used in current research appearing in peer-reviewed journals demonstrating efficacy (e.g., showing improved understanding of consent materials).

Three: Determine rights and responsibilities of those involved.

Four: Generate alternative decisions for each ethical dilemma, always including not doing anything or not using an ethical decision-making process such as this.

Five: Enumerate the positive and negative consequences (risks and benefits) of making each alternative decision and estimate the probability of occurrence. These consequences should include immediate, ongoing and long-term economic, psychological, social, or other effects upon the individuals involved, but primarily upon the participant.

Six: Determine the quality of the evidence on which enumeration of positive and negative consequences and their probability of occurrence is based. If little or no evidence exists or if the available evidence is not based upon the application of empirical methods, these are risks.

Seven: Make and implement the decision.

Eight: Evaluate whether the decision was successful and maintain information for future use and dissemination.

An Example in the Application of Ethical Decision Making: Informed Consent in Child Maltreatment Research

Questions surrounding informed consent in child maltreatment research, and whether parents and/or their children in fact are informed, continue to be raised (NRC, 1993). Do teen parents know what constitutes child maltreatment, for example? Do they fully appreciate what society expects them *not to do* in parenting even when that society does not provide them with guidance regarding what *to do* in parenting?

In fact, consent as it is now construed has been seen to be problematic in general, according to the Office for the Protection from Research Risks (Levine, 1981; OPRR, 1993; President's Commission for the Study of Ethical Problems in Medicine and Biomedical and Behavioral Research, 1981). Although a full discussion of consent will not be presented here, it is important for investigators to familiarize themselves with the rationale and justification for informed consent in all research, with the history of the development of informed consent (cf. Beecher, 1970), with the limitations of the current conceptualization of consent, and with the limitations of the methodologies and processes used in consent and the evidence on which these limitations are based (cf. President's Commission, 1981; Tymchuk & Ouslander, 1990).

The doctrine of informed consent seeks to protect the individual autonomy and right to self-determination of potential research participants (and of patients in a clinical setting). The intent of consent doctrine is to provide a format and a process for communication between the investigator and potential participants about specific information (e.g., that this is a research project, voluntariness, freedom to withdraw, certain risks and expected benefits and their probabilities of occurrence, and the evidence on which this is based). The goal of the consent process is to fully inform potential participants about their participation. Informed consent on the part of the individual requires the fulfillment of three requirements: the individual must be competent, must adequately understand the information, and must be free to consent without any real or believed coercion. Competence itself is a legal term which refers to being able to come to a reasonable decision based on adequacy of decision making with an understanding of the information about the decision to be made. See OPRR (1993) and 45 CFR 46 for more details.

The following vignette will be used to demonstrate the application of the ethical decision making process as it relates to some consent issues in child maltreatment research:

A researcher wishes to determine the relative efficacy of two similar parent educational strategies with young low-income English-speaking single mothers or mothers-to-be.

What Are the Ethical Dilemmas Facing the Researcher?

One of the most difficult aspects of ethical decision making often is being able to recognize that an ethical dilemma may, or actually does, exist, and what the components of that dilemma are. In this instance, although information about the study is incomplete, there are two dilemmas, each of which has several components. The dilemmas are

Dilemma 1

Are any of the potential participants teen parents? If so, are they emancipated for this purpose or do any of them live with parents or in facilities designed to provide them with support during pregnancy and after delivery?

Dilemma 2

Are all able to read and understand printed or spoken information in their primary language—information such as is usually found in consent material—and are all able to process the information, weigh it, and come to a reasonable decision? Can they remember the information so that they can be free to withdraw if they wish once the study has begun?

Each of these dilemmas must be addressed and the evidence on which a decision was made presented in order to ensure that the research is in fact conducted in an ethical manner; if not, the IRB will not approve the study. In the event that an investigator either does not address some part of the identified dilemmas or proceeds, even with piloting procedures, before IRB approval, they leave themselves open to criticism and legal consequences.

What Guides Are Available?

A number of guides are available. First, the investigator should consult the regulations for the conduct of human research (45 CFR 46) as well as interpretative information on those regulations supplied either by the OPRR or by their own IRB. This analysis will provide a base from which to start. Although investigators may wish to limit themselves only to parents who are adults, they may want to include teens, for whom consent status may shift even during the study. Such *consent shift* is an important element of which investigators must be aware.

On the one hand, the regulations provide requirements for the consent process, including criteria for establishing whether the teen is emancipated and thus able to consent. If the teen is not emancipated, but the parent or guardian is available, that person must consent on behalf of the teen unless it can be demonstrated that the parent or guardian would not act in the best interests of the teen. If the teen is living in a facility, the facility personnel may act in loco parentis. Teens must assent, however, and their wishes are superordinate. If the teen has an infant on which information will be gathered (e.g., birth history, weight, development over time), the circumstances remain the same for consent. If, however, there is information that might be seen to have potentially adverse effects on the child later in life, the IRB may desire that someone other than the parent consent on behalf of the child. An example of this might be when the child has been removed so that the court must consent on behalf of the child, although the parent would self-consent.

On the other hand, the regulations recognize that the teen's parents may not act in the best wishes of the teen or may be unavailable (e.g., teen is a runaway) and the regulations allow the investigator to look for the parent (Capron, 1982). Although criteria are not provided for how long such seeking should occur, other guides assume that the investigator would act responsibly. In the continued absence of a parent (or other relative), an advocate/witness is recommended.

A second guide is to review other similar research (cf. Rotheram-Borus & Koopman, 1992 and related chapters in *Social Research on Children and Adolescents* [Stanley & Sieber, 1992], which was based on the report of a specially constituted task force to OPRR; also see Capron, 1982), and/or to seek the advice of the IRB.

There are other issues, however. One issue relates to the possibility that even if the parents were adults, some may be considered vulnerable as defined by the

OPRR; the second issue relates to the shift in a teen's consent status. In the event of the former, if the person has a formal diagnosis of a disorder related to cognitive impairment, this diagnosis does not by itself mean that the person is incompetent to self-consent. However, extensive research evidence has indicated that a person with a diagnosis related to cognitive impairment may not understand all of the information necessary to make an informed decision whether to participate, or may not be able to maintain information in order to remain informed for the duration of the study. In addition, they may not weigh the risks and benefits of participating or of not participating. However, with adaptation to the consent process, both understanding and the adequacy of the decision making process will improve (Krynski, Tymchuk, & Ouslander, 1994; Tymchuk, Ouslander, & Rader, 1986; Tymchuk, Ouslander, Rahbar, & Fitten, 1988). Determining adequacy of understanding and decision making requires the investigator to assess these factors initially and during the study to ensure that the person remembers what they are participating in.

In the second situation, the teen's consent status may shift from the teen being seen as an emancipated minor, living on the street or in a shelter, and able to self-consent, to being legally unable to self-consent but required to assent if living with their parent or guardian. The investigator must be prepared for such a shift. However, the investigator also must consider the adequacy of understanding and decision making of the teen. To do this, again, requires assessment.

What Are the Alternatives Available?

There are a number of alternatives for each ethical dilemma, including not doing anything or not using an ethical decision making process such as this. In addressing the issue of ensuring informed consent, Table 2 contains a systematic process to ensure consent; this process was developed and tested in research both with adolescents and older people (Jacobs & Tymchuk, 1981; Tymchuk et al., 1988). The same process was used in developing the consent processes for a current project on improving self- and infant-healthcare and safety of high-risk young mothers approved by the UCLA IRB (Tymchuk, 1996). The alternatives then are to adhere to this process or use a traditional process for consent.

What Are the Consequences of Either Alternative?

All previous work has indicated that by matching information contained in the consent process to the comprehension abilities of the population for which the consent is meant will significantly increase their understanding as well as the quality of their decision making as compared with the use of a standard process. Although there has not been any research directly related to young mothers or mothers-to-be including teens, it is logical to assume that the same results would occur.

The methodologies used and the results obtained by Tymchuk and his colleagues are instructive, however. In a study of how well children and adolescents, hospitalized for treatment related either to their emotional disturbance or to their developmental disability, understood their rights as patients, 80 consecutive admissions were randomly assigned to one of four conditions after having been

Table 2. Suggested Process to Follow to Ensure Fairness and to Maximize Understanding in Consent Process

Step 1 Determine legal competency, guardianship status, and voluntariness status (e.g., implication of coercion for participation). In some instances both parent and child may be required to consent separately if it is deemed that parent would not act in best interests of child. If adult, self-consents. If adolescent parent lives with parent/guardian, latter receives information and consents while adolescent receives information and assents or dissents. In all instances adolescent's decision is respected. If adolescent parent has not attained age of majority and is responsible for own care, self-consents as emancipated minor. If adolescent parent lives in residential setting, designated individual in residence consents as in loco parentis and adolescent assents or dissents. If legally determined to be an incompetent adult, guardian receives consent and person assents or dissents. Persons with mental retardation are not, by definition, incompetent. Incompetence is adjudicated.

Step 2 Assess vision and hearing with corrective devices if needed.

Step 3 Assess potential participant's reading recognition and comprehension in primary language to determine level at which consent material would be presented. Consider whether reading abilities of parent-guardian should be assessed.

Step 4 Assess mental status including memory.

Step 5 Determine format in which consent information is to be presented including the use of large, uncluttered text with paragraphs demarcated read by or to participant, of sample illustrations, or of videotape, singly or in combination.

Step 6 Develop consent materials to be presented. Develop method for assessment of understanding of content, taking into consideration mental status and reading recognition and comprehension; that is, if person comprehends at grade 5, assessment to be at same grade level. Consider method for determining adequacy of decision-making process participant uses to weigh options and risks and expected benefits of each option.

Step 7 Determine need for alternative methodology for presentation, including repeated trials and allowing person to take home to examine and to discuss with others. All participants receive copy of signed consent form.

Step 8 Present information to person and to parent/guardian advocate individually if necessary.

Step 9 Assess choice, understanding and quality of decision making process (Table 6 contains example of quality of decision making rating).

Step 10 Regardless of choice, if understanding and quality of decision making are below criterion levels, either repeat information presentation or consider alternative method.

Step 11 Reassess. Continue to repeat process until either the criterion for understanding is met and quality of decision making is satisfactory, or process has been repeated for number of times preset for consideration of saying person is incapable of giving truly informed consent. Then a proxy must give consent.

Step 12 If proxy, then information is to be presented to them.

Step 13 If initial criteria for person's (or proxy's) understanding and quality of decision making are reached, accept choice and later, reassess understanding, quality of decision making and choice at pre-set time to determine whether person wishes to continue, to withdraw/change mind, or to be provided with additional information.

given the Patient's Bill of Rights in the standard format and manner (Jacobs & Tymchuk, 1981; Tymchuk, 1982b). These conditions included presentation of the Bill again (1) in the same standard format, (2) in a storybook form containing actual photographs of two children of staff accompanied by words simplified to the average reading comprehension level of a representative group of hospitalized children and using the same font as in the standard format, (3) in a simplified word format only, and (4) a videotaped depiction of the two children walking through the ward, demonstrating and verbally presenting each right. Immediately following admission and presentation of the Patient's Bill of Rights in the standard manner by hospital staff, the children, with their assent and parental consent, were asked individually what they thought their rights were, while they were on the ward; they then answered a set of true/false questions about those rights. The standard presentation did little to inform the children, who, on the average, could remember fewer than one. After the second presentation in any of the four formats, there was a significant improvement. This result suggested that repeated presentations of information may improve understanding for children. In a replication of this study with older residents of a long-term care facility, using elderly actors both for the photographs and for the videotape, the results were different (Tymchuk et al., 1986). The residents did not comprehend their rights presented in the standard format, and the videotape format seemed to confuse them, but the illustrated booklet format and the simplified format equally and significantly improved comprehension. Other studies built on this work have demonstrated that understanding and decision making improved after information about complex medical procedures was simplified to the older person's level of reading comprehension. The accuracy of the information was maintained through back-translation from the simplified format to the complex format (see e.g., Tymchuk et al., 1988; Krynski et al., 1994). These studies also showed that giving information within the consent process significantly affected understanding (Tymchuk & Ouslander, 1991), and the decision a designated proxy would make on behalf of their elderly relative or resident was not related to what the resident indicated their decision to be (Ouslander, Tymchuk, & Rahbar, 1989). There has not been any study of the degree of concordance of decision made by a proxy on behalf of a minor and what the minor would make related to healthcare or to research participation.

What Is the Decision and the Process for Implementation?

For the study in this vignette, after initial determination of the reading recognition and comprehension abilities, a consent process would be developed which would include printed materials in large print (14-point Times Roman) written at a grade 6 level of comprehension, as recommended by Tymchuk and his colleagues (1986). Each paragraph would be marked with a heading in bold, 18-point type, succinctly presenting the basic idea contained in the paragraph (see Table 3 for a possible template to follow for such headings). Each sentence would contain a single concept; the sentences would be short and use frequently used words. In order to determine the person's ability to read and understand the information related to OPRR's requirements, the UCLA Research Participation Reading Recognition Test (Tymchuk, 1993a) was developed (Table 4). It contains key words pertaining to the research consent process in general. Similarly, the UCLA Research Participation Reading Comprehension Test (Tymchuk, 1993b) was developed (Table 5). Both have expert validity and high test–retest reliability, but, most importantly, they can be used to educate the person about each word. Accompanying these lists is a dictionary containing the same words. Although nei-

Table 3. Headings for Use as Templates for Research Consent Forms

To Whom Consent is Given
Purpose of Research Project
What the Research Involves
Possible Immediate Discomforts, Hazards, Risks Involved If I Say Yes
Possible Long-term Discomforts, Hazards, Risks Involved If I Say Yes
Possible Immediate Benefits or Value If I Say Yes
    To Me
    To Others
Who Will Be Working with Me
My Choices
    I am free to take part or not.
    I am free to stop at any time.
    I am free not to answer any questions.
The Researcher May:
    Not want me to take part anymore
    Not tell me everything
What Will Happen With the Information about Me
Who Will Know What I Am Doing or Have Done
If I Have Any Questions
If I Have Any Concerns With What Has Been Done
If I Am Hurt or Become Ill

My Signature: Date:

Guardian (or other legally authorized representative):   Date:

Witness: Date:

Table 4. Words Contained in the Two Forms of the UCLA Research Participation Reading Recognition Test

Form 1	Form 2
risk	harm
health	study
subject	consent
research	physical
measure	coercion
longterm	immediate
benefits	placebo
medical	normative
assessment	alternatives
questionnaire	anonymous
evaluation	psychological
voluntary	confidential
validity	experimental
investigator	significance
hypothetical	remuneration

ther of these instruments pertains directly to child maltreatment issues, they can be helpful in determining the parent's knowledge of the OPRR concepts required of all consent processes.

Table 5. Sample Items within the UCLA Research Participation Reading Comprehension Test

What does *risk* mean?
    a) something that will harm you.
    b) something that will make you feel good.
    c) driving a car.
What does *benefit* mean?
    a) something that will be bad for you.
    b) something that will be good for you.
    c) something that the doctor does.
What does *experimental* mean?
    a) something that has not been tried before.
    b) something that is common.
    c) something that everyone can do.

Table 6. Quality of Decision Making Rating Scale (Tymchuk et al., 1988)

0 They were not able to make a decision or show any preference.

1 They were able to express what they want to do, BUT it was not based upon a full understanding of all the facts including the risks and benefits of the procedures involved.

2 They would be able to express what they want to do based upon a reasonable understanding of the facts including of the risks and the benefits BUT not with an adequate weighing of those risks and benefits.

3 They would be able to express what they want to do based upon a reasonable understanding of the facts AND with adequate weighing of the risks and benefits BUT WITHOUT a full consideration of all of the possible consequences to themselves. That is, their choice probably would not result in a reasonable and responsible outcome.

4 They would be able to express what they want to do based upon a reasonable understanding of the facts, upon reasonable weighing of the risks and benefits and a consideration of all potential outcomes, and this, therefore, probably would result in a reasonable and responsible outcome.

If resources were available, representative illustrations depicting key elements would be developed. Figures 1, 2, and 3 contain illustrations that are used in the current Wellness Project to explain the consequences of neglect through misuse of poisons (Tymchuk, 1996). Alternatively, a videotape could be developed. A script would be developed for presentation of the information contained in the consent process. A questionnaire containing items related to key elements of the process could be developed and administered after presentation of consent. If the person misses any information, this information would be repeated. Examples of such items might be the following: Once you join the study, you can never leave. Yes or No; All of your personal information can be shared with anyone outside of the study. Yes or No; You will be required to answer every question that we ask you. Yes or No.

What Are the Results of the Decision?

The final step in the EDM process would be to evaluate how effective the procedures were.

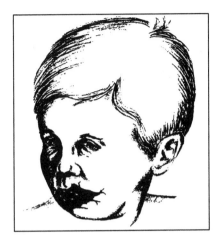

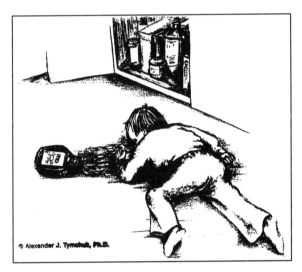

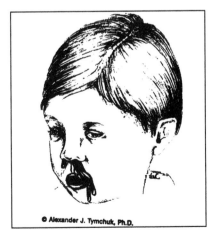

Figures 1, 2, and 3. Pictures used to illustrate the serious deleterious effects of neglect through misuse of household poisons.

SUMMARY AND CONCLUSIONS

As society becomes increasingly complex and as changes occur in service provision, it is apparent that more complex ethical dilemmas will arise. Child maltreatment researchers of today and tomorrow will have to be prepared to anticipate what those dilemmas will be and to develop strategies to respond to them, or in some instances, to prevent them from occurring.

There are a number of strategies to facilitate such preparation. First, as suggested by the NRC (1993), a research agenda on ethics in child maltreatment should be developed, implemented with adequate funding, and the results disseminated. Within this agenda, ethical decision making and how to best convey such skills about ethical decision making should be determined. Second, studies about consent with parents and children in child maltreatment along the lines of those done in other fields should be examined. Third, current journals in child maltreatment should establish a forum for discussion of ethical issues following a basic ethical decision-making process. Researchers should be encouraged to share their dilemmas, their ethical decision making, the end result of the process and how it all worked out. Fourth, a similar strategy can be implemented using various listservers available over the Internet. These recommendations also have applicability to administrative, policy, judicial, and clinical decision making in child maltreatment.

ACKNOWLEDGMENTS
The writing of this chapter was supported in part by grants from The California Wellness Foundation and SHARE, Inc., to Dr. Tymchuk. The author expresses his appreciation for that support.

REFERENCES

Association for Advanced Training in the Behavioral Sciences (AATBS). (1991). *Preparatory course for the psychology licensure examination.* Westlake, CA.: Author.

Bass, L., Dellers, S., Ogloff, J., Peterson, C., Pettifor, J., Reavers, R., Retfalvi, T., Simon, N., Sinclair, C., & Tipton, R. (1996). *Professional conduct and discipline in psychology.* Washington, DC: American Psychological Association.

Beecher, H. (1970). *Research and the individual.* Boston: Little, Brown, and Company.

Bok, S. (1989). *Lying–Moral choice in public and private life.* New York: Random House.

Bowie, G., Higgins, K., & Michaels, M. (1992). *Thirteen questions in ethics.* New York: Harcourt Brace Jovanovich College Publishers.

Canadian Psychological Association (CPA). (1991). *Companion manual to the Canadian Code of Ethics for Psychologists.* Ottawa, Ontario, Canada: Author.

Capron, A. (1982). The competence of children as self-deciders in biomedical interventions. In W. Gaylin & R. Macklin, (Eds.), *Who speaks for the child: The problem of proxy consent.* New York: Plenum Press.

Clemen, R. (1986). *Making hard decisions: An introduction to decision analysis.* Boston: PWS-Kent.

Corey, G., Corey, M., & Callahan, P. (1984). *Issues and ethics in the helping professions.* Pacific Grove, CA.: Brooks/Cole.

Dalglish, T. (1976). *Protecting human subjects on social and behavioral research: Ethics, law and the DHEW rules: A critique.* Berkeley, CA: Center for Research in Management Science.

Finkelhor, D. (1996). Introduction. In J. Briere, L. Berliner, J. Bulkley, C. Jenny, & T. Reid (Eds.), *The AP-SAC handbook on child maltreatment.* Thousand Oaks, CA: Sage.

Finkelhor, D., & Strapko, N. (1992). Sexual abuse and prevention education: A review of evaluation studies. In D. Willis, E. Holden, & M. Rosenberg, (Eds.), *Prevention of child maltreatment.* New York: Wiley.

Francoeur, R. (1983). *Biomedical ethics: A guide to decision making.* Philadelphia: Lippincott

Gawthrop, J., & Uhlemann, M. (1992). Effects of the problem-solving approach in ethics training. *Professional Psychology: Research and Practice, 23,* 38–42.

Gonsalves, M. (1989). *Right & reason: Ethics in theory and practice.* Columbus, OH: Merrill.

Halpern, D. (1989). *Thought and knowledge: An introduction to critical thinking.* Hillsdale, NJ: Lawrence Erlbaum Associates.

Harron, F., Burnside, J., & Beauchamp, T. (1983). *Health and human values: A guide to making your own decisions.* New Haven, CT: Yale University Press.

Jacobs, C., & Tymchuk, A. (1981). *Informed consent with children.* Paper presented at the annual meeting of the American Association on Mental Deficiency, Detroit, MI.

Janis, I., & Mann, L. (1977). *Decision making: A psychological analysis of conflict, choice and commitment.* New York: Free Press.

Joint Council on the Accreditation of Healthcare Organizations. (1994). *Accreditation standards.* Chicago; Author.

Keith-Spiegel, P., & Koocher, G. (1985). *Ethics in psychology: Professional standards and cases.* New York: Random House.

Krynski, M., Tymchuk, A., & Ouslander, J. (1994). How informed can consent be? *Gerontologist, 34,* 36–43.

Levine, R. (1981). *Ethics and regulation of clinical research.* Baltimore: Urban & Schwarzenberg.

Melton, G. (1992). Respecting boundaries: Minors, privacy, and behavioral research. In B. Stanley, & J. Sieber (Eds.), *Social research on children and adolescents: Ethical issues.* Newbury Park, CA: Sage.

Myers, J. (1992). *Legal issues in child abuse and neglect.* Newbury Park, CA: Sage.

National Commission for the Protection of Human Subjects of Biomedical and Behavioral Research. (1979). *The Belmont Report.* Washington, DC: Office for the Protection from Research Risks.

National Research Council (NRC). (1993). *Understanding child abuse and neglect.* Washington, DC: National Academy Press.

Office for Protection from Research Risks (OPRR). (1993). *Protecting human research subjects. Institutional Review Board guidebook.* Washington, DC: U.S. Department of Health and Human Services.

Ouslander, J., Tymchuk, A., & Rahbar, B. (1989). Health care decisions among elderly long term care residents and their potential proxies. *Archives of Internal Medicine, 149,* 1367–1372.

President's Commission for the Study of Ethical Problems in Medicine and Biomedical and Behavioral Research. (1981). *Protecting human subjects: The adequacy and uniformity of federal rules and their implementation.* Washington, DC: U.S. Government Printing Office.

Rae, W., & Worchel, F. (1991). Ethical beliefs and behaviors of psychologists: A survey. *Journal of Pediatric Psychology, 16,* 727–745.

Raines, M., & Tymchuk, A. (1993). Psychological factors in oncology nurses' ethical decision-making: Relationships among moral reasoning, coping style, and ethical stress. *Oncology Nursing Society Special Interest Newsletter, 4,* Parts 1 and 2 in Issues 2, 2–5 and 3, 1–5.

Rotheram-Borus, M. J., & Koopman, C. (1992). Protecting children's rights in AIDS research. In B. Stanley & J. Sieber (Eds.), *Social research on children and adolescents.* Newbury Park, CA: Sage.

Stanley, B., & Sieber, J. (Eds.). (1992). *Social research on children and adolescents.* Newbury Park, CA.: Sage.

Tymchuk, A. (1981). Ethical decision making and psychological treatment. *Journal of Psychiatric Treatment and Evaluation, 26,* 507–513.

Tymchuk, A. (1982a). Strategies for resolving value dilemmas. *American Behavioral Scientist, 26,* 159–175.

Tymchuk, A. (1982b, September). *Informed consent with vulnerable populations.* Invited paper to the joint NIH/FDA Conference on Human Subject Protection, University of California, Los Angeles.

Tymchuk, A. (1983a). *Ethical decision making and primary prevention.* Invited paper to the NIMH Conference on Ethics and Primary Prevention, Los Angeles.

Tymchuk, A. (1983b, May). *Guidelines for ethical decision making.* Invited address to the Canadian Psychological Association annual meeting, Winnipeg, Manitoba, Canada.

Tymchuk, A. (1985). Ethical decision making and psychology students' attitudes toward training in ethics. *Professional Practice of Psychology, 6,* 219–232.

Tymchuk, A. (1986). Guidelines for ethical decision making. *Canadian Psychology, 27,* 36–43.

Tymchuk, A. (1989). Anticipatory ethical and policy decision making in the community. *American Journal of Community Psychology, 17,* 361–365.

Tymchuk, A. (1990). Assent processes. In B. Stanley, & J. Sieber (Eds.). *Social research on children and adolescents.* Newbury Park, CA: Sage.

Tymchuk, A. (1993a). *Two forms of the UCLA Research Participation Reading Recognition Test—Experimental Version.* University of California, School of Medicine, Department of Psychiatry, Los Angeles.

Tymchuk, A. (1993b). *The UCLA Research Participation Reading Comprehension Test—Experimental Version.* University of California, School of Medicine, Department of Psychiatry, Los Angeles.

Tymchuk, A. (1996, 28–29 September). *The development, implementation and preliminary evaluation of a cross-agency, multi-locale self-healthcare and safety preparatory and prevention education program for parents with intellectual disabilities.* Invited address to the European Union Conference on Parenting with Intellectual Disability, Elsinore, Denmark. Published in the proceedings.

Tymchuk, A., Drapkin, R., Ackerman, A., Major, S., Coffman, E., & Baum, M. (1979). Survey of training in ethics in APA-approved clinical psychology programs. *American Psychologist, 34,* 1168–1170.

Tymchuk, A., Drapkin, R., Ackerman, A., Major. S., Coffman, E., & Baum, M. (1982). Ethical decision making and psychologists' attitudes toward training in ethics. *Professional Psychology: Research and Practice, 13,* 412–421.

Tymchuk, A., & Ouslander, J. (1990). Optimizing the informed consent process with elderly people. *Educational Gerontology, 16,* 245–254.

Tymchuk, A., & Ouslander, J. (1991). Does order affect recall of informed consent information? *Educational Gerontology, 17,* 11–19.

Tymchuk, A., Ouslander, J., & Rader, N. (1986). Informing the elderly: A comparison of four methods. *Journal of the American Geriatrics Society, 34,* 818–822.

Tymchuk, A., Ouslander, J., Rahbar, B., & Fitten, J. (1988). Medical decision making elderly people in long term care. *Gerontologist, 28*(Suppl.), 59–63.

Part VI

Conclusion

In this final chapter, I try to summarize the advances that are reported in this book in theory, research, treatment, and legal issues. I suggest that we have done a laudable job since the 1960s, when child abuse and neglect was first recognized professionally, and that the next century bodes well for tightening any areas of weakness in our current efforts.

24

Child Abuse and Neglect

Weaving Theory, Research, and Treatment in the Twenty-First Century

JOHN R. LUTZKER

As serious a societal problem as child abuse and neglect (CAN) is, it may be time to be somewhat laudatory about our accomplishments in addressing CAN in the last half of the 20th century. If we examine the history of science, or even the relatively young field of psychology, we become aware that most of science and psychology has had considerably more time to develop theory and effective treatments than has the field of CAN. Further, CAN may be more multidisciplinary than most other fields of human enterprise, and the field faces delicate legal and ethical issues.

Thus, in under 40 years we have come from virtually no recognition of CAN to laws, theories, treatments, and prevention programs, mostly from a multidisciplinary perspective. The chapters in this book should offer considerable optimism that the way is relatively clear toward improvement of assessment and treatment and awareness of what strategies may be more effective than others, what legal issues need further addressing, and what these advancements have allowed in the way of being able to create a coherent theory of the etiology of CAN.

THEORY

Again, rather than indict the CAN field for a lack of theory, we can look to history to suggest that despite the short time span in which CAN has been addressed, at this point we seem to be moving well toward an acceptable theory. Psychology spawned a number of theories of personality in the first half of the 20th century. The second half of the century brought an inundation of research on biological bases of behavior, learning theory and its applications, developmental, social, and cognitive

JOHN R. LUTZKER • Department of Psychology, University of Judaism, Los Angeles, California 90077-1599.

Handbook of Child Abuse Research and Treatment, edited by Lutzker. Plenum Press, New York, 1998.

areas, such that weaving it all together may have become a task so daunting that there currently is no widely held theory of personality in psychology today. Yet one may be more forthcoming in CAN.

Each chapter of this book provides substance for Azar and her colleagues' suggestion for a social/cognitive model of CAN. The meta-model that Azar and colleagues describe forms the basis for a model that could be generated from the chapters in this volume, because of their consistent theme of empiricism and social/ecological (and community) perspectives. Thus, there is reliability among the contributors here and, more broadly, in the published empirical literature on CAN regarding the multiple complex factors that contribute to its etiology. Lutzker, Bigelow, Swenson, Doctor, & Kessler (in press) have suggested that the only weakness in such a model is the limited data to date on the role of biological and intragenerational learned factors that may drive some of the impulsive and reckless behavior seen in many CAN perpetrators and their partners.

It appears from the literature that interpersonal skill deficits of adults, such as limited or poor parenting practices and inaccurate ideas about child development, and the subsequent disappointments resulting from the false expectations thus created, form one piece of the social/ecological model. Intertwined in the inappropriate expectations are false attributions that are the basis for the cognitive aspect of the theory. Further, as Yung and Hammond noted in Chapter 13, violence, in at least some subcultures, has become so prevalent that adolescents have become inured to it and cognitively accept it. This also could occur in some adult perpetrators of child maltreatment.

Do we have a coherent, practical theory of CAN? We are close. Azar and her colleagues' model represents a large step in the right direction. What may be missing is the biological piece and a better understanding of the etiology of CAN across socioeconomic status. That is, we know very little, from an empirical research perspective, about middle- and upper-class CAN. We know that it clearly seems less prevalent in those classes, but we know much less about it than we know about it in people of low SES, among whom it is most prevalent. One of the inherent problems in trying to research CAN from other than low SES is that it is very difficult to be funded to study it in those groups. Thus, in people of other than low SES, when CAN is reported, families seek private treatment and are seldom the subjects of empirical research. Thus, our theory of CAN might be very class bound. Nonetheless, we can speculate that families across the SES spectrum are affected by their unique social ecologies and that when CAN occurs, cognitive attributions as described by Azar and her colleagues play a role.

The social/cognitive model is the best that we have to date, and it will probably be embellished in the 21st century.

ASSESSMENT

A common theme runs through the majority of the chapters in this book regarding assessment. That is, some indirect assessments may be useful, especially as measures ancillary to direct behavioral assessment, but direct behavioral assessment is more often (or should be) the evaluation tool of choice in CAN. Many examples are shared in this volume; we reiterate a few. The HAPI–R (Home Accident Prevention Inventory–Revised) described by Lutzker, Bigelow, Doctor, Gershater, and Greene in this book, is a direct, actual count of hazards accessible to children in their homes. Rather than a rating, this direct assessment provides a clear frequency count of home safety hazards. Wurtele, in her chapter on child sexual abuse, reports that measures of children's skills, their actual behaviors, are critical in examining the effect of child sexual abuse prevention programs. Such measures give us a clearer picture of what a child might do when facing risk than do the results of a verbal test or other indirect assessments.

Fantuzzo and associates describe direct observation measures of children's social skills. In all of the chapters that describe parent training as the major component or one component of a program, again we see direct observation of parent–child interactions as the measures of choice. This is not to discount the role of indirect assessment; it is to say, however, that in CAN the indirect measures serve best as other interesting indices, but that direct behavioral assessment is the more reliable and useful approach to assessing parent and child behaviors that are germane to concerns about risk and to examine the effects of treatment. These measures more clearly reflect the social ecology of interest.

LEGAL ISSUES

Since the 1960s great strides have been taken in protecting children through the law. All states now have child protective services and reporting laws. As Portwood, Reppucci, and Mitchell note, however, definitions of CAN and standards of adequate parenting are still lacking careful, operational definition. Greene and Kilili argue that behavioral assessment and validation is needed in order to create such definition. The experts need to validate *behaviors* that define adequate parenting. Once adequate parenting is defined, criteria can be developed and subsequent behavioral assessment can be conducted with reported families, thus allowing courts and child protective services some operational measures by which to make judgments. These same protocols would greatly assist family courts in custody, placement, and parental rights termination issues.

If more definition came to the legal arena, many professionals, especially caseworkers, would themselves require performance-based training in how to utilize behavioral assessment strategies. It is presumed that this would be welcome, as many caseworkers express frustration at the rather random nature of decision-making at this point in CAN. Further, as noted in this book, data on their ability to accurately predict risk show no correlation in their ability to do so.

Finally, juvenile and family court judges need to become more aware of the importance of research and empirically based treatment programs. Unfortunately, most courts rely on clinicians who may have little or no research background and thus make their recommendations to courts based upon their own clinical intuitions, which have been found to be largely unsupported. Courts should be asking for data more than for opinions, or at least for opinions based on clear data, rather than the clinical speculations upon which they currently primarily rely.

TREATMENT

Is CAN treatable? To some extent, the answer to this question depends on what we mean by treatable. In every treatment chapter in this book there is evidence that behaviors associated with CAN risk can be changed for the better. Parents and children interact better. Parents can be taught to change negative attributions about their children. Children can learn new social skills. Children can learn to recognize and describe how they would behave if faced with sex abuse risk. Adolescents learn new attributions about violence and behave more positively in school. But, as Kolko and Ammerman and others have expressed, the big questions still need to be addressed. Specifically, do programs that demonstrate such behavior change actually reduce repeated CAN and even intragenerational CAN? Some program evaluation data exist, for example, the data reported from Project 12-Ways, but such reports are the exception rather than the rule.

Program evaluation data notwithstanding, again the CAN field should be applauded for the kind of data-driven successful treatment programs described in Section III of this book. Most of these programs clearly produce positive behavior change in children, adolescents, and parents. They most frequently do so with research design confidence that the interventions and not some other events are responsible for the behavior change. Also needed are treatment protocols that are so well defined and described that they can be replicated. It is most helpful when there is independent variable integrity. That is, when possible, data should be collected on the delivery of treatment services. For example, how often does the therapist conducting parent training provide models and reinforcers to the parent during a training session? Does the therapist make use of performance criteria for the parent before moving the parent from one stage of training to the next? These are issues of the integrity of the independent variable. When such data are gathered, it makes dissemination of successful programs more possible and more comfortable in that there is more confidence that when dissemination occurs the program will be conducted as it was designed.

CHILD SEXUAL ABUSE

CSA is not only a difficult topic because of its obviously sensitive nature, but it is a difficult area in which to conduct applied research. Teaching children to be safe, to recognize and report risk, to escape high-risk situations, and to avoid or allay guilt, blame or self-shame is no easy agenda. It is clear that training must be skill-based and that children must be taught behaviors. They can then role-play these behaviors with teachers. Of course, this kind of training must also be done with sufficient care so as to not make children overly afraid of all adults or so as to cause harm to their future sexuality. Probably the best suggestion for this work was that of Wurtele, who posited an idea of a multiyear curriculum on relationships. Embedded in such a curriculum could be the kinds of hands-on CSA prevention programs that have been described. These programs would, of course, need to have evaluation as a built-in component.

Another area that has had clinical, but limited, research attention is the long-term effects of CSA on young adults and older adults. It is clear that CSA can produce ongoing posttraumatic stress symptoms and many other psychological se-quelae that can affect several areas of social functioning in adults who were vic-tims of CSA. This area is in almost desperate need of empirical research.

PREVENTION

Primary prevention of CAN has fortunately become more prevalent. The Hawaii Healthy Start Program and other similar projects have served large num-bers of high-risk families. Tentative reports on home visiting programs show that they do serve a primary prevention function. These programs probably would be even more robust if they had school curricula built into them, so that while the parents and families receive services at home, the children are learning in school. This is the kind of multiyear curriculum proposed by Wurtele.

Given the kind of data shared by Pinkston and Smith on the increasing per-centage of American families with single parents who become entrapped in poverty, have many children, and are affected by high-risk social ecological fac-tors, it seems prudent to try to develop empirically based and active learning pro-grams in reproductive health that could be added to curricula for adolescents. Such programs are described by Yung and Hammond and by Pittman, Wolf, and Wekerle in adolescent violence prevention. Prevention should be seen as a con-tinuous developmental program that should proceed from birth into at least the early parenting years. Overall, if properly carried out, such an effort would un-doubtedly pay huge human and fiscal dividends in preventing family violence and reducing the enormous dollar and human costs to society that are the results of family violence.

ETHICS

Tymchuk drives home a concern that in an area as socially important as CAN research, it is surprising that we have accomplished so little in giving researchers and clinicians guidelines on how to make decisions about ethical issues. Although all human service providers, especially through their licensing bodies, are made aware of the broad ethical guidelines of their respective fields, Tymchuk points to the lack of practice and feedback in ethical decision making. This could be recti-fied through the very practice, feedback, and performance-based criteria that we use and admire in good treatment programs. Such work should cut across the multi-disciplinary fields that make up the professional CAN arena (e.g., psychology, psy-chiatry, social work, medicine, law, and education).

OTHER EOLOGICAL AND RESEARCH CONCERNS

The authors of this volume have made many contributions and suggestions, but, of course, they cannot be exhaustive. Neither can the following suggestions, but they are deserving of mention. For example, Donnelly (1997) has reported that there is evidence that the combined educational, treatment, media, and prevention efforts in CAN have apparently contributed to a decline in parental use and positive attribution of corporal punishment across the United States. Especially with the changing dynamics of the American family, this represents encouraging news.

Guterman (1997) suggests that the ecological base of our work needs expansion. The home, the community, the workplace, the extended family and friend networks all need to be considered in a comprehensive examination of CAN. Similarly, Willis (1995) argues that the community itself must be strengthened in order for us to provide comprehensive services. Wolfe, Reppucci, and Hart (1995) caution that prevention efforts must show reduced risks to children.

As Tymchuk and Feldman each reported in this book, parents with developmental disabilities are especially underserved by CAN research and services even though they are overrepresented in their numbers as CAN families. Bonner, Crow, and Hensley (1997) have also expressed concern that maltreated children with disabilities are quite underrepresented in our research and treatment efforts.

In a comprehensive review and summary of CAN research, Becker and colleagues (1995) have offered 13 well-conceived suggestions for improving our efforts. These bear review here.

1. Services must be culturally sensitive. As so well stated by Fantuzzo, the community must have a role in assessment, goals, process, and review of services and research efforts.
2. There is a need for incidence and prevalence studies across ethnic groups. I would add that we know very little about the nature of middle-class CAN. It may be that the predictor variables and etiology may be different across SES. Our research base basically derives from low SES and that is important, but it is also limiting our knowledge base.
3. Services should range from primary prevention to direct treatment for CAN and they need rigorous program evaluation.
4. "Research is needed to determine which factors separate sociocultural variables within ethnic–racial environments from issues of child maltreatment" (Becker, et al., 1995, p. 39).
5. A recurrent theme from chapters here . . . the field lacks behavioral definitions.
6. Assessments must include multiple culturally sensitive domains.
7. Control groups from random assignments or matched comparison groups must be utilized more frequently in treatment, prevention, and program evaluation research.
8. There is a considerable need for longitudinal studies of prevention and treatment programs. Needless to say, the very nature of CAN, which includes such problems as frequent relocation of families, makes this kind of effort difficult at best, but it would be very helpful to have more longitudinal data.
9. An extremely important issue is what Becker and colleagues (1995) call prophylactic factors. That is, we very much need to study successful families who have many of the known high-risk demographic, socioeconomic risk factors and do not engage in child maltreatment. There are far more such families than there are maltreating ones. If we were then successful in identifying some reliable prophylactic factors/variables, perhaps it

would be possible to create treatment services that incorporate these factors into treatment for families who have been reported for CAN or who are at the highest risk.

10. There needs to be more analysis of moderator variables such as age, sex, and ethnicity, and mediating variables such as the type of maltreatment, because these variables affect outcome.

11. We need to have a better sense of the integrity of the independent variable. That is, data should be available on what the mediators of treatment do in their sessions with families.

12. In addition to true longitudinal studies, there simply needs to be extended follow-up in smaller-scale treatment studies.

13. Becker and associates (1995) also suggest the need for a coherent and practical theory of CAN. As noted earlier, Azar and her colleagues appear close to offering this.

FINAL RECOMMENDATIONS, THOUGHTS, AND CONCLUSION

We have only begun to consider including the child in treatment services for the family. This is done by clinicians, but it has not been prevalent in the social/ecological research-based programs described here, with the exception of the work in CSA. Child victims of physical CAN or CSA should be assessed for anxiety and PTSD. They should receive cognitive/behavioral treatment, along with whatever other services their families are receiving. In addition, they should be actively taught how to avoid high-risk violence situations in their homes and how to safely escape and report such situations.

The role of genetic and biological predisposition to poor parenting may be demonstrated in tendencies toward aggressive behavior, recklessness, the role of any learning disabilities that may affect parenting . . . these are factors that deserve considerably more attention in the new century.

Psychology has recently begun to be much more aware of the role of religion and spirituality as helpful in family relationships and as adjuncts to mental health treatment services. The field of CAN has not even begun to address this possibility. Natural communities have much religion and spirituality. Thus, to ignore this in our understanding and treatment of CAN families may be a substantial oversight.

The amount of graphic violence in media, from news to television to movies, has received much attention, but its effect on family violence has not been well researched. Even if we learn that it has some of the deleterious effects we may fear, ways to control it is another issue that begs for consideration. Our standards of what is acceptable in the way of media violence have changed radically over the years, to the point that most people appear to accept without notice levels from which they would have turned away in disgust years prior. That is to say that we have become inured to media and community violence. Perhaps we all need a little adjustment of our viewpoints.

The idea of a multiyear human relations curriculum proposed by Wurtele is a provocative one. In an age of managed care and brief therapies, our thinking moves toward parsimony in our services. A multiyear educational curriculum, on the other hand, combined with weekly television programs and radio spots aimed at teaching human relations, in an entertaining fashion, might go a long way in changing the escalating problem of child maltreatment and family violence. In this light, for CAN families, consider the possibility of a 3-week camp during which there would be a virtual 24-hour indoctrination of human relations training that would include weekly follow-up in homes.

Several programs described here have used video as an adjunct or primary medium in teaching. The new century "calls" for increased use of technology, especially interactive types, in delivering effective human service programs.

These speculations about future possibilities aside, what does appear successful to date? Most in-home comprehensive prevention services appear to be effective. Programs that offer multiple services appear to be effective. Behavioral assessment strategies appear more practical than most indirect measures. Programs that are child centered and focus on language appear effective. Programs that teach with hands-on procedures and that teach behaviors (skills) are effective. Thus, we should be buoyed by the kinds of issues and programs presented in this book. The twenty-first century should see a positive outcome of the dissemination of these kinds of programs aimed at safer lives for children.

ACKNOWLEDGMENTS

The writing of this chapter was supported, in part, by a grant from the California Wellness Foundation. The assistance of Randi Sherman is gratefully acknowledged.

REFERENCES

Becker, J. V., Alpert, J. L., Bigfoot, D. S., Bonner, B. L., Geddie, L. F., Henggeler, S. W., Kaufman, K. L., & Walker, C. E. (1995). Empirical research on child abuse treatment: Report by the child abuse and neglect treatment working group, American Psychological Association. *Journal of Clinical Child Psychology, 24,* 23–46.

Bonner, B. L., Crow, S. M., & Hensley, S. D. (1997). State efforts to identify maltreated children with disabilities: A follow-up study. *Child Maltreatment,* 252–60.

Donnelly, A. C. (1997). We've come a long way, but the challenges ahead are mighty. *Child Maltreatment, 2,* 6–11.

Guterman, N. B. (1997). Early prevention of physical child abuse and neglect: Existing evidence and future directions. *Child Maltreatment, 2,* 12–34.

Lutzker, J. R., Bigelow, K. M., Swenson, C. C., Doctor, R. M., & Kessler, M. L. (in press). Problems related to child abuse and neglect. In S. Netherton, C. E. Walker, & D. Holmes (Eds.), *Comprehensive handbook of child and adolescent disorders.* New York: Oxford University Press.

Willis, D. J. (1995). Psychological impact of child abuse and neglect. *Journal of Clinical Child Psychology, 24,* 2–4.

Wolfe, D. A., Repucci, N. D., & Hart, S. (1995). Child abuse prevention: Knowledge and priorities. *Journal of Clinical Child Psychology, 24,* 5–22.

Author Index

Subject Index

ABOUT THE EDITOR

John R. Lutzker (Ph.D., University of Kansas) is the Ross Professor and Chair and Director of Graduate Training in Psychology at the University of Judaism. He is also Adjunct Professor of Human Development and Family Life at the University of Kansas. He is the author of two other professional books and more than 90 articles and chapters. Dr. Lutzker has been on numerous editorial boards and currently sits on five boards including that of the *Journal of Family Violence*. He is a Fellow in the American Psychological Association, the American Psychological Society, the American Association of Applied and Preventive Psychology, and the Behavior Research and Therapy Society. Dr. Lutzker created Projects 12-Ways and SafeCare, both comprehensive efforts aimed at the prevention and treatment of child abuse and neglect. In addition to child maltreatment, Dr. Lutzker's other research interests are in developmental disabilities.

Handbook of child abuse
research and treatment